In Vitro Methods
in Cell-Mediated
and Tumor Immunity

In Vitro Methods in Cell-Mediated and Tumor Immunity

Edited by

BARRY R. BLOOM

Departments of Microbiology and Immunology
and of Cell Biology
Albert Einstein College of Medicine
Bronx, New York

and

JOHN R. DAVID

Department of Medicine
Harvard Medical School
Robert B. Brigham Hospital
Boston, Massachusetts

With the Editorial Assistance of
Roberta David and Lenore Grollman

ACADEMIC PRESS   New York   San Francisco   London   1976
A Subsidiary of Harcourt Brace Jovanovich, Publishers

ACADEMIC PRESS, INC.
111 Fifth Avenue, New York, New York 10003

United Kingdom Edition published by
ACADEMIC PRESS, INC. (LONDON) LTD.
24/28 Oval Road, London NW1

Library of Congress Cataloging in Publication Data

Main entry under title:

In vitro methods in cell–mediated and tumor immunity.

    Includes bibliographical references and index.
    1.   Immunology–Technique.   2.   Cellular immunity.
3.   Tumor–Immunological aspects.   I.   Bloom, Barry R.,
Date   II.   David, John R.
QR183.I46   616.07'9   76-28700
ISBN 0–12–107760–8

CONTENTS

II. METHODS IN TUMOR IMMUNITY

A. CELL-MEDIATED CYTOTOXICITY

B. ANTIBODY-DEPENDENT CELL-MEDIATED IMMUNITY

C. BLOCKING

D. DETECTION OF IMMUNE COMPLEXES

E. LYMPHOCYTE TRANSFORMATION

F. MIGRATION INHIBITION AND CHEMOTAXIS

G. CULTURE OF TUMOR CELLS

H. FROZEN IMMUNE LYMPHOCYTES AND TUMOR CELLS

I. *IN VITRO* SENSITIZATION TO TUMORS

LIST OF CONTRIBUTORS

Numbers in parentheses indicate the pages on which the author's contributions begin. Affiliations listed are current.

Anthony C. Allison (395) Clinical Research Centre, Harrow, Middlesex, England

L. C. Andersson (309) Department of Immunology, Biomedical Center, Uppsala, Sweden

Robert D. Arbeit (143) Division of Infectious Disease, Department of Medicine, Beth Israel Hospital, Boston, Massachusetts

Fritz H. Bach (741) Immunobiology Research Center, Departments of Medical Genetics and Surgery, University of Wisconsin School of Medicine, Madison, Wisconsin

Charles M. Balch (105) Departments of Surgery and Microbiology, University of Alabama in Birmingham, The Medical Center, Birmingham, Alabama

R. W. Baldwin (541) Nottingham Cancer Research Campaign Laboratories, University of Nottingham, Nottingham, England

Michael A. Bean (27, 471) Virginia Mason Research Center, Seattle, Washington

Gunnar Bendixen (629) Laboratory of Clinical Immunology, Medical Department, Rigshospitalet University Hospital, Copenhagen, Denmark

Celso Bianco (407) The Rockefeller University, New York, New York

R. M. Blaese (359) National Cancer Institute, National Institutes of Health, Bethesda, Maryland

Barry R. Bloom (3, 27, 319) Department of Microbiology and Immunology, Albert Einstein College of Medicine, Bronx, New York

K. Theodor Brunner (423, 737) Swiss Institute for Experimental Cancer Research, Epalinges-sur-Lausanne, Switzerland

A. C. Campbell (511) Nuffield Department of Clinical Medicine, The Radcliffe Infirmary, Oxford, England

Grace B. Cannon (607) Department of Immunology, Litton Bionetics Research Laboratory, Kensington, Maryland

Jean-Charles Cerottini (27, 423, 737) Swiss Institute for Experimental Cancer Research, Epalinges-sur-Lausanne, Switzerland

Leonard Chess (255) Division of Tumor Immunology, Sidney Farber Cancer Center, Harvard Medical School, Boston, Massachusetts

Winthrop Hallowell Churchill (417) Robert B. Brigham and Peter Bent Brigham Hospitals, Boston, Massachusetts

Connie Clark (83) Departments of Laboratory Medicine and Pathology, University of Minnesota School of Medicine, and Veterans Administration Hospital, Minneapolis, Minnesota

Edward A. Clark (437) Department of Microbiology and Immunology, University of California School of Medicine, Los Angeles, California

Zanvil A. Cohn (3, 333, 341) The Rockefeller University, New York, New York

Robert J. Connor (481, 607) Biometry Branch, National Cancer Institute, National Institutes of Health, Bethesda, Maryland

Max D. Cooper (105) Department of Pediatrics, University of Alabama in Birmingham, The Medical Center, Birmingham, Alabama

Joyce M. Cox (363) Division of Hematology—Oncology, Children's Hospital Medical Center, Boston, Massachusetts

Peter Curtis (217) Imperial Cancer Research Fund, Tumour Immunology Unit, Department of Zoology, University College, London, England

John R. David (3, 27, 417) Department of Medicine, Harvard Medical School, Robert B. Brigham Hospital, Boston, Massachusetts

Jack H. Dean (607, 621) Department of Immunology, Litton Bionetics Research Laboratory, Kensington, Maryland

J. W. dePierre (353) Department of Biological Chemistry, Harvard Medical School, Boston, Massachusetts

Howard B. Dickler (143) Immunology Branch, National Cancer Institute, National Institutes of Health, Bethesda, Maryland

Frank J. Dixon (555) Scripps Clinic and Research Foundation, La Jolla, California

Paul J. Edelson (333) The Rockefeller University, New York, New York

Alfred G. Ehlenberger (113) Department of Pathology, New York University Medical Center, New York, New York

M. J. Embelton (541) Cancer Research Campaign Laboratories, University of Nottingham, Nottingham, England

Howard D. Engers (423, 737) Swiss Institute for Experimental Cancer Research, Epalinges-sur-Lausanne, Switzerland

Gregory P. Fischetti (613) Department of Immunology, Litton Bionetics Research Laboratory, Kensington, Maryland

Helle Fogh (677) Sloan-Kettering Institute for Cancer Research, Donald S. Walker Laboratory, Rye, New York

Jørgen Fogh (677) Sloan-Kettering Institute for Cancer Research, Donald S. Walker Laboratory, Rye, New York

A. Forsgren (193) Department of Clinical Bacteriology, University of Lund, Malmö General Hospital, Malmö, Sweden

Elwin E. Fraley (451) Department of Urologic Surgery, University of Minnesota, School of Medicine, Minneapolis, Minnesota

Michael M. Frank (203) Laboratory of Clinical Investigation, National Institute of Allergy and Infectious Diseases, National Institutes of Health, Bethesda, Maryland

Stig S. Frøland (137) Institute of Immunology and Rheumatology, Rikshospitalet University Hospital, Oslo, Norway

D. G. L. Gale (511) Nuffield Department of Clinical Medicine, The Radcliffe Infirmary, Oxford, England

Sidney H. Golub (731) Division of Oncology, Departments of Surgery and of Microbiology and Immunology, University of California School of Medicine, Los Angeles, California

Maureen Goodenow (677) Sloan-Kettering Institute for Cancer Research, Donald S. Walker Laboratory, Rye, New York

S. Gordon (341) Sir William Dunn School of Experimental Pathology, Oxford, England

Melvyn F. Greaves (3, 89, 217) Imperial Cancer Research Fund, Tumour Immunology Unit, Department of Zoology, University College, London, England

Ira Green (203) Laboratory of Immunology, National Institute of Allergy and Infectious Diseases, National Institutes of Health, Bethesda, Maryland

J. U. Gutterman (587) Department of Developmental Therapeutics, M. D. Anderson Hospital and Tumor Institute, The University of Texas System Cancer Center, Houston, Texas

Thomas R. Hakala (451) Department of Surgery, Division of Urological Surgery, University of Pittsburgh, Pittsburgh, Pennsylvania

W. J. Halliday (547) Department of Microbiology, University of Queensland, Brisbane, Queensland, Australia

Sten Hammarström (497) Department of Immunology, Wenner-Gren Institute, University of Stockholm, Stockholm, Sweden

P. Häyry (309) Transplantation Laboratory, Fourth Department of Surgery, University of Helsinki, Helsinki, Finland

Ingegerd Hellström (533) Fred Hutchinson Cancer Research Center, Seattle, Washington

Karl Erik Hellström (533) Fred Hutchinson Cancer Research Center, Seattle, Washington

Ulla Hellström (497) Department of Immunology, Wenner-Gren Institute, University of Stockholm, Stockholm, Sweden

Pierre A. Henkart (143) Immunology Branch, National Cancer Institute, National Institutes of Health, Bethesda, Maryland

Christopher S. Henney (429) Departments of Medicine and Microbiology, The Johns Hopkins University School of Medicine, and The Neill Memorial Research Laboratories of The Good Samaritan Hospital, Baltimore, Maryland

Ronald B. Herberman (27, 461, 481, 489, 607, 613, 621, 723) Laboratory of Immunodiagnosis, Division of Cancer Biology and Diagnosis, National Cancer Institute, National Institutes of Health, Bethesda, Maryland

E. M. Hersh (587) Department of Developmental Therapeutics, M.D. Anderson Hospital and Tumor Institute, The University of Texas System Cancer Center, Houston, Texas

Thomas Hoffman (71) The Rockefeller University, New York, New York

Howard T. Holden (489, 723) Laboratory of Immunodiagnosis, Division of Cancer Biology and Diagnosis, National Cancer Institute, National Institutes of Health, Bethesda, Maryland

C. Y. Hunter (587) Department of Developmental Therapeutics, M.D. Anderson Hospital and Tumor Institute, The University of Texas System Cancer Center, Houston, Texas

Elaine S. Jaffe (203) Laboratory of Pathology, National Cancer Institute, National Institutes of Health, Bethesda, Maryland

George Janossy (89, 217) Imperial Cancer Research Fund, Tumour Immunology Unit, Department of Zoology, University College, London, England

Larry F. Jerome (607) Department of Immunology, Litton Bionetics Research Laboratory, Kensington, Maryland

Mikael Jondal (3, 187, 241, 263) Department of Tumor Biology, Karolinska Institutet, Stockholm, Sweden

Anna Kadish (319) Department of Microbiology and Immunology, Albert Einstein College of Medicine, Bronx, New York

Manuel E. Kaplan (83) Department of Medicine, University of Minnesota School of Medicine, Minneapolis, Minnesota

Manfred L. Karnovsky (353) Department of Biological Chemistry, Harvard Medical School, Boston, Massachusetts

Mogens Kjaer (629) Laboratory for Clinical Immunology, Medical Department, Rigshospitalet University Hospital, Copenhagen, Denmark

Yoshihisa Kodera (471) Virginia Mason Research Center, Seattle, Washington

I. R. Koski (359) National Cancer Institute, National Institutes of Health, Bethesda, Maryland

Henry G. Kunkel (3, 71) The Rockefeller University, New York, New York

S. Labaume (155) Institut de Recherches sur les Maladies du Sang, Hôspital Saint-Louis, Paris, France

Peter Lachmann (369) Laboratory of Molecular Biology, The Medical School, Cambridge, England

Paul-H. Lambert (565) WHO Research and Training Centre, Hôpital Cantonal, Centre de Transfusion, Geneva, Switzerland

Paul H. Lange (451) Department of Surgery/Urology, Veterans Administration Hospital, and Department of Surgery, University of Minnesota School of Medicine, Minneapolis, Minnesota

H. Sherwood Lawrence (27) Department of Medicine, New York University Medical Center, New York, New York

Alexander R. Lawton (105) Department of Pediatrics, University of Alabama in Birmingham, The Medical Center, Birmingham, Alabama

James Loveless (677) Sloan-Kettering Institute for Cancer Research, Donald S. Walker Laboratory, Rye, New York

Diane Lowe (369) Laboratory of Molecular Biology, The Medical School, Cambridge, England

James L. McCoy (607, 621) Department of Developmental Therapeutics, M.D. Anderson Hospital and Tumor Institute, The University of Texas System Cancer Center, Houston, Texas

Ian C. M. MacLennan (27, 511) Nuffield Department of Clinical Medicine, The Radcliffe Infirmary, Oxford, England

Adel A. F. Mahmoud (387) Division of Geographic Medicine, Department of Medicine, Case Western Reserve University, and University Hospitals, Cleveland, Ohio

Bruce A. Maurer (613) Department of Immunology, Litton Bionetics Research Laboratory, Kensington, Maryland

G. M. Mavligit (587) Department of Developmental Therapeutics, M.D. Anderson Hospital and Tumor Institute, The University of Texas System Cancer Center, Houston, Texas

Christopher Meade (369) Clinical Research Centre, Harrow, Middlesex, England

E. Merler (279) Department of Pediatrics, Children's Hospital Medical Center, Boston, Massachusetts

Richard G. Miller (283) Department of Medical Biophysics, University of Toronto, and The Ontario Cancer Institute, Toronto, Ontario, Canada

Robert D. Nelson (663) Department of Pediatrics, University of Minnesota School of Medicine, Minneapolis, Minnesota

Kenneth Nilsson (713) The Wallenberg Laboratory, University of Uppsala, Uppsala, Sweden

S. Nordling (309) Third Department of Pathology and Fourth of Surgery, University of Helsinki, Helsinki, Finland

Myrthel E. Nunn (489) Laboratory of Immunodiagnosis, Division of Cancer Biology and Diagnosis, National Cancer Institute, National Institutes of Health, Bethesda, Maryland

Victor Nussenzweig (3, 113) Department of Pathology, New York University Medical Center, New York, New York

Robert K. Oldham (461, 481, 723) Division of Oncology, Department of Medicine, Vanderbilt University Hospital, Nashville, Tennessee

J. J. Oppenheim (231, 573) Cellular Immunology Section, Laboratory of Microbiology and Immunology, National Institute of Dental Research, National Institutes of Health, Bethesda, Maryland

John R. Ortaldo (723) Laboratory of Immunodiagnosis, Division of Cancer Biology and Diagnosis, National Cancer Institute, National Institutes of Health, Bethesda, Maryland

Carol O'Toole (437) Departments of Surgery/Urology and of Microbiology and Immunology, University of California School of Medicine, Los Angeles, California

M. B. Pepys (197) Department of Immunology, Royal Free Hospital School of Medicine, London, England

Hedvig Perlmann (497) Department of Immunology, Wenner-Gren Institute, University of Stockholm, Stockholm, Sweden

Peter Perlmann (27, 497, 523) Department of Immunology, Wenner-Gren Institute, University of Stockholm, Stockholm, Sweden

Willy F. Piessens (417) Department of Medicine, Harvard Medical School, Robert B. Brigham Hospital, Boston, Massachusetts

Marilyn Pike (651) Division of Rheumatic and Genetic Diseases, Departments of Medicine and of Microbiology and Immunology, Duke University Medical Center, Durham, North Carolina

Margaret J. Polley (123) Department of Medicine, New York Hospital-Cornell Medical Center, New York, New York

D. G. Poplack (359) National Cancer Institute, National Institutes of Health, Bethesda, Maryland

Carl O. Povlsen (701) Pathological-Anatomical Institute, Copenhagen Municipal Hospital, and Copenhagen County Hospital in Gentofte, Hellerup, Denmark

J. L. Preud'homme (155) Laboratoire de Immunochemie et Immunopathologie, Institut de Recherches sur les Maladies du Sang, Hôpital Saint-Louis, Paris, France

Paul G. Quie (663) Department of Pediatrics, University of Minnesota School of Medicine, Minneapolis, Minnesota

Heinz G. Remold (3) Department of Medicine, Harvard Medical School, Robert B. Brigham Hospital, Boston, Massachusetts

R. A. Robins (541) Nottingham Cancer Research Campaign Laboratories, University of Nottingham, Nottingham, England

Fred S. Rosen (405) Department of Pediatrics, Children's Hospital Medical Center, Boston, Massachusetts

D. L. Rosenstreich (231, 573) Cellular Immunology Section, Laboratory of Microbiology and Immunology, National Institute of Dental Research, National Institutes of Health, Bethesda, Maryland

Gordon D. Ross (123) Department of Medicine, New York Hospital-Cornell Medical Center, New York, New York

Jørgen Rygaard (701) Pathological-Antomical Institute, Copenhagen County Hospital, and Copenhagen County Hospital in Gentofte, Hellerup, Denmark

Stuart F. Schlossman (3, 255) Division of Tumor Immunology, Sidney Farber Cancer Center, Harvard Medical School, Boston, Massachusetts

Hiroshi Shiku (471) Human Cancer Serology, Memorial Sloan-Kettering Cancer Center, New York, New York

Ken Shortman (267) Walter and Eliza Hall Institute of Medical Research, Melbourne, Australia

Richard L. Simmons (663) Department of Surgery, University of Minnesota School of Medicine, Minneapolis, Minnesota

David F. Siwarski (613) Department of Immunology, Litton Bionetics Research Laboratory, Kensington, Maryland

Ralph Snyderman (651) Division of Rheumatic and Genetics Diseases, Departments of Medicine and of Microbiology and Immunology, Duke University Medical Center, Durham, North Carolina

Lynn E. Spitler (645) Laboratory of Cellular Immunology, Children's Hospital Medical Center, and University of California Medical Center, San Francisco, California

Ralph M. Steinman (379) The Rockefeller University, New York, New York

Jan Stjernswärd (597) Ludwig Institute for Cancer Research (Lausanne Branch), Swiss Institute for Experimental Cancer Research, Lausanne, Switzerland

Gerald Stoner (319) Department of Microbiology and Immunology, Albert Einstein College of Medicine of Yeshiva University, Bronx, New York

Thomas P. Stossel (363) Medical Oncology Unit, Massachusetts General Hospital, Boston, Massachusetts

Osias Stutman (27) Department of Cellular Immunology, Memorial Sloan-Kettering Cancer Center, New York, New York

Simon Sutcliffe (319) Department of Medical Oncology, St. Bartholomew's Hospital, London, England

A. Svedjelund (193) Department of Immunology, Uppsala University Biomedical Center, Uppsala, Sweden

Argyrios N. Theofilopoulos (555) Department of Immunopathology, Scripps Clinic and Research Foundation, La Jolla, California

Farkas Vánky (597) Department of Tumor Biology, Karolinska Institutet, Stockholm, Sweden

Christine Von Muller (645) Laboratory of Cellular Immunology, Children's Hospital Medical Center, and University of California Medical Center, San Francisco, California

S. M. Wahl (231) Laboratory of Microbiology and Immunology, National Institute of Dental Research, National Institutes of Health, Bethesda, Maryland

Birgitta Wåhlin (523) Department of Immunology, Wenner-Gren Institute, University of Stockholm, Stockholm, Sweden

Z. Werb (341) Laboratory of Radiobiology, University of California School of Medicine, San Francisco, California

Hans Wigzell (3, 193, 245) Department of Immunology, Uppsala University Biomedical Center, Uppsala, Sweden

Robert J. Winchester (3, 171) The Rockefeller University, New York, New York

Finn Wisløff (137) Institute of Immunology and Rheumatology, Rikshospitalet University Hospital, Oslo, Norway

Mildred Woodson (83) Department of Hematology, Veterans Administration Hospital, Minneapolis, Minnesota

Joyce M. Zarling (741) Immunobiology Research Center, Departments of Medical Genetics and Surgery, University of Wisconsin School of Medicine, Madison, Wisconsin

Rudolf H. Zubler (565) WHO Research and Training Centre, Hôpital Cantonal, Centre de Transfusion, Geneva, Switzerland

PREFACE

The cell-mediated immune response is known to be crucially involved in such diverse phenomena as resistance to intracellular parasites (including viral, bacterial, fungal, and protozoal infection), contact allergy, rejection of transplanted organs and tissues, autoimmune disorders, and rejection of tumors. In the five years that have elapsed since the publication of the first volume of *"In Vitro Methods in Cell-Mediated Immunity"* there has been an explosion of interest and knowledge in the field of cell-mediated immunity. *In vitro* methods have been vital at two levels: first, in providing appropriate models and tools for understanding the basic mechanisms which underlie the response *in vivo;* and second, at the clinical level, in establishing useful indices of the actual and potential immune responsiveness of patients. Many of the methods appearing in the first volume had been developed only for animal models and have now been adapted and refined for application to human systems. Many novel techniques, which would not have been dreamed of five years ago, have been introduced for characterizing, separating, and assaying functions of the cell populations involved in cell-mediated immunity.

As is the case in all fields of science, our understanding of cell-mediated immunity can proceed no further than the methods by which it is studied will permit. It is the purpose of this book to make available, as widely as possible, much of the recently developed methodology in cell-mediated immunity so that it may be applied to diverse problems of fundamental and clinical importance. The book should serve both as a guide to investigators who will rely on the methods presented and as a stimulus for development of better methods and wider application of available methods to human disease.

The scope of this volume reflects the tremendous progress made, particularly in two broad areas. The first encompasses the characterization and enrichment of lymphocyte and macrophage populations, the basic cell types mediating the cell-mediated immune response. The second is tumor immunology, which we believe to hold enormous potential clinical importance for vast numbers of people. Because of the complexities and subtleties associated with the various methods and their applications, two expert panels were convened, with the support of the National Cancer Institute, to review critically the "state of the art" in each of the major areas and to evaluate the strengths, limitations, and applications of the methods. Their contribution has been invaluable in providing a thoughtful and balanced perspective of the field.

We have indeed been privileged to have had such generous cooperation of the many scientists who have recorded their methods in detail for others to use. Because it was simply not feasible to include chapters from all of the many laboratories which have made significant contributions to methods in the field, we have had to select representative methods in a variety of areas, with the realization that those from other outstanding laboratories regrettably could not be included.

We wish to express our deep appreciation to the many people on whom this book depended. We thank Ms. Theodora Polihrom, Ms. Grace Sylvestri, and Ms. Karen Lahey for outstanding secretarial assistance. The expertise of the staff of Academic Press has been invaluable. We gratefully acknowledge the encouragement and advice of Dr. William Terry, the valuable assistance of Mr. William Fitzsimmons, and the support of the National Cancer Institute. We are indebted to Dr. Zanvil Cohn and The Rockefeller University for generously making available their outstanding facilities to the members of the expert panels. And, finally, we wish to express our sincere gratitude to all those contributors and expert panel members who generously agreed to give their valuable time and share their special knowledge with all who read this book.

Barry R. Bloom
John R. David

Contents of
IN VITRO METHODS IN CELL-MEDIATED IMMUNITY
Edited by Barry R. Bloom and Philip R. Glade

*Based on a Conference held May 28–29, 1970
at New York University—Bellevue Medical Center,
New York, New York*

Sessions

Methods

In Vitro Methods
in Cell-Mediated
and Tumor Immunity

Section A

Evaluations

I

Evaluation of *in Vitro* Methods for Characterization of Lymphocytes and Macrophages*

Barry R. Bloom, Zanvil A. Cohn, John David, Melvyn F. Greaves, Mikael Jondal, Henry G. Kunkel, Victor Nussenzweig, Heinz G. Remold, Stuart F. Schlossman, Hans Wigzell, and Robert J. Winchester

1. Lymphocyte Surface Markers: T Cells

A great many surface markers or receptors on human and animal mononuclear cells have been described in recent years, yet with the possible exception of surface immunoglobulin, all of these are relative rather than absolute criteria for identification of cells as B cells, T cells, or monocytes. In many cases the frequency of cells positive for a given marker may vary with the technique used; not all, but only a fraction of cells positive for one marker will share several of the other markers even in normal peripheral blood, and the lack of correlation may be more serious in studies on cells of patients with a variety of diseases. From studies on bursectomized fowl and thymectomized and nude mice, it is clear that there are two principal categories of lymphocytes—B cells and T cells. Apart from the two principal groups, there are cells not at the moment fitting into either category: these include K cells, which are operationally defined as cells capable of antibody-dependent, cell-mediated cytotoxicity and may not necessarily express markers distinct from T or B cells, and cells with none of the known surface markers. Only the latter are what are appropriately termed "null cells."

1.1. Preparation of Blood for Study

A few general comments relevant to characterizing cells by all methods can be made. Usually the more rapidly the blood is processed, the more consistent and meaningful are the results; there are suggestions that storage may alter the expression of some receptors and functional activities. It seems that blood or purified white cells are in general best maintained at room temperature prior to

*This evaluation was prepared at a meeting held on January 26–28, 1976, at The Rockefeller University, sponsored by Contract NIH-76-C-3 from the National Cancer Institute. The United States Government has a royalty-free, nonexclusive, irrevocable license to reproduce, translate, publish, and use Evaluations I and II for official government purposes.

3

study. It is necessary to monitor the purification by checking the recovery of cells; i.e., the number of lymphocytes in a small sample of the starting material should be counted to be certain that the recovery upon purification or fractionation is good. Low yields raise the question whether the recovered cells are representative of the original lymphocyte population.

In addition, it is important to determine the viability of cells recovered by any of the methods used, since dead cells may affect both the percentages of lymphocytes in various subpopulations and the reproducibility of the data. The procedures most commonly used for determining cell viability are the trypan blue (0.1–0.2%) staining of dead cells and fluorescein diacetate staining of viable cells (see Method 34), taken together with phase microscopy. Dead cells may be removed by Ficoll–Hypaque and albumin gradient centrifugation procedures (see Methods 21 and 22) and the low ionic strength filtration method of Williams and Shortman (36).

It must additionally be borne in mind that variations in the number and percentage of lymphocyte populations, even in healthy individuals, can vary with physiological changes. For example, it has been reported that there are marked diminutions in detectable T cells following exercise and in early pregnancy (40). Diurnal variations may also occur. Obviously, deviations from the normal distribution of lymphoid subpopulations have been observed in a number of immunological and nonimmunological disease states, following surgery and chemotherapy, etc.

It is possible, but treacherous, to enumerate T cells, B cells, null cells, and monocytes simultaneously on blood smears (17). There is one other method currently developed in which it is possible to stain whole blood for surface-membrane immunoglobulin (SmIg) and a T cell antigen with fluorochrome-conjugated reagents in suspension, and then make smears for counting (see Method 13) (31). In all other methods, some purification of mononuclear cells from blood is required. The most commonly used method is the Ficoll–Hypaque sedimentation of heparinized blood (3), which has the advantage of being simple, reproducible, fast, and, most important, giving high yields (approaching 100%) with minimal contamination with granulocytes. Disadvantages may be variable contamination with platelets and possible toxicity of the reagents attendant on standing or exposure to light. In general, for analytical work the Ficoll–Hypaque method is most convenient and useful, although in studies on cells of some patients with leukemia, cancer, anemia, and rheumatoid arthritis, there are suggestions that yields may be low and that other methods would be preferable. However, a note of caution is necessary. Heparin treatment may interfere with certain cellular functions, as it is known to bind to cell surfaces. For most functional assays, preservative-free heparin is commonly used, although commercial heparin preparations with benzyl alcohol preservative may be suitable as well. Further, Ficoll–Hypaque may alter some functions of cells, e.g., induce the production of chemotactic factors (38).

Sedimentation methods, either spontaneous or in the presence of 6% dextran or 3% gelatin are acceptable, although the contamination with granulocytes and erythrocytes is greater than with Ficoll–Hypaque. Further, some batches of dextran or gelatin are toxic. Sedimentation may be carried out on cells obtained from defibrinated blood, which has the advantage that most platelets are removed and that serum from the same sample can be recovered. There is some variation in yield of mononuclear subpopulations depending on the size of the beads used and on the duration and force of shaking to facilitate clotting.

For analytical as well as functional tests, in principle, it would be advantageous to remove the monocytes which share some surface markers with B lymphocytes and K cells. Methods commonly used include treatment with carbonyl iron and removal of phagocytic cells with a magnet (see Method 19), and adherence to glass surfaces, glass, plastic, or Sephadex G-10 bead columns, or nylon fibers. In general, it is found that such treatments deplete not only monocytes but also variable percentages of lymphocytes, particularly B cells, as well, so that they are not recommended for analytical work. A promising method of selective adherence for short times to deplete monocytes without removing B lymphocytes has been described (see Method 5) (43). For preparative experiments and functional tests, it is often necessary to employ one of the above techniques. It should be noted that the presence of monocytes may be obligatory for obtaining positive results in some functional assays, e.g., antigen stimulation. In general, for analytical tests, it is preferable to allow the monocytes to remain and to enumerate them by phagocytic and other tests for monocytes and macrophages.

In order to evaluate the significance of the data on lymphocyte subpopulations in clinical immunology, it is recommended that, in addition to recording the percentage of cells exhibiting various positive markers, an accurate absolute count of these cells be made.

1.2. Membrane Markers for T Lymphocytes

Table 1 lists all markers reported to be selective for human T lymphocytes. Some of these have been much more extensively analyzed than others, and the rosette test with sheep erythrocytes is perhaps the *only* one where specificity and reproducibility are now fairly well established.

1.3. E Rosette Tests

Rosette assays using sheep red cells have been extensively used in the past years for enumeration of human T cells. The data available suggest that rosette formation with sheep erythrocytes provides the best currently available marker for human T cells. Virtually every thymic lymphocyte ($> 99\%$) will form an E rosette, and in the blood (and tonsils) the majority of SmIg-negative cells make E rosettes. E^+ cells are absent or severely diminished in numbers in the blood of patients with thymic aplasia. Interestingly, this deficiency is largely corrected with remarkable speed (less than 2 days) after thymus transplantation. Although

TABLE 1
Summary of Reported Human T Lymphocyte Markers

Marker	References
E rosettes	
Sheep	Jondal *et al.* (18)
Rhesus monkey	Lohrmann and Novikovs (23)
Human	Kaplan and Clark (21), Yu (46), Gluckman and Montambault (9), Dewar *et al.* (7), Sandilands *et al.* (34), Baxley *et al.* (1); Methods 1, 2
B lymphoblasts	Jondal *et al.* (19)
Lectins: *Helix pomatia*[a]	Hammarström *et al.* (12); Method 46
Virus: Measles[b]	Valdimarsson *et al.* (42)
Ig: IgM (−RBC)	Moretta *et al.* (28), McConnell and Hurd (26)
IgG (−RBC)	Ross *et al.* (33), Brown and Greaves (4), Winchester *et al.* (44), Method 1
Anti-T sera (Anti-HuTLA)	See Methods 3 and 4

[a] A hemagglutinin from *Helix pomatia*; like all other carbohydrate-binding proteins, that from *Helix pomatia* binds a number of different sugars with different affinity. Greatest binding efficiency is to N-acetyl-D-galactosamine.
[b] Binding of T lymphocytes to cells infected with measles virus.

it can be shown that E^+ and $SmIg^+$ cells are almost entirely separate and distinct populations, there is no unequivocal proof that *every* T cell can make an E rosette or that every cell making an E rosette is indeed a T cell (by functional criteria). Clearly one needs to relate the membrane marker phenotype to functional capacity (see below).

It is generally recognized that a large number of variables can influence the results of E rosette assays (Table 2). Variation between individual sheep exists but is not pronounced. Nevertheless, wherever possible it is preferable to use a single donor. Old sheep cells give poor rosettes, and it is recommended that blood not be used after storage for more than 14 days (at 4°C). The rosetting capacity of sheep cells can be considerably modified by pretreating the red cells with various reagents (see Table 2). The effect of these maneuvers is to (1) increase the absolute number of rosette-forming cells in otherwise suboptimal conditions; (2) considerably increase the stability of rosettes; this may be particularly useful if rosette- and non-rosette-forming cells are to be physically separated (e.g., by centrifugation on Ficoll–Isopaque); (3) improve the rosetting capacity of aged sheep red cells.

TABLE 2
Potential Sources of Variation in Sheep Erythrocyte
Rosette Assay for Human T Cells

1. Erythrocytes
   a. Pretreatment of red cells, e.g., neuraminidase,[a] long-chain neutral polymers, e.g., dextran, Ficoll, sulfhydryl reagents (AET[b]) (see Method 2)
   b. Age of red cells (i.e., storage time at $4°C$)
   c. Sheep donor variation
2. Lymphoid cells
   a. Time out of body
   b. Pretreatment? e.g., neuraminidase,[a] phospholipase C ($\uparrow$), trypsin ($\downarrow$), papain ($\uparrow$)
3. Test
   a. Proportions and absolute levels of ingredients
   b. Presence of fetal calf serum, human serum, or serum proteins (e.g., bovine serum albumin)
   c. Protocol: centrifugation (time, g force, temperature), period left (and temperature), method of resuspension and preparation for counting
   d. Criteria for positives (3+, ?)
   e. Fixation to stabilize rosettes? (e.g., glutaraldehyde or paraformaldehyde)

[a]Treatment with neuraminidase should be defined at pH below 7.0 to activate the enzyme without cell lysis; optimum pH of neuraminidase is 5.1, but it is usually necessary to use somewhat higher pH to maintain the integrity of cells under study.
[b]AET, 2-S-aminoethylisothiouronium bromide.

Pretreatment of lymphocytes with neuraminidase can increase the *proportion* of rosette forming cells. After such treatment the percentage of E-rosetting cells may reach 90% (see Method 1) (43). The "additional" cells that have become reactive include cells that were previously either SmIg⁻ or were "labile" IgG positive (i.e., IgG bound via Fc receptors). It is difficult at this stage to know whether these "enhancible" E rosetting cells are in fact functional thymus-derived lymphocytes, and this should be borne in mind when this modification is used. Treating lymphocytes with phospholipase C also increases the proportion of E rosettes. Since this procedure also converts cells from B lymphoid cell lines into E rosette formers, it seems possible that this modification alters some B (SmIg⁺?) lymphocytes to become E⁺. If this were to happen, then the proportion of T lymphocytes in blood would obviously be overestimated.

If one works on the premise that the E⁺ and SmIg⁺ lymphocytes are exclusive, separate populations (see Method 1), then parallel or simultaneous testing for E and SmIg provides a form of "internal" control.

The details of the E test system itself also vary considerably in different published reports (see Methods 1 and 2), and it may be that some of these differences (e.g., time, temperature) are of minimal importance if care is taken in resuspending the rosettes once they are formed. Pretreatment of erythrocytes with aminoethylisothiouranium bromide has been found to increase the number of erythrocytes bound to the T cells without any increase in the number of E-rosetting cells. The binding appears to be stronger than with untreated cells, making it a useful procedure for preparative removal of E-rosetting lymphocytes (see Method 2). It is generally agreed that the addition of protein (either fetal calf serum or albumin) increases the reproducibility of the assays and also increases the stability of rosettes. All sera used for rosettes should be absorbed with RBC.

The number of red cells bound per individual T cell varies considerably—an observation that may be of interest in relation to T cell subsets; a "threshold" value of 3 red cells seems to be a reliable criterion for T cell enumeration. Some workers fix the rosetted cells with glutaraldehyde (0.5%) or paraformaldehyde (2%) before final enumeration. This may be of use when there is a need to store the cell suspensions for subsequent analysis, as dissociation of rosettes will presumably not occur.

There has been no systematic study on the rosetting capacity of T lymphocytes at different times after taking blood or harvesting cells from tissues. However, since the capacity of T cells to make rosettes is dependent upon their being viable and metabolically active, it is advisable to perform the assay as soon as possible *and* simultaneously to assess viability using, for example, trypan blue. Dead cells, therefore, should not be scored as E-negative cells, as this could lead to an underestimate of the T cell proportion.

There have been two reports on the use of nonhuman primate red cells for rosette assays. Lohrmann and Novikovs (23) have presented evidence which suggests that rhesus monkey red cells may give essentially the same result as sheep erythrocytes (i.e., T cell specific). Different cell surface receptors may, however, be involved. In contrast to red cells from rhesus monkeys, erythrocytes of the Japanese ape (*Macaca speciosa*) make rosettes preferentially around B rather than T cells (30). However, granulocytes and monocytes also make rosettes with these and other monkey cells (e.g., pig-tailed monkey), as do a number of non-B malignant cells, e.g., acute lymphoblastic and acute myelogenous leukemia (M. F. Greaves, unpublished observations). At present there seems to be no particular advantage to be gained from using these various monkey red cell—rosette systems. It should also be pointed out that many primate species, including *Macaca speciosa,* may carry organisms that are very pathogenic for man.

Rosette tests have also been used to a limited extent as assays for T cells in a few animal species (see Method 16). Thus, rabbit red cells rosette selectively with T cells of guinea pigs, human red cells give T rosettes in dogs, and sheep RBC give T cells in New World monkeys.

1.4. Autorosettes

Several groups have recently reported that some human lymphocytes can rosette with autologous or homologous red cells. Thymus cells react better than blood lymphocytes, and the proportion of reactive cells can be considerably increased by pretreating the lymphocytes with neuraminidase. In double-rosette assays using both sheep and human cells effectively, every cell binding human red cells also made an E rosette, but not every sheep E binder also had human red cells attached (46); this result suggests that rosette tests with human red cells may identify a T cell subset (see below). The rosettes formed in this system may be very weak, although activated T cells [e.g., phytohemagglutinin (PHA)-activated lymphoblasts] may give stronger reactions. The test is nevertheless more fickle than sheep RBC rosetting, and some difficulty has been found in reproducing these observations (R. J. Winchester and M. F. Greaves, unpublished observations).

1.5. Anti-T Cell Sera

Numerous attempts have been made to produce antisera to human T cell antigens (anti-HuTLA). A wide variety of cellular immunogens, immunization protocols, absorption procedures, and assay systems have been employed (see Method 3) and at present it is not possible to "distill" from all this information which regimen is the best. As has been described (see Methods 3 and 4), rabbit antisera to monkey thymus *can* provide good sera. It may also be possible to obtain anti-T cell sera from patients with autoimmune and other disorders (see Methods 3 and 10).

It appears to be a general experience that extensive absorption of anti-T sera with either CLL cells (i.e., SmIg$^+$ malignant B cells) and/or B lymphoid cell lines is essential and that the majority of antisera raised against T cells may not provide workable reagents (i.e., a high failure rate is to be anticipated). Some human sera from patients with a variety of pathological conditions may contain anti-T antibodies (see Methods 3 and 10); however, such sera may still require extensive absorption, and at present they do not appear to provide a reliable source of anti-T sera. A promising new approach appears to be the production of antibodies against rhesus monkey thymocytes, which after only a few absorptions with human B cells, have excellent specificity by immunofluorescence for human T cells (see Method 4). The critical point to be considered is clearly the precise sensitivity of the antisera, whether the specificity is absolute or relative; then, if it is relative, by what criteria should one assign positive and negative cells. Different workers have adopted a variety of criteria for specificity (see Methods 3 and 4). It is usually considerably more difficult to make such sera specific by immunofluorescent tests (or other binding assays) as compared with cytotoxicity. We suggest that the most relevant and reliable criterion for T cell specificity is the reciprocal reactivity vis-à-vis $SmIg^+$ cells (see Method 3). In other words, double or simultaneous testing with anti-HuTLA and anti-SmIg should ideally reveal two exclusive and nonoverlapping populations. It is also important to determine whether or not the anti-T cell sera can react at all with non-T non-B cells (e.g., monocytes, granulocytes, stem cells). The possibility of reactivity with activated B cells should also be tested (i.e., on B lymphoid cell lines or on "normal" B cells activated *in vitro* with staphylococcal mitogen) (see Method 12).

Although one or more of the procedures for producing anti-T sera (see Methods 3 and 4) may eventually be found to provide a reproducible protocol, they will continue to be laborious and pose logistical problems. Perhaps the ultimate aim should be to use whatever T cell-specific sera are available to purify the putative T cell-specific antigens—and to immunize with these.

TABLE 3
Classification of Mouse T Cells

Property	Subset[a]	
	$T_H{}^b$	$T_{C,S}{}^b$
Ly phenotype[c]	$1+$	$2,3^+$
Ontogeny	Late	Late
Atx[d]	Resistant	Resistant
Recirculation[e]	+	+
Histamine receptor		+
Ia phenotype	?+	?+
Phytohemagglutinin response	+	+
Concanavalin A	+	?
Cytotoxic precursor		+
Cytotoxic effector		+
Proliferation in MLC[f]	+	−
Specific T helper	+	
Specific T suppressor		+

[a]This table does not include another T-cell subset, Ly $1,2.3^+$. These cells constitute a large proportion of peripheral T cells; however, their functions have not yet been clearly delineated. They appear early in ontogeny and have been referred to as T_E for T "early" cells.
[b]T_H is a T helper, $T_{C,S}$ is T cytotoxic, suppressor.
[c]Ly phenotype is defined in C57BL/6 mice and is not necessarily applicable in other strains.
[d]Atx = athymic or thymectomized.
[e]Recirculation = presence in thoracic duct lymph.
[f]MLC, mixed leukocyte culture.

1.6. T Cell Subsets

In the mouse there is now considerable evidence for T cell subsets based on both functional assays and membrane markers—particularly the Ly antigens (see Table 3). The precise relationship of the subsets is not yet established (i.e., are they parallel lines of postthymic development or sequential derivatives of one line?).

It is highly probable that analogous T cell subset heterogeneity exists in man, and this is likely to be of considerable importance in relation to immunological competence in normal and disease states. At present, there is no unequivocal membrane marker that clearly delineates a functional T cell subset in man. However, there are a number of hints that such subsets do indeed exist and that they may be identifiable through differential reactivity with a variety of T cell markers. These preliminary observations are listed in Table 4. As yet, the functional repertoire of these different T cells has not been assessed.

In addition to these differences, thymus lymphocytes are distinguished from peripheral T cells by both surface antigens (see Method 3) and by their content

TABLE 4
Preliminary Evidence Suggesting Heterogeneity of
Human T Lymphocytes

1. Heterogeneity of E_s rosettes	
"Early" or "active" versus "late"	Wybran and Fudenburg (45), Yu (47)
Number of bound RBC population A 2–8 population B>10	Brown and Greaves (4)
Neuraminidase-dependent subset	See Method 1
2. Autorosettes (see Table 1)	
Only a proportion of sheep E rosette formers react	
3. Weak or strong staining or subset staining only with anti-T sera	See Method 3
4. Differential elution from *Helix pomatia* absorbent columns using N-acetyl-D-galactosamine[a]	Hellström *et al.* (14)
5. Differential reactivity with wheat germ agglutinin (WGA)	Hellström *et al.* (13)
6. IgM-RBC rosettes; subset of sheep E-rosetting cells reactive	See Table 1
7. IgG-RBC or AggIgG binding T-cell subset	See Table 1

[a]Elution from *Helix pomatia* (HP) column with 1.0 mg of D-GalNAc per milliliter gives a highly T-enriched fraction, >90% HP⁺. Of these "T cells," 5–10% are both HP⁺ and SmIg⁺, but the Ig is all externally adsorbed IgG. These cells also have Fc and C receptors. (See Method 46.)

of the enzyme terminal deoxynucleotidyltransferase (25). It seems very likely that definition of markers of human T cell subsets will take place during the next year or two, and while this adds a "complication" to the clinical immunologist's technical repertoire, it offers an important potential for more detailed analysis of this immunological status of patients.

1.7. Other Markers

A variable proportion of human T cells may have cell-surface binding sites for immunoglobulins. As in the mouse, it appears that up to 10% of T cells in human blood can bind IgG when this is in a cross-linked or aggregated form. Recent studies in the mouse (22) and in man (see Table 1) also suggest that a proportion of T cells may have receptors for IgM. In man these are at present demonstrable only after incubation of blood lymphocytes for 24 hr *in vitro.* Most of the cells binding IgM (e.g., IgM-coated red cells) also make E (sheep) rosettes, but as yet there is no unequivocal evidence that some SmIg$^+$ B cells are not also reactive in this assay.

Lectins in general (e.g., PHA, Con A, lentil) bind to all lymphocytes. Hammarström *et al.* (12) have presented evidence that agglutinin from albumin glands of the snail *Helix pomatia* (HP) has T-cell specificity. Binding to T cells requires pretreating the lymphocytes with neuraminidase. A considerable proportion of the SmIg$^+$ CLL cells bind HP, but the nature of the HP receptor is not known (it may be different from the HP receptor in normal blood lymphocytes). Neither do we know the nature of the Ig on the double-staining CLL cells (15).

In the mouse, wheat germ agglutinin (WGA) reacts weakly with normal lymphocytes but strongly with myeloid cells, lymphoblasts, and a variety of leukemic cells (10). In man, however, all blood lymphocytes bind WGA (13). T cells obtained by passage through Wigzell-type columns consist of two subpopulations; one (approximately 15%) binds WGA weakly, the other (majority of the cells) binds WGA strongly.

Jondal *et al.* (19) have reported that all blood T lymphocytes can bind B lymphoblasts from continuous cell lines (rosette assay). The nature of the cell-surface site that T cells recognize on B lymphoblasts has not been determined.

It has been observed that mitogen and antigen activated lymphocytes are capable of replicating a variety of RNA viruses, and in the mouse replication of vesicular stomatitis virus appears to be selective for activated T cells (20). By the use of a virus plaque assay, it is possible to enumerate antigen- or mitogen-activated lymphocytes (see Method 15). Before the method can be usefully applied to clinical problems, however, it remains to be established whether virus production is selective for T cells in human lymphoid populations and whether all activated cells or only a portion or subpopulation of them are detected by this assay.

2. Lymphocyte Surface Markers: B Cells

The B lymphocyte is defined as a cell with membrane bound, intrinsicially produced surface Ig, comprising 5—15% of the blood lymphocytes. This definition does not include at present Ig-negative precursor cells or the surface Ig-negative plasma cells, although these cells are considered part of the B-cell series. There is general agreement among investigators that a typical B lymphocyte expresses other markers, such as complement and Fc receptors. Other markers summarized in Table 5 are also demonstrable on B lymphocytes.

T lymphocytes are recognized by the formation of rosettes with sheep erythrocytes (E rosettes), a property not shared by B lymphocytes. Such T cells comprise approximately 80% of peripheral blood lymphocytes (PBL). This broad division of PBL into typical T and B cells thus accounts for all but perhaps 5—15% of PBL.

There is some difference of opinion about the nature and characteristics of the cell populations comprising this remainder, with evidence for heterogeneous populations that cannot be classified as either B or T cells. For example, a number of findings demonstrate a lymphoid cell population characterized by readily demonstrable Fc receptors, an absence of SmIg, but the property of forming E rosettes (see Method 1) and K-cell activity (see Method 46).

Two different problems are associated with the methods for separation and analysis of B lymphocytes. The first is the reliability of the method in unambiguously measuring a given marker without technical interference. Recent developments in many of the techniques have, to a considerable degree, altered the interpretation of some of the initial findings. Second, there is a conceptual problem that concerns the proper inference that is to be made from the demonstration of the given marker regarding the lymphocyte class. In this respect a number of difficulties present themselves. These include: the existence of functional and molecularly defined subsets of both T and B cells; the fact that differentiating cells may express only some of their repertoire of markers, and last, the possibility that well defined but minor classes of lymphocytes will be recognized that are neither T nor B cells.

For enumeration of B cells, an important concern must be the adequacy of monocyte identification. Since the monocyte shares markers with the B lymphocytes (see Table 5), it is possible that they could be erroneously counted as B lymphocytes.

Another technical point of great importance in the enumeration of B cells is to exclude the adsorption of complexes containing IgG to Fc-positive non-B cells. Such cells otherwise appear as surface Ig-positive "B" cells. The most reliable procedure to this end is to use Fab_2 anti-Ig antibodies (see Methods 9 and 10). Also, overnight incubation at $37°C$ (in the absence of human IgG) results in release of most or all adsorbed IgG, and short-term culture after trypsin treatment has the same effect.

TABLE 5

Surface Markers on Human Peripheral Blood B Lymphocytes

Surface marker	Approximate frequency	Distribution	Technique	Presence on non-lymphoid cells
Intrinsic S Ig Predominantly IgDκ and IgMκ with lesser numbers of IgG, IgA, and λ-positive cells	2–15%	The basic definition of the B lymphocyte	Immunofluorescence (Methods 9, 10) mixed agglutination; immunoperoxidase; immunoautoradiography	Monocytes and granulocytes by virtue of cytophilic IgG receptors under staining conditions with anti-IgG reagents
Complement receptors C3d and C3b (C4b)	5–15%	Present on most or all B lymphocytes and on a number of SmIg cells, such as the K cell population	Rosette formation (EAC) (Methods 5 and 6), immunofluorescence	Monocytes have both C3b and C3d receptors; granulocytes and erythrocytes have only C3b receptors
IgG Fc receptors	10–20%	Present on most or all B lymphocytes and on a number of non-B cells, such as the K cell population and possibly on a subset of T cells	Rosette formation: ox, Ripley (Method 7); immune complexes or aggregated IgG (Method 8)	Monocytes and granulocytes have Fc receptors

EBV receptor[a]	5–15%	Newly introduced; present on most or all B lymphocytes	Immunofluorescence; rosette formation (Method 11)	No
Mouse red blood cell receptor	5–15%	Newly introduced; present on most or all B lymphocytes	Rosette formation	Not ascertained
LB alloantigens[b]	5–15%	Newly introduced; present on all B lymphocytes and on a small number of non-B cells	Indirect immunofluorescence; cytotoxicity (Method 10)	Monocytes express the antigen
Heteroantigens		Newly introduced	Immunofluorescence; cytotoxicity [Greaves and Brown (11)]	Not ascertained
P 23,30[c]	15–25%	Present on all B cells	Schlossman et al. (35)	—

[a] EBV, Epstein-Barr virus.
[b] LB, lymphocyte B antigens.
[c] P 23,30, B lymphoblast cell lines.

Owing to such problems, the percentage of cells staining with anti-immuno-globulin reagents, in certain older literature, was sometimes considerably higher. It is now clear that IgD and IgM constitute the major membrane Igs of blood B cells. Most B cells have both IgM and IgD although roughly one-fourth of the cells have only either one or the other class detectable. IgA- and IgG-bearing cells together account for about 1% of peripheral blood lymphocytes in the average normal person.

Cells with Fc receptors are found in at least two lymphocyte populations: the typical B cell, and a second cell type that lacks SmIg but has, to a considerable degree, the property of forming E rosettes as mentioned in the introduction.

The complement-receptor lymphocytes mostly coincide with Ig-bearing cells in normal human peripheral blood; however, C receptors are also present on some SmIg cells that have Fc receptors and frequently adsorbed IgG. True null cells are difficult to enumerate in normal peripheral blood using analytic techniques, and they require isolation followed by the use of multiple marker experiments once they lack SmIg, Fc, and complement receptors, and fail to form E rosettes.

The problem of autologously reacting anti-lymphocyte antibodies merits par-ticular comment. These antibodies, by adhering to the surface of the lympho-cyte, can confer positive surface staining to an otherwise Ig-negative cell (see Methods 9 and 10). The presence of these antibodies can usually be recognized when the sum of surface staining plus E rosettes exceeds 100%. These anti-lymphocyte antibodies may occur in a number of diseases, such as infectious mononucleosis, systemic lupus erythematosus, mycoplasma pneumonia, rheuma-toid arthritis, and various other lymphoproliferative diseases. The fact that in most instances they are primarily of the IgM class also contributes to their being confused with SmIg. The bulk of the antibodies can be removed by washing the cells at 37°C. The sensitivity of the SmIg method to this type of interference can, however, be turned to good advantage by performing the staining reaction for surface Ig at 4°C on samples of cells incubated in patients' serum; the finding of an elevated proportion of positive cells in the former situation indicates the presence of antilymphocyte antibodies (see Methods 9 and 10).

Recently, several laboratories have described differentiation alloantigens ex-pressed on B lymphocytes but not on the vast majority of T lymphocytes. Pregnancy sera and heterosera have been used in fluorescent antibody or cyto-toxicity assays to demonstrate these antigens. These antigens are expressed in the absence of surface Ig and have been used as a marker of a B cell precursor.

3. Purification of T and B Cells

There are a number of approaches to the problem of fractionation of human lymphocytes into T and B subpopulations. The methods available vary widely from being simple and inexpensive to requiring sophisticated technology and equipment presently available only in a few laboratories in the world (e.g., a cell sorter). The latter will not be considered here; however, the reader is referred to the publications of Hertzenberg and his co-workers (2, 24) and Greaves (10) for details of technology and applications. When considering other techniques, the choice of method will largely depend on the requirements of the problem and of the investigators, as the methods vary in complexity, recovery of cells, purity of cellular subpopulations, and applicability to testing various functional properties.

One of the simplest and yet quite efficient methods of fractionating human T and B lymphocytes is by rosetting with sheep RBC (see Method 16). Rosetting techniques have both vices and virtues. They are especially suitable when fractionating samples from several donors. Cell losses during fractionation are comparatively minor compared to some column filtration procedures. However, with regard to the purity of the subfractions obtained, rosetting techniques are frequently inferior to column techniques. Further procedures to remove the RBC bound to lymphocytes in the rosetted population, such as lysis with ammonium chloride (if necessary), may lead to changes in the functional capacity of the lymphocytes (16). Red blood cells from several species have been suggested for use in the separation of T and B lymphocytes (see Method 16). In this context, one should consider the potential hazard of dangerous infections when using monkey RBC.

Special applications of rosetting techniques involve the selective depletion or enrichment of a minor subgroup of cells in a population. These techniques have been found quite useful, for example, for the depletion of naturally cytotoxic cells (see Method 20) or for the isolation of T cells (containing specific killer cells) from larger masses of tumor cells (see Method 17).

There are several disadvantages of the E rosette depletion method. The volume of lymphoid cells that can be handled is limited. Repeated rosettings lead to relatively low yields of recovered cells, and there is usually a small contaminating fraction of residual cells that cannot be removed and could influence functional tests.

Column fractionation procedures, especially those utilizing affinity chromatography, are especially useful for separating large numbers of cells. Their main application has been in the separation of cells with Ig on their surfaces. Column techniques separate lymphocytes according to two principles: (1) removal of the more adherent cells via poorly defined interactions, and (2) removal of cells carrying surface structures with specific affinity for the material on the column. It is likely that cells bound by this latter principle will be subject secondarily to nonspecific forces, and thus, cells that were originally bound for specific reasons are now also retained for reasons of "adhesiveness."

There are presently three types of column techniques in use: nylon fiber columns (see Method 15), Degalan glass-bead columns (see Method 18), and

Sephadex anti-Ig columns (see Method 19). Comparison of their advantages and disadvantages can be summarized as follows.

The nylon fiber technique is, of the three, the simplest, and it is the most efficient for removing adherent cells. When human peripheral blood is passed over such columns in the presence of 50% serum or plasma, monocytes are retained and there is almost complete recovery of T and B lymphocytes. If the cells are passed in low serum concentrations (10%), moncytes and some adherent T and B cells are retained. The cells that come through in that case represent a subpopulation of T lymphocytes (approximately 50% of total) and a subpopulation of B cells programmed for IgG synthesis. Also, with low concentrations of serum some monocytes may come through.

Degalan glass-bead, anti-Ig columns do not remove adherent cells to the same extent as nylon fiber columns, yet they are at least as efficient in removal of surface Ig-positive cells. Such columns will also remove cells with receptors for the Fc of IgG. They also remove a sizable proportion of the T cells. The adherent cells can be recovered via mechanical elution.

The Sephadex anti-Ig columns used with EDTA show a low degree of retention of adherent cells and a high yield. They will remove surface Ig-positive cells and will leave in the population passing through the column most of the T cells as well as a subset of Ig-negative and E-negative cells destined to differentiate into B cells. The surface Ig-positive cells can be recovered quantitatively by a combination of specific and mechanical elution procedures. Compared to the glass or Degalan beads, the anti-Ig Sephadex columns are somewhat more elaborate, requiring larger quantities of purified reagents. To further ensure that anti-Ig columns selectively remove Ig-positive cells, it may be advantageous to use $(Fab)_2$ anti-Ig when preparing such columns.

There are two potential disadvantages of the anti-Ig column method. It is possible that cells might be adsorbed by virtue of surface immunoglobulins bound to their Fc receptors. These cells might then be eluted with Ig and stained by anti-SmIg reagents if the Ig were not removed from their Fc receptors. Second, adsorption of B cells to the anti-Ig columns could lead to a membrane perturbation that may render them more susceptible to subsequent activation by other stimuli.

Table 6 shows some of the functional activities of human blood lymphocytes obtained by Ficoll–Hypaque and separated by various fractionation procedures.

4. Purification of Monocytes/Macrophages

One of the most important problems in macrophage or monocyte purification is distinguishing them from lymphocytes and polymorphonuclear leukocytes. A variety of approaches that have different advantages and drawbacks, can be used (see Methods 26, 28, 29, 34, and 36).

TABLE 6 Preliminary Response Profiles

	Unseparated	Nylon fiber passed	E rosette depleted	Sephadex anti-Fab, bound and eluted	Sephadex anti-Fab, passed and E rosette depleted	Sephadex anti-Fab passed	Degalan/glass anti-Ig, passed
Proliferation							
A. Polyclonal mitogens							
1. PHA[a] and Con A[a]	+++	++	-	+	+	+++	+
2. PWM[a]	++	+	-	+	+	+	+
3. Staphylococcal A protein	+	?	++	?	?	?	-
B. MLC[a]							
1. Responding cell	+++	+++	-	-	-	+++	+++
2. Stimulating cell	+++	+++	+++	+++	+++	+	+
Stimulation by antigen							
1. ^{3}H-Thymidine incorporation	+	+	-	-	-	+	?
2. MIF[a] production	++	+	++	++	+	++	?
3. Mitogenic factor production	++	++	-	-	-	++	?
4. Chemotactic factor production	++	?	++[b]	?	?	?	?
Cytotoxicity							
1. Ab-independent specific CMC[a]	++	++	-	-	-	++	++
2. Ab-dependent CMC[a]	++	++	+++	++	+++	+	-
3. Spontaneous non-specific CMC[a]	++	+	+++	?	?	?	+
Immunoglobulin synthesis	+	-	+	+	+	-	-
Virus replication							
1. VSV[a] myxovirus, and paramyxovirus	+	+	-	?	?	?	?
2. EBV[a]	+	-	+	+	?	-	-

[a]PHA, phytohemagglutinin; Con A, concanavalin A. PWM, pokeweed mitogen; MLC, mixed lymphocyte culture; MIF, migration inhibitory factor; CMC cell-mediated cytotoxicity; VSV, vesicular stomatitis virus; EBV, Epstein-Barr virus.

[b]E rosetted cells also make chemotactic factor.

4.1. Histochemistry

The use of myeloperoxidase and nonspecific esterase for staining phagocytic vesicles is useful for determining phagocytic cells and for the exclusion of lymphocytes (see Method 29). These methods are especially valuable for differentiating macrophages and monocytes from lymphoid cells coated with erythrocytes. On the other hand, polymorphonuclear leukocytes will also show positive reactions. In the presence of polymorphonuclear leukocytes, additional morphological criteria have to be included.

4.2. Morphology

Whereas the ability to phagocytize and pinocytize may well be used to differentiate between lymphoid cells and monocytes/macrophages, the latter cannot be differentiated by these methods from polymorphonuclear cells. The simplest and, in many cases, most reliable method to differentiate lymphocytes, macrophages, and polymorphonuclear leukocytes is microscopic examination of a stained smear or examination using phase-contrast microscopy. Although, in certain cases, it is impossible to differentiate monocytic cells from large lymphocytes, morphological criteria seem to be the most reliable means to differentiate macrophages and polymorphonuclear leukocytes.

4.3. The Concept of Macrophage Activation

A number of different methods to obtain activated monocytes and macrophages are available. This implies also that the term "activation" is defined differently by different investigators. We can basically describe two types of "activated" macrophages.

4.3.1. Macrophages elicited by intraperitoneal injection of certain irritants behave as activated in terms of certain physiological functions in comparison to peritoneal exudate washout cells. For example, macrophages obtained by thioglycolate injection produce plasminogen activator (41) whereas peritoneal washout cells do not.

4.3.2. Casein- or oil-induced peritoneal exudate cells, when stimulated *in vitro* with lymphocyte mediators, are activated in terms of increased bacteriostasis, tumor cell killing, glucose C-1 oxidation, and phagocytosis of dead tubercle bacilli (5) (see Method 37). This effect can be enhanced by direct incubation of macrophages with intact sensitized and stimulated lymphocytes (37). Peritoneal exudate cells from bacillus Calmette-Guérin (BCG)-sensitized animals also exhibit an increased ability to kill bacteria, such as *Listeria monocytogenes* (27).

It should be borne in mind that different modes of activation may lead to different biochemical, morphological, and functional changes, and that macrophages activated by one stimulus may thus not be identical to those activated by another. Further studies will be required to clarify these differences.

4.4. Purification of Monocytes and Macrophages

Further purification of monocytes and macrophages following Ficoll–Hypaque or albumin density-gradient centrifugation, which eliminates polymorphonuclear cells, can be achieved in a number of ways. Adherence of the macrophage- or monocyte-enriched fraction for 1 hr at 37°C eliminates most of the lymphocytes; however, a small number of lymphocytes will also adhere to the plate. The adherent cells then can be obtained by (a) trypsinization in the presence of EDTA, which does not remove all cells quantitatively; (b) scraping the plate using a rubber policeman, which might break up an unknown number of cells; and (c) using anesthetics, such as lidocaine (32).

4.5. *In Vitro* Cultivation

In most instances blood monocytes and tissue macrophages can be maintained *in vitro* under simple culture conditions on the surface of plastic or glass (see Method 26). These cells do not normally divide although the addition of conditioned medium leads to one or two rounds of replication. It should be pointed out, however, that there is a considerable variation in cell survival in long-term cultures which depends in part upon the source and species of cells employed. In general, oil-induced peritoneal cells from the rabbit and guinea pig as well as alveolar macrophages from both man and rodents demonstrate a progressive detachment from the substrate and subsequent loss into the medium. Similar observations have been made with equine monocytes, whereas mouse peritoneal cells are more stable. In addition, human monocytes can be maintained alive for 2 weeks on cover slips in Medium 199 containing 10% heat-inactivated autologous serum (8). The variability of cellular survival in culture requires that appropriate methods be employed for the quantitation of cell numbers or the analysis of cell components. This can be accomplished by direct photographic analysis of cell numbers (see Method 26) or the determination of DNA or cell protein (see Method 37). Factors that influence cell loss in culture include fastidious nutritional requirements or selection from a heterogeneous starting population of cells. An additional complication results from the presence of contaminating fibroblasts and mesothelial cells, which actively divide and may, on prolonged cultivation, represent a substantial proportion of the culture. These cells are particularly prominent in macrophage cultures obtained from inflammatory exudates, but may be removed selectively by brief trypsinization. Monocytes and macrophages are usually more resistant to treatment with trypsin and/or EDTA and remain attached to the substrate.

Finally it should be pointed out that polymorphonuclear leukocytes (PML) detach after plating for 18 hr whereas monocytes/macrophages remain adherent. This is a useful and simple method of eliminating polymorphonuclear leukocytes when Ficoll–Hypaque gradient separation cannot be employed. On the other hand, PML in suspension will survive 24 hr of incubation.

4.6. Phagocytosis

A number of useful methods are available to measure the endocytic activity of mononuclear phagocytes (see Methods 30–32). These vary in complexity and specificity, and a few comments on their usefulness under different experimental conditions seem appropriate. One of the most rigorous is described by Stossel *et al.* (39) (Method 30) and is most helpful in quantitating the extent and rate of interiorization of cells maintained in suspension culture. It should be apparent that both granulocytes and mononuclear phagocytes interiorize the lipid emulsion, so that the homogeneity of the population should be carefully evaluated. In addition, some difficulty is experienced with cells attached on a monolayer since the low-density particles float in the aqueous environment. The specificity of phagocytosis is also a consideration when dealing with heterogeneous populations or in characterizing transformants. The stable Fc receptor is particularly useful in that it is invariably expressed on both monocytes and macrophages (see Methods 35 and 36). The receptor for EA is also quite protease resistant, although the receptor for monomeric Ig is sensitive to trypsin. Phagocytosis of latex particles presumably occurs by nonimmunological mechanisms and is a property shared by macrophages and fibroblasts alike. The latex particle, however, is quite useful in examining the monocyte contamination of peripheral blood lymphoid cells obtained by Ficoll–Hypaque methods in which granulocytes are not a serious problem. In addition, it requires only short experience with the phase microscope to distinguish intracellular from surface-bound latex beads.

4.7. Sources

Mononuclear phagocytes can be obtained from a number of sources and differ in both morphological and biochemical properties. This functional heterogeneity is in part the result of local environmental conditions, which in time govern such properties as endocytosis and the storage of slowly degradable substances. Not all such cells are described here because of limitations of space. One should mention, however, that in man alveolar macrophages obtained by bronchoscopic lavage are particularly useful cells. Similarly, the alveolar macrophages from rabbit and guinea pig are a rich source in normal or BCG-activated states and have proved to be useful for biochemical, cell-fractionation, and suspension culture techniques. More recently a number of investigators have reported on the isolation of hepatic Kupffer cells after destruction of the hepatocytes by pronase digestion (29). These can be cultivated *in vitro* and should be excellent tools for both labeling and functional studies. It is apparent that the source of human cells is still quite limited, and cells from serious cavities, i.e., ascitic and pleural fluid, should be exploited in the future.

Since macrophages do not divide actively *in vitro* and since they are often minor components in tissues, cell numbers become limiting for more sophisticated analyses. This situation may change in the near future as continuous cell lines with macrophage properties are described and through the use of replicating transformants. Careful characterization of these lines is underway in many laboratories and should result in useful materials for genetic analysis, receptor isolations, etc.

4.8. *In Vivo* Ablation

The ability to destroy both circulating and resident mononuclear phagocytes would be a most useful technique to examine many problems of immunology, transplantation biology, and infectious diseases. Unfortunately, this area is still in its infancy and requires considerable investigation in terms of the extent and specificity of the cell destruction. Allison and co-workers report on one approach (see Method 34) in which silica destroys the cells that ingest it (6). The procedure appears to be most efficient within the confined limits of the peritoneal cavity and less efficient via the bloodstream. The situation points out a major defect in our knowledge, namely, the preparation of specific antisera that react with the surface of mononuclear phagocytes. Such procedures have been successfully employed in destroying cells of the granulocyte series, but much less is known in the case of macrophages. Although anti-macrophage antisera have been raised, detailed studies of their specificity are lacking. Such a reagent would also be most useful in identifying monocytes and macrophages in mixed-cell populations by fluorescent techniques.

EDITOR'S NOTE

Because this meeting was primarily concerned with the evaluation of methods, it was not possible to review all the applications of the methods to a variety of disease states. Several reviews have, however, recently appeared on this subject, and the reader is referred to the following:

Greaves, M. F., Immunodeficiency diseases, *Prog. Haematol.* IX, 255 (1975).
Greaves, M. F., Brouet, J.-C., Preud'homme, J.-L., and Seligman, M., Leukemia and lymphoproliferative disease, *Blood Cells* 1, 81 (1975).
Hayward, A., and Greaves, M. F., *in* "Recent Advances in Clinical Immunology" (R. A. Thompson, ed.). Pergamon, Oxford, 1976.
"A.A.I. Manual of Clinical Immunology" (N. R. Rose and H. Freidman, eds.). Amer. Soc. for Microbiology, Washington, D.C., 1976.
"Immunodeficiency in Man and Animals" (D. Bergsma, ed.). Sinauer, Sunderland, Massachusetts, 1975.
Immunodeficiency (G. Möller, ed.) *Transplant. Rev.* 16 (1973).

In addition, we have not discussed in any detail the new and exciting work on Ly antigens in the mouse. In this case we refer you to the original papers as follows:

Shiku, H., Kisielow, P., Bean, M. A., Takahaski, T., Boyse, E. A., Oettgen, H. F., and Old, L. J., *J. Exp. Med.* 141, 227 (1975).
Cantor, H., and Boyse, E. A., *J. Exp. Med.* 141, 1376 (1975).
Cantor, H., and Boyse, E. A., *J. Exp. Med.* 141, 1390 (1975).
Hirst, J. A., Beverly, P. C. L., Kisielow, P., Hoffman, M. K., and Oettgen, H. F., *J. Immunol.* 115, 1555 (1975).

REFERENCES

1. Baxley, G., Bishop, G. B., Cooper, A. G., and Wortis, H. H., *Clin. Exp. Immunol.* **15**, 385 (1973).
2. Bonner, W. A., Hullett, H. R., Sweet, R. G., and Herzenberg, L. A., *Rev. Sci. Instrum.* **43**, 404 (1972).
3. Böyum, A. A., *Scand. J. Clin. Lab. Invest.* **21**, 51 (1968).
4. Brown, G., and Greaves, M. F., *Eur. J. Immunol.* **4**, 302 (1974).
5. David, J. R., *Fed. Proc.* **34**, 1730 (1975).
6. Davies, P., Page, R. C., and Allison, A. C., *J. Exp. Med.* **139**, 1262 (1974).
7. Dewar, A. E., Habershaw, J. A., Young, G. A., Stuart, A. E., Parker, A. C., and Wilson, C. D., *Lancet* **1**, 216 (1974).
8. Einstein, L. P., Schneeberger, E., and Colten, H. R., *J. Exp. Med.* **143**, 114 (1976).
9. Gluckman, J. C., and Montambault, P., *Clin. Exp. Immunol.* **22**, 302 (1973).
10. Greaves, M. F., *Prog. Haematol.* **IX**, 255 (1975).
11. Greaves, M. F., and Brown, G., *Nature (London)* **246**, 116 (1973).
12. Hammarström, S., Hellström, U., Perlmann, P., and Dillner, M. L., *J. Exp. Med.* **138**, 1270 (1973).
13. Hellström, U., Dillner, M. L., Hammarström, S., and Perlmann, P., manuscript submitted.
14. Hellström, U., Hammarström, S., Dillner, M. L., Perlmann, H., and Perlmann, P., *Scand. J. Immunol.* Suppl. 5 (1976) in press.
15. Hellström, U., Mellstedt, H., Holm, G., and Perlmann, P., *Clin. Exp. Immunol.* (1976) in press.
16. Herberman, R. B., unpublished observations.
17. Holm, G., Petterson, D., Mellstedt, H., Hedfors, E., and Bloth, B., *Clin. Exp. Immunol.* **20**, 443 (1975).
18. Jondal, M., Holm, G., and Wigzell, H. J., *J. Exp. Med.* **137**, 1532 (1972).
19. Jondal, M., Klein, E., and Yefenof, E., *Scand. J. Immunol.* **4**, 259 (1975).
20. Kano, S., Bloom, B. R., and Howe, M. L., *Proc. Natl. Acad. Sci. U.S.A.* **70**, 2299 (1973).
21. Kaplan, M. E., and Clark, C., *J. Immunol Methods* **5**, 131 (1974).
22. Lamon, E. W., Whitten, H. D., Lidin, B., and Fudenberg, H. H., *J. Exp. Med.* **142**, 542 (1975).
23. Lohrmann, H. P., and Novikovs, L., *Clin. Immunol. Immunopathol.* **3**, 99 (1974).
24. Loken, M. R., and Herzenberg, L. A., *Ann. N. Y. Acad. Sci.* **254**, 163 (1975).
25. McCaffrey, R., Harrison, T. A., Parkman, R., and Baltimore, D., *N. Engl. J. Med.* **292**, 775 (1975).
26. McConnell, I., and Hurd, C. M., *Immunology* **30**, 835 (1976).
27. Mackaness, G. B., *J. Exp. Med.* **120**, 105 (1964).
28. Moretta, L., Ferrarini, M., Durante, M. L., and Mingari, M. C., *Eur. J. Immunol.* **3**, 565 (1973).
29. Munth-Kass, A. C., Seglen, P. O., and Seljelid, R., *J. Exp. Med.* **141**, 1 (1975).
30. Pellegrino, M. A., Ferrone, S., and Theofilopoulos, A. N., *J. Immunol.* **115**, 1065 (1975).
31. Pepys, M. B., Sategna-Guidetti, C., Mirjah, D. D., Wansbrough-Jones, M. H., and Dash, A. C., *Clin. Exp. Immunol* in press.
32. Rabinowitz, M., and DeStefano, M. J., *J. Exp. Med.* **143**, 290 (1976).
33. Ross, G. D., Rabellino, E. M., Polley, M. J., and Grey, H. M., *J. Clin. Invest.* **52**, 377 (1973).
34. Sandilands, G. P., Gray, K., Cooney, A., Browning, J. D., and Anderson, J. R., *Clin. Expt. Immunol.* **22**, 493 (1975).

616.079 Inlv
c. 1

35. Schlossman, S., Chess, L., Humphrey, R. E., and Strominger, J., *Proc. Natl. Acad. Sci. U.S.A.* **73**, 1288 (1976).
36. Shortman, K., Williams, N., and Adams, P., *J. Immunol. Methods* **1**, 273 (1972).
37. Simon, H. B., and Sheagren, J. N., *J. Exp. Med.* **133**, 1371 (1975).
38. Snyderman, R., and Stahl, C., *in* "The Phagocytic Cell in Host Resistance" (J. A. Bellanti and D. H. Dayton, eds.), pp. 280–281. Raven, New York, 1975.
39. Stossel, T. P., Alper, C. A., and Rosen, F. S., *J. Exp. Med.* **137**, 690 (1973).
40. Strelkauskas, A. J., Wilson, B. S., Dray, S., and Dodson, M., *Nature (London)* **258**, 331 (1975).
41. Unkeless, J., Gordon, S., and Reich, E., *J. Exp. Med.* **139**, 834 (1974).
42. Valdimarsson, H., Agnarsdottir, G., and Lachmann, P. J., *Nature (London)* **255**, 554 (1975).
43. Weiner, M. S., Bianco, C., and Nussenzweig, V., *Blood* **42**, 939 (1973).
44. Winchester, R. J., Fu, S. M., Hoffman, T., and Kunkel, H. G., *J. Immunol.* **14**, 1210 (1975).
45. Wybran, J., and Fudenberg, H. H., *J. Clin. Invest.* **52**, 1028 (1973).
46. Yu, D. T. Y., *Clin. Expt. Immunol.* **20**, 311 (1975).
47. Yu, D. T. Y., *J. Immunol.* **115**, 91 (1975).

II

Evaluation of *in Vitro* Methods for
Assaying Tumor Immunity*

*Michael A. Bean, Barry R. Bloom, Jean-Charles Cerottini, John A. David,
Ronald B. Herberman, H. Sherwood Lawrence, Ian C. M. MacLennan,
Peter Perlmann, and Osias Stutman*

1. General Considerations

One of the central problems in evaluating tumor immunity *in vitro*, particularly in man, is the methodology itself. Most of the methods are newly introduced, often adapted from simpler animal models, and their application to human cancer has been fraught with unforeseen difficulties. Some of the methodological difficulties confronting the investigator include (a) development of methods that are highly reproducible and standardizable; (b) determination of the sensitivity in human systems where the level of cellular immunity may be far lower than that in commonly studied animal systems; (c) correlation of the effector populations with defined lymphocyte subpopulations of known surface and functional markers; (d) quantitation of the number of effector cells or strength of response; and (e) correlation of the reactivity *in vitro* with the clinical course of the disease and prognosis of the patients. Evaluation of the last point is hampered by many practical limitations. For example, most cellular immunological studies in man are carried out on peripheral blood lymphocytes; study of lymphocytes from lymph nodes draining the tumor, or indeed invading the tumor itself to study their reactivity, should be encouraged.

Before proceeding it is worth pointing out that immunologists and oncologists alike must recognize the possibility, as is the case in numerous spontaneous and artificially induced tumors, that there will be some tumors that express *no* tumor-specific transplantation antigen of any kind, and that all problems may not merely be methodological ones.

1.1. The Problem of Specificity

Another general problem in evaluating the immunological status of cancer patients concerns the specificity of the responses of their lymphocytes *in vitro*.

*This evaluation was prepared at a meeting held on January 29–31, 1976, at The Rockefeller University, sponsored by Contract NIH-76-C-3 from the National Cancer Institute. The United States Government has a royalty-free, nonexclusive, irrevocable license to reproduce, translate, publish, and use Evaluations I and II for official government use.

The nature of the specific tumor antigens recognized by lymphocytes is, at present, unknown. Indeed there may well be more than a single antigen involved in immune recognition of a tumor, both because different subpopulations of lymphocytes may be active in different *in vitro* systems and because induction and effector stages in these reactions, even mediated by the same lymphocyte subpopulation, may exhibit different requirements for antigen recognition. It has been difficult, even in animal systems, to distinguish between reactivity to tumor-specific antigens which lead to rejection, reactions to tumor-associated antigens, oncofetal antigens, endogenous or adventitious viral antigens, or mycoplasma which may modify the surfaces of tumor cells, differentiation antigens which are organ or histological cell-type specific, and minor histocompatibility antigens (42). In this regard it is noteworthy that in studies on tumor immunity in man, lymphocytes of patients often react with tumors of a given histological type obtained from different individuals, whereas in experimental animals, such cross-reactivity to allogeneic tumors of the same histological type is not usually found. In this regard, it must be borne in mind that different tumor cells or cell lines of the same histological type may differ qualitatively in the types of antigenic determinants and quantitatively in the amount of antigen expressed, and may also differ widely is susceptibility to killing by cytotoxic lymphocytes or antibody-dependent mechanisms.

Recent studies in animals on lymphocyte-mediated cytotoxicity of virus-infected cells (24, 31, 59) and chemically modified cells (104) and even killing across minor histocompatibility antigens (7) have indicated that in many systems, in order to obtain specific T cell-mediated cytotoxicity, there is a requirement that the target cell exhibit at least one major serologically detectable histocompatibility antigen that the effector cell either shares or recognizes as "self" (25). These results support the hypothesis proposed by Lawrence (61) that cell-mediated immunity was directed at "self + X" determinants, where the exogenous antigen "X" could be derived from a virus, bacterium, fungus, or parasite, etc. In view of the recent experiments, T cells may recognize an antigen complex consisting of the foreign determinant complexed with major histocompatibility antigens. There is indirect evidence to support this view, for example, failure to inhibit cytotoxicity with excess virus-infected allogeneic cells or with excess syngeneic uninfected cells (7, 25), and cocapping of a murine leukemia virus antigen and H2 (103). However, there is at present no direct evidence on the chemical nature of the antigen actually recognized by the T lymphocytes. There are suggestions that the H2 or HLA restriction on T cell killing may not be absolute, in that killing of some virus-induced tumors may occur across histocompatibility barriers or following immunization with allogeneic tumors. In addition, there are recent reports that tumor cells in inbred mice may exhibit histocompatibility antigens not normally found on cells of that strain (32, 50), raising the possibility that rejection of tumor cells could occur across these "inappropriate" histocompatibility determinants. The data supporting the "self + X" or altered-self hypothesis emphasize the subtlety of discrimination required to ward off autoimmune disease by natural mechanisms that serve to regulate or block cell-mediated immunity, and the need to understand and to modulate them in order to augment specific tumor immunity in the cancer patient. In any case, it is vitally important that studies on tumor immunity *in vivo* take into consideration the HLA types of the donor and target cells to ascertain whether failure to detect responses *in vitro* in some instances may reflect not a lack of immunocompetent cells but an inability to detect them. While this histocompatibility restriction may be relevant to T cell killing, all evidence on K cell killing (see Section 5) would indicate that there is no HLA antigen restriction on killing of tumor cells in antibody-dependent, cell-mediated cytotoxicity.

In spite of the immunologist's fixation on specificity, one must not overlook the likelihood that there may be important mechanisms that are nonspecific, at least in the usual sense, for restricting the growth of tumor cells, and that, for example, may in part explain the resistance of athymic nude mice to carcinogenesis. There is an ever-increasing body of evidence to indicate that there are "spontaneous" killer lymphocytes, obtainable from normal individuals, that can kill tumor cells *in vitro* (40, 55). In the past, those cells have been largely ignored or considered as "background" in cytotoxicity assays. Additionally, macrophages, particularly "activated" macrophages, have been observed to inhibit growth or kill tumor cells (1, 28, 46, 65). In these instances there appears to be some selectivity for affecting tumor cells but not normal cells, although there is not the same degree of specificity as is generally expected of immunological reactions. These phenomena may be of real significance *in vivo* and demand further study (see Section 6).

Nevertheless, despite the fact that many of the problems involving the question of tumor specificity remain to be clarified, it should be emphasized that the *in vitro* tests presently available serve as practical and useful assays for monitoring the degree of nonspecific immunosuppression imposed on cancer patients by their disease or by therapeutic intervention, for example, by studying *in vitro* responses to common bacterial antigens and mitogens.

1.2. Problems of Patient and Control Populations

One of the major variables, it must be acknowledged, in all *in vitro* studies on tumor immunity is the patient. The level of study to date has been primarily that of patient populations with a given type of cancer, often not truly random but selected unintentionally on the basis of availability, general state of health, age, and other nonmedical factors. Within these classified populations, marked differences usually exist in the patients studied, in terms of histological type of lesion, degree of lymphocyte infiltration of the tumor and inflammation, stage and extent of disease, particularly extent of metastases, time after surgery, anticancer therapy and medication, transfusions, age, and sex. These factors are often difficult to control for or to standardize, but they are known to influence the immunological tests. Until recently, it would have been difficult to design experimental protocols otherwise, but with the introduction of improved techniques for freezing and storing both tumor cells and lymphocytes (see Methods 67 and 68) it may be possible to follow individual patients in horizontal studies over considerable periods of time and to approach the question directly of whether different *in vitro* tests correlate with the clinical course of disease.

It is no less difficult to decide what the most appropriate control populations ought to be. While most studies on cellular immunity in cancer patients utilize effector cell preparations from healthy individuals as controls, it is also necessary to compare cells from patients with other forms of cancer, cells from patients with benign diseases of the same organ, cells from noncancer patients with inflammatory processes, contacts, and family members.

As will be emphasized repeatedly in the discussions that follow, it is essential not only to establish reproducible immunological phenomena by these *in vitro* techniques, but also to attempt to relate these *in vitro* responses to the clinical status of the patient. The *in vitro* results are of interest at three levels. They offer the possibility of providing useful diagnostic and prognostic tests for cancer. Second, they may provide useful measures of general immunological status of the patients and their degree of immunosuppression which may render them susceptible to infection. Last, the simplified *in vitro* systems permit the analysis and evaluation of the fundamental mechanisms of tumor immunity, which one hopes will provide the basis for future approaches to the immunoprophylaxis and immunotherapy of cancer.

2. Isotope Release and Incorporation Methods

Several radioisotopic assays have been developed to assess the lytic potential of effector cell populations. Ideally, the following criteria should be fulfilled by an isotopic label: (a) the amount of isotope incorporated into target cells should be sufficient to allow adequate labeling of relatively small numbers of cells without toxicity; (b) the isotope should be evenly distributed among the individual target cells, irrespective of their metabolic activity or cell cycle stage; (c) the incorporated isotope should be released in the supernatant fluid only when irreversible damage of the target cells has occurred; (d) release should be rapid and complete; and (e) once released, the isotope should not be reutilized by target cells or lymphocytes. It should be emphasized that none of the currently used isotopes fulfill all these criteria.

Assays using prelabeling of cells with different radioactive compounds have been developed, the most commonly used being ^{51}Cr, ^{125}I-iododeoxyuridine (IUdR), and ^{3}H-proline. These prelabeling procedures are designed to measure primarily direct lytic events (either as release of label from the damaged cells and/or loss of adherent target cells), without interference by cytostatic and other cell growth-related phenomena. In some systems, target cell loss (i.e., detachment) has been demonstrated to correlate with cell lysis in these tests (see Method 42). The above-mentioned, as well as other isotopes, have also been used in postlabeling assays (i.e., labeling of the target cells remaining after incubation with lymphocytes). However, especially in long-term incubations, postlabeling cannot differentiate lysis from cytostasis. and the contribution of remaining effector cells in isotope incorporation becomes difficult to evaluate.

2.1. ^{51}Cr Release Assay

In this assay, target cells are labeled with ^{51}Cr, which, as chromate ion (^{51}CrO$_4$$^{2-}$), diffuses into the cytoplasm, where it apparently binds to macromolecules that remain ill-defined. Little is known about the actual fate of the isotope, except that there is no reutilization after release of the label into the supernatant fluid. From limited studies designed to evaluate the relationship between ^{51}Cr release and cell death, it appears that the assay primarily measures irreversible alterations of the cell membrane characterized by an efflux of intracellular macromolecules preceding actual lysis. However, interpretation of results may be complicated by the occurrence of spontaneous release of the isotope from target cells incubated without effector cells. Although little is known about the significance of this spontaneous release, several factors influencing the rate of spontaneous release have been delineated, and, hence, appropriate procedures can be used to reduce it to an acceptable level (for further discussion, see Method 38). Although in many instances the assay has to be limited to a 6-hr incubation period, several studies indicate that a 24-hr incubation period is feasible in selected systems.

The assay can be performed with target cells in suspension or in monolayers, and it has been used successfully to detect the lytic activity of T cells, K cells, spontaneous killer cells, monocytes, macrophages, and polymorphonuclear cells (14a) (see Method 38). It is thus evident that cytolysis as assessed by the short-term ^{51}Cr release assay in general cannot be attributed to a single mechanism involving only one particular effector cell type. It should be noted that the mechanism of lysis at the molecular level is yet to be defined. In model systems of alloantigen-reactive cytotoxic T lymphocytes (CTL), there is evidence that ^{51}Cr release from a labeled target cell may occur several minutes to a few hours after the target cell has been irreversibly damaged by the relevant effector cell. Hence, the rate of ^{51}Cr release does not necessarily reflect the kinetics of target-cell damage and may, particularly in very short-term assays, give an underestimate of the number of target cells actually damaged. While these findings have been documented in model systems using target cells highly susceptible to cell-mediated lysis, further work is needed to investigate the behavior of target cells with a relatively low susceptibility.

With appropriate ^{51}Cr-labeled target cells, a quantitative estimation of the lytic potential of a given effector cell population can be obtained by using varying effector-to-target cell ratios. Dose–response curves have been used to evaluate the relative number of CTL or K cells under appropriate conditions (see Methods 38, 46, and 47). The amount of cytotoxic activity in a given lymphocyte preparation can be compared with the activity in other preparations by measuring the number of lymphocytes that must be added to produce a specified level of target-cell lysis. For such comparisons to be valid it is essential that the slope of the dose–response curves, i.e., percent cytotoxicity versus log effector cell number, be parallel for the different sample populations. Another useful application of the ^{51}Cr assay is the development of an inhibition assay using mixtures of unlabeled and labeled target cells (Method 45). Although the usefulness of this method has been documented in several CTL systems, it should be noted that the various factors involved in the inhibition assay have yet to be defined. In particular, it is unclear whether or not the major factor is the amount of relevant antigen present on the surface of the unlabeled target cell. However, the use of well-defined inhibition assays may lead to a better characterization of the membrane-bound antigens recognized by CTL. Along this line, it should be noted that, although specific and effective inhibition can be obtained with unlabeled target cells, attempts to use membrane particulate or soluble extracts have met with little, if any, success in inhibition studies using the ^{51}Cr assay to measure CTL-mediated lysis.

2.2. Other Isotope Release Assays

Prelabeling of target cells with ^{3}H-proline, ^{3}H-thymidine, or ^{125}IUdR is especially applicable to long-term assays (i.e., 24 hr or more), where spontaneous release of ^{51}Cr from prelabeled cells would be too great a problem. With ^{3}H-proline, high levels of label (both nuclear and cytoplasmic) are incorporated with relatively low toxicity whereas spontaneous release is usually low (5) (see Method 43). This technique has been mainly applied in systems using adherent target cells. Since ^{3}H-TdR and ^{125}IUdR are incorporated only in the nucleus of cells undergoing DNA synthesis, these isotope methods can only be applied to dividing target cells. Another limitation of these labels is their relative toxicity for target cells, although spontaneous release is usually low. The ^{125}IUdR technique has been used with both suspension and adherent target cells (see Method 42).

In general, these assays using prelabeled allogeneic adherent target cells in mice have shown comparable results to those observed in ^{51}Cr release assays with cells in suspension, although the kinetics and phenomenology of these responses are still less defined (51, 105, 112, 114). It should be pointed out that release of nuclear labels from damaged target cells is delayed for several hours when compared to ^{51}Cr or other cytoplasmic labels. On the other hand, comparison of ^{51}Cr-release tests with visual microcytotoxicity assays (which measure both lysis and cytostasis) have shown differences in timing and kinetics (30, 62), although some of these differences might be due to technical variables. Assays using syngeneic adherent tumor cells, which have not been selected for high susceptibility to lysis, usually require longer incubation times and probably measure additional differentiation steps besides the direct lytic event at the effector cell level (105, 112). However, the amount of target cell lysis still appears to be proportional to the number of lymphocytes present in the cultures. In man, the few studies comparing ^{51}Cr release and visual counting in microcytotoxicity assays showed no apparent important differences between the two methods (44, 109).

2.3. T Cell Killing in Animal Syngeneic Tumor Systems Measured by Isotopic Techniques

There is increasing evidence that cytotoxic T lymphocytes are formed during the response to tumor-associated antigens in mice (41, 91, 123). Similar studies using rat (23, 121) or guinea pig (6) syngeneic tumor systems have also documented the formation of cytolytic effector cells belonging to the T cell lineage, although the specificity of the antisera used to characterize the nature of the effector cells has not been established as extensively as in the mouse. In some systems, generation of CTL has been obtained *in vitro* using mixed leukocyte tumor cell cultures (MLTC) (90, 123) (see Methods 69 and 70). Furthermore, there is evidence that immunity is accompanied by the potential for an anamnestic CTL response upon secondary challenge with the relevant tumor-associated antigens either *in vivo* or *in vitro*.

Although several studies have documented the appearance of CTL in spleen, lymph nodes, peritoneal cavity, and peripheral blood during the primary response to tumor-associated antigens, more recent data indicate that CTL can be detected in the tumor mass itself (39, 93). Time-course analysis of the appearance of CTL after injection of Maloney sarcoma virus (MSV) or transplantation of mammary virus-induced tumor cells indicated that the effector cells could be first detected in the regional lymph nodes, then in spleen and blood, while peak activity within the tumor occurred concomitantly with the onset of tumor regression (93, 112).

It has been a general finding that CTL activity in lymphoid organs declines gradually as a function of time in tumor-immune animals. While similar findings have been reported in allogeneic systems, they have been interpreted as suggestive evidence against the participation of CTL in the effector mechanisms involved in long-term immunity. However, it is now evident that immune animals, although they contain few, if any, detectable numbers of CTL, possess the ability to mount an anamnestic CTL response suggesting the development of increased numbers of CTL progenitor cells as a result of primary immunization

(90). In functional terms, these progenitor cells can be defined as "memory" cells, although little is known about their relationship with the actual effector cells induced during the primary response; i.e., they represent the progeny of such CTL or they are derived from a different lineage of antigen-reactive T cells. Additionally, the possible effects of suppressor T cells must be considered.

In vitro studies of the differentiation pathway of CTL generated in allogeneic mixed leukocyte cultures strongly suggest that CTL, once formed, are not necessarily end cells, but may further differentiate into inactive small lymphocytes, which, under appropriate antigenic stimulation, can rapidly enlarge and regain lytic activity before undergoing extensive proliferation (70). Similar studies using syngeneic tumor systems have yet to be performed. It is evident, however, that CTL formed *in vivo* in the MSV system appear to follow the same differentiation pathway. Moreover, studies of the physical characteristics of CTL generated in MLTC using immune spleen cells as the source of CTL progenitor cells demonstrate a striking similarity in size transition as a function of time among effector cells generated against tumor-associated or allogeneic antigens (92). Although it is tempting to speculate that "memory" T cells formed *in vivo* are indeed the progeny of the CTL detected during the primary response, direct evidence for such a relationship awaits the demonstration of specific markers for CTL that are expressed also in their progeny. In the mouse, there is evidence that alloantigen-reactive CTL from C57BL/6 mice belong to a subset of Ly 1^-, Ly $2,3^+$ T cells (14, 106) and Ly $1,2,3^+$ T cells (107), and the antisera to lymphocyte differentiation antigens could provide powerful reagents for characterizing functional lymphocyte subpopulations (14, 106).

2.4. Isotope Release Studies in Man

In man, very few attempts have been made to characterize the nature of the effector cells active against prelabeled target cells. Studies of the cytotoxic cells generated in mixed lymphocyte cultures have indicated that T cells are predominantly responsible for the lytic activity (67, 84). Additional characterization by velocity sedimentation at unit gravity indicated that the effector cells in cell-mediated lysis was part of a relatively heterogeneous population of rapidly sedimenting (i.e., medium to large-sized) cells, albeit derived from small progenitors (69). However, the relationship of these findings to antitumor responses in man remains to be defined.

As assessed by isotope release, lymphocytes from normal donors have been shown to possess lytic activity against different tumor target cells. Recent studies indicate that this activity is mediated by non-E-rosetting cells (44, 88, 94). Similarly, the effector cells present in peripheral blood of bladder tumor patients which lyse ^{51}Cr-labeled bladder tumor cells belong to the K population (117). On the other hand, cytotoxic T cells active against ^{51}Cr-labeled cells have been detected in biopsy cell populations derived from a case of Burkitt's lymphoma (53). Clearly characterization of the cell types involved in cell-mediated cytotoxicity of human tumor cells remains an urgent problem in evaluating the assays and their relevance to tumor immunity in man.

3. Microcytotoxicity Assays

A considerable number of cytotoxicity assays are currently in use, and the modifications introduced by many different investigators have tended to highlight or emphasize various facets of the assay that are considered most important by each investigator. Consequently, the many assays now in use appear to measure, or at least tend to select, different functions of effector cells (e.g., lysis, cytostasis). There are many methodological differences of equal or greater importance than the length of the assay in determining the kind(s) of effector cell function detected. The following discussion attempts to point out some of the major differences in these techniques and to clarify what the various assays may be measuring.

3.1. Visual Microcytotoxicity Test

Takasugi and Klein (113) introduced this assay, subsequently modified by the Hellstroms (38), in which the number of target cells remaining adherent to the bottom of a microwell after incubation with effector cells was considered to be the number of target cells surviving exposure to lymphocytes (see Methods 40, 41, and 49). This assay takes advantage of the fact that the majority of solid tumors from animals and man attached to the culture surface and grew as "monolayers." When cells are killed, they generally detach from the substrate. However, it is now clear that most target cells divide during the assay (24–48 hr) so that, in addition to cell destruction, effects on cell growth and adherence to the substrate may influence the end result. Therefore, apparent cytotoxicity may include, not only target cell destruction, but also a wide variety of other phenomena such as inhibition or stimulation of division due to immunologically specific and nonimmunological factors, or loss of surface adherence. Metabolism of the target cells may be altered by contact with effector cells, by conditions in the medium, density of cells, etc. And there may be problems in quantitating the number of target cells at the end of the assay. For example, does one count only the cells that appear healthy and disregard the pycnotic-looking cells? Does one count the clusters of cells as a colony or as individual cells? In some types of plates, there may be more cells on the walls of the wells, which are not scored, than on the flat bottom, which are counted.

3.2. Cytotoxicity Assays Utilizing Isotope Labeling at the Termination of the Assay (Postlabeling)

There have been a number of different isotopes used to quantitate the number of target cells remaining after treatment with effector cells. Superficially, this would seem to provide an easier method than visual counting to quantitate these cells. Nevertheless, many of the same factors that enter into the interpretation of the visual microcytotoxicity test also apply here. Postlabeling will aid in determining the number of cells at the end of the assay but will not discriminate between effects on growth (e.g., cytostasis) and target cell death. However, the various protocols may in fact measure many different things. For example, technetium-99 (3) appears primarily to label the cell surface, whereas ^{51}Cr, ^{3}H-proline nicotinamide, and rubidium label cytoplasm and ^{3}H-thymidine (51) and ^{125}IUdR (19) label DNA (see Methods 38, 39, 42, 43). It is easy to visualize a circumstance where there would be little or reduced incorporation of DNA precursors when the target cells are contact-inhibited but metabolically otherwise intact. On the other hand, cell membrane labels, such as technetium-99, would not distinguish between intact dead and live cells. In addition, the various labels may be incorporated to a variable degree by the effector cells remaining attached to the substrate and to the target cells. It is difficult to remove completely all the effector cells by washing without disturbing some of the target cells as well.

3.3. Cytotoxicity Assays Utilizing Isotope Labeling prior to the Addition of Effector Cells (Prelabeling)

The rationale for prelabeling target cells with isotope prior to the addition of effector cells is that this will reduce the influence of cell division on the results, giving a truer estimate of target-cell lysis or destruction. Most of the same isotope-labeled agents mentioned previously have also been used for prelabeling. At the termination of the assay, the amount of residual or released isotope is determined. Again the choice of label will affect the test results. If one looks at release, the cytoplasmic labels appear to give a more sensitive estimate of toxicity whereas release of DNA labels may discriminate later stages in the death of the cells. Release of isotopic label (especially DNA labels) from dead cells may be enhanced by enzyme treatment of the target cells. On the other hand, spontaneous release of the isotope in assays over 24 hr may be a problem. ^{51}Cr has been used extensively with short-term assays but is less satisfactory in long-term assays employing monolayer target cells. At the other extreme, ^{125}IUdR and ^{3}H-thymidine are less subject to spontaneous release. Reutilization of the released isotope may be a problem that can influence the results. Reutilization is a problem with ^{3}H-thymidine and ^{3}H-uridine (37), but not with ^{51}Cr, or ^{3}H-proline, or ^{125}IUdR.

The question of which assay is the best cannot be simply answered. In many respects it may be more logical to take advantage of the differences and use a combination of assays, e.g., pre- and postlabeling, in such a manner as to have an estimate of both cell death and cytostasis.

3.4. Choice of Target Cells For Assays

There are both significant advantages and disadvantages to the use of target cells fresh from the patient compared to cells from short-term and long-term tissue culture. Tumor cells taken directly from the patient are the most representative of the *in vivo* condition and will probably have suffered the least from antigenic loss or gain due to selection of cells capable of growing *in vitro* and to contamination by infectious agents. That one is dealing with tumor cells can usually easily be confirmed by microscopic examination of the specimen. However, there may be host humoral factors and cellular infiltrates present, inadequate yields of tumor cells, low viability of the tumor cells, bacterial or fungal contamination, and technical difficulties in making cell suspensions or labeling them with isotopes, e.g., a low mitotic rate. Of considerable importance, tests may not be repeatable over time with the patient's effector cells at various stages during the course of the disease. Cryopreservation of some tumors (notably leukemias) is both feasible and useful for such studies. Many of these problems relate to the type and location of the tumor. Use of tumor cells from effusions, e.g., ascites, may obviate the difficulties in making suspensions of cells from solid tumors, but conversely restricts the study to metastatic tumors, which may differ in important ways from primary tumors (for example, antigenicity).

Short-term tissue culture offers some advantages as the antigen expression of the cells, in contrast to cells from long-term culture, may be more representative of the original tumor. Also, antigens that have been "blocked" or modulated *in vivo* may be detectable in short-term cultures. Manipulation of culture conditions can often enrich for tumor cells relative to contaminating host immunocytes and stromal elements. However, again quantity of materials and reproducibility may be problems, as may be characterization of the growing cells and antigenic changes. Assays using cells from short-term cultures may be more susceptible to some technical variation, such as feeder effects, if they have not fully adapted to culture. Last, use of DNA precursor labels may be more limited owing to these same considerations.

Long-term culture target cells have several advantages in that well-characterized cells may be grown in large quantities and used in many assays. Characterization implies not only histological confirmation at one end of the spectrum, but also immunologically useful information about the antigen(s) expression of the cells at the other extreme. However, antigen loss or gain may be major problems, as is the acquisition of exogenous antigens, due to viral or mycoplasmal contamination, thus raising the question of how relevant to the *in vivo* situation are the results of assays using such cells. Another major concern is the question of quality control. Mix-ups and contamination of cell lines with infectious agents do occur, and rigid controls are required for the maintenance of cultures.

3.5. Effector Cells

The effector cells most studied in man, in contrast to the mouse, are contained in venous blood rather than lymph node, spleen, or peritoneal cavity. They are prepared by a variety of means that include more variables in technique than the cytotoxicity assays themselves. Coagulation of the venous blood may be accomplished by defibrination or by the addition of heparin. Defibrination reduces technical problems caused by the presence of platelets in the preparations but could potentially remove a subpopulation of lymphoid cells, while heparin (and preservatives contained in commercial preparations of it), gelatin or dextran, as well as Ficoll and Isopaque (or Hypaque), may not be innocuous extrinsic influences. It seems clear that different protocols may produce quite different yields of different types of lymphoid and nonlymphoid cells (4).

The effects of the preparative manipulations on the activity of the cells present in the final cell suspension are not yet totally clear and must constantly be considered. For example, it has recently been reported by two groups (58, 126) that under certain conditions Tris-NH_4Cl treatment of human effector cells will significantly inhibit their ability to function in antibody-dependent, cell-mediated lysis of human target cells.

The effector-to-target cell ratio is another variable of importance for understanding the assay results. The term effector-to-target (or attacker-to-target) ratio implies that all the cells in the leukocyte suspension are effector cells, which is clearly not the case. The absolute numbers of cells used and the geometry of the system may profoundly influence the results; therefore, absolute numbers of cells used must be indicated. The actual percentage of active cells is not known, making comparisons difficult but not impossible. Another consideration is the geometry of the assay. Rocking assays in which both target and effector cells are in suspension facilitate cell–cell interaction. On the other hand, when the target is adherent, such treatments may reduce binding of free-floating effector cells. Increasing the number of target cells while holding the absolute number of effector cells constant will result in better contact in isotope prelabel, monolayer target-cell assays, giving an apparent reduction in the minimum effector-to-target cell ratio necessary to demonstrate cytotoxicity (105). The presence of a dose-response effect observed by titration of the effector cells can also serve to establish the validity of the cytotoxic response.

Few data are as yet available on the functions of isolated subpopulations of human lymphocytes in the various cytotoxicity assays. What few data are available have been derived primarily from experiments where the residual activity of effector cell preparations was measured after depletion of cell population(s). It is important to realize that such depletion experiments indicate the dependence of the reaction on certain subpopulations of cells but do not necessarily identify the actual effector cell(s).

It would seem important that more attention be devoted to the characterization of effector cells being used in the assays by different groups to clarify the relationship of the observed effects to the type and proportion of the various cell types present (4).

3.6. Experimental Design

Results obtained in any assay are very dependent on the design of the individual experiments. Some of the concerns related to this are indicated below, relating to the target cells to be included, the types of effector cells, and the various possible baseline controls.

3.6.1. *Target Cells*

The desired variety of target cells to be included in cytotoxicity assays can most easily be described for well-defined animal tumor systems. In those models, control target cells of various types, with known differences in tumor-associated antigens or alloantigens from those of the test cells, can be tested as specificity controls. Each of these control target cells should be expected to give a positive result with the appropriate immune effector cell. It is not satisfactory to use control target cells that are resistant to the type of cytotoxicity under study. For example, normal fibroblasts may be useful specificity controls, particularly for detection of nonselective or non-tumor-associated cytotoxicity, but they must be shown to be susceptible to cytotoxicity in the assay.

In human studies, the selection of the appropriate target cells for specificity control is more difficult. The minimum requirement would seem to be the use of a number of target cells derived from tumors of various histological types. As noted above, each of these target cells must be shown to be susceptible to cytotoxicity by some batches of effector cells. To determine whether the detected antigens are tumor associated, it is desirable to include cells from normal tissues. However, negative results with such normal cells may be misleading because of resistance of many normal target cells, e.g., fibroblasts, to cytotoxicity.

3.6.2. *Effector Cells*

Effector cell preparations from a variety of individuals need to be included in each assay. To establish normal reactivity, cells from more than one normal individual should be included. It is usually very important to use normal individuals of both sexes, of various ages including ones in the same range as the tumor-bearing individuals, and to be aware of the possible effects of drugs and other factors. In clinical studies, the availability of a large pool of appropriate normal donors often presents a logistical problem. In this regard, it is important to recognize the deficiencies in comparisons between elderly cancer patients and young laboratory workers. Further, one should avoid the selection of normal controls based on knowledge of their previous lack of reactivity or reactivity in the assay. Such a procedure would obviously bias the results. Repeated testing of some normal controls may be quite useful in determining the reproducibility of the tests, but multiple determinations on the same individual should not be accumulated in population data.

In studies of animal tumor systems, it is desirable to use effector cells from animals immunized against two different tumors, which have been shown to be antigenically distinct. One can then perform experiments with reciprocal specificity controls, by testing against both tumor cells as targets. In addition, when reactivity in an unknown test population is being examined, it is very helpful to include effector cells from animals with known reactivity as positive effector cell controls. Cryopreserved effector cells are very useful for this purpose.

In man, the types of patients to be included in the tests must be carefully considered. Patients with cancer of various histological types and comparable stages of disease and therapy should be included. In addition, patients with benign diseases of the same organ systems as the cancer patients, and patients with inflammatory diseases, should be tested.

3.6.3. *Controls for Effector Cells*

Various base line controls have been used in cytotoxicity assays. The selection of the base line control requires careful consideration, since judgments regarding "positive" results in an experiment are entirely dependent upon the particular base line selected. The three types of baseline controls which have been used are: media controls, immunologically inert cell controls, and normal controls.

Medium controls, i.e., target cells cultured in the absence of any added effector cells, are a commonly used baseline controls. However, there are major potential problems with the use of the medium control as a baseline. Target cells cultured by themselves at low density often behave quite differently from when they are mixed with large numbers of other cells. The addition of other cells may either produce feeder effects and thus give cytotoxicity below the media control, or may have adverse, nonimmunological effects on the target cells and thus give results considerably above the medium controls. In order to use the medium control as base line, it must be shown, in the particular assay and with the particular target cell, that the medium control is a stable and valid base line.

In order to correct for the cell density present in groups with effector cells, base line controls with immunologically inert cells, in place of effector cells, have been used by some investigators. The autologous control, i.e., the use of unlabeled target cells, has been useful as a base line in the short-term ^{51}Cr-release assay and in the ^{125}IUdR and proline assays with some target cells. However, this control is not applicable to the visual microcytotoxicity assays and may not be suitable for some target cells in long-term isotopic assays, presumably because of effects related to their active proliferation. Nonreactive lymphoid cells, e.g., thymocytes, also have been used as base line controls, once they are shown to be negative against the given set of cell lines.

Preparations of lymphoid cells from normal individuals are commonly used as baseline controls. However, these often present a problem since some normal individuals have been previously sensitized against alloantigens (e.g., by pregnancy, transfusions) on the target cells and since natural cytotoxicity has been demonstrated in cytotoxicity assays in several species (see Method 45). Perhaps the best compromise is to use as base line the least reactive of a group of normal individuals tested at the same time or the normal individual with the median reactivity. Alternatively, a large preparation of cells from a normal individual may be cryopreserved and used repeatedly as the standard base line.

It should be noted that although the choice of baseline control is a critical issue in analysis of results in cytotoxicity assays, there is by no means general agreement as to the most satisfactory baseline control.

3.7. Delineation of Effector Mechanisms

It must be borne in mind that cytotoxicity may be produced by a variety of effector mechanisms and that results obtained by one preparation of cells may not be due to the same mechanism as those obtained with another batch, even when the same target cells are used. The analysis of the subpopulation of effector cells in each preparation which is responsible for the cytotoxicity is one major method for looking for this heterogeneity. The cytotoxicity produced by one individual may be dependent on T cells, whereas that of another may be T-cell independent but require macrophages, for example.

In addition to analysis of the nature of the effector cells, it would be helpful to have other procedures for discriminating among different mechanisms for cytotoxicity. However, few procedures are readily available for this purpose. The most approachable question is whether the effector mechanism involves antibody-dependent, cell-mediated cytotoxicity (ADCMC) since there are several methods that will inhibit ADCMC but do not appear to affect other types of CMC.

3.8. Evaluation of Specificity of Results

The most commonly used method for evaluation of specificity is the description of patterns of reactivity of effector cells against various target cells. A convenient way to categorize positive results has recently been suggested (4), and this is indicated in Table 1. The type of results obtained is largely dependent on the experimental design of the tests, as discussed above. To clarify further the pattern of reactivity, repeat tests may be performed against different sets of

TABLE 1
Classification of Results in Microcytotoxicity Assays

1. Diseased-related cytotoxicity: cytotoxicity solely for the specific tumor tissue target cells by leukocytes from patients with that form of cancer
2. Selective cytotoxicity: cytotoxicity for some test target cells of other histological types, but not for all test target cells
3. Nonselective cytotoxicity: killing of all or most test target cells unrelated and related to the patient's histological tumor cell type
4. Nonreactivity: no cytotoxicity

target cells. It may be pointed out that there are two major problems with this approach to evaluation of specificity. One is that reactivity of a given effector cell population against two target cells may be due to reactions against two distinct antigens. Furthermore, some target cells may be negative on direct testing, not because of absence of the relevant antigens but rather because of subthreshold amounts of antigen. Again, the possibility that histocompatibility antigens must be shared between effector cells and targets should be considered in detail.

For more detailed evaluation of specificity, inhibition assays may be very helpful. One can perform these by addition of either intact tumor cells, cell extracts, or sera to the assay mixtures and assaying for decreased cytotoxicity. It should be noted that this method is applicable only to the prelabeling isotopic assays, since the unlabeled inhibitor cells must be distinguished from the labeled target cells. This approach has been shown to be applicable to ^{125}IUdR-release assays and to the proline assay, as well as in the short-term ^{51}Cr-release assay.

Subcellular extracts have also been tested for inhibition of cytotoxicity. In general, it has not been possible to detect specific inhibition of cytotoxic T cells by extracts. In contrast, extracts have been shown to be effective inhibitors in ADCMC and in visual microcytotoxicity assays. They have not yet been adequately evaluated in the long-term isotopic assays.

Sera from various individuals, those bearing different types of tumor and controls, can be tested for specific inhibition. If sera are shown to be positive, their specificity can be further evaluated by absorptions with different cell types. It should be noted that one needs to be aware of nonspecific inhibition by serum factors, and careful use of sera for specific inhibition offers the opportunity to compare the specificities of different assays or of assays performed in different laboratories, by determining whether the same sera are inhibitory in each assay. Inhibition by serum factors is a potentially powerful approach to evaluation not only of specificity, but also of mechanisms and of factors that operate *in vivo* and affect the development and expression of cell-mediated immunity against tumors.

4. Calculation and Analysis of Data: General Considerations

Two different formulas have most frequently been used to describe the results in the cytotoxicity assays. The first is an expression of percent cytotoxicity taking into account the increment in reactivity in the experimental group above the baseline control, relative to the total number of cells (or counts per minute of isotope incorporated in the cells) or to the maximal cytotoxicity that can occur in the system (e.g., by multiple freezing and thawing of target cells).

$$\% \text{ Increase in cytotoxicity} = [(cpm_{exp} - cpm_{bc}) / cpm_t] \times 100$$

where cpm_{bc} is the counts per minute of isotope released into the supernatant for the baseline control, cpm_t is the total counts per minute incorporated into the cells at the onset of the experiment (or the maximal cytotoxicity), and cpm_{exp} is the counts per minute released into the supernatant for an "experimental" individual tested in the experiment. The second is the cytotoxic index, which is an expression of the difference in cytotoxicity between the experimental group and the baseline control divided by the number of cells, or counts per minute remaining in the cells, at the end of the assay in the baseline control

$$\text{Cytotoxic index} = (cpm_{exp} - cpm'_{exp})/cpm'_{bc}$$

where cpm'_{exp} is the counts per minute *remaining* in cells at the end of the incubation period of an "experimental" individual and cpm'_{bc} is the counts per minute remaining in cells of the baseline control. This formula may be related to the first formula, since $cpm_x + cpm'_x = cpm_t$. A common variant of this measure is the percent reduction

$$\% \text{ reduction} = \frac{cpm'_{bc} - cpm'_{exp}}{cpm'_{bc}}$$

It should be noted that the method used for calculation of percent cytotoxicity by Brunner and Cerottini

$$\frac{cpm_{exp} - cpm_{bc}}{cpm_t - cpm_{bc}} \times 100$$

gives a result identical to the formula for percent reduction.

For tests in which the baseline control cytotoxicity is low, the differences in results between the two formulations are small. However, with high baseline controls, i.e., poor survival of cells in the baseline control, the numbers obtained by the cytotoxic index appear considerably larger than those obtained by the formula for percent cytotoxicity (see Methods 41, 45, and 47 for more detailed discussion). The problems that may occur when the cytotoxic index or percent reduction formulas are used may be illustrated by some frequent problems in the visual microcytotoxicity assays. Although lymphocyte:target cell ratios are often calculated relative to the number of target cells added to the well, the cpm_t for the experiment would actually be the number of cells which actually were *adherent* to the wells at the onset of the experiment. This number is often not determined. (It is desirable to use target cells with a high plating efficiency, so that cpm_t is close to the number of cells added, but this has often not been the case.) If the cpm_t in an experiment was 100, the cpm'_{bc} was 30, and the cpm'_{exp} was 15, then the percent reduction would be 50%, whereas the percent increase in cytotoxicity would be only 15%. The large difference in numbers in this case is entirely due to the relatively poor survival of cells in the base line control.

In well-defined test systems in which the baseline controls have low cytotoxicity and dose–response titrations are performed, calculations of percent reduction have been quite useful in the determination of lytic units (see Methods 38 and 39). Careful dose–response titrations should be more widely performed in these assays, since they allow quantitative estimations of relative numbers of effector cells. However, the dose–response curves in many of the long-term assays, particularly the visual microcytotoxicity assay, are often erratic and not susceptible to this form of analysis. This presumably reflects technical problems in assays, which would have to be corrected before such quantitative estimations could be made.

Regardless of which formula is used for expression of results, it is always important to provide the data regarding cpm_{bc} and cpm_t in reporting of results, so that the reader can adequately evaluate the experiments.

It should be noted that the formulas discussed above are used only for descriptive purposes and are not used in the statistical analysis of the data. For analysis, the most commonly accepted methods are the students' t test carried out on raw data or the Welch or similar modifications of students' t test, in which the log-transformed raw data (cpm_{exp} or cpm'_{exp}) of the experimental group and the baseline control (cpm_{bc} or cpm'_{bc}) are compared. The commonly accepted definition of a positive test is significant difference between the experimental group compared to the baseline control. (The most commonly used is $p < 0.05$, but perhaps more stringent criteria, e.g., $p < 0.01$, should be used for these assays with multiple variables.) A difference in the direction of less target cell survival is considered cytotoxicity or inhibition, and increased survival in the experimental group is usually defined as "stimulation."

Results between different experiments can then be pooled or summarized by the proportion of tests within each experimental group that gave cytotoxicity or stimulation. By using multiple normal individuals in each experiment, one can get an estimate of the amount of normal reactivity. Similarly, one can describe the proportion of positive results in each patient group. It must be emphasized that all this information will be entirely dependent on the baseline control used for analysis of the data. If the baseline control is too low, all groups may show a high incidence of reactivity, regardless of diagnosis.

For clinical studies, it may not be sufficient to compare results by disease category alone, but rather, to minimize effects of variables, such as kinetics, it may be necessary to subclassify according to stage of disease, therapy, etc.

5. Antibody-Dependent Cell-Mediated Cytotoxicity

5.1. General Considerations

Antibody-dependent cell-mediated cytotoxicity covers a large number of effector cell systems, many of which are defined in some detail. The type of effector system(s) operative in any experimental situation depends upon the nature of the target cell and the species from which the effector cells are derived.

The effector cells currently recognized include: lymphocytes, macrophages, neutrophils, and eosinophils.

5.1.1. *Effector Cells*

Lymphocytes *K Cells.* K cell is the operational term for a lymphocyte which is particularly active in human peripheral blood and cannot easily be classified as belonging to either the myeloid series or to the majority of immunologically competent cells (69, 73, 87, 116). They do not attach to glass or plastic surfaces and are not phagocytic. Killing is induced by binding to IgG on the target; although activated C3 may augment the reaction in certain circumstances, IgG is essential to trigger lysis (85) (see Methods 46–48).

There has been a considerable volume of work carried out on the surface marker properties of K cells, although a clear-cut picture of a single, homogeneous, cytotoxic population has not yet emerged. Table 2 lists some of the principal characteristics of human K cells.

All K cells carry receptors for the Fc portion of IgG, yet it is important to note that not all cells with Fc receptors show K-cell activity. There is evidence that K cells can be distinguished from the bulk of other Fc$^+$ cells by the high avidity of the receptor for Fc (98).

While the majority of human lymphocytes that form rosettes with sheep red blood cells (E+ cells) are inactive in K cell assays, some, perhaps all, appear to have low-affinity E receptors when neuraminidase-treated lymphocytes or, in preliminary studies, sheep erythrocytes are used. Further evidence showing coincidence with a marker predominantly associated with T cells is provided by the fact that some of the K cell activity of neuraminidase-treated human lymphocytes is retained on columns carrying A hemagglutinin from *Helix pomatia*. This activity can be eluted from the columns by using *N*-acetylgalactosamine, which competes for the active A hemagglutinin determinant. It does not necessarily follow from this that K cells are a subfraction of T lymphocytes (86).

On the other hand, most data suggest that K cell activity is not found on cells with high-density surface immunoglobulin. Many K cells appear to have receptors for C3b and C3d but by no means all cells with such receptors have K cell

TABLE 2
Properties of Human K Cells

Adherence to plastic or glass	None
Phagocytosis	Not seen
Fc binding	High-affinity receptors for altered IgG1, 2, and 3, some binding to IgG4
Binding to activated C3	Many K cells bind activated C3
Binding to sheep erythrocytes (SRBC)	Some K cells or neuraminidase-treated K cells show low avidity binding to neuraminidase-treated SRBC
Binding A-hemagglutinin of *Helix pomatia*	Some neuraminidase-treated K cells bind this agent
Surface immunoglobulin	K cells do not have easily demonstrable surface immunoglobulin
Distribution in the body	
Splenic lymphocytes	Strong activity
Blood lymphocytes	Strong activity
Bone marrow cells	Some activity
Lymph node cells	Slight activity
Thoracic duct lymphocytes	Little or no activity
Thymocytes	Little or no activity
Rheumatoid arthritis joint fluid	Strong activity

activity. The avidity of these receptors for complement seems to be relatively weak on K cells (86).

Recently, direct evidence has been provided indicating that K cell activity against chicken RBC is shown by at least 5% of phagocyte-depleted human peripheral blood lymphocytes and that one K cell can kill a number of sensitized target cells (see Method 48). There are reports showing that bystander target cells are not killed and that the cytotoxic reaction requires contact between K cell and the target (70, 83).

T Cells. Some evidence has now been provided to show that murine T cells may cooperate with target cell-specific IgM to induce target-cell lysis (60).

Macrophages and Neutrophils. Phagocytic cells can kill a number of target cells sensitized with antibody. This may follow phagocytosis and phagolysosome formation but also may occur outside the effector cell. One mechanism for extracellular lysis is through the release of lysosomal enzymes, such as peroxidase, from the phagocytic cells (17). This mechanism can be activated in the test tube by immune complexes and does not require direct contact with the target cell. The susceptibility of different target cells to lysosomal lytic systems varies greatly, erythrocytes, many bacteria and fungi being most susceptible. However, tumor cells have been shown to be lysed by phagocytes and antibody. Both these mechanisms can also be triggered by activated C3. IgG can also cooperate with C3 in the activation of phagocytes (75). Phagocytosis itself, however, does not inevitably result in cell lysis. Finally, it is possible that phagocytic cells may damage antibody-sensitized target cells by a direct cell-to-cell cytotoxic mechanism analogous to that seen by cytotoxic T cells and K cells. Firm evidence for this mechanism has not yet been forthcoming.

Eosinophils. Recently, Butterworth and his colleagues (13) have shown that eosinophils can damage sensitized schistosomula. This finding would provide the most clear-cut function for eosinophils yet put forward in this regard.

5.2. Susceptibility of Different Target Cells to Different Effector Cells

It is now clear that different target cells show different susceptibility to lysis by different effector cells. This fact can be used to devise assays in which only one effector system appears to be operative. The number of systems that have been fully worked out are still restricted. Table 3 lists some of the best characterized examples using human peripheral blood effectors.

It should be noted that certain nonlymphoid target cells, such as *Herpes simplex* virus (HSV)-infected cells (95) or tumor cells (115) display Fc receptors and can form EA rosettes. In this regard, it has been found that high levels of spontaneous cytotoxicity of HSV-infected targets by normal lymphocytes in the absence of antibody have been observed which have been attributed to cross-linking effector cells and target cells through aggregated Ig or complexes in sera, even fetal calf serum (96).

5.3. The Nature of Sensitizing Antibody

With the exception of the T cell–IgM system briefly mentioned above, all the effector systems described rely on IgG for activation.

TABLE 3
Effector Cells Active against Different Sensitized Target Cells

Cells Killed by K Cells	
Chang human liver cells[a] (73)	Sensitized with rabbit or human antibody
P815 mouse mastocytoma (68)	Sensitized with rabbit antibody
Human lymphoblastoid line (116)	Sensitized with HLA antibody
Cells Killed by K Cells, Macrophages, and Neutrophils	
Chicken RBC's (69, 87)	Sensitized with mouse, rabbit, or human antibody
Cells Killed by Macrophages and Neutrophils, But Not K Cells	
Human group A RBC (49)	Sensitized with human anti-A IgG

[a]These cells show some spontaneous lysis when exposed to peripheral blood lymphocytes from many individuals in the absence of sensitizing agents (see Method 47). These examples are chosen because they are well defined, but information is now available on a large range of target cells regarding their susceptibility to various types of effector cells.

EVALUATION II

TABLE 4
IgG Subclasses Active in Antibody-Dependent
Cell-Mediated Toxicity

Cells	IgG_1	IgG_2	IgG_3	IgG_4
1. K cells	++	++	++	+
2. Macrophages	++	−	++	−
3. Neutrophils	++	++	++	−
4. Eosinophils	IgG but subclasses unknown			
5. C1q	++	++	++	−

Table 4 summarizes the subclasses of IgG that can be active with the different systems. The binding of IgG to the complement factor C1q is added for comparison. Apart from C1q activation it should be noted that these data were derived previously from inhibition assays using aggregated myeloma proteins.

A single IgG_1 or IgG_3 myeloma protein is capable of reacting with neutrophils, K cells, and C1q, indicating that determinants for all these effector systems are found on the same molecule. Investigation of the location of the active determinants have shown that these sites are not identical for all effector mechanisms. The C1q determinant is on the C_H2 domain, while both macrophage and neutrophil phagocytosis can be inhibited by isolated C_H3 domain. The K cell determinant is present on whole Fc, but isolated C_H3 has little or no capacity to block K cell cytotoxic activity. Paradoxically IgG minus the C terminal domain is also inactive, so the precise location of this determinant remains obscure but must be assumed to be in the C_H2–C_H3 area.

Native IgG antibody has little or no affinity for K cells, and K cell lysis will occur in physiological concentrations of native IgG. Aggregated IgG or immune complexes, however, will bind to the K cells. Macrophages may additionally have some ability to bind native IgG.

5.4. Species Differences

There are marked differences between species in the capacity of their leukocytes to kill antibody-sensitized target cells. This activity is particularly prominent in man, where K cells will lyse a wide variety of freshly explanted cells and cell lines. Activity against lymphocytes and other cells sensitized with HLA antibodies is strong.

In the rat, while many cell lines are lysed by cells resembling human K cells, activity is weak against allogeneic lymphocytes sensitized with anti-AgB antibody. In mice, the range of target cells susceptible to lysis by allogeneic leukocytes when sensitized with antibody is more restricted than in the rat. Target cells sensitized with anti-H2 antibody are generally unharmed by mouse leukocytes. These statements relate to the chromium release assay, and there is good evidence in mouse systems that a considerable range of sensitized cells is damaged in long-term assays. Nevertheless, the fact remains that in relation to antibody-induced cytotoxicity there are very considerable differences between mice and men.

5.5. Relation to Neoplasia

There are several reasons for the oncologist to consider antibody-dependent cytotoxic systems, and some of these are listed and discussed below.

1. Clearly these cytotoxic mechanisms could be operative against tumors with recognizably new antigens. For example, in human bladder cancer there is evidence for ADCMC (80). There are two possibilities to consider here. One is the production of sensitizing antibody by the patient himself. The second is the possibility of tumor treatment by passive transfer of allogeneic or xenogeneic antisera raised against the tumor. There are a number of instances in which antibody transfer has been successful in causing regression of animal tumors (21, 33, 43, 77, 122), treatment of lymphoreticular neoplasms being particularly successful. Paradoxically, many successful experiments *in vivo* have been carried out in mice, which appear to have rather poor antibody-dependent cytotoxic systems in culture. The role of complement in these experiments *in vivo* was investigated by Hersey, who showed the C3 depletion with cobra venom was not associated with loss of the antileukemic effect of an xenogeneic serum given to rats (43). Obviously it is very difficult in such *in vivo* experiments to ascertain the nature of the effector mechanism.

While the ideal may be to obtain a tumor-specific antibody for passive transfer, it may be possible in some cases to use antibody raised against normal tissue antigens. Some tumor cells may show considerably greater sensitivity to antibody-dependent lysis than many normal tissues.

2. Antibody-dependent cellular mechanisms are also of importance to the oncologist in that they may play an important role in physiological defense systems against infections. For example, neutrophils and macrophages are essential in the body's defenses against bacterial and fungal infection. There is some evidence that K cells may have a role to play in viral infections (35, 95). The relationship of eosinophils to parasitic infection has already been mentioned (13, 74).

Chemotherapy and radiotherapy used in the treatment of neoplasia can markedly reduce the number of various different antibody-dependent effector cells, and so may compromise resistance to infection. This has particular importance in some of the neoplastic diseases where chemotherapy and radiotherapy are most successful. Unhappily in some series of acute lymphoblastic leukemia patients with good prognosis, deaths in complete remission from infections are almost as common as deaths following relapse.

3. Antibody-dependent cytotoxic activity can be reduced by immune complexes competing for Fc receptors. Immune complexes have been found in the inoculation of tumor-bearing animals (12), and these may exist in certain patients with neoplasms. In many chronic inflammatory diseases, such as rheumatoid arthritis and ulcerative colitis, patients may have substantial quantities of circulating immune complexes which can block K cell activity *in vitro* (52).

The considerations listed above make it desirable that antibody-dependent cytotoxic activity be measured at a variety of levels in patients with neoplasia.

5.5.1. *Effector Cell Quantitation*

It is clearly of interest to measure effector cell activity. It is probably best to choose assay systems that more or less exclusively detect one effector cell type, for example, the lymphoblastoid line used by Trinchieri (116) or Chang cells for human K cells and group A red cells sensitized with anti-A for macrophages and neutrophils. In the second case separation of neutrophils from monocytes is essential. While the chicken red cell has given much valuable information about K cells their vulnerability to lysis by macrophages and neutrophils makes careful purification of lymphocytes an essential preliminary step.

5.6. Detection of Cytotoxicity Mediated by Antibody and/or Leukocytes from Immune Animals or Patients

Antibody-dependent, cell-mediated cytotoxicity may be an important tissue-damaging mechanism occurring during different phases of the immune response against a tumor. Thus, when effector cells from immune donors are incubated with the relevant target cells, the resulting cytotoxicity may reflect the activity of antibody-dependent effector cells. When this is the case, then the *in vitro* reaction reflects a cell cooperation between antibody-releasing cells that are not cytotoxic by themselves and effector cells that utilize the released antibody but do not produce it (72, 102). In this case, the time of appearance of significant (and measurable) target cell damage is usually prolonged.

Assay procedures to show the presence of antibody-dependent cell-mediated cytotoxicity in immune systems are utilized to establish the nature of the effector cells that are operative during different phases of disease, or, alternatively, for establishing the presence or absence of antibodies mediating cell-mediated cytotoxicity. The choice of target cells and/or the assay system depends on which of these aspects is being investigated.

5.6.1. *Target Cells*

Freshly explanted cells from normal tissue, from solid tumors or cells grown in culture for a short time are used in some instances. Such cells have the advantage of well-preserved original antigenicity. It may also be possible to use effector cells and target cells in autologous combinations. However, target cells taken from fresh explants are often highly heterogeneous in regard to the cell types surviving in tissue culture. In this case, it can be difficult to establish the specificity of a given response. Moreover, freshly explanted cells are generally more fragile and do not withstand the conditions of the *in vitro* assay. They may also be coated with immunoglobulin, leading to false-positive or false-negative results in the cytotoxicity test.

This statement relevant to freshly implanted cells from solid tumors is not valid for lymphoid target cells. These cells (e.g., leukemic cells) are more stable *in vitro* and may also be utilized after storage in the frozen state. The rather strong expression of antigens determined by the MHC locus on lymphoid target cells may be disadvantageous when the effector cell and/or serum donor are allogeneic in relation to the target cells.

Cells from established tissue culture cell lines are usually more stable under the conditions of the cytotoxicity assay, and are also frequently, but not invariably, better defined than freshly explanted cells as to histogenetic cell types. However, such cells are in most instances allogeneic in relation to the effector cells or the serum donor, and this may give either false-negative or false-positive results in the cytotoxicity assay. Furthermore, such cells may have lost some of their original antigenicity, or may have gained new antigens, for example, because of viral transformation, mycoplasma infection or altered growth patterns.

In those instances in which the relevant antigen is available in a soluble form, it is possible to couple it to the surface of sheep or chicken erythrocytes, which then can be used as target cells. These cells are stable under the conditions of the assay and are susceptible to antibody-mediated phagocytosis or lysis by a much larger variety of effector cells than tissue culture target cells. These targets, therefore, tend to be highly sensitive agents, and this sensitivity may not necessarily reflect the capacity to kill tumor cells *in vivo*.

5.6.2. *Assay Procedures*

Available assay procedures are essentially of two types: (a) procedures that directly measure target cell lysis, and (b) procedures that record the combined lytic and cytostatic effect of effector cells (e.g., microcytotoxicity assay).

Isotope Release. The most common procedures involve measurements of the release of isotopic tracer from prelabeled target cells (see Methods 46–48). The time of incubation needed to show significant target-cell damage may vary but is generally considerably shorter than in the second type of assay. When the cytotoxicity-inducing potency of patients' serum is investigated using effector cells from healthy donors, 1–8 hr incubation may be sufficient, depending on the nature and concentration of the antibodies present. Mouse tumors, sensitized with mouse antibody, may be damaged by human effector cells in situations where mouse lymphocytes are inactive. When the assay is used to study the antibody-dependent cytotoxic activity of various effector cells from an immune donor, the incubation time needed will be longer, since target-cell lysis usually will depend on release of antibody during the assay.

Effector cell fractionations show that K cells are the predominating antibody-dependent effector cells in cytotoxic reactions against tumor cells.

While direct incubation of effector cells and target cells is used to establish the cytotoxic activity of effector cells from immune donors, release or production of antibodies may also be determined by sensitive inhibition assays. They rely on the fact that sensitized target cells of one type can interfere with antibody-dependent cell-mediated cytotoxicity against a second sensitized target. For example, if effector cells from a tumor bearer are mixed with tumor cells and antibody sensitized ^{51}Cr-labeled chicken red cells, lysis of the chicken red cells will be inhibited if tumor-specific IgG is produced. This assay was initially developed for detecting mouse transplantation antigens (34).

Microcytotoxicity Assay. The results obtained with procedures that measure the net results of target-cell lysis and growth inhibiton may frequently be the same as those obtained with the procedures measuring lysis only. However, the results have also been shown to differ in several systems. In the microcytotoxicity assay, release of target cells from the monolayer often occurs before lysis, and different types of effector cells may predominate in the two types of assay systems. In addition to K cells, other antibody-dependent effector cells, such as monocytes or macrophages, may be active in the microcytotoxicity assay. The microcytotoxicity assay usually requires longer incubation times that allow *in vitro* sensitization or activation of effector cells.

When patients' sera are investigated for antibodies or inhibitory complexes, ^{51}Cr release assays should be used in preference to microcytotoxicity assays. Addition of a serum antigen to an incubation mixture may nonspecifically promote target cell growth (feeder effect) in the microcytotoxicity assay.

5.6.3. Discrimination between Different Cell-Mediated Mechanisms for Cytotoxicity

When effector cells are obtained from immune donors and are added to target cells without addition of immune serum, the resulting cytotoxicity may be antibody-dependent or may be caused by cytotoxic T cells. One way to discriminate between different systems is to fractionate effector cells on the basis of surface markers or other effector cell properties before assaying (see Method 46).

Other methods to discriminate between effector mechanisms make use of the addition of various agents to the assay system.

1. Antibodies to effector cells (e.g., anti-T, anti-θ) inhibit cytotoxic T-lymphocyte (CTL)-dependent systems but not K cells if added with complement

and the lysed cells are removed. If added without complement, the complexes formed on the surface of T cells competitively inhibit K cell activity (34). Similarly, addition of anti-immunoglobulin may inhibit K cells by forming complexes on the surface of B cells, which become competitive target cells.

2. Antibodies to effector cell antigens, such as HLA, H2, inhibit K cell cytotoxicity, but affect CTL very little.

3. Anti-immunoglobulin inhibits K cell activity by neutralizing sensitizing antibody but does not affect CTL. F(ab) fragments are used to avoid cross-linking of target cells that may interfere with cytotoxicity. Whole anti-immunoglobulin could also give false-positive ADCC by reacting with target cell-bound immunoglobulin.

4. Antibodies to target-cell surface antigens inhibit CTL when of relevant specificity. IgM antibody has been shown to inhibit K cell-mediated lysis in this way.

5. Soluble antigens inhibit K cell cytotoxicity by competing for sensitizing antibody. Such antigen has been found to be remarkably inefficient in inhibiting CTL.

6. Aggregated IgG inhibits K cells but not CTL.

7. Immune complexes involving the relevant surface antigen of target cells may inhibit K cell cytotoxicity and CTL activity, but under appropriate conditions they may potentiate K cell cytotoxicity.

The agents used in 3 and 5 will also inhibit spontaneous cytotoxicity in many systems in which lymphoid cells added to nonsensitized targets produce some killing. It may well be that this "spontaneous cytotoxicity" actually reflects a K cell activity, at least to some degree.

6. Macrophages and Tumor Immunity

While considerable emphasis has been placed on the role of lymphocytes in tumor cytotoxicity, the role of macrophages must also be considered. There is increasing evidence that macrophages may have an important effector function to play in cell-mediated immunity both to infectious agents and tumors. It is quite clear that infiltration of tumors by macrophages or histiocytes is a very general phenomenon and in some cases may be associated with better prognosis (1, 26, 101).

Of particular interest is the finding that a number of immunological processes alter the morphology, metabolism, and function of macrophages. Much of this information derives from the important animal models for resistance to intra cellular parasites, such as listeria and toxoplasma (2, 72). In these systems it has been demonstrated that an interaction between specifically sensitized lymphocytes and macrophages *in vivo* is crucial to effect resistance to infection. There is a requirement both for specific sensitization and for challenge with specific antigen in order to generate resistance, but, once the macrophages are "activated," they are commonly found to be resistant to many organisms and antigens unrelated to the specific immunological sensitization and challenge.

The term "activated macrophage" has been used in a wide variety of different contexts and with various meanings to describe such *in vitro* properties as increased ability (a) to attach and spread on glass, (b) to phagocytose certain particles, (c) to exhibit increased levels of lysosomal hydrolases, (d) to secrete a variety of enzymes, and (e) to exert a cytotoxic or cytostatic effect on microorganisms or tumor cells (see Methods 26–37). It is important to note here that many of these changes indeed can occur independently of one another. For example, in the mouse, induction of peritoneal exudates with thioglycolate broth has been found to yield macrophages that attach and spread to a greater degree than normal macrophages, have high levels of lysosomal hydrolases, and enhanced ability to produce extracellular proteases, yet exhibit no greater ability to kill several types of infectious agents than uninduced macrophages. It remains a vital problem to characterize those biochemical morphological and metabolic events that are directly related to their function in resisting infectious agents and in destroying or limiting growth of tumor cells (119, 119a).

There is accumulating evidence that macrophages, for example obtained from the peritoneal cavity of mice previously infected with BCG or *Toxoplasma gondii,* have the capacity to inhibit growth and/or kill tumor cells to a greater degree than primary somatic cells in culture (27, 45–47). However, the methodology chosen is often of critical importance to interpretation of such experiments. In many systems it has been found that activated macrophages will cause a marked inhibition of cell proliferation or incorporation of tritiated thymidine, for example without concomitantly causing a release of radioactivity from isotopically prelabeled cells (118). Since macrophages are metabolically active but divide relatively infrequently, growth inhibition of some tumor cells has been attributed simply to release of thymidine into the medium. It is likely, therefore, that some of the observed "cytotoxic" effects of "activated" macrophages reflect growth inhibition rather than actual destruction of tumor cells. On the other hand, there are clearly situations in which nonspecifically or specifically activated macrophages can bring about the release of isotopic label from syngeneic tumor cells, but not non-neoplastic cells (89). Many of the *in vitro* studies attempting to demonstrate cytotoxicity of macrophages even for ingested bacteria or protozoa as well as tumor cells have indeed failed to show more than a cytostasis or growth-inhibitory activity *in vitro*. This stands in contrast to the ease of demonstrating the ability of activated macrophages to clear infections *in vivo*. This disparity raises the question whether the dramatic effects seen *in vivo* are solely a property of metabolically altered individual macrophages or perhaps reflect an enhanced ability to generate and mobilize increased numbers of such cells at the site of insult *in vivo*. This is a problem that has perhaps received too little attention and requires clarification in a variety of different systems.

The molecular mechanisms by which macrophages acquire the various attributes of activation remain obscure. It is of interest that macrophages which have been cultured with products of activated lymphocytes have recently been shown to kill syngeneic tumor cells as measured by release of radiolabel from these cells more efficiently than nonactivated macrophages, and their cytotoxicity is greater on neoplastic cells than on untransformed cells (15, 16). The effect of this "macrophage activating factor" (MAF) appears to be nonspecific, in that cells treated with this factor are capable of killing a variety of distinct syngeneic tumor cells. The characteristics of MAF appear to be quite similar to those of the factor responsible for inhibition of migration (MIF) (79).

There are other experiments in which it is possible to demonstrate that sensitized lymphocytes produce a specific macrophage "arming" factor (SMAF) which imparts an ability to macrophages to inhibit the growth or to kill specific tumor cells, but not a variety of other tumor cells (27, 28, 65, 82). In contrast to the nonspecific SMAF, the specific arming factor appears to be cytophilic and can be absorbed by macrophages as well as the specific tumor. It remains to be clarified whether the specific arming factor is indeed antibody, whether it acts by mediating an antibody-dependent, cell-mediated cytotoxicity on the part of the macrophages, or by activating them nonspecifically by means of an immune complex formed between the tumor-cell antigen and the specific arming factor through a receptor on the macrophage cell surface, or by other mechanisms. The evidence for direct contact-dependent killing by macrophages of antibody-coated target cells, similar to the K cell system, is not great and is a potentially important mechanism requiring considerably more study.

Many questions remain unanswered. To what extent are the bacteriocidal and tumorcidal properties in the host intrinsic to the metabolic state of individual macrophages and to what extent do they reflect an ability to generate and mobilize increased numbers *in vivo*? What are the mechanisms by which activated macrophages exert growth-inhibitory effects on tumor cells? Is the major function of such activated macrophages *in vivo* primarily cytotoxic or growth inhibitory? What are the relative roles of nonspecific and specific MAF found *in vitro*? How do activated macrophages discriminate between neoplastic and non-neoplastic cells?

7. *In Vitro* Lymphocyte Blastogenesis with Tumor Antigens

7.1. General Considerations

The difficulties encounted in evaluating host responses to tumor antigens in the *in vitro* lymphocyte blastogenesis assay arise not from the paucity of data, but rather from problems of interpretation. In this sense, tumor-associated antigen (TAA) induced lymphocyte blastogenesis suffers from the same inadequacies that hamper work using microbial and other soluble antigens, namely: the contribution of the proliferative response in the overall cascade of interrelated events that lead to the final expression of cell-mediated immunity (i.e., relationship to mediator production, cytotoxicity); the relationships to defined lymphocyte populations (T, B, or other). In addition, the TAA system introduces unique problems that involve separation of effects initiated by native or altered HLA antigenic mosaics from those initiated exclusively by tumor-specific determinants.

This view could be critical to our understanding the vagaries of the *in vitro* lymphocytes blastogenesis assay for tumor immunity and its slender connection to *in vivo* events and the clinical status of the tumor-bearing patient.

In reviewing the pertinent literature on this assay, it will be useful to keep in mind the following distinctions: (a) Are we recording an MLC-type of response when either whole viable or mitomycin-treated allogeneic tumor cells are used as antigen? (b) When extracts of tumor cells are employed, does this lymphocyte proliferative response detect an antigen unique to the tumor or is it a variant of an MLC response launched by cell extracts?

With these caveats in mind reflection on the growing literature on TAA-induced lymphocyte proliferation as an assay for CMI to tumors may provide some hints as to the pressing question of what precisely is being measured.

Since most of this work has been accomplished in tumor-bearing patients, it is fraught with the additional variable of the human condition: nature, extent, and duration of disease; prior therapy; and the most uncontrollable variable, a rapidly changing relationship between host, tumor, and environment. We will consider the experimental results in humans first and then look to those obtained in controlled experimental animal models (see Methods 54–56).

7.1.1. *Mixed Lymphocyte-Tumor Interaction (MLTI)*

Stjernswärd and his colleagues were among the first to employ lymphocyte blastogenesis as a potential measure of host immunological reactivity to autochthonous tumor antigens (110). This group has reported evidence for positive results using autochthonous tumor cells over a period of several years in a diverse group of patients suffering from a wide variety of tumors. Of 105 patients studied, 40 (38%) expressed a positive response by the "mixed" lymphocyte target interaction (MLTI) test and 27/40 had greater than 2-fold lymphocyte blastogenesis, although the 2-fold increment must be regarded as of questionable biological significance. This group also demonstrated a blocking effect of autologous sera on autochthonous tumor cells, and circulating lymphocytes were more often stimulated by tumor cells than lymph node lymphocytes (111).

There is some suggestion of the detection of prior sensitization to melanoma antigens in a pair of monozygotic twins, excluding the contribution of HLA differences to the blastogenic response observed (78). However, when these studies were extended to a random population, this suggestion was not borne out.

7.1.2. *Response to Solubilized Tumor Extracts*

Studies measuring lymphocyte blastogenesis triggered by intact tumor cells leave the nagging doubt that one may be detecting a primary immune response analogous to that detected in the mixed leukocyte culture assay rather than revealing a preexisting state of immunity to TAA. Efforts have been made, to partially resolve this doubt by the preparation and use of solubilized tumor antigens to stimulate lymphocytes in culture. In the histocompatibility system soluble HLA antigens are generally not thought to induce lymphocyte blastogenesis unless the subject tested has been subjected to prior active sensitization to the same antigens (54). However, more recently Dean *et al.* (22) have reported allogeneic stimulation using KCl extracts of normal lymphocytes. Hence, the finding that soluble KCl extracts of tumor antigens stimulate lymphocyte blastogenesis in tumor-bearing patients suggests either prior sensitization to such antigens or the presence of functional MLC antigens in the extracts.

Analogous results have been reported using KCl extracts and a diverse array of human tumors (120). In this study, lymphocyte blastogenesis triggered by autochthonous tumor cells was compared *pari passu* with that triggered by KCl extracts of the same tumor antigens, and the results were concordant in 10 of 18 patients. In control studies only 1 of 18 nonmalignant tissue-cell suspensions, and 1 of 10 nonmalignant KCl extracts simultaneously tested, gave positive results. The concordant results of intact tumor cells and KCl extracts also correlated well with delayed-type hypersensitivity responses *in vivo* in skin tests performed with tumor extracts, but no correlation could be established between *in vitro* or skin test responses and the extent or stage of the disease.

Preliminary studies suggest the possibility of a correlative trend between a clinical response and positive blastogenesis to melanoma antigen following BCG immunotherapy (64). Further studies are required to verify this.

In other systems, it has been difficult to demonstrate significant blastogenesis with tumor extracts. Carefully controlled studies of this type comparing intact tumor cells, KCl extracts, and nonmalignant tissue responses *in vitro* and *in vivo* promise to clarify the origins of the variability of the results encountered.

Studies of syngeneic tumors (line 1 and line 2 diethylnitrosamine-induced hepatomas) in inbred guinea pigs have shown correlations between acquisition of cutaneous delayed-type hypersensitivity reactivity, macrophage migration inhibition, and lymphocyte blastogenesis to KCl tumor extracts. There was good correlation between the tests, and the responses were shown to be tumor-line specific and dose dependent (76).

The study presents an example of the promise afforded by the study of tumor systems in inbred animal models to evaluate the nature and significance of *in vitro* assays, their relationship to *in vivo* events, and the natural clinical course of the disease as well as monitoring immunotherapy.

7.2. Methodology

The lymphocyte blastogenesis assay has been standardized and a vast experience has been accumulated with mitogens and soluble microbial antigens (see Method 54). However, the adaptation to soluble tumor extracts is more recent and presents pitfalls in respect to toxicity of the preparations used and the possibility of contamination with antigens (microbial, viral, fungal, HLA) other than tumor-associated antigens.

Moreover, the goal of a 2-fold increase in thymidine incorporation of experimental over control lymphocyte stimulation has crept into the literature. There is no guarantee that a 2-fold increase is any more or less significant than a lesser stimulation, and even the relationship between statistical significance and biological significance remains obscure. The problem of interpretation of published results is compounded when only stimulation indices are given in the absence of raw data.

The current availability of microtechniques for lymphocyte blastogenesis should help to resolve this problem in that many more tests and controls can be done simultaneously. This in turn will provide an adequate volume of data for statistical analyses and evaluation of the significance at least of the assay if not the results achieved.

7.3. Problems of Interpretation and Immunological Significance

A critical question in this area relates to the nature and significance of the limited sampling of lymphocyte subpopulations isolated from the circulation for assay. It is possible, even likely, that the tumor target cell mass can act as an *in vivo* antigen adsorbent to deplete selectively the circulation of specifically reactive lymphocytes thought to form the basis of this and other *in vitro* assays. Such a mechanism could explain the increase in the number of reactive lymphocytes in the circulation following extirpation of the tumor mass and decrease with extensive metastases. It is also possible, as in the mouse MLC, that the human system may reflect a dissociation of proliferating T cells from killer T cells. Finally, there is no formal evidence concerning which cell is responding in the tumor cells, whether T, B, or other subpopulations, to varying degrees. Nor is there any hint of which of the myriad of individual, organ, or tumor-specific antigens in the tumor extract are triggering the event that is recorded.

Nevertheless, the easy availability of a continuous supply of blood lymphocytes and the need for only small quantities of the patient's tumor, coupled with automated machines to register thymidine incorporation, all conspire to make lymphocyte blastogenesis a most popular assay of tumor immunity despite the problem surrounding its significance. However, unless autochthonous tumor is employed as a source of antigen, when KCl extracts are used, this assay may measure merely an elaborate MLC response.

Having eliminated this source of error, as with most other types of tests, there is as yet no assurance that tumor immunity is being detected by this technique or that the results reflect the clinical status of the patient or can serve to monitor the effects of therapy.

8. Assays of Inhibition of Cell Migration

A number of techniques utilizing the principles of inhibition of cell migration have been used to detect lymphocytes sensitized to tumor antigens (see Methods 57–61). The methods are based on the finding that sensitized lymphocytes, when stimulated by specific antigen, produce a number of soluble mediators, including migration inhibitory factor (MIF), which inhibits the migration of macrophages/monocytes, and leukocyte inhibitory factor (LIF), which inhibits the migration of polymorphonuclear leukocytes (9, 20, 100). In man, these two mediators are produced by T and B lymphocytes (81, 99). The mechanisms of the direct inhibition of buffy-coat leukocytes by antigen is based on this latter principle (108). In the direct assay, buffy-coat leukocytes are placed in either microcapillary tubes (29, 66), agarose plates (18), or agarose droplets (36), and the cells are allowed to migrate in the presence and in the absence of various antigens. In the indirect assay, lymphocyte-rich populations are incubated with the antigens in question, and the supernatant obtained from these cultures is tested for the presence of LIF, using normal PMN, or of MIF, using normal macrophages or monocytes. Studies in which a variety of microbial antigens were used have shown clearly that the production of both MIF and LIF by cells from normal persons correlates well with the presence or the absence of delayed hypersensitivity skin reactions to these antigens by the donor.

Both direct (see Methods 57, 60, and 61) and indirect (see Methods 58 and 59) inhibition of migration assays have been used to detect lymphocyte sensitivity to a variety of tumor antigens.

To obtain tumor antigen preparations suitable for testing, tumors have either been homogenized and extracted with saline (9) or extracted with 3 M KCl (97). The choice of control antigens is often difficult. Controls in various studies have included benign tumors of a related organ, normal tissue from the same organ as the tumor, fetal tissues and carcinomas from different organs. Extracts of normal and malignant tissues from the same organ and the same individual are preferable when it is possible to obtain them.

From the results of a number of clinical studies, the use of allogeneic tumor extracts seems feasible (see below). Since large amounts of most tissue extracts may inhibit or cause stimulation of the migration of cells, it is necessary to determine the dose of each antigen preparation that will not significantly affect the migration of normal cells. Such an optimal dose will frequently inhibit the migration of leukocytes obtained from patients bearing the tumor in question, the two best-studied human systems being breast (66) and renal carcinoma (56). It is most helpful to carry out dose—response titrations using a wide range of protein concentrations with each extract on cells from patients and controls at the same time. In addition, it is advisable to determine the general reactivity of the patient's cells at the same time by using a microbial antigen, such as streptokinase-streptodornase (SK-SD) to be sure that a negative result is not simply secondary to general depression of the immune response. Such immuno-suppression can obviously be due either to the disease or the therapy or to a combination of the two.

In addition to inhibiting the leukocytes of patients directly, these antigen preparations can also be used to stimulate the production of MIF by cells from tumor-bearing patients (15, 48).

Some workers have used puromycin to differentiate the inhibition by antigen due to mediator production from that due to nonspecific toxic effects of the antigen preparation. Puromycin will counteract the effect of specific antigen by preventing the production of the mediator, but will not affect inhibition due to a nonspecific toxic effect (29).

There are a number of clinical studies which suggest that the inhibition of leukocyte migration by tumor antigens may bear some relation to the clinical state of the patient. For instance, in a study on patients with renal carcinoma, patients with distant metastasis had significantly less-positive tests with the leukocyte migration assay than patients without distant metastasis (57).

The finding that the *in vitro* migration of leukocytes from patients with breast carcinoma was inhibited by extracts of allogeneic breast tumors suggests that the different breast carcinomas possess at least some common antigens (66). Similar suggestions for common antigens in renal carcinoma and other tumors have been found (56). The further purification of these antigens may aid in standardizing these assays and making them more reproducible and reliable. Of note, allo-geneic extracts can be used without the problems encountered when these are used in lymphocyte proliferative assays.

Although most studies have employed the direct assay of leukocyte inhibition of migration, the indirect assay (involving the production of MIF and LIF and other mediators) has also been used to detect tumor-sensitized lymphocytes.

When particulate antigens are used, there is the advantage that the antigens can be removed by centrifugation prior to assay on the target cell. The indirect assay may also have advantages in horizontal studies, as lymphocytes can be frozen and stored during a clinical study and all samples tested at the same time. The indirect assay has the disadvantage of requiring more cells and taking more time than the direct assay. However, microassays are being developed to measure human mediators; these include the agarose-plate, microcapillary-tube, and agarose-drop assays, all of which require fewer cells. Further, these assays can be useful in monitoring the activity of different fractions of tumor antigens in chemical purification studies. One hopes that other assays for different products of activated lymphocytes will be examined in terms of tumor immunity (e.g., Methods 61–63).

One of the serious problems in interpreting results of migration inhibition assays derives from numerous observations that MIF (11, 81, 125) and LIF (99) as well as other products of activated lymphocytes (124) can be produced by activated B cells as well as by T cells. And in the case of mediator production by T cells, it is not yet clear whether these factors are produced by specific functional subpopulations, such as helper cells, killer cells, or suppressor cells. In the guinea pig, while there is no question that MIF is produced by non-T lymphocytes, there is evidence that such cells require the presence of some sensitized T lymphocytes in order to produce MIF (10). In contrast, in man the evidence suggests that B cells have the capacity to produce MIF in the absence of T cells, suggesting that MIF and LIF may not be T cell-dependent at all (99). Therefore, interpretation of migration inhibition data in terms of the quantitative, or even qualitative, functioning of human lymphocyte subsets at present remains problematic.

In summary, the following problems are frequently encountered with the inhibition of migration assays in tumor immunity: (a) the assays have proved to be useful for a number of tumor antigens, but have not detected sensitivity to all such antigens used; (b) technical problems are not infrequent involving toxicity of antigens, irregular mediator production, or indicator cell migration and difficulties in quantification; and (c) the relationship to functions of lymphocyte subsets remains unclear.

However, when comparing the various assays for the detection of tumor-sensitized lymphocytes, the assays employing the principle of inhibition of migration may have advantages over several others, particularly where primary or continuous tumor-cell cultures are difficult to obtain. In some studies they appear to correlate with the clinical state of the patient; if this can be verified, it would seem especially important to develop methods using these principles, which are more reliable and reproducible than many of the present assays. It is hoped that the use of more purified antigens will also aid in this endeavor, as these antigens may well allow greater discrimination between the cells obtained from patients and normal subjects than do the present crude tumor antigen preparations. Extracts of well-established and characterized tissue culture lines may be especially useful.

REFERENCES

1. Alexander, P., Evans, R., and Grant, C. K., *Ann. Inst. Pasteur* **122**, 645 (1972).
2. Anderson, S., and Remington, J. S., *J. Exp. Med.* **139**, 1154 (1974).
3. Barth, R. F., and Gillespie, G.-Y., *Cell Immunol.* **10**, 38 (1974).
4. Bean, M. A., Bloom, B. R., Herberman, R. B., Old, L. J., Oettgen, H. F., Klein, G., and Terry, W. D., *Cancer Res.* **35**, 2902 (1975).
5. Bean, M. A., Pees, H., Rosen, G., and Oettgen, H. F., *Natl. Cancer Inst. Mongr.* **37**, 41 (1973).
6. Berczi, I., and Sehon, A., *Int. J. Cancer* **16**, 665 (1973).
7. Bevan, M. J., *Nature (London)* **256**, 419 (1975).
8. Blair, P. B., and Lane, M. A., *J. Immunol.* **115**, 184 (1975).
9. Bloom, B. R., Bennett, B., Oettgen, H. F., McLean, E. P., and Old, L. J., *Proc. Natl. Acad. Sci. U.S.A.* **64**, 1176 (1969).
10. Bloom, B. R., and Shevach, E., *J. Exp. Med.* **142**, 1306 (1975).
11. Bloom, B. R., Stoner, G., Gaffney, J., Shevach, E., and Green, I., *Eur. J. Immunol.* **5**, 218 (1975).
12. Bowen, J. G., Robins, R. A., and Baldwin, R. W., *Int. J. Cancer* **15**, 640 (1975).
13. Butterworth, A. E., Sturrock, R. F., Houba, V., Mahmoud, A. A. F., Sher, A., and Rees, P. H., *Nature (London)* **256**, 727 (1975).
14. Cantor, H., and Boyse, E. A., *J. Exp. Med.* **141**, 1376 (1975).
14a. Cerottini, J.-C., and Brunner, K. T., *Adv. Immunol.* **18**, 67 (1974).
15. Churchill, W. H., and Rocklin, R. E., *J. Natl. Cancer Inst. Monogr.* **37**, 135 (1973).
16. Churchill, W. H., Jr., Piessens, W. F., Sulis, C. A., and David, J. R., *J. Immunol.* **115**, 781 (1975).
17. Clark, R. A., and Klebanoff, S. J., *J. Exp. Med.* **151**, 1442 (1975).
18. Clausen, J. E., *J. Immunol.* **110**, 546 (1973).
19. Cohen, A. M., Millar, R. C., and Ketchum, A. S., *Transplantation* **13**, 57 (1972).
20. David, J. R., *Proc. Natl. Acad. Sci. U.S.A.* **56**, 72 (1966).
21. Davies, D. A. L., and O'Neill, G. J., *Br. J. Cancer* **28**, Suppl. I, 285 (1973).
22. Dean, J. H., Silva, J. S., McCoy, F. L., Leonard, C. M., Middleton, M., and Herberman, R. B., *J. Natl. Cancer Inst.* **54**, 1295 (1975).
23. Djeu, J. Y., Glaser, M., Kirchner, H., Huang, K. Y., and Herberman, R. B., *Cell. Immunol.* **12**, 164 (1974).
24. Doherty, P. C., and Zinkernagel, R. M., *J. Exp. Med.* **141**, 502 (1975).
25. Doherty, P. C., and Zinkernagel, R. M., *Transplant. Rev.* **19**, 84 (1974).
26. Evans, R., *Transplantation* **14**, 468 (1972).
27. Evans, R., and Alexander, P., *Nature (London)* **228**, 620 (1970).
28. Evans, R., Grant, C. K., Cox, H., Steele, K., and Alexander, P., *J. Exp. Med.* **136**, 1318 (1972).
29. Federlin, K., Maini, R. N., Russell, A. S., and Dumonde, D.-C., *J. Clin. Pathol.* **24**, 533 (1971).
30. Fossati, G., Holden, H. T., Herberman, R. B., *Cancer Res.* **35**, 2600 (1975).
31. Gardner, I. D., Bower, N. A., and Blanden, R. V., *Eur. J. Immunol.* **5**, 122 (1975).
32. Garrido, F., Schirrmacher, V., and Festenstein, H., *Nature (London)* **259**, 228 (1976).
33. Gorer, P. A., and Amos, D. B., *Cancer Res.* **16**, 338 (1956).

34. Halloran, P., Schirrmacher, V., and Festenstein, H., *J. Exp. Med.* **140,** 1348 (1974).
35. Harfast, B., Andersson, T., and Perlmann, P., *J. Immunol.* **114,** 1820 (1975).
36. Harrington, J. T., and Stastmy, P., *J. Immunol.* **110,** 752 (1973).
37. Hashimoto, Y., and Sudo, H., *Gann* **62,** 139 (1971).
38. Hellstrom, I., and Hellstrom, K. E., *in "In Vitro* Methods in Cell-Mediated Immunity" (B. R. Bloom, and P. R. Glade, eds.), p. 409. Academic Press, New York, 1971.
39. Herberman, R. B., Kirchner, H., Holden, H. T., Glaser, M., and Bonnard, G. P., *Proc. Am. Soc. Microbiol. Symp.* in press.
40. Herberman, R. B., Nunn, M. E., Holden, H. T., Lavrin, D. H., *Int. J. Cancer* **16,** 230 (1975).
41. Herberman, R. B., Nunn, M. E., Lavrin, D. H., and Asofsky, R., *J. Natl. Cancer Inst.* **51,** 1509 (1973).
42. Herberman, R. B., Ting, C. C., Kirchner, H., Holden, H., Glaser, M., Bonnard, G. D., and Lavrin, D. H., *Prog. Immunol. II* **3,** 285 (1974).
43. Hersey, P., *Nature (London), New Biol.* **244,** 22 (1973).
44. Hersey, P., Edwards, J., Edwards, A., Adams, E., Kearney, R., Milton, G. W., *Int. J. Cancer* **16,** 169 (1975).
45. Hibbs, J. B., Jr., *Nature (London), New Biol.* **235,** 48 (1972).
46. Hibbs, J. B., Jr., *Science* **180,** 868 (1973).
47. Hibbs, J. B., Jr., Lambert, L. H., and Remington, J. S., *Science* **177,** 998 (1972).
48. Hilberg, R. W., Balcerzak, S. P., and LoBuglio, A. F., *Cell. Immunol.* **7,** 152 (1973).
49. Holm, G., *Int. Arch. Allergy Appl. Immunol.* **43,** 671 (1973).
50. Invernizzi, G., and Parmiani, G., *Nature (London)* **254,** 713 (1975).
51. Jagarlamoody, S. M., Aust, J. C., Tew, R. H., and McKhann, C. F., *Proc. Natl. Acad. Sci. U.S.A.* **68,** 1346 (1971).
52. Jewell, D. P., and MacLennon, I. C. M., *Clin. Exp. Immunol.* **14,** 219 (1973).
53. Jondal, M., Svedmyr, E., Klein, E., and Singh, S., *Nature (London)* **255,** 405 (1975).
54. Kahan, B. D., *in* "Transplantation Antigens" (B. D. Kahan and R. A. Reisfeld, eds.), p. 411. Academic Press, New York, 1972.
55. Kiessling, R., Klein, E., Pross, H., and Wigzell, H., *Eur. J. Immunol.* **5,** 117 (1975).
56. Kjaer, M., *Eur. J. Cancer* **10,** 523 (1974).
57. Kjaer, M., *Eur. J. Cancer* **11,** 281 (1975).
58. Kodera, Y., and Bean, M. A., *Int. J. Cancer* **16,** 579 (1975).
59. Koszinowski, U., and Ertl, H., *Nature (London)* **257,** 597 (1975).
60. Lamon, E. W., Whitten, H. D., Skurzak, H. M., Andersson, B., and Lidin, B., *J. Immunol.* **115,** 1288 (1975).
61. Lawrence, H. S., *Physiol. Rev.* **39,** 811 (1959).
62. Leclerc, J. C., Gomard, E., Plata, F., Levy, J. P., *Int. J. Cancer* **11,** 426 (1973).
63. Levinthal, B. G., Mann, D. L., and Rogentive, G. N., Jr., *Transplant. Proc.* **3,** 243 (1971).
64. Lieberman, R., Wybran, J., and Epstein, W., *Cancer* **35,** 756 (1975).
65. Lohmann-Matthes, M. L., Schippea, H., and Fischer, H., *Eur. J. Immunol.* **2,** 45 (1972).
66. McCoy, J. L., Jerome, L. F., Dean, J. H., Carmon, G. B., Alfred, T. C., Doering, T., and Herberman, R. B., *J. Natl. Cancer Inst.* **53,** 11 (1974).
67. MacDermott, R. P., Chess, L., Schlossman, S. F., *Clin. Immunol. Immunopathol.* **4,** 415 (1973).
68. MacDonald, H. R., and Bonnard, G. D., *Scand. J. Immunol.* **4,** 129 (1975).
69. MacDonald, H. R., Bonnard, G. D., Sordat, S., and Zawodnik, S. A., *Scand. J. Immunol.* **4,** 487 (1975).

70. MacDonald, H. R., Sordat, B., Cerottini, J.-C., and Brunner, K. T., *J. Exp. Med.* **142** 622 (1975).
71. Mackaness, G. P., *J. Exp. Med.* **129**, 973 (1969).
72. MacLennan, I. C. M., and Harding, B., *Immunology* **18**, 405 (1970).
73. MacLennan, I. C. M., *Transplant. Rev.* **13**, 67 (1972).
74. Mahmoud, A. F., Warren, K. S., and Peters, P. A., *J. Exp. Med.* **142**, 805 (1975).
75. Mantovani, B., Rabinovitch, M., and Nussenzweig, V., *J. Exp. Med.* **135**, 780 (1972).
76. Meltzer, M. S., Oppenheim, J. J., Littman, B. H., Leonard, C. J., and Rapp, H. J., *J. Natl. Cancer Inst.* **49**, 727 (1972).
77. Milleck, J. von, and Pasternak, G., *Arch. Geschwulstforsch.* **42**, 192 (1973).
78. Nagle, G. A., St. Arneault, G., Holland, J. F., Kirkpatrick, P., and Kirkpatrick, R., *Cancer Res.* **30**, 1828 (1970).
79. Nathan, C. F., Remold, H. G., and David, J. R., *J. Exp. Med.* **137**, 275 (1973).
80. O'Toole, C., Stejskal, V., Perlmann, P., and Karlsson, M., *J. Exp. Med.* **139**, 457 (1974).
81. Papageorgiou, P. A., Henley, W. L., and Glade, P. R., *J. Immunol.* **108**, 494 (1972).
82. Pels, E., and DenOtter, W., *Cancer Res.* **34**, 3089 (1974).
83. Perlmann, P., and Perlmann, H., *Cell. Immunol.* **1**, 300 (1970).
84. Perlmann, P., Wigzell, H., Golstein, P., Lamon, E. W., Larsson, A., O'Toole, C., Perlmann, H., and Svedmyr, E. A., *Adv. Biosci.* **12**, 71 (1973).
85. Perlmann, P., Perlmann, H., and Müller-Eberhard, H. J. J., *J. Exp. Med.* **141**, 287 (1975).
86. Perlmann, P., Biberfeld, P., Larsson, A., Perlmann, H., and Wahlin, B., *in* "Membrane Receptors of Lymphocytes" (M. Seligmann, J. L. Preud'homme, and F. M. Kourilsky, eds.), p. 161. North-Holland Publ., Amsterdam, 1975.
87. Perlmann, P., *in* "Clinical Immunobiology" (F. H. Bach and R. A. Good, eds.), Vol. 3, pp. 107–131. Academic Press, New York, 1976.
88. Peter, H. H., Pavie-Fischer, J., Friedman, W. H., Aubert, C., Cesorini, J. P., Roubin, R., and Kourilsky, F. M., *J. Immunol.* **115**, 539 (1975).
89. Piessens, W. F., Churchill, Jr., and David, J. R., *J. Immunol.* **114**, 293 (1975).
90. Plata, F., Cerottini, J.-C., and Brunner, K. T., *Eur. J. Immunol.* **5**, 227 (1975).
91. Plata, F., Gomard, E., Leclerc, J. C., and Levy, J. P., *J. Immunol.* **111**, 667 (1973).
92. Plata, F., MacDonald, H. R., and Engers, H. D., *J. Immunol.* in press.
93. Plata, F., MacDonald, H. R., and Sordat, B., *Proc. Int. Symp. Comp. Res. Leukemia Related Dis., 7th, 1976,* in press.
94. Pross, H. F., and Jondal, M., *Clin. Exp. Immunol.* **21**, 226 (1973).
95. Rager-Zisman, B., and Bloom, B. R., *Nature (London)* **251**, 542 (1974).
96. Rager-Zisman, B., Grose, C., and Bloom, B. R., *Nature (London)* **260**, 380 (1976).
97. Reisfeld, R., Pellegrino, M. A., and Kahan, B. D., *Science* **172**, 1134 (1972).
98. Revillard, J. P., Samarat, C., Carolies, G., and Brodies, J., *in* "Membrane Receptors of Lymphocytes" (M. Seligmann, J. L. Preud'homme, and F. M. Kourilsky, eds.), p. 171. North-Holland Publ., Amsterdam, 1975.
99. Rocklin, R. E., MacDermott, E. P., Chess, L., Schlossman, S. F., and David, J. R., *J. Exp. Med.* **140**, 1303 (1974).
100. Rocklin, R. E., Meyer, O., and David, J. R., *J. Immunol.* **104**, 95 (1970).
101. Russell, S. W., Doe, W. F., and Cochrane, C. G., *J. Immunol.* **116**, 164 (1976).
102. Schirrmacher, V., Rubin, B., and Pross, H., *J. Immunol.* **112**, 2219 (1974).
103. Schrader, J. W., Cunningham, B., and Edelman, G. M., *Proc. Natl. Acad. Sci. U.S.A.* **72**, 5066 (1975).
104. Shearer, G. M., Rehn, T. G., and Garbarino, C. A., *J. Exp. Med.* **141**, 1388 (1975).

105. Shiku, H., Bean, M. A., Old, L. J., and Oettgen, H. F., *J. Natl. Cancer Inst.* **54**, 415 (1975).
106. Shiku, H., Kisielow, P., Bean, M. A., Takahashi, T., Boyse, E. A., Oettgen, H. F., and Old, L. J., *J. Exp. Med.* **141**, 227 (1975).
107. Shiku, H., Kisielow, P., Bean, M. A., Takahashi, T., Oettgen, H. F., and Old, L. J. *Proc. Am. Assoc. Cancer Res.* **16**, 67 (1975).
108. Søborg, M., and Bendixen, G., *Acta Med. Scand.* **181**, 247 (1967).
109. Steele, G., Sjögren, H. O., Lannerstad, O., and Stadenberg, I., *Int. J. Cancer* **16**, 682 (1975).
110. Stjernswärd, J., Clifford, P., Singh, S., and Svedmyr, E., *East Afr. Med. J.* **45**, 484 (1968).
111. Stjernswärd, J., Vánky, F., and Klein, E., *Br. J. Cancer* **28**, Suppl. I, p. 72, (1973).
112. Stutman, O., *Cancer Res.* **36**, 739 (1976).
113. Takasugi, M., and Klein, E., *Transplantation* **9**, 219 (1970).
114. Ting, C., Bushar, G. S., Rodrigues, D., and Herberman, R. B., *J. Immunol.* **115**, 1351 (1975).
115. Tønder, O., Morse, P. A., and Humphrey, L. J., *J. Immunol.* **113**, 1162 (1974).
116. Trinchieri, G., Bauman, P., deMarchi, M., and Tokes, Z., *J. Immunol.* **115**, 249 (1975).
117. Troye, M., Perlmann, P., and Perlmann, H., in preparation.
118. Unanue, E., *Proc. Natl. Acad. Sci. U.S.A.* **71**, 4273 (1974).
119. Van Furth, R. (Ed.), "Mononuclear Phagocytes." Blackwell, Oxford, 1975.
119a. Nelson, D. (ed.), "Immunobiology of the Macrophage." Academic Press, New York, 1976.
120. Vánky, F., Klein, J., Stjernswärd, J., and Nilsson, U., *Int. J. Cancer* **14**, 277 (1974).
121. Veit, B. C., and Feldman, J. D., *Int. J. Cancer* **13**, 367 (1975).
122. Voisin, G. A., Kinsky, R., Jansen, F., and Bernard, C., *Transplantation* **8**, 618 (1969).
123. Wagner, H., Rollinghof, M., and Nossal, G. J. V., *Transplant. Rev.* **17**, 3 (1973).
124. Wahl, S. M., Iverson, G. M., and Oppenheim, J. J., *J. Exp. Med.* **140**, 1631 (1974).
125. Yoshida, T., Sonazaki, H., and Cohen, S., *J. Exp. Med.* **138**, 784 (1973).
126. Yust, I., Smith, R. W., Wunderlich, J. R., and Mann, D., *J. Immunol.* **116**, 1170 (1976).

Section B

Methods

1

The E Rosette Test

Thomas Hoffman and Henry G. Kunkel

1. Introduction

Human lymphocytes and sheep erythrocytes will become bound together when brought into close contact *in vitro*. Since lymphocytes with adherent sheep red blood cells (SRBC) (E) give the appearance of a rosette (Fig. 1) when viewed under the microscope, the term "E rosette" has become an accepted description for the combined unit.

The discovery of this phenomenon arose from the study of receptors on lymphoid cells for antigen or antigen—antibody complexes. With widespread use of sheep cells as antigen or as indicator cells coated with antibody, a number of observers independently noted that nonimmune lymphocytes reacted with washed, unsensitized sheep erythrocytes (1–4).

Only a varying proportion of human peripheral blood lymphocytes demonstrates this capability. Monocytes, granulocytes, and B lymphocytes do not, under the usual conditions employed in testing, form spontaneous sheep erythrocyte rosettes.

Accumulated evidence from diverse sources has established spontaneous RBC rosette formation as a marker of T lymphocytes (5, 6). Human thymic cells at 15 weeks of gestation form rosettes, but peripheral fetal lymphocytes do so only with progressive gestational age; almost all mature thymocytes form rosettes (7). Rosette formation is inhibited by anti-thymocyte or specific anti-T lymphocyte antisera, but not by anti-immunoglobulin antisera (1, 8). Long-term lymphoid cell lines with characteristic B cell markers uniformly do not rosette; only the rare lines derived from malignant T cells may do so. Chronic lymphocytic leukemia (CLL) lymphocytes, considered to be prototypes for B cells in normal peripheral blood, generally do not form rosettes. Studies of normal lymphocyte subpopulations usually show complementarity between the number of rosette-forming cells and those bearing markers for B cells (Fc and complement receptor, membrane immunoglobulin) and only rare or unusual instances of overlap.

The basic, straightforward simplicity of the technique has lent itself to immediate wide application in different clinical and experimental settings (Section

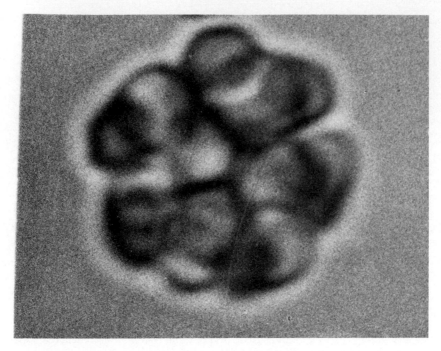

Fig. 1. Sheep red blood cells (E) viewed under the microscope. Note "rosette" appearance.

4). Paradoxically, along with the proliferation of information derived from the method and its application, a parallel body of literature has emerged demonstrating the vagaries of the E rosette assay (Section 3.2).

2. Materials

2.1. Sheep Erythrocytes. Sheep blood is obtained sterilely from a peripheral vein (usually external jugular) directly into transfer packs containing ACD. The same sheep is always bled and is not used in any other experiments, including immunization.

Blood is stored at 4°C between uses. "Aging" does not necessarily precede use; blood stored more than 4 weeks is generally not employed. An appropriate aliquot is removed from the pack, discarding the initial few milliliters of blood flow. Cells are washed four times in 5–10X volume with isotonic saline or Hanks' balanced salt solution. The erythrocytes are resuspended at 0.5% (v/v) in Hanks' balanced salt solution, PBS, or medium (RPMI 1640 or other commercially available tissue culture solutions are equivalent for this purpose).

Packed red cells, 0.1 ml in 20 ml of salt solution (approximately 10^8 RBC/ml), provide a convenient supply for average day-to-day requirements of this reagent. Fresh suspensions are made at least every other day; they too are stored at 4°C between uses.

2.2. Serum. Fresh human type AB serum (pooled, preferably from non-transfused male donors) is employed after suitable decomplementation and absorption against packed sheep erythrocytes. Serum is heated at 56°C for 30 min and filtered through a Millipore filter. Packed cells, 1/3–1/2 volume, are mixed with serum and incubated at room temperature for 30 min (absorption may be carried out at 4° and 37°C as well). The mixture is pelleted, the supernatant serum is removed, and the process is repeated with a new aliquot of washed, packed cells. Serum from these absorptions is Millipore-filtered, divided into volumes of 1–2 ml, and stored at −70°C for future use. Understandably, serum should be tested for completeness of absorption by routine tests for hemagglutination or C'-dependent lysis in any standard system. No additives, antibiotics, or azides are employed in preservation of sera.

2.3. Lymphocytes. Mononuclear cell suspensions obtained from buoyant density-gradient separation (Ficoll–Hypaque) are washed 3 times in phosphate-buffered saline (PBS) and resuspended in PBS, Hanks', or RPMI with added calcium and magnesium. Cells, 1×10^7, and one drop of 5% latex particle suspension per 5-ml volume, are incubated with occasional agitation at 37°C for 1 hr. The cells, washed twice more in PBS, are resuspended at 2×10^6 lymphocytes per milliliter of medium or salt solution.

2.4. Solutions. Phosphate-buffered saline, Hanks' balanced salt solution, and tissue culture media are readily available as ready-mixed solutions or as prepackaged powders suitable for reconstitution with distilled water (DIFCO, GIBCO, Microbiologic Associates). They also can be prepared from standard chemical reagents available in all labs. For cell viability testing, 1:10 dilution of 1% stock trypan blue, centrifuged prior to use, or 0.1% toluidine blue, is used.

2.5. Equipment. Round-bottom plastic test tubes (12 × 75 mm, Falcon No. 2054) are used extensively but may be substituted for with different-volume plastic containers as dictated by availability or quantities needed. Rosettes are read in a hemocytometer (Neubauer, etc.), using an ordinary light microscope in standard use in hematologic or histologic technique. Short-format, wide-bore Pasteur pipettes are used to transfer rosette suspensions.

In summary, aside from usual laboratory materials, including calibrated pipettes, centrifuges, refrigeration and incubation sources, and common chemical reagents, the following are the essentials for assaying sheep erythrocyte rosettes:

1. A source of sheep cells
2. Relatively pure lymphocyte suspension

3. AB serum
4. PBS or common physiologic solutions
5. Microscope and hemocytometer

3. Technique

3.1. Method. Lymphocyte suspension, 0.1 ml (2×10^5 total cells) and 0.1 ml of 0.5% sheep erythrocyte suspension (1×10^7 cells) are added to 12×75 mm round-bottom plastic test tubes, preferably in duplicate. Twenty microliters of absorbed, heat-inactivated AB serum are added to designated tubes. The mixture is agitated by vortexing briefly or by scraping the tube along a test tube rack with a wrist-flicking motion. Each tube is centrifuged at 50 g for 5 min at room temperature. Short-incubation rosettes are read immediately; long incubation lasts overnight (18 hr) at 4°C.

Resuspension of the sheep RBC–lymphocyte pellet is accomplished by gentle tilting of the test tube held between the thumb and forefinger. This rocking motion disrupts the pellet as the meniscus edges over the rounded tube bottom. This action, accompanied by a firm but cautious, coordinated swirling motion ensures the most complete dispersion of individual rosettes, unclumped, into the original medium. A drop of trypan or toluidine blue is added after complete suspension is attained. Approximately 10 μl are drawn up into a Pasteur pipette by simple capillary action and likewise loaded into the hemocytometer chamber in sufficient quantity to fill the counting stage area.

The suspension is viewed through the 45X objective using conventional optics. Scoring the number of rosette-forming cells is done by tabulating the number of lymphocytes with three or more adherent red cells and the number of lymphocytes without. Dead cells or latex-ingesting cells are not entered into the count. Results are expressed as percentage of rosettes over total cells counted (usually 200). Optimally, percentages of rosettes are obtained for both short and long incubation, with and without AB serum, and may be correlated with the total lymphocyte count to yield an absolute number of rosette-forming cells.

3.2. Procedural Modifications. As mentioned above, discordant results have been obtained in enumerating numbers of E rosetting cells in human peripheral blood. Although the exact basis for this divergence has not been identified, there is widespread agreement that seemingly minor changes in methodology are responsible. The following discussion focuses on aspects of the technique that introduce or modulate variability.

3.2.1. Sheep Cells. Erythrocytes from different sheep may evince greater or lesser affinity for lymphocytes, or vice versa (9). Although genetic differences may underlie this disparity, they have not yet been adequately studied.

Comparison between sheep erythrocytes from different commercial sources and lots may show considerable differences. Also, storage additives might impart differences to sheep cell sources. Duration of storage minimally may affect usability in the assay; most often aged (beyond 4–6 weeks) cells show greater tendency to clump or hemolyze.

3.2.2. Lymphocytes. Although density-gradient separation has become the most prevalent technique for isolation of mononuclear cells, other methods are still in use and could conceivably alter yields of a particular cell type. Data are available on comparison of rosette-forming cells using lymphocytes isolated by different techniques (9, 10). In light of information on the effect on rosette formation of charged compounds, anticoagulants, polysaccharides, etc. (see below), or other reagents in use in preparing blood for density gradients, their use at any stage of separation should be evaluated critically.

Since energy dependence and protein-synthesizing capacity are vital determinants for rosetting (5, 10, 11), possible perturbations of these, especially during handling or incubation, should be considered as sources of "error" or differences in results.

3.2.3. Serum. AB serum definitely enhances the adherence of sheep erythrocytes (SRBC's) to the lymphocyte in that both the number of cells participating in the reaction and the number of sheep cells adherent per lymphocyte increase (10). Other serum sources, FCS, FBS, even sheep or other species' serum share this property to varying degrees (2). Differences in final serum concentration from 1% to 25% show only slight effect. The serum component responsible for this enhancing property, as well as mechanisms underlying it, remain unknown.

3.2.4. Medium. At extremes of pH, rosette formation is impaired (12). Conflicting evidence exists regarding dependence on Ca and Mg ions, but by the above method similar results are obtained when the assay is performed in calcium and magnesium-free solution.

3.2.5. Cell Concentrations and Proportions. Ratios of 20–100 erythrocytes per lymphocyte in the reaction mixture ensure reliability of the assay. At extremes of concentration of either cell type, tendency to clump interferes with resuspension, and thickness of the preparation precludes adequate visualization during counting. Although, theoretically, adherence between lymphocytes and sheep cells take place in the pellet, potentially allowing for use of reagents in differing concentrations as long as total cell numbers remain constant, one should be aware that large pellets or large supernatant volumes may make resuspension difficult or might yield insufficient or inappropriate numbers of cells for final counting.

3.2.6. Incubation Conditions. As lymphocytes and SRBC's are incubated for longer periods of time, rosettes gradually increase quantitatively and qualitatively (4, 6). Numbers of short-incubation ("early," "STAT") rosettes range from 20 to 80% of "late" or long-incubation (overnight) rosettes; the difference is less dramatic in the presence of serum (14).

Many conflicting data exist on the temperature sensitivity of the rosette test (2, 4–6, 9, 12–14). Most investigators now agree that rosette formation by peripheral blood cells is optimal at temperatures between 4° and 25°C, and that rosettes form poorly at 0°C and disintegrate at 37°C (4, 5, 14). Practically, a short period of 37°C preincubation after mixing and prior to centrifugation, once thought beneficial to rosette stability, is probably less important, if not deleterious to the outcome of the assay (9).

A majority of thymocytes, in contrast to PBL, form stable E rosettes at 37°C (5–6).

3.2.7. Lymphocyte Viability and Selection. Loss of specific cell populations during isolation, incubation, or enumeration, will result in obvious aberrations in percentages of rosette-forming cells. For example, selective adherence of B cells to glass or plastic tubes, or their differential viability during incubation, will result in observed "high" levels or rosette-forming cells (RFC) in a heterogeneous original population. Should metabolic impairment, short of cell inviability, result from any manipulation, RFC from that population of cells tested will be "falsely low."

3.2.8. Resuspension. Rosettes, once formed, are to a greater or lesser degree, fragile. Shearing forces applied through vortexing, pipette mixing, or shaking will disrupt or abolish the rosette (9).

Counting errors or bias apply irrespective of the technique used to count. Although some investigators advocate sealed cover slip preparations, or dried stained slides, these give lower RFC percentages, in comparison to the hemocytometer method. Excessive agitation, drying, delays in counting, all will impair accurate enumeration of rosette numbers and type. Most important, failure to adequately identify monocytes will result in spurious values for total RFC, as monocytes are inaccurately scored as nonrosetting lymphocytes. Identification of rosettes is less of a problem as experience is gained, but definition by arbitrary criteria (i.e., the number of adherent sheep cells qualifying a rosette) is important when rosettes are less stable, as, for example, in counting short-incubation rosettes, when "low affinity" sheep cells are employed, or in the absence of serum or enhancer substances.

Toluidine blue added to the suspension immediately before counting helps in identifying mononuclear cells, distinguishing dead (purple-staining) from live (blue-staining) lymphocytes, and detecting lymphocytes beneath "morulae" of surrounding sheep cells. Glutaraldehyde fixation prior to counting is probably not useful (18).

3.2.9. Stabilizers and Inhibitors. Assorted treatments of the cells involved in rosetting may alter their propensity to participate in the reaction, or their detectability in the scoring procedure. For example, treating the lymphocyte with papain enhances rosette formation whereas trypsin or phospholipase A treatment decreases or abolishes it (18). Curiously, phospholipase A from cobra venom, but not from other sources, induced the ability to form E rosettes in human lymphoblastoid (B cell) lines (19). Neuraminidase will enhance rosetting if used to treat either the lymphocytes or the red cells, or both (20, 21). Papain treatment of RBC's will increase percentages of rosettes at certain concentrations under specific conditions (22). Trypsin treatment of the red cells abolishes rosette formation (23). Aminoethylisothiouronium (AET) bromide, a sulfhydryl reagent used to treat red cells, increases sheep rosette stability in a fashion similar to neuraminidase (24, 25). This reagent appears to minimize differences noted in the use of sheep cells from different sources.

Polycations (DEAE-dextran, polybrene, poly-L-lysine, spermadine) increase proportions of early rosettes, whereas polyanions, heparin, and dextran sulfate induce the opposite effects (26). Ficoll, like dextran, increases rosettes (27).

Metabolic poisons, such as sodium azide, iodoacetamide, 2,4-dinitrophenol, cytocholasin B, inhibit rosettes (5, 6, 10, 11, 28). Dead cells, frozen and thawed cells, and heavily X-irradiated cells (unpublished) will not rosette optimally. Antimetabolites have been shown to have various effects. Puromycin and cycloheximide increased "active" rosettes (29), but puromycin, as well as α-amanitin and actinomycin D, inhibit the ability of thymocytes to regain the capacity to form rosettes subsequent to trypsin treatment (30). Dibutyryl cyclic AMP (cAMP), or drugs that elevate intracellular cAMP, will inhibit the rosetting reaction (31, 32).

These technical variables reflect on and contribute to the ignorance of the essential biophysical interactions governing spontaneous sheep erythrocyte–lymphocyte rosetting. This deficiency underlies our lack of understanding of the basic biologic or physiologic principle which the phenomenon represents. Standardization of procedures and reagents will, it is hoped, hasten the resolution of the problem.

3.3. Applications

3.31. Density-Gradient Separation. The differential in density between lymphocytes with and without adherent SRBC's permits separation of those cells by density gradients in a manner analogous to mononuclear cell isolation. Pellets prepared in the same manner as for counting, but often in larger proportions (100X), are resuspended and gently layered in entirety directly over aliquots of Ficoll–Hypaque. Cells without adherent RBC's will be collected at the interface after centrifugation at 200 g for 40 min in the cold; rosette-forming cells will be found in the pellet and may be employed in standard analyses subsequent to red cell removal or hypotonic lysis. Obviously, the technical caveats employed for counting apply for separation also. Principally, caution must be exercised not to disrupt rosettes during manipulation; serum or a stabilizer (e.g., AET) is virtually mandatory. Controls to ensure relative purity are necessary; rosette and nonrosette fractions must be subject to "re-rosetting" and other marker tests.

3.3.2. Other E Rosettes. Red blood cells from different species also form rosettes with human lymphocytes when tested by analogous techniques. Monkey, pig, goat, dog, horse, chicken, and cat RBC's may demonstrate rosette formation with variable percentages of lymphocytes, notably under conditions of serum or neuraminidase enhancement (33).

Rosette formation with mouse (34) or *Macaca speciosa* (35) RBC's has been advocated as a marker of B lymphocytes. Of particular interest is the description of autologous rosette formation in human subjects (30, 36–38) on the order of 2–5%. This population is also enhanced by serum or neuraminidase treatment (30, 37).

4. Comment

4.1. Interpretation. Using the method described above in detail, optimally 88 ± 6% of human peripheral blood lymphocytes form E rosettes (Table 1). Different laboratories have reported widely divergent results (in a range from 20% to 90%), probably as a reflection of those variables considered above, principally, differences in handling techniques, sources of sheep cells, and variation in scoring. In the absence of an absolute T cell marker analogous to alloantigens of the mouse (θ, Ly), these number differences cannot be easily reconciled or evaluated by any absolute reference standard.

The pressing central issue of interpretation of these differences relates to the question of how a given procedural change may alter the measurement of specific populations of cells. For example, do any reagents advocated for stabilizing rosettes (serum, enzymes, AET, etc.) increase the apparent proportion of RFC by protecting fragile rosettes already formed, or do they lead to rosette formation on the part of mononuclear cells that would not bind E in their absence?

Although the ability to form E rosettes is at present an established marker for T cells in the human, it is important not to lose sight of the heterogeneity of subclasses of lymphocyte populations arbitrarily assigned as T or B. Many studies have shown cells having double markers, capable of binding E as well as EA, EAC, or RBC's of other species (21, 39–42). Notably treatment of PBL with neuraminidase includes a new population in the rosetting reaction. Even without neuraminidase, cells with Fc receptors have been shown to participate in

TABLE 1

E Rosette Formation by Human
Peripheral Blood Lymphocytes

	Medium	AB serum
"STAT"	63 ± 15	83 ± 6
Overnight	70 ± 9	88 ± 6

spontaneous E rosetting under conditions of optimal serum enhancement and long incubation (43).

Evidence is accumulating that in man, as in the mouse, subpopulations of T lymphocytes exist with different functions. Possibly these are mirrored by variations of E rosette technique. For example, fractionation procedures have demonstrated differential response to mitogen in PBL separated on the basis of their ability to rosette with or without serum (14). As mentioned above, thymocytes differing in their ability to rosette at 37°C show differing functional properties as well. In addition, interaction to varying degrees with autologous or other species' RBC's characterizes subsets of the broader T lymphocyte population defined by sheep rosettes.

Despite general acceptance of the E rosette test, caution must still be exercised in interpreting the precise nature of the E-rosetting cell.

4.2. Use. Clinical and laboratory knowledge has benefited from this very basic procedure. Our understanding of the cell origin of a number of malignancies and proliferative disorders has evolved from studies employing E-rosette assays in conjunction with other marker systems. Acute and chronic lymphocytic leukemia, Sezary syndrome, leukemic reticuloendotheliosis, mycosis fungoides, malignant lymphoma, and infectious mononucleosis are among the proliferative disorders that have lent themselves to this analysis (44–46).

A corollary functional utilization of E rosettes has been as a measure of cell-mediated immunity. However, in this area considerable caution in interpretation is still required. Numbers of E rosettes have been correlated with mitogen responsiveness and T cell function in certain situations. In disease states associated with depressed cellular immunity (cancer, autoimmune disease, viral or bacterial infection) aberrations of number of circulating rosette-forming cells sometimes have been noted (31, 47–52).

Concepts about immune deficiency have been considerably augmented from marker analysis and enumeration. T-cell deficiencies (severe combined immunodeficiency, Nezeloff syndrome, DiGeorge syndrome, Wiskott–Aldrich syndrome, chronic mucocutaneous candidiasis) have been associated with diminished numbers of E rosettes, and their reconstitution was accompanied by restoration of this function (53). Knowledge of the various forms of immunoglobulin deficiency has also been enhanced by identification of cell types represented in peripheral blood, as well as interactions between them which contribute to pathogenesis. For example, T cells have been identified (by E rosetting) that suppress immunoglobulin synthesis in certain cases of common variable immunodeficiency (CVID, formerly acquired hypogammaglobulinemia) (54).

Evaluation of the clinical efficacy of anti-lymphocyte or anti-thymocyte sera has been aided considerably by comparing inhibiting effects in the rosette assay (1, 9). Effect on rosettes of other biologic products [thymosin (30), α-fetoprotein (55), immunoregulatory α-globulin (IRA) (56), the lipoprotein rosette inhibitory factor (RIF) (57), etc.] has also been employed as an indicator for the functional integrity for the respective system producing these substances.

The affinity of cells for sheep erythrocytes remains most useful in sorting cell populations. Whether applied to enumerating or isolating T and B cells in peripheral blood, lymphoid organs, or tissue infiltrations, or to marking cells in tissue culture, this characteristic reaction, despite its limitations, functionally identifies a particular cell or population. The general problems involved in cell—cell interactions are clearly manifest in this system, and it well may serve further as a model for future study in this difficult area.

REFERENCES

1. Bach, J. F., Dormont, J., Dardenne, M., and Balner, H., *Transplantation* 8, 265 (1969).
2. Brain, P., Gordon, J., and Willets, W. A., *Clin. Exp. Immunol.* 6, 681 (1970).
3. Coombs, R. R. A., Gurner, B. W., Wilson, A. B., Holm, G., and Lindgren, G., *Int. Arch. Allergy Appl. Immunol.* 39, 658 (1970).
4. Lay, W. H., Mendes, N. F., Bianco, C., and Nussenzweig, V., *Nature (London)* 230, 531 (1971).
5. Jondal, M., Holm, G., and Wigzell, H. J., *J. Exp. Med.* 137, 1532 (1972).
6. Froland, S. S., *Scand. J. Immunol.* 1, 269 (1972).
7. Wybran, J., and Fudenberg, H. H., *Trans. Assoc. Am. Phys.* 84, 239 (1971).
8. Wortis, H. H., Cooper, A. G., and Brown, M. C., *Nature (London), New Biol.* 243, 109 (1973).
9. Steel, C. M., Evans, J., and Smith, M. A., *Br. J. Haematol.* 28, 245 (1974).
10. Bentwich, Z., Douglas, S. D., Siegal, F. P., and Kunkel, H. G., *Clin. Immunol. Immunopathol.* 1, 511 (1973).
11. Whittingham, S., and MacKay, I. R., *Cell. Immunol.* 6, 362 (1973).
12. Chaves, M. A. and Arranhado, E., *Lancet* 1, 42 (1972).
13. Sasaki, M., Sekizawa, T., Takahoshi, H., Abo, T., and Kimagai, K. *J. Immunol.* 115, 1509 (1975).
14. Mendes, N. F., Tolnai, M. E. A., Selveira, N. P. A., Gilbertson, R. B., and Metzgar, R. S., *J. Immunol.* 111, 860 (1973).
15. Mendes, N. F., Saraiva, P. J., and Santos, O. B. O., *Cell. Immunol.* 17, 560 (1975).
16. Galili, V., and Schlesinger, M., *J. Immunol.* 115, 827 (1975).
17. Evans, J., Smith, M. A., and Steel, C. M., *J. Immunol. Methods* 7, 371 (1975).
18. Chapel, H. M., *Transplantation* 15, 320 (1973).
19. Hanaumi, K., Abo, T., and Kunnagai, K. *Nature (London)* 259, 124 (1976).
20. Bentwich, Z., Douglas, S. D., Skutelsky, E., and Kunkel, H. G., *J. Exp. Med.* 137, 1532 (1973).
21. Galili, U., and Schlesinger, M., *J. Immunol.* 112, 1628 (1974).
22. Wilson, A. B., Haegert, D. G., and Coombs, R. R. A., *Clin. Exp. Immunol.* 22, 177 (1975).
23. Weiner, M. S., Bianco, C., and Nussenzweig, V., *Blood* 42, 939 (1973).
24. Kaplan, M. E., and Clark, C., *J. Immunol. Methods* 5, 131 (1974).
25. Pellegrino, M. A., Ferrone, S., Dierich, M. P., and Reisfeld, R. A., *Clin. Immunol. Immunopathol.* 3, 324 (1975).
26. Yu, D. T. Y., and Pearson, C. M., *J. Immunol.* 114, 788 (1975).
27. Brown, C. S., Halpern, H., and Wortis, H. H., *Clin. Exp. Immunol.* 20, 505 (1975).
28. Kersey, J. H., Hom, D. J., and Buttrick, P., *J. Immunol.* 112, 862 (1974).

29. Wybran, J., Belohradsky, B. H., and Fudenberg, H. H., *Cell. Immunol.* **14**, 359 (1974).
30. Bushkin, S. C., Pantic, V. S., and Good, R. A., *J. Immunol.* **114**, 866 (1975).
31. Chisari, F. V., and Edgington, T. S., *J. Exp. Med.* **140**, 1122 (1974).
32. Galant, S. P., and Renno, R. A., *J. Immunol.* **114**, 512 (1975).
33. Slankard, M., and Kunkel, H. G., unpublished observations (1974).
34. Braganza, C. M., Stathopolous, G., Davies, A. J. S., Elliot, E. V., Kerbel, R. S., Papamichail, M., and Holborow, E. J., *Cell* **4**, 103 (1975).
35. Pellegrino, M. A., Ferrone, S., and Theofilopoulos, A. N., *J. Immunol.* **115**, 1065 (1975).
36. Sandilands, G. P., Gray, K., Cooney, A., Browning, J. D., and Anderson, J. R., *Clin. Exp. Immunol.* **22**, 493 (1975).
37. Gluckman, J. C., and Montambault, P., *Clin. Exp. Immunol.* **22**, 302 (1975).
38. Sheldon, P. J., and Holobrow, E. J., *J. Immunol. Methods* **7**, 379 (1975).
39. Dickler, H. B., Adkinson, N. F., and Terry, W. D., *Nature (London)* **247**, 213 (1974).
40. Dewar, A. E., Habeshaw, J. A., Young, G. A., Stuart, A. E., Parker, A. C., and Wilson, C. D., *Lancet* **1**, 215 (1974).
41. Chiao, J. W., Pantic, V. S., and Good, R. A., *Clin. Exp. Immunol.* **18**, 483 (1974).
42. Ross, G. D., Rabellino, E. M., Polley, M. J., and Grey, H. M., *J. Clin. Invest.* **52**, 377 (1973).
43. Winchester, R. J., Fu, S. M., Hoffman, T., and Kunkel, H. G., *J. Immunol.* **114**, 1210 (1975).
44. Seligmann, M., *N. Engl. J. Med.* **290**, 1483 (1974).
45. Edelson, R. L., Kirkpatrick, C. H., Shevach, E. M., Schein, P. S., Smith, R. W., Green, I., and Lutzner, M., *Ann. Intern. Med.* **80**, 265 (1974).
46. Pattengale, A. K., Smith, R. W., and Perlin, E., *N. Engl. J. Med.* **291**, 1146 (1974).
47. Wybran, J., and Fudenberg, H. H., *J. Clin. Invest.* **52**, 1026 (1973).
48. Gross, R. L., Latty, A., Williams, E. A., and Newberne, R. M., *N. Engl. J. Med.* **292**, 439 (1975).
49. Messner, R. P., Lindstrom, F. D., and Williams, R. C., *J. Clin. Invest.* **52**, 3046 (1973).
50. DeHoratius, R. J., Strickland, R. G., and Williams, R. C., *Clin. Immunol. Immunopathol.* **2**, 353 (1974).
51. Lisak, R. P., Levison, A., Zweiman, B., and Abden, N., *Clin. Exp. Immunol.* **22**, 30 (1975).
52. Dwyer, J. M., Bullock, W. E., and Fields, J. P., *N. Engl. J. Med.* **288**, 1036 (1973).
53. Wybran, J., Levin, A. S., Spitler, L. E., and Fudenberg, H. H., *N. Engl. J. Med.* **288**, 710 (1973).
54. Waldman, T. A., Broder, S., Blaese, R. M., Durm, M., Blackman, M., and Strober, W., *Lancet* **1**, 609 (1974).
55. Gupta, S., and Siegel, F. P., *N. Engl. J. Med.* **293**, 302 (1975).
56. Menzoian, J. D., Glasgow, A. H., Nimberg, R. B., Cooperband, S. R., Schmind, K., Saporeshetz, I., and Mannick, J. A., *J. Immunol.* **113**, 266 (1974).
57. Chisari, F. W., Routenberg, J. A., and Edgington, T. S., *J. Clin. Invest.* **57**, 1227 (1976).

2

Detection of Human T Lymphocytes by Rosette Formation with AET-Treated Sheep Red Cells

Manuel E. Kaplan, Mildred Woodson, and Connie Clark

1. Introduction

Selective, nonimmune cytoadherence of sheep red blood cells (SRBC) to human thymus-derived lymphocytes (T-L), resulting in formation of rosettes, was independently described by three groups of investigators in 1972 (1–3). Since that time, this phenomenon has been utilized extensively to identify and quantitate T-L in human peripheral blood and, to a more limited extent, to detect T-L obtained from solid tissues (thymus, lymph nodes, spleen, etc.). Early reports from different laboratories showed marked variation (4–70%) in the percentage of T-L among peripheral blood lymphocytes from normal human volunteers (1–6). It subsequently became apparent that a number of procedural variables could profoundly influence the speed and strength of interaction of T-L with sheep erythrocytes (SRBC's), e.g., age of sheep cells used, duration of incubation of T-L with SRBC's, protein content of the incubation medium (7–12). Thus, modifications designed to minimize the variability in results inherent in the originally proposed rosetting procedures have been described (13–15). The assay we developed (15) utilizes SRBC treated with the sulfhydryl compound 2-*S*-aminoethylisothiouronium bromide (AET). Using AET-treated SRBC (SRBC-A), maximal rosette formation occurs in less than 1 hr; the rosettes are large, stable, and quite resistant to mechanical disruption.

2. Materials and Equipment

2.1. 12 X 75 mm polypropylene test tubes (Falcon Plastics, Oxnard, California; Catalogue No. 2063)

2.2. Allopolymer centrifuge tubes, 29 X 104 mm, 50-ml capacity (International Centrifuge Division of Damon Corporation, Needham Heights, Massachusetts; Catalogue No. 2828). Wash thoroughly and dry. Cover with aluminum foil and steam sterilize.

2.3. Polycarbonate centrifuge tubes, 15-ml, conical with plug seal cap, sterile (Falcon Plastics, Oxnard, California; Catalogue No. 2095)

2.4. Graduated glass culture tubes, round bottom, 20 × 150 mm, 25-ml capacity (Corning Glass Works, Corning, New York; Catalogue No. 400834). Wash thoroughly and dry. Siliconize. Cover with aluminum foil and steam sterilize.

2.5. Graduated glass culture tubes, 25 × 100 mm, 50-ml capacity (Corning Glass Works, Corning, New York; Catalogue No. 400835). Wash thoroughly and dry. Siliconize. Cover with aluminum foil and steam sterilize.

2.6. Vacutainer tubes, 10 ml containing powdered EDTA (Becton, Dickinson Corp., Rutherford, New Jersey; Catalogue No. 4713)

2.7. Vacutainer tubes, 10-ml, containing 143 units of heparin (Becton, Dickinson Corp., Rutherford, New Jersey; Catalogue No. 4716)

2.8. Sterile disposable plastic pipettes, 5-ml (Falcon Plastics, Oxnard, California; Catalogue No. 7543)

2.9. Sterile disposable plastic pipettes, 10-ml (Falcon Plastics, Oxnard, California; Catalogue No. 7551)

2.10. Sterile disposable plastic syringes, 5-ml (Plastipak, Becton, Dickinson Corp., Rutherford, New Jersey; Catalogue No. 805L/S)

2.11. Sterile disposable plastic syringes, 50-ml (Plastipak, Becton, Dickinson Corp., Rutherford, New Jersey; Catalogue No. 5663)

2.12. Nalgene filter unit containing 0.45μm grid membrane (Nalge, Sybron Corp., Rochester, New York; Catalogue No. 245-0045)

2.13. Siliclad solution (Clay Adams, Division of Becton-Dickinson Corp., Parsippany, New Jersey)

2.14. Trypan blue solution, 0.4% (Grand Island Biological Co., Grand Island, New York; Catalogue No. 525)

2.15. 2-S-Aminoethylisothiouronium bromide (AET) (Aldrich Laboratories, Milwaukee, Wisconsin; Catalogue No. A5460-1)

2.16. Sterile sheep blood in Alsever's solution (Grand Island Biological Co., Grand Island, New York). Sheep blood obtained from other suppliers may also be used.

2.17. RPMI 1640 (RPMI) tissue culture medium (Grand Island Biological Co., Grand Island, New York, or alternatively from Associated Biomedical Systems, Buffalo, New York)

2.18. Fetal calf serum (FCS) (Grand Island Biological Co., Grand Island, New York; or Rehatuin, Armour Pharmaceutical Co., Phoenix, Arizona). As required, an aliquot of sterile FCS is heated for 1 hr at 56°C. Nine volumes of heated FCS are mixed with 1 volume of packed, saline-washed SRBC's, incubated for 30 min at 37°C, then centrifuged at 850 g for 15 min at 4°C. The absorbed FCS is transferred to a Nalgene filter unit (2.12) and filter-sterilized by water suction. The sterile FCS is divided into aliquots, which are frozen and stored at −80°C; as needed, 20 ml of sterile, heat-inactivated absorbed FCS are added to 80 ml of RPMI (RPMI- FCS).

2.19. Hypaque, sodium diatrizoate solution, 50% (Winthrop Division, Sterling Drugs Inc., New York, New York; Cat. No. H272). As needed, a 30-ml bottle of 50% Hypaque is diluted to 34% by adding it aseptically to 14.1 ml of glass-distilled water.

2.20. Ficoll-400 (Pharmacia Fine Chemicals, Piscataway, New Jersey). A solution of 9 g per 100 ml of distilled water is filter-sterilized and stored aseptically at 4°C. A Ficoll–Hypaque solution is prepared by mixing 5 volumes of 34% Hypaque with 12 volumes of 9% Ficoll; the solution is filter sterilized and stored aseptically in the dark at 4°C for no longer than 1 week before it is used.

2.21. Dextran T150 (Pharmacia Fine Chemicals, Piscataway, New Jersey). A 3 g/100 ml solution of Dextran T150 is prepared in isotonic saline, sterilized by filtration, and stored aseptically at 4°C.

2.22. Technicon Lymphocyte Separating Reagent (Technicon Corp., Ardsley, New York)

2.23. Technicon Lymphocyte Separator Mixer (Technicon Corp., Ardsley, New York)

2.24. Technicon Lymphocyte Separator Magnetic Processor (Technicon Corp., Ardsley, New York)

2.25. Technicon sterile transfer tube and plastic plug (Technicon Corp., Ardsley, New York; Catalogue No. P/N 197-B006)

3. Detailed Methodologies

3.1. Preparation of AET Solution. AET, 402 mg, is dissolved in 10 ml of deionized or glass-distilled water to yield a 0.143 M solution. The pH is carefully adjusted, using a pH meter, to 9.0 by dropwise addition of 4 N NaOH (usually 9–10 drops are required). The alkaline AET solution must be prepared immediately before use and the excess discarded.

3.2. Preparation of SRBC-A. Sheep blood is removed sterilely from the storage bottle using a 5-ml sterile plastic syringe with a 21-gauge disposable needle. The blood is gently transferred to a 15-ml sterile graduated conical polycarbonate centrifuge tube and centrifuged at 750 g for 5 min at room temperature. Diluted plasma and buffy coat are removed, and the red cells are washed 5 times in approximately 20 volumes of sterile isotonic saline at room temperature by repeated centrifugations. After the last saline wash, the volume of packed red cells is noted and the cell pellet is gently dispersed by swirling. To each volume of the washed, packed SRBC's, 4 volumes of freshly prepared AET solution, pH 9.0, are added. The cells are mixed thoroughly by repeated gentle tilting and inversion of the capped tube and incubated at 37°C for 15 min, mixing every 5 min. Cold, sterile isotonic saline is added to fill the conical tube, which is then lightly centrifuged (400 g) for 5 min to minimize the increased cell "stickiness" that follows AET treatment. The SRBC-A cell pellet is washed 5 times in cold, sterile isotonic saline, thoroughly resuspending the packed erythrocytes after each centrifugation. Little, if any, hemolysis should be observed after the last saline wash. The packed, washed cells are suspended in 10–15 ml of cold RPMI and centrifuged at 400 g for 5 min. Sufficient RPMI-FCS is added to the measured red cell pellet to yield a 10% suspension. SRBC-A in RPMI-FCS may be used for rosetting immediately or can be stored at 4°C for as long as 5 days without affecting the rosetting properties.

3.3. Isolation of Lymphocytes. Lymphocytes may be isolated from the peripheral blood or from solid tissues by one of several well-established methods (12). The technique used in this laboratory is described in detail since the percentage of rosetting cells may vary depending upon the lymphocyte isolation procedure utilized. Blood, 10–50 ml, is drawn from the antecubital vein into heparinized or EDTA-containing Vacutainers. The anticoagulated blood is mixed with one-half volume of 3% Dextran T150 in sterile 25- or 50-ml graduated, siliconized, round-bottom glass culture tubes, which are covered with Parafilm and incubated at 37°C in an upright position for 30 min. The leukocyte-rich plasma is layered over an equal volume of Ficoll–Hypaque in sterile round-bottom, allopolymer centrifuge tubes, which are then centrifuged at 600 g for 30 min at 20°C. The supernatant plasma is discarded, and interface cells are carefully harvested with a 5- or 10-ml sterile disposable pipette and centrifuged at 500 g for 15 min at room temperature. The pelleted cells are resuspended in 32 ml of Technicon Lymphocyte Separating Reagent and aspirated into a sterile 50-ml plastic syringe through a sterile 20-gauge hypodermic needle, which is sealed by embedding the tip in a plastic plug (2.25). The syringe is constantly rotated by inversion at 37°C for 30 min, using a Technicon Lymphocyte Separator Mixer. The syringe contents are passed through a Technicon Lymphocyte Separator Magnetic Processor via a sterile transfer tube at room temperature. The effluent cells are collected into 15-ml sterile polycarbonate centrifuge tubes, which are capped tightly. These tubes are centrifuged at 500 g at room temperature for 15 min. The supernatant wash fluids are discarded, then the cells are pooled in RPMI and washed three times in RPMI at room temperature. After the final wash, the cells are suspended in 1–2 ml of RPMI-FCS, counted, and examined for viability by trypan blue exclusion. The recovered cells should be comprised of essentially pure lymphocytes ($\geq$ 99%) having at least 95% viability. The cell concentration is adjusted with RPMI-FCS to 2×10^6 lymphocytes per milliliter. Rosetting need not be performed immediately; the cells may be stored at 4°C for up to 18 hr without significantly affecting their viability or rosetting properties.

3.4. Rosetting Procedure. An aliquot of the 10% SRBC-A suspension in RPMI-FCS is sterilely diluted 1:20 in this medium to yield a 0.5% cell suspension. Then 0.4 ml of 0.5% SRBC-A and 0.4 ml of lymphocyte suspension ($2 \times$

10^6 cells/ml) are added to 12×75 mm round-bottom polystyrene test tubes. The tubes are covered with Parafilm, mixed thoroughly, placed in a $37°C$ bath for 15 min, and mixed every 5 min. The tubes are centrifuged at 200 g for 10 min. at room temperature and placed in crushed ice for a minimum of 45 min. The cell pellets are resuspended by gentle, repetitive (10 times) tilting of the test tubes. Usually a small, compact red cell pellet remains unsuspended. One drop of the cell suspension is transferred to a clean microscope slide with a Pasteur pipette, covered with a clean cover slip, which is blotted gently by pressing the inverted slide on a clean cotton towel, and sealed with clear fingernail polish. The slides may be read immediately or may be left at $4°C$ for 3–4 hr without affecting the results. Using Nomarski (interference) or phase-contrast optics, 200–400 lymphocytes are counted. Lymphocytes having 3 or more adherent red cells are recorded as "positive."

4. Critical Comments

4.1. The percentage of rosetting cells detected in normal human volunteers has been found to range from 67 to 86%. For a given normal subject, this percentage is usually quite constant (±5%). In approximately 50 patients with chronic lymphocytic leukemia (untreated and treated), the percentage of rosetting lymphocytes has been found to range from <1 to 45%. Characteristically, however, the percentage detected in untreated patients is <15%.

4.2. As purchased, solid AET is stable indefinitely (for at least one year) at room temperature. It does not require refrigeration or desiccation. However, the reagent bottle should be tightly closed during storage.

4.3. Rare batches of commercial sheep cells have been observed to rosette suboptimally after AET treatment (i.e., <60% with normal human lymphocytes). The reasons for this are not known. Consequently, each time a new shipment of sheep blood is received, lymphocytes from a previously studied donor should be examined. The variation in percentage of rosetting cells for a given normal subject should not exceed ±5–7% with different batches of sheep blood.

4.4. Although some batches of sterile sheep blood may be kept as long as 8–10 weeks at $4°C$ and still yield stable rosetting percentages after treatment with AET, a maximum of 3 weeks of storage at $4°C$ is recommended to ensure maximum reproducibility of results.

4.5. Once slides are prepared for counting of rosettes, they may be read immediately or left at $4°C$ for as long as 3–4 hr without affecting the percentage of rosettes visualized. However, slides should not be warmed to $37°C$, since many rosettes will dissociate at elevated temperatures.

4.6. During the counting procedure, small clumps of red cells that appear as morulae are occasionally encountered. If a central lymphocyte cannot be clearly visualized, such clumps are disregarded and not counted as rosettes.

4.7. Only viable T-L will rosette. If there is a question of lymphocyte viability, one drop of eosin Y may be added to the resuspended rosetted cell mixture containing lymphocytes and SRBC-A. Dead lymphocytes will be stained red and should not be counted.

REFERENCES

1. Froland, S. S., *Scand. J. Immunol.* **1,** 269 (1972).
2. Jondal, M., Holm, G., and Wigzell, H., *J. Exp. Med.* **136,** 207 (1972).
3. Wybran, J., Carr, M. C., and Fudenberg, H. H., *J. Clin. Invest.* **51,** 2537 (1972).
4. Papamichail, M., Holborow, E. J., Keith, H. I., and Currey, H. L. F., *Lancet* **2,** 64 (1972).
5. Mendes, N. F., Tolnai, M. E. A., Silveira, N. P. A., Gilbertsen, R. B., and Metzgar, R. S., *J. Immunol.* **111,** 860 (1973).
6. Ross, G. D., Rabellino, E. M., Polley, M. J., and Grey, H. M., *J. Clin. Invest.* **52,** 377 (1973).
7. Yata, J. Tsukimoto, I., and Tachibana, T., *Clin. Exp. Immunol.* **14,** 319 (1973).
8. Heier, H. E., *Scand. J. Immunol.* **3,** 677 (1974).
9. Bach, J. F., and Dardenne, M., *Lancet* **1,** 633 (1972).
10. Wybran, J., Carr, M. C., and Fudenberg, H. H., *Clin. Immunol. Immunopathol.* **1,** 408 (1973).
11. Jonsson, V., *Scand. J. Haematol.* **13,** 361 (1974).
12. IUIS Report, *Clin. Immunol. Immunopathol.* **3,** 584 (1975).
13. Weiner, M. S., Bianco, C., and Nussenzweig, V., *Blood* **42,** 939 (1973).
14. Bentwich, Z., Douglas, S. D., Siegal, F. P., and Kunkel, H. G., *Clin. Immunol. Immunopathol.* **1,** 511 (1973).
15. Kaplan, M. E., and Clark, C., *J. Immunol. Methods* **5,** 131 (1974).

Antisera to Human T Lymphocytes*

Melvyn F. Greaves and George Janossy

1. Introduction

In mice, thymocytes and T lymphocytes can be identified by their expression of the cell-surface alloantigen θ; an antigen shared with brain and fibroblasts (1). Part of the same molecular structure can be recognized by heteroantisera to brain, and there is considerable evidence for a structurally related T axis-associated molecular entity in rats (2). The best biochemical data available suggest that θ-like antigen in the rat is a glycoprotein (3). Some evidence has also been presented which the authors interpret to suggest that θ antigen(s) can be associated with glycolipids, in particular gangliosides (4, 5). θ is considered to be absent from the T lineage prior to the thymus stage. However, studies on nude mice and θ conversion of spleen or marrow cells by thymic "hormone" extracts/ factors have suggested that prethymocyte cells may exist with a limited θ expression and that θ expression can be rapidly elicited (6). Alternatively, some of these results might reflect responses of immature *postthymic* cells.

T-axis cells also express the alloantigens TL, Ly1, Ly2, and Ly3, and along with θ these antigens serve as valuable markers of T cell differentiation and probably immunocompetent T cell subsets (7). A fairly comprehensive picture is therefore emerging of the T cell membrane antigenic phenotype in rodents. Current experience with antisera to human T lymphocytes is much more limited and largely anecdotal. In this chapter we summarize the published reports of various attempts to produce anti-T sera for man. Our experience at University College has involved screening a considerable variety of sera, and although some success is recorded we have not so far found a "guaranteed" method for producing effective human T lymphocyte-specific sera. Part of these studies have been published previously (8).

*Abbreviations used: T, thymus derived (lymphocyte); B, "bursa equivalent" derived (lymphocyte); Ig, immunoglobulin; FACS, fluorescence activated cell sorter; RBC, red blood cells; ALL, acute lymphoblastic leukemia; AML, acute myeloid leukemia; CLL, chronic lymphocytic leukemia; CFA, complete Freund's adjuvant; s.c., subcutaneous; i.v., intravenous; i.m., intramuscular; SmIg, surface-membrane immunoglobulin; HuTLA, human T lymphocyte antigen; PHA, phytohemagglutinin.

2. Materials

2.1. Cells. Lymphocytes were prepared from blood and tonsils as described elsewhere in this volume (see Method 15). Thymus tissue was obtained either through abortions (12–22 weeks) or from infants (1–8 years) undergoing thoracic surgery. Leukemia cells were obtained from untreated or relapsed patients attending St. Bartholomew's Hospital, Hammersmith Hospital, The Hospital for Sick Children, or University College Hospital (UCH) London. Adult brain and liver tissue was obtained at postmortems (UCH). Red cells for absorptions were obtained from the UCH blood bank (outdated blood).

In some experiments blood lymphocytes were prepared by a simple modification of the Böyum Ficoll–Isopaque method.*

2.2. Antisera and Membrane Markers. The methods used to raise anti-T cell sera are detailed in Section 3. Several other membrane markers of T and B lymphocytes were used to evaluate the specificity of anti-T sera. The details of these additional reagents are given in relation to separation on nylon fiber columns (see Method 15). All antisera were heat inactivated ($56°/30$ min). Adsorptions were carried out with 1:3 packed cell volume:serum by rotation at $4°C$ for 2 hr. After final absorption, cell sera were ultracentrifuged at $100,000\,g$ at $4°C$ for 90 min.

2.3. Immunofluorescence Analysis. Binding of anti-T cell sera was assessed empirically by indirect immunofluorescence using either a Vickers Photoplan UV microscope with incident light or a Zeiss microscope with an epifluorescence condenser.

Later sera in the series were also analyzed using the fluorescence activated cell sorter (FACS). Details of the FACS machine and its applications can be found in references 9 and 10.

The results shown are Polaroid photographs of the oscilloscope screen portraying histograms of the stained cell populations. The machine was operated under standard conditions with respect to laser power (100 mW) and photomultiplier tube amplification (600 V). Sensitivity was varied, however, in particular experiments by altering the fluorescence gain, as indicated in results. In all experiments the histograms based on light-scattering signals were first used to "gate out" all

---

*Separation of human mononuclear cells from blood by density centrifugation. Layer 0.5 ml of heparinized blood + 0.5 × 2 ml of Earle's saline on top of 0.6 ml of Ficoll–Isopaque (density 1.077 g/ml) in a polyethylene tube. Centrifuge at 14,000 g for 1 min in a microcentrifuge. Red cells and granulocytes will sediment to the bottom of the Ficoll: lymphocytes and monocytes will stay at the interface. Carefully remove interface cells and wash (once at 1500 rpm for 10 min and twice at 1000 rpm for 10 min). Resuspend in an appropriate volume of Earle's saline and count cells in a hemocytometer. This is a modification of the Böyum method (N. Rapson, C. Percy, and M. F. Greaves, unpublished observations).

fluorescent signals derived from particles much larger or much smaller than the cell population of interest.

2.4. Cell Population Purification. T lymphocytes were purified from tonsil or blood by nylon column filtration as described elsewhere in this volume (see Method 15). In a few experiments they were also purified by filtration through anti-Ig Degalan columns (8) (see Method 18). B lymphocytes were purified by E rosette sedimentation in Ficoll—Isopaque as previously published (11).

3. Detailed Protocols for Raising and Assessing Anti-human T Cell Sera and Their Evaluation

3.1. Strategies and Summarized Experience. In Tables 1 and 2 we have documented details on all antisera that we have attempted to assess for T cell specificity. As can be seen at a glance a large variety of cellular immunogens have been tried, but our immunization schedules and absorption procedures have been relatively standard. In all, 18 animal sera and 31 human sera have been tested. As indicated in the Tables 1 and 2 we were totally unsuccessful in detecting T cell-specific activity in any of the human sera, and in the animal sera only 7 had usable activity. All 7 had operational selectivity for T cells; however, in none would we claim that specificity was absolute. Indeed, in the 4 sera analyzed by FACS it is clear that residual anti-B cell activity can persist after extensive absorption with chronic lymphocytic leukemia (CLL) cells from up to 10 separate donors (see below).

3.2. Anti-brain Sera. Our experience with anti-brain sera has already been published (8), but note that most sera raised against cerebrum with an identical protocol had little or no activity. The selectivity of sera 1 and 2 for thymus and T cells, however, was quite convincing (see Ref. 8 and Table 3).

> 3.2.1. The sera stained the presumed appropriate number of cells from various cell populations (see Table 2).
>
> 3.2.2. In simultaneous or double-marker tests the sera preferentially reacted with the SmIg negative cells (8).
>
> 3.2.3. The sera showed good selectivity when tested on various purified cell suspensions (Table 3).

Although we did not test the anti-brain sera using FACS, we noted that only one-third of blood T cells stained reasonably brightly and that the remaining two-thirds of the T cells reacted very weakly. These observations are in accord with recent observations by Brouet and Tobin (12) who found that rabbit anti-fetal brain sera appeared to stain only a T cell subset, possibly corresponding to our "brighter" cells. None of our anti-brain sera had any selective cytotoxicity for T cells, and the two sera that appeared to be specific

TABLE 1

Summary of Attempts to Produce T Cell-Specific Antisera

Species immunized	Cellular immunogen	Immunizing schedule	Absorption schedule	Serum No.	Properties of sera
Rabbit	Human cerebrum	CFA i.m.+s.c. (6 sites), days 0 and 14; bled days 21–26	RBC (2×), Liver (2×) CLL (4–10×)	1	Appeared T-cell specific (see text and Ref. 8)
				2	Same properties as serum 1
				3	Only 1/3 T cells stained, very weakly; not used further
				4	No detectable T cell staining after
				5	absorption with CLL
				6	
Rabbit	Rat or mouse brain	As above	None	7	No detectable reactivity with human lymphocytes
				8	
Rabbit	Human infant thymus	10^8–10^9 CFA 2–5× (every other week)	RBC (2×), Liver (2×) CLL, (3–10×)	9	Very high binding titers to T+B cell, but no residual T cell specificity after extensive absorption with CLL
				10	
				11	
				12	Discriminate between T and B, but some weak residual anti-B staining (see text)
				13	
Rabbit	T-Leuk (ALL)	2×10^8 i.v., days 0 and 14	As above	14	As sera 9–11
		2×10^8 i.v., days 0 and 40	As above	15	As sera 9–11
Rabbit	Monkey thymus	2×10^8 i.v., days 0 and 14	RBC (3×)	16	Good staining against T cells
			CLL (3×)	17	+weak residual anti-B activity (see text)
Pig	Fetal thymus	7×10^9 CFA i.m., s.c., i.p., day 0 7×10 i.m., s.c., i.p., day 14 (no CFA); bled, days 21–28	RBC (2×) Tonsil (4×)	18	Stained thymocytes and T lymphoblasts, but had no detectable activity against B or T lymphocytes from tonsil and blood (see text)

TABLE 2
Human Sera with Potential Anti-T Lymphocyte Activity[a]

Sera or Ig assayed	Number	Previously reported positives
SLE patients	15	Lies *et al.* (29)
Cold agglutinins		
Anti-i	6	Thomas (30)
Anti-I	2	
Schizophrenia patients	10	Luria and Domashneva (31)

[a]All sera were analyzed by indirect fluorescence against thymus cells using antihuman Ig reagents. No staining was observed with any of the sera from patients with systemic lupus erythematosus (SLE) or schizophrenia. All anti-i and anti-I antibodies tested were equally reactive with T and B cells as assayed by I antibody-binding tests, cytotoxicity, and inhibition of E or EAC rosettes (32, 33) (see also Method 1 for description of sera that contain anti-T activity).

by indirect fluorescence had no demonstrable cytotoxicity (tested with guinea pig and rabbit complement). Although this observation might reflect anticomplementary effects resulting from the extensive absorptions, it corresponds with the failure of others to demonstrate lymphocytotoxic antibodies in anti-human brain sera (13, 14).

One interesting side issue of the anti-brain sera was their content of antibodies reactive with nonlymphoid cells. Golub had previously recorded that rabbit anti-mouse brain sera contained antibodies to red cells and myeloid stem cells (15). When testing anti-brain sera for reactivity with various leukemias, we found that virtually all acute myeloid leukemias were reactive with CLL-absorbed (i.e., T "specific") sera as well as two erythroleukemias. Limited cross absorption studies indicated that *different* antigens shared with brain existed on T cells (and T leukemias) and on non-T cells in the hematopoietic system (Table 4).

We concluded from this limited series of experiments on anti-brain sera that, as in other mammalian species, there is an antigen shared between brain and the T cell axis. The expression of this antigen appears to be much weaker than is θ in mice and differs also in being expressed better on peripheral T cells than on thymus lymphocytes (1). In view of the suggestions that θ determinants might be expressed on ganglioside glycolipids (4, 5), we considered this possibility also for the human T cell determinant. Cholera toxin, which binds selectively to G_{M1} (16) gangliosides, binds equally well to human T and B cells as assayed by FACS with fluorescent antitoxin antibodies (17, 18). Five rabbit antiganglioside sera (kindly provided by Dr. E. Thompson) were tested against human and mouse lymphocytes; although two of these did bind to lymphocytes, there was no indication of T cell specificity. Finally when we analyzed CLL and thymus cell

TABLE 3

Reactivity of Human Lymphocytes with Rabbit Anti-brain Sera[a,b]

Cells	No. tested	Reactivity[c]		
		Anti-brain (%)	E+ (%)	SmIg+ (%)
A. Normal cells				
Thymus				
fetal 15–22 wk	3	55,98,85	85,82,88	2,3,1
infant 1–8 yr	6	>99	99.5	0.5
Tonsils	12	52.8±1.9	59.4±1.7	42.4±1.5
Spleen	2	30.0 35.0	25.0,37.0	40.2,48.0
B. Malignant cells				
Thymoma	1	97.2	94	0.9
Non-T, non-B ALL	17	0.1±0.1	1.9±0.8	1.5±0.6
T-ALL	4	84.5±4.1	91.6±2.6	1.1±0.5
CLL	9	<1.0	4.1±2.1	91.5±0.6
IgG myeloma	1	8.3	10.4	41.0

[a]See Brown et al. (34).
[b]Sera 1 and 2 in Table 1.
[c]Indirect immunofluorescence.

TABLE 4

Anti-T Plus Antimyeloid Activity in Anti-brain Sera[a]

Cells	None	Reactivity of anti-brain sera (absorbed by CLL) after additional absorptions with		
		Thymus	AML	Brain
Thymus	+	−	+	−
T cells	+	−	+	−
B cells	−	−	−	−
CLL	−	−	−	−
AML	+	+	−	−
ALL-T[b]	+	−	+	−
ALL-Non T, Non B,[c]	−	−	−	−
Erythroleukemia	+	NT	NT	−

[a]Taken from Brown et al. (34) plus unpublished observations.
NT, not tested.
[b]E+ SmIg−.
[c]E−, SmIg−.

extracts for charged glycolipid pattern in thin-layer gel chromatography (R. K. Murray and M. F. Greaves, unpublished observations), no unique bands were observed. In view of the reported wide species cross-reactivity of anti-brain sera (19), we also tested the capacity of strong antisera to mouse and rat brain to bind to human lymphocytes. No reactivity could be demonstrated by indirect fluorescence testing.

3.3. Anti-thymus Sera. Antiserum 18, pig anti-fetal thymus, was of particular interest since after absorption with peripheral T and B cells (tonsil) it still

TABLE 5

Reactivity of Human Lymphocytes from Various Sources
with Anti-T Sera 16 and 17

Cells		% Positive[a]		
		Anti-thymus[b]	Anti-SmIg	E
Blood (B)	1	65	27	−
	2	74	22	70
	3	75	−	−
	4[c]	76	10	78
	5[c]	80	11	80
	B[d]	1	78	1
	T[e]	95	2	94
Tonsil (T)	T and B	53	−	−
		51	44	48
		32	55	31
	T[e]	97	1.0	96
		99[f]	<0.2	95
		87	5.7	83
	B[d]	4	72	<1
		8	85	9
Thymus, infant		70		
Bone marrow		3	6	4
CLL		<1	94	2
		<1	96	2
		5.4	90	4

[a]Monocytes that had phagocytosed latex were ignored in the enumerations.
[b]At 1:10 or 1:20 dilution.
[c]Warmed at 37°C prior to testing in order to elute "labile" cell surface IgG (35, 36).
[d]Purified by E-rosette sedimentation (11).
[e]Purified by nylon column filtration (see Method 15).
[f]Purified by nylon fiber column filtration + E-rosette sedimentation (i.e., pelleted E rosettes used after ammonium chloride lysis of red cells).

stained thymus but very few blood or tonsil T cells. However, when T lymphocytes were stimulated by PHA the E^+ lymphoblasts stained well with the
anti-thymus serum. Similar sera have been reported by Thomas and Phillips (20)
and Schlossman *et al.* (21), although ours differed from Schlossman's in being
poorly reactive with T cell ALL's (i.e., brain antigen +, E^+).

Antisera 12, 13, 14, and 17 were all raised against either human infant thymus
or rhesus monkey thymus. We adopted the latter source of immunogen after the
comment to us by Dr. Charles Balch that in his hands this appeared to be a good
method to produce strong antisera that were T cell specific by indirect immunofluorescence (see Method 4). Our results suggest that this may be the case and
presumably relates in some way to the partial sharing of cell-surface antigens
within primates. Extensive absorption of the sera plus uniform positivity against
all T cell donors appears to rule out that we are looking at a T cell alloantigen.
All 4 sera (sera 12, 13, 16, and 17) behaved rather similarly when tested against
purified cell populations and analyzed by FACS. Detailed data on serum 17 are
given here. Analysis of various lymphocyte cell suspensions (Table 5) suggested
that the serum was T cell selective. These observations were confirmed by FACS
analysis (Fig. 1). Both FACS analysis and direct visual observations indicated
that some slight but definite residual B-cell staining remained. We have not yet
determined the source of this reactivity. There are several possibilities, including
incomplete adsorption and interaction with Fc receptors. Separation of $SmIg^+$

TABLE 6
Simultaneous Testing with T and B Cell Markers[a]

Cells	Anti-thymus	Anti-SmIg	E	EAC[b]	Anti-thymus[c] + Anti-SmIg		Anti-thymus + EAC	
					Double	Null	Double	Null
1. Blood[d]	65	17	68	–	4	11	–	–
2. Tonsil	32	55	34	–	1	14	–	–
3. Tonsil	51	40	56	46	9.2[e]	2	8.6	5.4

[a]"Double" assay for evaluating the specificity of anti-T cell sera. (i) Reagents must be
cross-absorbed, i.e., anti-SmIg with sheep or ox E, antirabbit Ig with human Ig. (ii) Labile
IgG^+ cells are avoided; i.e., preincubate cells at $37°C$ or, better still, use $F(ab')^2$ reagents in
all tests. (iii) Ultracentrifuge all antisera.
[b]Ox red cells + anti-Ox IgM + mouse complement.
[c]Rabbit anti-monkey thymus → goat anti-rabbit Ig-rhodamine + goat anti-human Ig-fluores-
cein.
[d]Separated on Ficoll–Isopaque. phagocytic; monocytes enumerated with 0.1-μm latex
particles.
[e]All weakly stained with anti-T; i.e., compare with population (1) in Fig. 3.

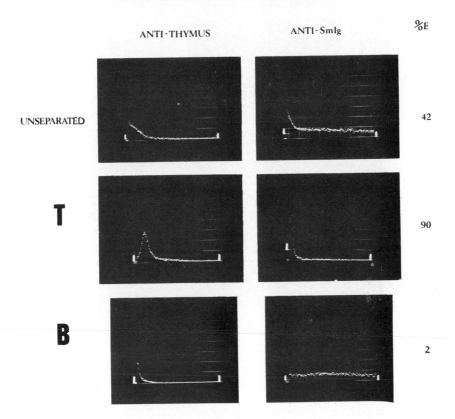

Fig. 1. Fluorescence-activated cell sorter (FACS) analysis of anti-T cell serum (No. 17). Vertical axis: relative number of cells; horizontal axis: relative fluorescence intensity. T cells were purified by nylon column filtration (see Method 15); B cells were purified by E rosette sedimentation (11). FACS operating conditions: Laser 100 mW, PMT 600 V; scatter gain = 1/0.5; fluorescence gain = 8/0.5. Note typical blood range of intensity observed with anti-SmIg. A much narrower distribution is seen with monoclonal malignant B cells, i.e., CLLs (M. F. Greaves and D. Capellaro, to be published) Similar results have been obtained with sera 12 and 13 (see Table 1).

and SmIg$^-$ tonsil lymphocytes by the FACS resulted in the expected reciprocal distribution of HuTLA$^+$ cells (Fig. 2). Double-labeling experiments provide additional evidence for the T cell specificity of anti-thymus sera (Table 6). These experiments also indicate the existence of "null" cells.

FACS analysis of purified T cells with anti-monkey thymus serum (No. 17) has also suggested a potentially important heterogeneity (Fig. 3). Two reactive populations appear to exist: one (corresponding to two-thirds of total) with

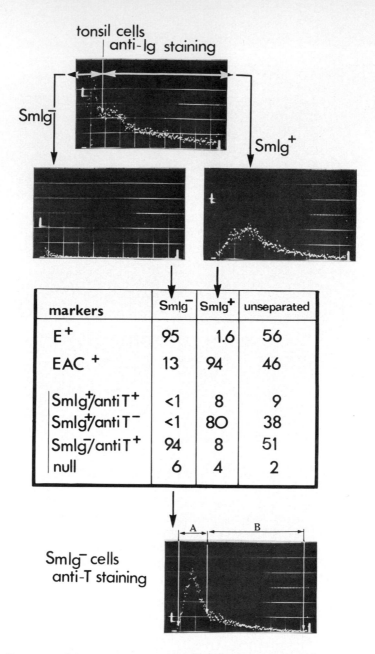

Fig. 2. Human tonsil lymphocytes were stained with anti-Ig and separated by FACS into SmIg⁻ and SmIg⁺ fractions. These fractions were further analyzed by FACS for the purity of samples and by additional membrane markers as shown. When SmIg⁻ cells were restained with anti-monkey T-cell serum (No. 17) the FACS analysis revealed a considerable heterogeneity of T cells. Of SmIg⁻ cells, 62% were weakly positive (A) and the rest were strongly positive (B).

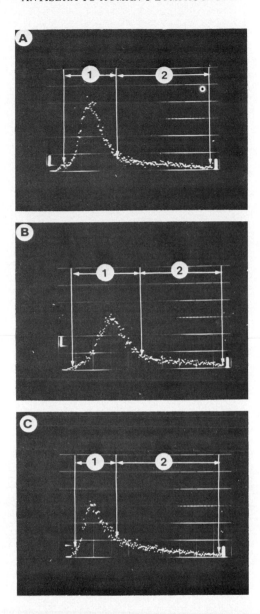

Fig. 3. FACS analysis of T cell heterogeneity. Axes as in Fig. 1. (A) T cells purified from tonsil (87% E). (B) T cells purified from tonsil (97% E). (C) T cells purified from blood (94% E). FACS operating conditions as in Fig. 1. Positive cells (93–96% in all cases) were divided into two populations as shown: (1) uniformly and moderately stained, (2) well stained but with wide spread of intensity. Proportions in the two populations were as follows: In (A), 1 = 66%, 2 = 34%; In (B), 1 = 71%, 2 = 29%; In (C), 1 = 65%, 2 = 35%.

TABLE 7

Summary of Published Data on Anti-T Cell Sera

Animals	Cells	Schedule	Absorptions	No.	Evaluation[b]		Evidence for specificity	References
					Assay system[c]			
Rabbits	Thymus	6 × 10^7 cells, CFA s.c. 1 per week, 6 wk	CLL (5×)		F		A, E	Williams et al. (37)
Rabbits	Fetal or infant thymus	10^9 cells, CFA f.p. day 14, 10^9 cells i.v.; bled day 21	B-LCL (?)	Pool of sera	C		C, D, E, G	Smith et al. (38)
Rabbits	Fetal or infant thymus	As above	B-LCL (12×) serum		C		D, G, E, F	Woody et al. (39)
Goat	Thymus	?	E, CLL	1	C		D	Kersey et al. (40)
Rabbits	XL-A donor blood B cells	8.5×10^6 i.v. 3×/week, alternate weeks	B-LCL (2×), CLL,[a] adherent cells	2/6	C		A, B, C, H, F, E, G	Touraine et al. (41)
	As above	1.4×10^7 CFA s.c. 3×/week, alternate weeks (frozen cells used for boosters)	As above	3			Sera too weak	Touraine et al. (41)
Goat	As above	4.5×10^7 i.v., boosted with same alternate weeks (6×)	B-LCL (4×)	1	C		Sera too weak	Touraine et al. (41)
Rabbits	As above	9×10^6 i.v., boosted with same alternate weeks (5×)	As above	1	C		High titer still killed B cells	Touraine et al. (41)
Rabbits	Infant thymus	Homogenized cells CFA, s.c., boosted 2-week intervals, 2× CFA cells 1× saline cells	Brain, liver CLL	?	C		B, G, E, F	Ishii et al. (42)

Species	Immunogen	Immunization protocol	Absorbents				Reference
Rabbits	19-week fetus	1×10^8 CFA f.p., day 14 1.9×10^8 i.v.	bc (1×), fetal liver (2×), CLL (3×)	(?)	F	E, G, D	Aisenberg et al. (43)
Rabbits	XL-A donor blood B cells	3×10^7 i.v., 1×/week, 4 weeks	None	3	C	H, F, B (diluted serum)	Aiuti et al. (44)
Goat	Infant thymus	5×10^9 cells CFA s.c. (8 sites), booster days 14, 21 (5×10^9/saline)	RBC (6×), CLL (4 ml serum absorbed with 28×10^{10} CLL cells)	1	C	B, E, G, D, F	Bobrove et al. (45)
Rabbit	Fetal cerebrum	Homogenate CFA s.c., days 0, 14	RBC (3×), liver (3×), serum (1×), insol. Ig (1×), CLL (2×)	1		A, D; Blood T subsets only (thymocytes -ive)	Brouet and Toben (12)
Rabbits	Infant thymus 18 Week fetal thymus	5×10^8 CFA f.p.; after 5 months, booster: 25×10^8 i.p.	RBC (4×), B-LCL (1×), Marrow (1×), CLL (1×)	1	F	E, G, D	Mills et al. (46)
Rabbits	Infant thymus	5×10^8 CFA s.c. monthly injection	LCL	1	B	X	Zimmerman (23, 24)
Goat	Infant thymus	10^9 cells in CFA s.c. 1× every 8 weeks for 14 months	RBC (2×), insol. Ig (1×), CLL (1×)	1		F, E	Owen and Fanger (47)
Rabbit	Blood T cell, SRBC receptor, 65,000 and 30,000 MW	Soluble antigen CFA s.c., 3×, 3-week intervals		1		F, E	Owen and Fanger (47)
Rabbit	Antibody, monkey thymus						See Balch et al. (Method 4)

[a]B-lymphoid cell lines are possibly better absorbents than CLL.

[b]Sera raised against thymocytes may also define antigen(s) present on thymus cells but absent from blood T cells [Ablin and Morris (48); Thomas and Phillips, (29); see also Table 1].

[c]C = cytotoxicity. F = fluorescence.

[d]Evidence for specificity: A, Double or simultaneous tests, e.g., E + anti-SmIg fluorescence; B, purified T and B cells studies; C, lymphocytes from patients with well-defined selective immunodeficiencies studies; D, T or B cell leukemias studied; E, titration to "presumed" T or B cell level; F, inhibition of T or B cell functions, e.g., E rosetting, PHA response, MLR; G, thymocytes, MLR response, PHA response, MLR; G, thymocytes, B lymphoid cell lines studied; H, additivity of T and B tests (i.e., sequential assays).

moderate intensity of staining, and another (corresponding to one-third of total) with a broad spectrum of bright fluorescence. These observations are similar to earlier observations with antibrain sera (Nos. 1 and 2, see above).

4. Conclusions

We have not yet tested sufficient numbers of antithymus sera to suggest that the schedule adopted for antisera 12/13 or 16/17 provides a reliable, reproducible procedure for producing anti-human T cell sera. Our experience is clearly anecdotal, and we can only conclude that these methods can work. The longer-term objective should be to use such sera to isolate T cell-specific antigens and to immunize with these. This has been achieved with some success in mice (22), and there are encouraging results in this direction from Zimmerman's work (23, 24) on human lymphocytes.

The general published experience with anti-human T cells sera is summarized in Table 7. While it is possible that some human sera may have considerable potential as anti-T reagents (see Method 1), convincing evidence for T cell specificity of animal sera is scanty. This, however, applies to immunofluorescence assays, not to cytotoxicity, where T cell specificity is more readily demonstrable. This distinction, which is we believe a general experience, remains a puzzle. We have tested anti-thymus sera (provided by Dr. J. Woody, National Institutes of Health), which, although quite T cell specific by cytotoxicity, did not appear to distinguish between T and B cells at all by fluorescent binding criteria.

Any method for predicting, prior to extensive absorption, that anti-T sera did indeed contain antibodies specific for T cells could be a great help. It has been suggested that this might be possible using either E rosette inhibition (25) or immunosuppresive potency *in vivo* (26). Our experience here has been again on the negative side, since by the E rosette-inhibiting criteria two anti-CLL sera had fairly high titers comparable to those of anti-T cell sera. However, this system should be further studied, particularly in view of the work of Owen and Fanger (27, 28). These workers have shown that goat antibodies raised against thymus cells may cocap the T cell binding site for sheep erythrocytes and that isolated E receptors can be used to produce effective anti-T cell sera. Although antisera may have several advantages over rosette systems, it will be disappointing if anti-HuTLA and E rosettes are not independent markers for T cells. It will be helpful in this respect if other workers using these two marker systems would investigate their possible interrelationship.

ACKNOWLEDGMENTS

This work was supported by the Imperial Cancer Research Fund and the Medical Research Fund. Many colleagues participated in various aspects of the studies reported. We should particularly like to acknowledge the collaboration of Dr. G. Brown, Mr. D. Sutherland, Mr. D. Capellaro, Mr. K. Adams, Drs. M. K. Zeylemaker, A. Lister, R. K. Murray, K. Shumak, W. Prusanski, R. Falk, M. Pepys, D. Doniach, and R. Binns.

REFERENCES

1. Greaves, M. F., Owen, J. J., and Raff, M. C., "T and B Lymphocytes: Their Origins, Properties and Roles in Immune Responses." Excerpta Medica Foundation, Amsterdam, 1973.
2. Clagett, J., Peter, H. H., Feldman, J. D., and Weigle, W. O., *J. Immunol.* **110**, 1085 (1973).
3. Morris, R. J., Letarte-Muirhead, M., and Williams, A. F., *Eur. J. Immunol.* **5**, 282 (1975).
4. Esselman, W. J., and Miller, H. C., *J. Exp. Med.* **139**, 445 (1974).
5. Vitetta, E. S., Boyse, E. A., and Uhr, J. W., *Eur. J. Immunol.* **3**, 446 (1973).
6. Scheid, M. P., Goldstein, G., Hammerling, U., and Boyse, E. A., *in* "Membrane Receptors of Lymphocytes" (M. Seligmann, J. L. Preud'homme, and F. M. Kourilsky, eds.), p. 353. North-Holland Publ., Amsterdam, 1975.
7. Medawar, P. B., and Simpson, E., *Nature (London)* **258**, 106 (1975).
8. Brown, G., and Greaves, M. F., *Eur. J. Immunol.* **4**, 302 (1974).
9. Loken, M. R., and Herzenberg, L. A., *Ann. N. Y. Acad. Sci.* **254**, 163 (1975).
10. Greaves, M. F., *Prog. Haematol.* **IX**, 255 (1975).
11. Greaves, M. F., and Brown, G., *J. Immunol.* **112**, 420 (1974).
12. Brouet, J.-C., and Toben, H., *J. Immunol.* **116**, 1041 (1976).
13. Thiele, H. G., Stark, R., Keeser, D., and Zunpel, H., *Lancet* **2**, 1447 (1973).
14. Kongsharn, P. A. L., Gold, P., Shuster, J., Colquhoun, B., and Freedman, S. O., *Clin. Immunol. Immunopathol.* **3**, 1 (1974).
15. Golub, E. S., *J. Exp. Med.* **136**, 869 (1972).
16. Cuatrecasas, P., *Biochemistry* **12**, 3558 (1973).
17. Revesz, T., Greaves, M. F., Capellaro, D., and Murray, R. K., *Br. J. Haematol.* in press (1976).
18. Revesz, T., Greaves, M. F. in "Membrane Receptors of Lymphocytes" (M. Seligmann, J.-L. Preud'homme, and F. M. Kourilsky, eds.), p. 403. North-Holland Publ., Amsterdam, 1975.
19. Golub, E. S., *J. Immunol.* **109**, 168 (1972).
20. Thomas, D. B., and Phillips, B., *J. Exp. Med.* **138**, 64 (1973).
21. Schlossman, S. F., Chess, L., Humphreys, R. E., and Strominger, J. L., *Proc. Natl. Acad. Sci. U.S.A.* **73**, 1288 (1976).
22. Sauser, D., Anckers, C., and Bron, C., *J. Immunol.* **113**, 617 (1974).
23. Zimmerman, B., *J. Immunol.* **113**, 625 (1974).
24. Zimmerman, B., *J. Immunol.* **115**, 701 (1975).
25. Wortis, H. H., Cooper, A. G., and Brown, M. C., *Nature (London) New Biol.* **243**, 109 (1973).
26. Smith, R. W., and Woody, J. N., *Transplantation* **17**, 503 (1974).
27. Owen, F. L., and Fanger, M. W., *J. Immunol.* **113**, 1138 (1974).
28. Owen, F. L., and Fanger, M. W., *J. Immunol.* **115**, 765 (1975).
29. Lies, R. B., Messner, R. P., and Williams, R. C., *Arthritis Rheum.* **16**, 369 (1973).
30. Thomas, D. B., *Eur. J. Immunol.* **3**, 824 (1973).
31. Luria, E. A., and Domashneva, I. V., *Proc. Natl. Acad. Sci.* **71**, 235 (1974).
32. Prusanski, W., Farid, N., Keystone, E., Armstrong, M., and Greaves, M. F., *Clin. Immunol. Immunopathol.* **4**, 248 (1975).

33. Shumak, K. H., Rachkewich, R. A., and Greaves, M. F., *Clin. Immunol. Immunopathol.* **4**, 241 (1975).
34. Brown, G., Greaves, M. F., Lister, T. A., Rapson, N., and Papamichael, M., *Lancet* **ii**, 753 (1974).
35. Kumagai, W. A., Abo, T., Sekizaga, T., and Suzaki, M., *J. Immunol.* **115**, 982 (1975).
36. Winchester, R. J., Fu, S. M., Hoffman, T., and Kunkel, H. G., *J. Immunol.* **114**, 1210 (1975).
37. Williams, R. C., De Board, J. R., Mellbye, O. J., Messner, R. P., and Lindstrom, F. D., *J. Clin. Invest.* **52**, 283 (1973).
38. Smith, R. W., Terry, W. D., Buell, D. N., and Sell, K. W., *J. Immunol.* **110**, 884 (1973).
39. Woody, J. N., Ahmed, A., Knudsen, R. C., Strong, D. M., and Sell, K. W., *J. Clin. Invest.* **55**, 956 (1975).
40. Kersey, J., Nesbit, M., Hallgren, H., Sabad, A., Yunis, E., and Gajl-Peczalska, K., *Cancer* **36**, 1348 (1975).
41. Touraine, J. I., Touraine, F., Kiszkiss, D. F., Choi, Y. S., and Good, R. A., *Clin. Exp. Immunol.* **16**, 503 (1974).
42. Ishii, Y., Koshiba, H., Uneo, H., Imai, K., and Kikuchi, K., *Clin. Exp. Immunol.* **19**, 67 (1975).
43. Aisenberg, A. C., Block, K. J., Long, J. C., and Colvin, R. B., *Blood* **41**, 417 (1973).
44. Aiuti, F., and Wigzell, H., *Clin. Exp. Immunol.* **13**, 171 (1973).
45. Bobrove, A., Strober, S., Herzenberg, L., and De Pamphilis, J., *J. Immunol.* **112**, 520 (1974).
46. Mills, B., Sen, L., and Borella, L., *J. Immunol.* **115**, 1038 (1975).
47. Owen, F. L., and Fanger, M. W., *J. Immunol.* **113**, 1128 (1974).

4

Preparation of Heterologous Antisera Specific for Human T Cells*

Charles M. Balch, Alexander R. Lawton, and Max D. Cooper

1. Introduction

The detection of differentiation antigens on thymus-dependent lymphocytes has been useful in elucidating their biological properties. Alloantisera and hetero-antisera prepared against rodent T cells, for example, have been used to define the function, distribution, stages of differentiation, and even subpopulations of T cells (1–3).

Antigens used for preparing heterologous antisera reactive with human T cells have included: human thymocytes, soluble extracts of thymocytes, brain, leukemic lymphocytes bearing T cell markers, and peripheral lymphocytes from boys with X-linked agammaglobulinemia (XLA). The dose schedules, routes of administration, and use of adjuvants varied widely, and no immunization protocol emerged as clearly superior to others. Virtually all these antisera required extensive absorptions with combinations of human kidney, liver, erythrocytes, malignant B cells, and cultured B lymphoid cells to be rendered T cell specific. With indirect immunofluorescence or cytotoxicity assays, these reagents have been used to define the distribution and certain functional attributes of T cells in normal humans and in various pathological conditions, such as immunodeficiency diseases and lymphoproliferative malignancies (4–16).

We have developed a relatively simple method for preparing anti-human T cell antiserum of sufficiently high titer and specificity to be used in a direct immunofluorescence assay on lymphocyte suspensions. The distinctive feature of this method is the use of monkey thymocytes as an antigen source. Rabbit anti-monkey thymocyte serum required far fewer absorptions to render it specific for human T cells than other antisera produced in our laboratory against human thymus, thymocyte membranes, or peripheral T cells from an XLA patient (16). The rationale for using cross-reactive antisera, an approach that is applicable also to other species combinations, is described elsewhere (17).

*This study was supported by the National Cancer Institute, NIH (Nos. CA 16673 and CB-23882).

2. Materials

2.1. Antisera Preparation

2.1.1. Adult rabbits 3–4 kg weight

2.1.2. Rhesus monkey thymus

2.1.3. BSS: Hanks' balanced salt solution or phosphate-buffered saline, calcium and magnesium free (International Scientific Industries)

2.1.4. Sodium heparin, 1000 units/ml (Abbott Laboratories)

2.1.5. Syringes, 1 ml and 60 ml; and needles, 20 gauge and 26 gauge

2.1.6. Centrifuge tubes, 50 ml (Falcon)

2.1.7. Petri dishes, 100 × 15 mm (Falcon)

2.1.8. Dialysis tubing with 12,000 MW cutoff

2.1.9. Sodium sulfate

2.1.10. Other equipment: fine metal screen, 150–200 mesh; fine scissors and forceps; scalpel; Pasteur pipettes; 56°C water bath; hemocytometer or Coulter counter; refrigerated centrifuge

2.2. Fluorochrome Conjugation

2.2.1. Fluorescein isothiocyanate (FITC) isomer I (Baltimore Biological Laboratories)

2.2.2. Celite (J. T. Baker Chemical Co.)

2.2.3. NaOH, 1.0 N

2.2.4. Borate-saline, 0.15 M, pH 8.2: 8.48 g of H_3BO_3, 9.54 g of $Na_2B_4O_7 \cdot 10\ H_2O$, 4.38 g of NaCl made up to 1 liter with water

2.2.5. Phosphate buffer, 0.01 M, pH 7.5 and aliquots containing 0.05, 0.1, 0.2, and 0.5 M NaCl

2.2.6. Sephadex G-10 or G-25 (Pharmacia) and DEAE-cellulose (Whatman DE-52) with columns of appropriate size

2.2.7. UV lamp (Mineralight, UVS11)

2.2.8. Other equipment: pH meter (with microcombination electrode); magnetic stirrer; glass scintillation vials; protein concentrating device; UV spectrophotometer

2.3. Cell Preparations

2.3.1. Ficoll–Hypaque: 6.3 g of Ficoll 400 (Pharmacia) and 11 ml of Hypaque-M-90% (Winthrop) made up to 100 ml with distilled water

2.3.2. Hanks' BSS containing 5% heat-inactivated fetal calf serum (FCS) and 0.1% sodium azide

2.3.3. Eppendorf micro test tubes, 1.5 ml (Brinkman)

2.3.4. Pipettor, 10 μl, and tips

2.3.5. Other materials as listed in Section 2.1

2.4. Immunofluorescence

2.4.1. Rhodamine-labeled anti-human immunoglobulin

2.4.2. Microscope slides; glass cover slips, 22 mm

2.4.3. 1:1 mixture of paraffin and petroleum jelly, melted for sealing cover slips

2.4.4. Fluorescent microscope with phase-contrast optics

2.5. Absorptions

2.5.1. Fetal liver, kidney, or other human tissues not containing T cells, obtained from fresh autopsy specimens

2.5.2. Cultured cell lines (e.g., B lymphoid cells, fibroblasts, tumors) not bearing T cell markers

2.5.3. Pooled erythrocytes

3. Methods

3.1. Preparation of Antisera. Cell suspensions of rhesus monkey thymocytes are prepared by teasing fresh thymus into cold BSS, after all fat, connective tissue, and parathymic lymph nodes have been carefully dissected away. Alternatively, minced 3–5 mm cubes of thymus are gently pressed through a fine-mesh metal screen using a scalpel. The dispersed cells are filtered through gauze or a nylon-mesh cell filter into a 50-ml plastic centrifuge tube and centrifuged at 800 rpm (170 g) for 5 min. The pellet is *gently* resuspended in a small volume of BSS, washed twice with 10–20-ml volumes, and resuspended in a final cell concentration of 2 to 5 X 10^8 thymocytes per milliliter. One hundred microliters (100 units) of heparin are added for each milliliter of the immunizing cell suspension. This method should yield a greater than 90% viability by trypan blue exclusion assay.

Adult rabbits, screened for the absence of naturally occurring cytotoxic antibodies (18), are immunized with 2 to 5 X 10^8 thymocytes injected slowly (10–20 sec) into an ear vein on days 0, 14, and 21. On days 27, 28, and 29, 30–40 ml of blood are obtained by cardiac puncture twice daily.

The blood is allowed to clot at room temperature for 1 hr or kept overnight at 4°C. After centrifugation, the immune serum is collected and heat-inactivated at 56°C for 45 min.

γ-Globulin is precipitated from the serum using Na_2SO_4. Crystalline Na_2SO_4 (18 g/100 ml) is added slowly (over 30 min) to the serum at room temperature with gentle stirring. When the crystals are dissolved, the precipitated γ-globulin is recovered by centrifugation at 6000 rpm (4630 g) for 20 min at room temperature and dissolved in borate-saline totaling one-half of the starting serum volume. The precipitation is repeated with 14% Na_2SO_4 (w/v). The γ-globulin is dialyzed overnight against large volumes of borate-saline, changed at least three times.

Precautions: Avoid denaturing the protein by stirring too vigorously during the precipitation. The entire procedure must be conducted at room temperature to avoid crystallization of Na_2SO_4.

3.2. Fluorochrome Conjugation. An aliquot of the dialyzed γ-globulin fraction is diluted with borate-saline to a protein concentration of 10 mg/ml, and the pH is adjusted to 9.5 with 1 N NaOH. Glass scintillation vials are convenient containers for this adjustment as well as for the conjugation procedure. Fluorescein isothiocyanate (FITC) and Celite are mixed in a 1:9 (w/w) ratio and ground thoroughly with a glass rod. (This mixture should be stored in a desiccator at 4°C and mixed well by vortexing prior to use.) FITC-Celite mixture is added to stirred gamma globulin at a ratio of 2 mg/10 mg of protein and allowed to react for 30 min at room temperature with gentle stirring. (Lower F/P molar ratios can be obtained by using 1 mg/10 mg protein.) Celite is removed by pelleting at 1500 rpm (600 g) for 10 min. Unreacted fluorescein is separated from the conjugate by passage over a Sephadex G-25 column in 0.01 M phosphate buffer. This can be done in a darkened room with a UV lamp to monitor passage of the fluorescein conjugate through the column. The first fluorescent peak, which contains the conjugated protein, is further fractionated by passage over a DEAE-cellulose column equilibrated to pH 7.5 with 0.01 M phosphate buffer. Fractions are eluted with 0.01 M phosphate buffer containing 0.05, 0.1, 0.2, and 0.5 M NaCl.

Fluorescein/protein (F/P) ratios are calculated by reading the optical density of each elution fraction at 276 and 493 nm and plotting these on a nomogram (19). Conjugates with molar F/P ratios between 3 and 6 are suitable for surface labeling of lymphocyte suspensions while those with F/P ratios of 1–2 may be more suitable for tissue immunofluorescence. The relevant conjugates are concentrated to 8–10 mg/ml, and the borate–saline buffer is removed by dialysis against PBS before absorbing for specificity. (Addition of 0.1% sodium azide to the conjugates prevents bacterial growth.)

3.3. Preparation of Cells. Purified peripheral blood lymphocytes are isolated using standard methods. Using the Ficoll–Hypaque method, we have found that lymphocytes comprise 80–95% of the harvested cells, the remaining cells being monocytes. (We have not used iron filings for removing phagocytes because they introduce a nonspecific fluorescence with rhodamine filters under UV light.) Human lymphoid tissues are prepared by the method described above for obtaining thymocyte suspensions. All lymphoid cells are washed twice in BSS (containing 5% fetal calf serum and 0.1% sodium azide), counted, and kept on ice.

3.4. Immunofluorescence. Lymphoid cells, 1.5×10^6, are pelleted in a 1.5-ml plastic tube, and the medium is aspirated with a Pasteur pipette (previously drawn out to a fine tip over a flame). The pellet is resuspended with 10 μl of FITC-labeled anti-T cell antiserum (centrifuged just prior to use to remove any precipitates). The mixture is incubated for 30 min with intermittent agitation. The cells are washed 3 times, then the pellet is resuspended with 30 μl of medium. Aliquots, 10 μl, are placed on glass slides, cover-slipped, and sealed with melted paraffin. The slides should be examined within 2–4 hr and are kept cold prior to examination. At least 100 nucleated cells are enumerated under the fluorescence microscope, first by phase microscopy and then under ultraviolet light for FITC-labeled lymphocytes. It is preferable to examine viable cell suspensions because alcohol fixation diminishes the staining intensity.

3.5. Absorptions. Unabsorbed antisera generally stain all cells in lymphocyte suspensions. To determine absorption strategy, the antiserum is tested to a panel of cell types not containing T cells. These might include cultured human B lymphoid cells (e.g., RAJI), tumor cells, or fibroblasts, as well as viable washed cells from fetal liver, kidney, and B leukemia cells. The antiserum is absorbed with the most reactive (and the most available) of these until negative staining is obtained for that absorbing cell source. (Note: Absorptions with chronic lymphatic leukemia cells, which usually contain a minor T cell population, might diminish the T cell antibody titer). The antiserum is tested again with the cell panel, and absorptions are continued until it is nonreactive with the entire panel, but retains the capacity to stain peripheral blood T cells. In general, four or more absorptions employing several different tissues will be necessary.

Absorptions are carried out by incubating with one-third to one-fifth packed volume of the absorbing material at room temperature for 30–40 min with intermittent agitation. The absorbing tissue is removed by centrifugation at 2000 rpm (1000 g) for 10 min. In addition, the antiserum is absorbed with equal volumes of human erythrocytes until all hemagglutinating antibodies are removed. (Note: T lymphocytes should be removed first from the erythrocytes by careful aspiration of the buffy coat or passage over Ficoll–Hypaque gradients). Some preparations may require absorptions with insolubilized human serum, although we have not found this to be necessary.

Specificity for T lymphocytes is conveniently determined by a double fluorochrome assay, in which rhodamine-conjugated anti-immunoglobulin is used to label B lymphocytes. Lymphocytes (1.5×10^6) are first incubated alone with 10 μl of FITC anti-T cell serum as described above. After 10 min, 10 μl of RITC-conjugated anti-human immunoglobulin is added to the mixture, and the incubation is continued on ice for 30 min. The cells are then washed three times and prepared for fluorescence microscopy. Selective filtration for fluorescein and rhodamine excitation is used to determine whether the two reagents discriminate for different lymphocyte populations.

Serial 2-fold dilutions of the fully absorbed antiserum are tested against peripheral blood T lymphocytes for an end point where the percentage of positive cells declines by >20% from plateau values. The entire batch of antiserum is then diluted to a point 2 dilutions from this end point, aliquoted into 0.5–1.0-ml volumes, and stored frozen.

4. Comments

4.1. Antisera prepared by this method react with 95–100% of normal human thymocytes, 70–80% of peripheral blood lymphocytes, 35–45% of spleen cells, 5–10% of bone marrow cells and completely block formation of non-immune E rosettes in these populations. Typical nonphagocytic B lymphocytes bearing surface immunoglobulin and labeled with RITC conjugates of anti-immunoglobulins do not stain. Phagocytes may contain ingested conjugates. Some monocytes may have a patchy surface stain, possibly because of non-specific binding to Fc receptors, but this pattern of staining is clearly distinguish-able from that on T lymphocytes.

4.2. Specific staining of T lymphocytes is manifest by ring fluorescence. Suspensions of thymocytes have a fairly uniform, and usually bright, pattern of fluorescence. Peripheral T cells show considerable variation in staining intensity, probably reflecting differences in concentrations of antigen(s) expressed on their surface. The best correlation of percentages of cells forming E rosettes and of cells staining with anti-T has been obtained by enumerating even the most weakly stained cells.

4.3. Optimal conditions for fluorescence microscopy are needed. The use of incident-light fluorescence excitation in conjunction with phase-contrast optics is highly advantageous, since this system provides a convenient means of viewing cells sequentially with either visible or UV light. High-intensity light sources (mercury or xenon), narrow band-pass excitation filters (KP490 or KP500), and the use of low power (6X) oculars with objectives of high numerical aperture all serve to increase fluorescence intensity and contrast.

5. Specificity of AMT for Human T Cells

5.1. Distribution of reactive cells in human lymphoid compartments (% ± SD): thymus, 96.1 ± 3.48; lymph node, 55.7 ± 6.2; peripheral blood lymphocytes, 75.7 ± 5.6; bone marrow, 12.5 ± 8.0; spleen, 39.8 ± 8.3.

5.2. Lack of reactivity with human cells of nonthymic origin: cultured B cell lines (RAJI, GOLAN), fibroblasts, Burkitt lymphoma, fetal liver, chronic lymphocytic leukemia cells, peroxidase-labeled macrophages, and Ig-bearing B cells in peripheral blood and spleen.

5.3. Reactivity with cultured T cells (MOLT, 8402) and T-cell leukemias.

5.4. Removal of *all* T cell reactivity by absorption with thymocytes.

5.5. Blocking of E rosette formation; conversely, blood lymphocytes de-pleted of E rosette-forming cells are not stained by AMT.

REFERENCES

1. Balch, C. M., and Feldman, J. D., *J. Immunol.* **112**, 79 (1974).
2. Balch, C. M., Wilson, C. B., Lee, S., and Feldman, J. D., *J. Exp. Med.* **128**, 1584 (1973).

3. Greaves, M. F., Owen, J. J. T., and Raff, M. C., "T and B Lymphocytes: Their Origins, Properties and Roles in Immune Response." Excerpta Medica Foundation, Amsterdam, 1973.
4. Toben, H. R., and Cooper, M. D., *Clin. Res.* **20**, 797 (1972).
5. Aiuti, F., and Wigzell, H., *Clin. Exp. Immunol.* **13**, 171 (1973).
6. Smith, R. W., Terry, W. D., Buell, D. N., and Sell, K. W., *J. Immunol.* **110**, 884 (1973).
7. Williams, R. C., deBoard, J. R., Mellbye, O. J., Messner, R. P., and Lindstrom, F. D., *J. Clin. Invest.* **52**, 283 (1973).
8. Touraine, J. L., Touraine, F., Kiszkiss, D. F., Choi, Y. S., and Good, R. A., *Clin. Exp. Immunol.* **16**, 503 (1974).
9. Brown, G., and Greaves, M. F., *Scand. J. Immunol.* **3**, 161 (1974).
10. Owen, F. L., and Fanger, M. W., *J. Immunol.* **113**, 1128 (1974).
11. Bobrove, A. M., Strober, S., Herzenberg, L. A., and DePamphilis, J. D., *J. Immunol.* **112**, 520 (1974).
12. Mohanakumar, T., and Metzgar, R. S., *Cell. Immunol.* **12**, 30 (1974).
13. Ishii, Y., Koshiba, H., Ueno, H., Imai, K., and Kikuchi, K., *Clin. Exp. Immunol.* **19**, 67 (1975).
14. Yata, J., Gatti, R. A., Klein, G., Good, R. A., and Tsukimoto, I., *Clin. Immunol. Immunopathol.* **2**, 519 (1974).
15. Husby, G., Strickland, R. G., Caldwell, J. L., and Williams, R. C., *J. Clin. Invest.* **56**, 1198 (1975).
16. Balch, C. M., Dagg, M. K., Lawton, A. R., and Cooper, M. D., *Fed. Proc., Fed. Am. Soc. Exp. Biol.* **34**, 994 (1975).
17. Balch, C. M., Dagg, M. K., and Cooper, M. D., *J. Immunol.* **117**, 447 (1976).
18. Mittal, K. K., Ferrone, S., Michey, M. R., Pellegrino, M. A., Reisfeld, R. A., and Terasaki, P. I., *Transplantation* **16**, 287 (1973).
19. Wells, A. F., Miller, C. E., and Nadel, M. K., *Appl. Microbiol.* **14**, 271 (1966).

5

Identification of Cells with Complement Receptors*

Alfred G. Ehlenberger and Victor Nussenzweig

1. Introduction

A common property of macrophages, monocytes, neutrophils, and B lymphocytes is their ability to bind antigen (Ag)–antibody (Ab) complexes or Ag–Ab–complement complexes. On the basis of binding assays, membrane receptors that interact with specific components of the immune complex (C3, Fc) have been operationally defined. The properties of these receptors are discussed elsewhere (1–5). Two different receptors for C3 products have been identified. The first recognizes cell-bound or fluid-phase C3b, generated by the reaction between $C\overline{1,4,2}$ enzyme complex and C3. The second receptor recognizes C3d, a much smaller fragment which remains on the cell after cleavage of C3b by a serum enzyme, C3b inactivator. Human red cells, polymorphs, lymphocytes, and monocytes all bind C3b, but only lymphocytes and monocytes bind C3d (6).

Many systems have been used to determine the presence of complement receptors on leukocytes using various soluble or particulate antigens. Sheep erythrocytes (E) sensitized with antibody (A) and complement (C) remain, however, the most convenient, quantifiable, and reliable reagent for this purpose for the following reasons: (a) the presence of receptors is shown by the formation of "rosettes," where the sensitized red cells bind to the leukocyte in a fashion that can be readily seen in a light microscope; (b) products of the reaction between E, A, and C components have been well characterized—it is possible to prepare defined EAC intermediates to study the effects of different classes of antibody and of different C components; and (c) E coated with IgG antibody and C3 is a good reagent to assay for the presence of viable phagocytes in cell preparations. Although C3 bound to a particle does not directly induce phagocytosis, it enhances the effect of opsonizing antibodies from 30 to 1000 times, depending on experimental conditions (6). Thus, red cells coated with both C3 and IgG are ingested most avidly by monocytes and neutrophils either in suspension or adhered to glass, and again only a light microscope is needed to identify the phagocyte.

*Work supported by NIH Grants Nos. AI-08499 and CA 16247.

We present here some techniques for the preparation of EAC, and convenient means of carrying out the rosette and phagocytosis assays.

2. Materials

Plastic capsule, Beem (Ernest F. Fullum, Schenectady, New York; Catalogue No. 5206)

RPMI 1640; (40 ml of 0.25 M HEPES, pH 7.4 is added to 1 liter of RPMI) (Grand Island Biological Co., Grand Island, New York; Catalogue No. H-18)

Trypsin, A grade (Calbiochem, La Jolla, California; Catalogue No. 6502)

Soybean trypsin inhibitor (Worthington Biochemical Corp., Freehold, New Jersey; Code SI, Catalogue No. 3570 or 3571)

Gentian violet (Harleco, Gibbstown, New Jersey; Catalogue No. 227)

MacNeal's tetrachrome stain (Allied Chemical, Morristown, New Jersey)

Sheep erythrocytes in Alsever's; cells used are at least 1 week old, but no more than 4 weeks old (Animal Blood Center, Syracuse, New York; Catalogue No. 2025)

Antiserum: 19 S antibodies to sheep red cells (Cordis Laboratories, Miami, Florida; Catalogue No. 768-990); 7 S antibodies to sheep red cells (Cordis; Catalogue No. 768-970)

Human complement components (Cordis Laboratories, Miami, Florida); C1 (Catalogue No. 755-510); C2 (Catalogue No. 755-520); C3 (Catalogue No. 755-530); C4 (Catalogue No. 755-540)

3. Methods

3.1. Preparation of Buffers

3.1.1. DGVBS^{++} (dextrose-gelatin-veronal-buffered saline with calcium and magnesium added). This buffer should either be prepared fresh daily or may be kept frozen until use. It is prepared as follows:

For 100 ml of buffer, use (a) 10 ml of 5x Isover solution (see below), (b) 2.5 g of dextrose, (c) 0.1 ml of Ca$^+$, Mg^{2+} stock solution (see below), (d) 0.1 g of gelatin, (e) glass-distilled water. The gelatin should be added to 20 ml of cold water, and this should be heated gently until the gelatin dissolves. Other components are then added and the volume is made up to 100 ml with water.

3.1.2. 5x Isover solution. This stock solution is stable at least 6 months at 4°C. For 2 liters of stock solution, use (a) 83 g of NaCl, (b) 10.19 g of Na-5, 5-diethyl barbiturate, (c) glass-distilled water. Dissolve solute in 1.5 liters of water and adjust the pH to 7.35 ± 0.05 with 1 N HCl. Bring the volume to 2 liters with water.

3.1.3. Ca^{2+}, Mg^{2+} stock solution (1.0 M Mg^{2+} + 0.15 M Ca^{2+}). This solution is prepared by mixing equal volumes of 2 M $MgCl_2 \cdot 6H_2O$ and 0.3 M $CaCl_2 \cdot 2H_2O$. These solutions are most accurately prepared using specific gravity measurements. Specific gravities of 2 M $MgCl_2$ and 0.3 M $CaCl_2$ may be found by interpolation of published values in the "Handbook of Chemistry and Physics."

3.1.4. EDTA, 0.1 M, pH 7.4. The pH is adjusted with I N NaOH.

3.1.5. Veronal-buffered saline (VBS). Dilute 5X Isover solution 1:4 with glass-distilled water.

3.1.6. EDTA-VBS. Add 1 volume of 0.1 M EDTA to 9 volumes of VBS.

3.1.7. Modified Turk's solution. Combine 10% acetic acid in water + 0.001% gentian violet

3.1.8. Isotonic red cell lysing solution. For 1 liter add: (a) 8.3 g of NH_4Cl, (b) 1.0 g of $KHCO_3$, (c) 1 ml of 0.1 M EDTA (pH 7.4), (d) glass-distilled water to 1 liter, (e) 1 N NaOH to adjust pH to 7.4. The pH of this solution rises with storage owing to loss of CO_2. Therefore it should either be used immediately or the pH be restored by bubbling 5% CO_2 through the solution before use. Phenol red may be added as a pH indicator.

3.2. Preparation of E E should be used between 1 and 3 weeks after bleeding in rosette assays. In studies involving phagocytosis, E should be as fresh as possible, because "aged" E will be ingested by some phagocytes. When dealing with activated mouse macrophages, for example, E used 3 or 4 days after bleeding will be ingested by about 5–10% of the phagocytes without opsonization. Some investigators avoid E in rosette assays for the identification of complement receptors in human lymphoid cells because of the binding of unsensitized E to human T cells. This binding is easily eliminated by trypsin treatment of the red cell as below. After trypsinization, no rosettes form between human T cells and E even if the cells are centrifuged together and incubated at 0°, 25°, or 37°C. In species other than human, no pretreatment of E is required.

Trypsinization of E (in RPMI–HEPES, pH 7.4). Wash E three times with RPMI and prepare a 5% suspension by volume in RPMI. Each milliliter of this suspension contains approximately 10^9 red cells. Prepare a solution of trypsin in RPMI at 2 mg/ml. Mix equal volumes of 5% E and trypsin and incubate 1 hr at 37°C, agitating occasionally. Prepare a solution of soybean trypsin inhibitor (STI) at 10 mg/ml concentration. Add 1 ml of STI solution to 10 ml of red cell–trypsin suspension; mix and wash 4 times in RPMI.

3.3. Antibody Sensitization. E which have either been trypsin treated (as above) or washed 4 X in RPMI are suspended at 5% (v/v). IgM anti-E antibody is diluted to the maximum dose which is not agglutinating (with the Cordis preparations usually 1:80), and equal volumes of E and antibody solution are mixed. Studies with radiolabeled antibody show that this represents about 2000 molecules of IgM per red cell.

Incubate E and antibody 15 min at 37°C, shaking occasionally. The red cells are now spun down, washed once in DGVBS⁺⁺, and resuspended at 5% (v/v) (for sensitization with mouse complement) or at 1% (v/v) (for purified human complement components), in DGVBS⁺⁺. These cells are called E IgM or EA.

3.4. Complement Fixation: Mouse Complement. Because mouse complement is poorly lytic, serum from any strain of mouse may be used. In theory, it is better to use C5-deficient mice such as A/J, or DBA/2J, but this is not critical. A list of C5-deficient mice is given by Cinader *et al.* (7).

Preparation of Mouse Complement

a. Anesthetize mouse with ether.

b. Collect blood by cutting the axillary vessels.

c. Allow blood to clot at room temperature for 10 min and then place in ice for 60 min.

d. Centrifuge 10 min at 700 g at 4°C.

e. Use preferably fresh or store at −70°C until use.

Mouse complement may contain antibodies to E that could cause rosette formation through the Fc receptor, as indicated elsewhere in this text. If Fc binding is suspected (see Section 3.8), the complement may be absorbed as follows: Serum at 0°C is mixed with one-tenth its volume of packed, washed E, also at 0°C, and incubated for 5 min in ice. The red cells are spun out in the cold, and the serum is used immediately.

To prepare EAC, dilute mouse serum 1:10 in DGVBS⁺⁺ and add an equal volume of 5% E IgM. Mix and incubate for 40 min at 37°C, occasionally agitating the suspension to prevent red cells from settling. Dilute 5 times with cold DGVBS⁺⁺ and spin down the red cells. Wash the red cells 3 times in RPMI and suspend at a concentration of 5% for storage. EAC prepared in this way presumably have C3 present mainly as C3d. Red cells with predominantly C3b can probably be prepared by shortening the incubation to 5–10 min. However, in order to deal with well characterized EAC intermediates, purified human (or guinea pig) complement components have to be used as indicated below.

3.5. Complement Fixation: Human Complement. The red cell-bound enzyme C3 convertase formed by C1, C4, and C2, cleaves C3 into two fragments, C3a and C3b. C3b binds to the membrane of E in a rather nonspecific manner, and probably hundreds of C3b molecules can be deposited around one C1,4,2 site.

C3b is converted to another cleavage product, C3d, by a heat-stable enzyme, called C3b inactivator, which is found in normal human serum.

3.5.1. Preparation of C3b-Coated E

a. Suspend E IgM at 2×10^8/ml in DGVBS⁺⁺ at 0°C.

b. Reconstitute C1, C4, C2, and C3 (Cordis) from the lyophilized state according to instructions.

c. Add 2000 U of C1 per milliliter of E IgM and incubate at 0°C for 1 hr, shaking occasionally.

d. Spin down and resuspend cells at 2×10^8/ml in DGVBS^{++} that has been warmed to 30°C. Add 200 U of C4 per milliliter of EA$\overline{C1}$ and incubate 25 min at 30°C.

e. Spin down and resuspend red cells at 2×10^8 in DGVBS^{++}. Add 200 U of C2, and 200 U of C3 per milliliter. Incubate 45 min at 30°C.

f. Wash 3 times in RPMI.

g. These red cells have C1, C4, C2, and C3 bound to their surfaces. Although cell-bound C4 reacts with the C3b receptors (8), there are not enough C4 molecules on the red cells to cause adherence. Controls made with IgM, C1, C4, and C2 (without C3) will show no rosette formation. C1 and C2 can be removed from the red cell surface if desired, although no role is known for them in immune adherence. C1 may be eluted by washing in EDTA-GVB. C2 will decay if the washed cells are incubated for 1–2 hr at 37°C.

3.5.2. Conversion of C3b-Coated Red Cells (EAC4, 3b) to C3d-Coated Red Cells (EAC4, 3d)

a. Normal human serum, preferably pooled from 4 or more donors, is heat inactivated (56°C for 30 min).

b. The heat-inactivated serum is absorbed 3 times, each time using one-third the serum volume of packed sheep red cells, and finally diluted 1:1 with DGVBS^{++}

c. The C3b-coated red cells, with C1 and C2 removed as above, are suspended in the diluted, heat-inactivated, absorbed serum at a concentration of 2×10^8/ml. The cells are incubated for 2 hr at 37°C, then washed twice in DGVBS^{++}, washed once with RPMI, and finally suspended in RPMI at a concentration of 2×10^8/ml.

d. Conversion of C3b into C3d can be controlled as follows: EAC are prepared at 0.25% (5×10^7/ml) and human red cells are prepared at 1% in DGVBS^{++}. Equal volumes are mixed, and the cells are allowed to settle at room temperature for a few hours. (This is done most conveniently in microtiter plates using 0.1 ml of each suspension.) Settling patterns, indicating immune adherence, can be read by eye. All tests should be done in triplicate, and positive control with EAC4, 3b included.

3.6. Preparation of Red Cells Coated with C3 and IgG (EIgM C4, C3-IgG)

a. Suspend EAC4, 3b or EAC4, 3d at 10^9/ml in RPMI.

b. Dilute antisheep IgG in RPMI to the minimum nonagglutinating dilution (usually a dilution of 1:100 for the Cordis IgG preparation).

c. Add equal volumes of diluted IgG and red cells and incubate 30 min at 37°C, mixing occasionally.

d. Wash twice and suspend at 2×10^8/ml in RPMI.

3.7. Rosette Assay

3.7.1. EAC Rosettes with Lymphocytes. Lymphocytes are washed 3 times in RPMI and suspended at 2×10^6/ml. Complement-coated red cells are suspended at 10^8/ml (0.5%) in RPMI. (These concentrations may be varied, but at all times the red cell concentration should be 50 times the white cell concentration in order to prevent the formation of large red cell–lymphocyte aggregates.) Equal volumes (0.3 ml) of lymphocytes and red cells are added to small plastic capsules. The capsules are sealed with hot paraffin and cooled immediately in water after sealing. The capsules are rotated around a horizontal axis at about 20 rpm for 30 min at 37°C. A small air bubble should remain free to assure proper mixing during incubation. The capsules are then removed and the rosettes counted directly on a hemocytometer; a rosette is defined as a lymphocyte with 3 or more red cells bound.

The concentrations given above provide optimum cell concentrations for counting in a hemocytometer. For precise results with low rosette counts, both sides of the hemocytometer chamber should be filled and all 18 squares counted.

Capsules waiting to be counted may continue to rotate at room temperature. If set aside, the capsule should be inverted gently a dozen times before counting to assure a uniform distribution of rosettes in the suspension.

White cells should be counted in a separate preparation after red cell lysis. This is accomplished by mixing 5 parts of cell suspension with 1 part Turk's solution. The percentage of rosettes is then defined as the rosette concentration divided by the white cell concentration in the sample (the dilution caused by the Turk's solution is accounted for by multiplying the apparent white cell concentration by 1.2).

3.7.2. Macrophages, Monocytes, and Polymorphs. These cells are handled most conveniently when adhered to glass cover slips. We recommend using about 50,000 cells on an 18 × 18 mm No. 2 thickness cover slip. Red cells are prepared at 10^8/ml, and 0.2 ml is overlaid on the cover slip containing the phagocytes. The cover slips covered with red cells are incubated for 30 min at 37°C in a CO_2 incubator and gently washed until nonadherent red cells are removed by dipping the cover slips repeatedly into beakers containing RPMI at room temperature. Rosettes may be counted after fixation with 2% glutaraldehyde in saline. Cover slips with fixed rosettes are placed face-up on slides and counted, keeping the preparation wet at all times.

3.8. Detection of Phagocytes in Human Lymphoid Cell Preparations. The use of red cells to detect phagocytes has several advantages over other means used to detect these cells. First, it defines a phagocyte in terms of its ability to phagocytose a large particle. Second, attachment of the particle can be distinguished from ingestion by lysing red cells which are external to the phagocyte. In the case of latex and other particles, it is sometimes difficult to distinguish ingestion from attachment; furthermore, some cells that are not recognized as phagocytic may be able to internalize a few latex particles. The following protocol presents methods for detecting viable phagocytes in adherent or suspended lymphoid preparations:

Incubate leukocytes with EAC as indicated above, either in suspension or with cells adherent to glass. However, EAC bearing both C3 and IgG (EIgM C4,

C3b·IgG) should be used. Incubate for 45 min at 37°C, and then assay for ingestion by lysing red cells that have not been internalized, by one of the following procedures:

3.8.1. Cells in Suspension. Centrifuge cells into a pellet at 4°C. Resuspend the cells in their initial volume, but in isotonic lysing solution. Incubate at 4°C for 4 min. This will lyse all noningested red cells. White cells are stable in this solution for at least 10 min. Cells may then be smeared and stained or, preferably, may be deposited on slides in a concentrated fashion using the cytocentrifuge (Shandon Scientific Company, Inc., Sewickley, Pennsylvania) and then stained. Ingested red cells will be clearly visible, but no free red cells should be present.

3.8.2. Adherent Cells. External red cells may be lysed by soaking cover slips in the isotonic red cell lysing solution as above. A quicker method is to soak the cover slips for 15 sec in a mixture of 3 parts of water and 1 part of 0.15 M NaCl. Isotonicity is then restored by soaking in RPMI medium for 5 sec. Cover slips can then be dried, with hot air provided by a hair blower, fixed, and stained with MacNeal's tetrachrome.

3.9. Controls. Controls in rosette formation should include the following:

a. Rosettes with E alone—as stated previously, red cells, unless trypsinized, can form rosettes with human T cells.

b. Rosettes with E IgM–IgM preparations may be contaminated by IgG. Binding may thus occur through the Fc receptor. In addition, receptors for IgM have been reported on mouse macrophages (9).

c. Rosettes with E IgM, which have been incubated with decomplemented serum. The serum used as a source of complement may contain 7 S antibodies to E. Therefore spurious rosette formation could occur through Fc receptors. This is rarely a problem with the reagents described above, but may be controlled as follows: the sensitization with complement is carried out as described above, but EDTA-VBS is substituted for DGVBS^{++}. Chelation of calcium and magnesium will prevent complement fixation. As an alternative, heat-inactivated (56°C for 30 min) complement may be used.

3.10. Problems in Identification of Complement Receptor Lymphocytes (CRL). Some of the problems involved in the identification of CRL among human PBL are (a) that T lymphocytes bind E, (b) that EA (IgG) bind to Fc receptors, and (c) that human neutrophils and erythrocytes have membrane receptors for C3b. (In our laboratory we use trypsin treated E, and IgM antibodies, to prepare EA. When these cells are coated with C3d they do not bind to human neutrophils, erythrocytes or T lymphocytes.) (d) Another problem is counting errors. As mentioned previously, we prefer to count the rosettes and leukocytes separately. The advantages are that between 10^3 and 2×10^3 lymphocytes can be easily screened and that the number of lymphocytes within clusters are counted more precisely after lysis of erythrocytes. (e) Human monocytes have membrane receptors for both C3b and C3d and should be selectively removed from the preparation of mononuclear cells. (f) Lymphocytes from PBL should be *very carefully washed* to remove C3 or C3b which may be bound to the cell membrane and inhibit rosette formation.

The following procedure can be used to obtain from human PBL a preparation of lymphocytes which is almost free of monocytes or platelets and without apparent selective losses of T or B cells.

3.10.1. Materials.

Ficollpaque, Pharmacia, catalogue No. 78402.

RPMI–HEPES

Heat inactivated ($56°C$ for 1 hr) fetal calf serum (FCS).

Heparin, 1000 $\mu m/ml$.

50 ml plastic conical tubes, Falcon plastics, Catalogue No. 2070.

Washed slides (3 X 1 inches)

Note: It is important to keep the pH of the RPMI–HEPES at 7.4. If necessary the pH is adjusted by blowing 10% CO_2 on the slides or tubes with cell suspensions. The tubes containing cells should be capped when not in use.

3.10.2. Method

1. Fifty milliliters of venous blood are drawn in a plastic syringe. Ten milliliters are transferred to a glass tube without heparin to obtain serum; 40 ml are mixed with about 500 μl of heparin, and diluted with an equal volume of RPMI–HEPES.

2. Carefully overlay the diluted blood on to 30 ml of Ficollpaque equally distributed into two 50 ml plastic tubes. Centrifuge at 400 g for 35 min at room temperature.

3. Harvest the interface with a Pasteur pipette, taking out about 15 ml of fluid from each tube. Dilute to 50 ml with RPMI–HEPES. Count and calculate yield. About 12×10^7 cells should be recovered from 40 ml of blood from a normal individual. Centrifuge at 250 g for 15 min at room temperature.

4. Resuspend in 40 ml RPMI–HEPES containing 5% FCS. Centrifuge at 250 g for 15 min at room temperature.

5. Resuspend the pellets in 10 ml of 12% autologous serum in RPMI–HEPES.

6. Overlay the cells onto 6 microscopic slides and incubate in a CO_2 incubator for 30 min at $37°C$.

7. Fill one 50 ml tube with RPMI–HEPES containing 5% FCS. Immerse the slides one by one 20 times into the tube and subsequently agitate the slides in the tube as vigorously as possible for a few seconds. Count and calculate yield. About 60% of the cells should be recovered at this step.

8. Centrifuge at 200 g at room temperature for 15 min.

9. Resuspend cells in 10 ml of RPMI–HEPES + 5% FCS. Incubate at $37°C$ for 5 min. Centrifuge at 200 g for 15 min.

10. Repeat step 9.

11. Resuspend in RPMI–HEPES + 5% FCS. Count and adjust concentration to 2×10^6/ml. Approximately 30–40% of the nucleated cells obtained in step 3 are recovered.

12. The rosette assay is performed as described, *but incubation at 37°C is prolonged to 1 hr.*

The above method was adapted from Koller *et al.* (10) and has the advantage that the cells that are removed can be examined and identified. We found that 98% or more of the adherent cells were monocytes (mononuclear phagocytic cells that did not bear tightly bound surface immunoglobulin). On the other hand, less than 1% of nonadherent cells were phagocytic, and they contain about 10% CRL. These results were obtained with *normal* human peripheral blood; under pathological circumstances different results might be obtained. Using these techniques, we have recently shown that CRL and B cells are coincident in the circulation (11).

REFERENCES

1. Nussenzweig, V. N., *Adv. Immunol.* **19,** 217 (1974).
2. Shevach, E. M., Jaffe, E. S., and Green, I., *Transplant. Rev.* **16,** 3 (1973).
3. Bianco, C., *in* "Biological Amplification Systems in Immunity." Plenum, New York, in press.
4. Grey, H. M., Anderson, C. L., Heusser, C. II., and Kurnick, J. T., *in* "Membrane Receptors of Lymphocytes," (M. Seligmann, J. L. Preud'homme, and F. M. Kourilsky, eds.), p. 185. North-Holland Publ., Amsterdam, and American Elsevier, New York 1975.
5. Dickler, H. B., and Kunkel, H. G., *J. Exp. Med.* **136,** 191 (1972).
6. Ehlenberger, A. G., and Nussenzweig, V., *Fed. Proc., Fed. Am. Soc. Exp. Biol.* **34,** 854 (1975).
7. Cinader, B., Dubiski, S., and Wardlaw, A. C., *J. Exp. Med.* **120,** 897 (1964).
8. Ross, G. D., and Polley, M. J., *J. Exp. Med.* **141,** 1163 (1975).
9. Lay, W. H., and Nussenzweig, V. N., *J. Immunol.* **102,** 1172 (1972).
10. Koller, C. A., King, G. W., Hurtubise, P. E., Sagone, A. L., and Lo Buglio, A. F., *J. Immunol.* **111,** 1610 (1973).
11. Ehlenberger, A. G., McWilliams, M., Phillips-Quagliata, J. M., Lamm, M. E., and Nussenzweig, V. N., *J. Clin. Invest.* **57,** 53 (1976).

6

Detection of Complement-Receptor Lymphocytes (CRL)*

Gordon D. Ross and Margaret J. Polley

1. Introduction

Human CRL have two different types of C receptors, the immune adherence receptor and the C3d receptor (1, 2). Most normal CRL have both types of C receptors, but in normal blood, a few CRL occasionally can be detected which have one receptor or the other; and in normal tonsils, 10–20% of lymphocytes contain only the C3d receptor (1). The two types of C receptors are antigenically distinct (1, 2), cap independently, and have specificities for different regions of C4 or C3 molecules (1). The immune adherence receptor is shared with erythrocytes, granulocytes, and monocytes and reacts with C4b or the C3c region of C3b. The C3d receptor is shared only with monocytes (3) and eosinophils (4) and reacts with either C3d or the C3d region of C3b.

Mouse leukocytes have the same two types of C receptors, as do human cells. Mouse C3d receptors react with mouse C3d (5) and, to a lesser extent, with human C3d (6). Mouse immune adherence receptors react well with mouse or guinea pig C3b, but are unreactive with human C3b (5–7). As with human CRL, some binding of C3b to C3d receptors can also be demonstrated (7). The C receptors of other mouse leukocytes have also been studied. The majority of peritoneal macrophages apparently contain only the immune adherence receptor (7, 8) while bone marrow derived colony macrophages grown *in vitro* usually have both types of C receptors (7, 9). Mouse blood neutrophils have both types

*Abbreviations used: A, antibody; C, complement; CRL, complement-receptor lymphocytes; E, erythrocytes; EA, sheep E sensitized with rabbit IgM anti-E antibody; EAC, erythrocyte–antibody–complement complex; C4b, immune adherence receptor-reactive form of C4; C4c and C4d, C receptor-inactive fragments of C4b produced by cleavage with the C4b-C3b inactivator(s) (C4b-C3b INA); ^{oxy}C2, I$_2$ oxidized C2; C2i, hemolytically inactive C2; C3b, fragment of C3 that is reactive with both types of C receptors; C3c, fragment of C3b that is released from EAC1-3b after cleavage by the C4b-C3b INA; C3d, fragment of C3b that remains bound to EAC1-3b after cleavage of C3b by the C4b-C3b INA; GVB, gelatin Veronal buffer; HBSS, Hanks' balanced salt solution; EDTA, ethylenediamine tetraacetate; 0.01 GVBE or 0.04 GVBE; 0.01 M EDTA or 0.04 M EDTA in Ca^{2+}-Mg^{2+} free GVB; mo, mouse; hu, human.

of C receptors, whereas mouse bone marrow-derived colony eosinophils grown *in vitro* have neither type of C receptor (7, 9).

Many different methods have been reported for detecting CRL. Of these, the method reported by Bianco *et al.* (5) seems to be the simplest and most reliable. Sheep E are coated with antibody (A) and C, yielding EAC that form rosettes with CRL.

Human E should not be used to prepare EAC. Human E have immune adherence receptors, and C-coated human E may form rosettes among themselves. Second, human E are larger than sheep E and similar in size to small lymphocytes. This means that a lymphocyte rosetted by human EAC may be difficult to distinguish from the surrounding human E. Finally, human E are valuable as immune adherence receptor indicator cells for testing EAC for their content of C4b or C3b, and could not be used as such if the EAC were also formed from human E.

In addition to the various methods of rosette formation, CRL have also been detected with soluble radiolabeled immune complexes (10) and soluble complement fragments labeled by immunofluorescence (1, 11) or radioactivity (11). These methods have a high degree of specificity and can be used for double-label studies in which another type of receptor is labeled by rosette formation.

The following scheme lists the complement reactions relevant to the formation of EAC for detection of CRL. Also refer to the list of abbreviations on the first page of this chapter.

$$E + A \longrightarrow EA \xrightarrow{\ C1\ } EAC1 \xrightarrow{\ C4\ } EAC14b$$

$$EAC14b \underset{C4b\text{-}C3b\ INA}{\overset{C2}{\searrow}} EA\ C14b2 \xrightarrow{\ C3\ } EAC14b23b$$
$$EAC14d + C4c$$

$$EAC14b23b \xrightarrow{C4b\text{-}C3b\ INA} EAC14b23d + C3c$$

$$EAC14b23d \underset{C1}{\overset{EDTA}{\searrow}} EAC4b23d \xrightarrow{37°C,\ 30\ min} EAC4b3d + C2i$$

$$EAC4b3d \xrightarrow{C4b\text{-}C3b\ INA} EAC4d3d + C4c$$

Because of the C4b-C3b INA contained in serum, EAC formed by addition of whole serum to EA contain variable amounts of C4b, C3b and C3d and, therefore, are not specific for either type of C receptor. If purified C components or C reagents are utilized, EAC14b or EAC14b23b (EAC1-3b) can be produced that contain no C3d. EAC14b are specific for immune adherence receptors, whereas EAC1-3b react with both types of receptors. EAC1-3b, however, do not react as strongly with C3d receptors as do EAC1-3d, which are specific for C3d receptors. EAC1-3b cannot be used to detect all CRL since they do not react with cells containing only weak C3d receptors.

2. Materials

2.1. Buffers and Solutions

2.1.1 5X Veronal buffer: (a) Dissolve 4.6 g of barbituric acid, 2 g of sodium barbital, and 83.8 g of NaCl in 2 liters of boiling water. (b) Cool and add water to 2 liters. (c) Check that a 1:5 dilution with water has a pH of 7.2–7.4 and a conductance of 14–16 millimhos/cm (isotonic with normal saline).

2.1.2. Ca^{2+}–Mg^{2+} solution: Dissolve 0.44 g of $CaCl_2 \cdot 2H_2O$ and 2.03 g of $MgCl_2 \cdot 6H_2O$ in 100 ml of water.

2.1.3. Gelatin, 2%: (a) Dissolve 40 g of gelatin powder in 2 liters of boiling water (stir slowly until dissolved). (b) Cool and add water to 2 liters. (c) Dispense in 50-ml volumes and autoclave. (d) Store at 4°C.

2.1.4. EDTA, 0.2 M pH 7.2: (a) Dissolve 37.23 g of disodium EDTA and 38.02 g of tetrasodium EDTA in 1 liter of boiling water. (b) Cool and add water to 1 liter. (c) Check that pH = 7.2–7.4.

2.1.5. Gelatin Veronal buffer (GVB): (a) Melt 50 ml of 2% gelatin at 37°C. (b) Add the gelatin to 200 ml of 5X Veronal buffer and 5 ml of the Ca^{2+}–Mg^{2+} solution. (c) Add water to 1 liter total volume. (d) Check that pH = 7.2–7.4 and conductance = 14–16 millimhos/cm.

2.1.6. EDTA-GVB, 0.01 M (0.01 GVBE): (a) Prepare 1 liter of GVB, but omit the Ca^{2+}–Mg^{2+} solution. (b) Dilute 50 ml of 0.2 M EDTA, pH 7.2, to 1 liter with the Ca^{2+}–Mg^{2+}-free GVB.

2.1.7. EDTA–GVB, 0.04 M (0.04 GVBE): Dilute 200 ml of 0.2 M EDTA, pH 7.2, to 1 liter with Ca^{2+}–Mg^{2+}-free GVB.

2.2. Sheep E.
Sheep blood in Alsever's solution can be purchased from many different suppliers (Animal Blood Center, Syracuse, New York; Colorado Serum Co., Denver).

2.3. Antisheep E antibody.
The IgM fraction of rabbit antisheep E serum can be purchased from Cordis Laboratories, Miami, Florida. This antibody has been titrated by the manufacturer and is supplied with information concerning the amount required for formation of EA.

2.4. C1.
Ice-cold, fresh human serum is adjusted to pH 7.0 with 1 N HCl and then diluted 1:3 with ice-cold distilled water. After 30 min stirring at 0°–4°C, the precipitate (functionally pure C1) is pelleted by centrifugation at 1000 g for 30 min at 4°C. The supernatant is discarded, and the precipitate is washed by careful resuspension in 5 times the original serum volume of ice-cold 5X Veronal

buffer diluted 1:15 with water, followed by centrifugation at 1000 g for 30 min at 4°C. The washed precipitate is dissolved by carefully resuspending in one-fourth the original serum volume of ice-cold 5X Veronal buffer diluted 1:2.5 with water and containing one-tenth part of Ca^{2+}–Mg^{2+} solution. After stirring for 15 min at 4°C, an equal volume of water is added; the C1 is stored at −70°C in 0.5-ml volumes (12). C1 should be thawed rapidly and maintained on ice until added to the EA.

2.5. C4. C4 is purified by anion-exchange cellulose column chromatography followed by Pevikon block electrophoresis (13). Functionally pure C4 can be purchased from Cordis Laboratories. Heat-inactivated (56°C, 30 min) human serum, absorbed three times at 0°C with one-tenth volume of packed sheep E, can also be used as a C4 source. Some heat-inactivated sera may be unsatisfactory as a source of C4 because the ratio of C4 to C4b-C3b INA is too low.

2.6. C2. C2 is purified from human serum by cation-exchange column chromatography followed by Pevikon block electrophoresis and hydroxyapatite column chromatography (14). Functionally pure C2 may be purchased from Cordis Laboratories. Before use, the C2 is treated with iodine to form oxidized C2 (^{oxy}C2), which forms a stable complex with EAC14 (EAC14^{oxy}2) and fixes 20–30 times more C3 than does native C2 (15).

Alternatively, an ^{oxy}C2 reagent may be prepared by treatment of fresh human serum with iodine (16) and potassium thiocyanate (KSCN) (17). An iodine stock solution is prepared in a 100-ml volumetric flask by mixing 250 mg of iodine and 8.3 g of potassium iodide (KI) in 4 ml of 0.09 M phosphate buffer pH 6. This yields a saturated solution of KI in which the iodine is readily soluble. Addition of the same buffer to 100 ml total volume, dissolves the remaining KI (16). The iodine stock solution should be stored in a brown bottle at 4°C and discarded after 1 week. The amount of iodine required will vary somewhat with different batches of serum and must be determined by treating small samples of serum with different dilutions of the iodine stock solution: 1.0 ml samples of serum are mixed with equal volumes of iodine stock solution, diluted 1:5, 1:7, 1:10, 1:12, or 1:15 in 0.09 M phosphate buffer, pH 6, and maintained at room temperature for 5 min. Next, the iodine-treated serum is dialyzed overnight at 4°C against 10 liters of Veronal buffer (GVB prepared without gelatin). The iodine-treated serum samples are then compared for enhancement of C hemolytic activity relative to the control serum treated with phosphate buffer, pH6, without iodine. Into 5-ml glass tubes standing in an ice bath are pipetted 0.4 ml of EA (5 × 10^8/ml in GVB; see Section 3.1) and 0.4-ml dilutions (in GVB) of iodine-treated serum. Several different dilutions of each of the iodine-treated sera and the control serum are tested. Dilutions of 1:25, 1:50, 1:75, and 1:100 are suggested. The EA and serum dilutions are then incubated at 37°C for 1 hr, with shaking to keep the EA suspended. The tubes are then placed in an ice-bath, 2 ml of ice-cold saline are added to each, and after centrifugation the hemoglobin in the supernatants is quantitated by measuring the OD_{541}. For the OD_{541} blank, 0.4 ml of EA is incubated with 0.4 ml of GVB instead of serum and processed in the same manner. The OD_{541} equivalent to 100% hemolysis is determined by lysing a 0.4-ml sample of EA with 2.4 ml of water. From this test, the iodine treatment producing the greatest enhancement of C hemolysis is determined. Suitably oxidized serum should produce 3–6 times more hemolysis than the control serum at the same dilution (16). The remaining untreated serum is then treated with the optimal dilution of iodine for 5 min at room temperature and then dialyzed overnight against Veronal buffer at $4°C$.

The iodine-treated serum is then mixed with an equal volume of $2\,M$ KSCN and incubated overnight at $4°C$. Next, the KSCN-treated serum is dialyzed overnight at $4°C$ against 100 times the serum volume of Veronal buffer. The dialysis bag should not be filled more than 50%, in order to allow water uptake. Finally, the treated serum is concentrated (Amicon PM-10 or PM-30 membrane) down to the original serum volume (approximately 5-fold) and frozen in 1-ml volumes at $-70°C$.

The I_2–KSCN-treated serum should be tested to determine the extent of C2 oxidation by tests for C2 hemolytic activity and the stability of the EAC142 complex. To determine C2 hemolytic activity, 0.2-ml volumes of I_2–KSCN-treated serum dilutions in GVB (try 1:100–1:800) are added to 0.2 ml of EAC14 (5×10^8/ml in GVB) and incubated at $32°C$ for 12 min. Similar dilutions of the untreated serum control should be tested in parallel. Next, 0.2 ml of whole human serum diluted 1:2 with 0.2 M EDTA at pH 7.2 (EDTA–serum) is added to each tube, and incubation is continued at $32°C$ for 1 hr. Then 2 ml of ice-cold saline are added, and hemolysis is quantitated as before. The EAC14 utilized for the assay of I_2–KSCN-treated serum should be prepared with an excess of C4 in a similar manner as those prepared for detection of C4-dependent rosette formation (see Section 3.2). Also, C1 should be readded to the EAC14 just before use in a similar manner as when $EAC14^{oxy}2$ are being prepared (see Section 3.2). For the OD_{541} blank, an additional reaction mixture tube should be included in which 0.2 ml of GVB is substituted for 0.2 ml of I_2–KSCN-treated serum dilution. The OD_{541} equal to 100% lysis is determined from the supernatant of a reaction mixture diluted with 2 ml of water instead of 2 ml of saline. From this assay the amount of I_2–KSCN-treated serum producing approximately 63% hemolysis can be determined. This amount of I_2–KSCN-treated serum supplies one effective molecule of C2 per EAC14 (18). (see Section 3.2). Oxidation of serum is considered suitable if the enhancement of C2 hemolytic activity is 10- to 15-fold (16).

Next, the I_2–KSCN treated serum is tested for the stabilization of EAC142 as determined by a kinetic assay for C2 fixation and decay. Five milliliters of EAC14 are mixed with 5 ml of a dilution of I_2–KSCN-treated serum in GVB and incubated at $32°C$. The appropriate dilution of the I_2–KSCN-treated serum is calculated from the previous C2 hemolytic assay and should be an amount that will produce a maximum of 50–70% hemolysis in this system (supplies approximately one effective molecule of C2 per EAC14). At zero time and at 1, 3, 5, 7, 10, 12, 15, 30, and 60 min after mixing, 0.4-ml samples of the cell suspension are removed and pipetted into tubes containing 0.2 ml of EDTA–serum and further incubated at 32°C for 1 hr. As each sample tube completes the final period of incubation, it is transferred to an ice-bath, 2 ml of ice cold saline are added, and the degree of hemolysis is determined as before. In this manner the formation and decay of EAC142 are determined. Maximal formation of EAC142 from EAC14 is usually 10–12 min when C2 is used in its oxidized form as compared to 3–5 min for native C2 (15, 16). Oxidation of the C2 in whole serum is considered suitable if the half-life of the EAC142 complex is more than 60 min as compared to 8 min when the complex is prepared with untreated C2 (16).

2.7. C3. C3 is purified from human serum by TEAE-cellulose column chromatography followed by hydroxyapatite column chromatography and Pevikon block electrophoresis (19). Functionally pure human C3 can be purchased from Cordis Laboratories. This commercially available C3 has been reported by others (3) to be satisfactory for the production of EAC1-3b for detection of complement receptors.

2.8. Suramin. The drug suramin, also known as Antrypol, can be purchased from FBA Pharmaceuticals, New York, New York.

2.9. C5-Deficient Mouse Serum. Many strains of mice are genetically deficient in C5. A list of C5(MuB1 antigen) deficient and normal strains of mice was published by Cinader *et al.* (20). Some examples of C5-deficient strains are: AKR, A/HeJ, DBA/2J, and A/J. When mice are bled for C, the blood should be collected in an ice-cold glass tube and clotted on ice for not more than 3 hr. The mouse serum should then be absorbed 3 times at 0°C for 10 min with one-tenth volume of packed sheep E and frozen in 4-ml volumes at −70°C. Commercially available mouse serum is usually not suitable as a source of C.

2.10. C4b-C3b Inactivator(s) (C4b-C3bINA). Protease activity in serum which cleaves both C4b (21) and C3b (22) may be the same enzyme. This C4b-C3b INA can be partially purified from human serum by DEAE- and CM-cellulose column chromatography (23). Alternatively, a whole serum reagent can be prepared by first treating human serum with an equal volume of 2 *M* potassium thiocyanate (KSCN, see third paragraph of Section 2.6) and then heating it at 56°C for 2 hr. After these treatments, the serum must also be absorbed 3 times for 10 min at 37°C with one-tenth volume of packed sheep E and stored at −70°C.

2.11. Latex Particles. Latex particles 1.1 μm in diameter for labeling contaminating phagocytic cells can be purchased from Dow Diagnostics, Indianapolis, Indiana, as a 10% suspension. These should be washed 5 times in PBS with centrifugation at 15,000 g for 10 min and stored as a 5% suspension in PBS.

2.12. Microscope. For counting CRL rosettes and distinguishing these from rosettes of contaminating human E, granulocytes, or monocytes, a good phase contrast microscope is required. A Nikon L-KE microscope equipped for phase contrast (Ehrenreich Photo Optical Industries, Garden City, New York) has been found to be highly suitable for this purpose. A Leitz microscope (Ernst Leitz, Inc., Rockleigh, New Jersey) equipped with Zernike-type phase contrast also works well.

2.13. Rotator. A tissue culture-type test tube rotator is required for the CRL rosette assay to keep the cells in suspension and to promote cell–cell contact. A unit with 9-inch radius which rotates at 6–60 rpm has been found to be both satisfactory and reliable (Catalogue No. R4171, Scientific Products).

3. Methods

3.1. Preparation of EA. Sheep E from 10 ml of sheep blood are washed three times with 50 ml of ice-cold saline (10 min, 1000 g, 4°C). The sheep leukocyte layer ("buffy coat") on top of the E pellet is aspirated from the E pellet (along with some of the E) and discarded after the first centrifugation step. After the last wash, the sheep E are resuspended at a concentration of 5% (v/v) in 0.01 GVBE and warmed to 37°C. The concentration of the sheep E should be checked spectrophotometrically. For this purpose, a 0.5-ml sample of the approximate 5% sheep E suspension is lysed by addition of 14.5 ml of water (1:30 dilution). Following centrifugation, the OD_{541} of this lysed sample in a standard 1-cm cuvette should be 0.350 if the sheep E are correctly suspended at 5% (v/v). If the optical density indicates a different cell concentration, the volume of the cell suspension should be appropriately adjusted.

The IgM antisheep E antibody is diluted (with Cordis antibody, a concentration three times higher than that recommended by the manufacturer should be used) in 0.01 GVBE and warmed to 37°C. Equal volumes of sheep E and antisheep E antibody appropriately diluted are mixed, incubated at 37°C for 30 min, and then washed once with ice-cold 0.01 GVBE and twice with ice-cold GVB.

3.2. Preparation of EAC^{hu}. EAC1 are prepared by addition of 0.5 ml of C1 to 10 ml of EA suspended at 2.5% (5×10^8/ml) in GVB, followed by incubation at 37°C for 15 min. The generated EAC1 are washed twice at room temperature with 40 ml of GVB warmed to 37°C, resuspended at 5×10^8/ml in 37°C GVB, and used immediately for preparation of EAC14.

In order to prepare EAC14 to detect C4-dependent rosettes, 75–150 μg of purified C4 (or 0.1–0.2 ml of heat-inactivated serum) are added to 10^9 EAC1 (5×10^8/ml). However, when EAC1-3b and EAC1-3d are prepared, it is important to use less C4 (5–10 μg of purified C4 or 10–25 μl of heat-inactivated serum per 10^9 EAC1) for the formation of the EAC14 intermediate, so that the finally generated EAC form rosettes that are dependent on C3b or C3d and independent of C4. EAC1-3b prepared with excess C4 cannot be converted to C3d receptor-specific EAC1-3d because the excess C4b they contain is resistant to C4b-C3b INA owing to the protective effort of ^{oxy}C2. For this reason the C4 (either pure C4 or heat-inactivated serum) must be previously tested to determine the maximum amount that can be added to EAC1 without generating EAC14 that are reactive with either human E or CRL. A single titration of the C4 should be carried out in which a wide range of C4 amounts (3–200 μg pure C4 or 0.01–0.3 ml of heat-inactivated serum) are added to tubes containing 2 ml of EAC1 (5 × 10^8/ml). With purified C4, the incubation to form EAC14 is 30 min at 37°C. When heat-inactivated serum is used as a C4 source, the incubation period is reduced to 15 min to reduce inactivation by the serum C4b-C3b INA. Immediately at the end of the incubation period with heat-inactivated serum, the EAC14 are diluted and washed twice with ice-cold GVB. If purified C4 is utilized, the washes are performed instead with GVB warmed to 37°C in order to help preserve C1 sites. Each of the different batches of EAC14 generated are then tested for human E rosette formation. The maximum amount of C4 that will produce EAC14 that are unreactive in immune adherence is used for preparation of EAC1-3b. On the other hand, in order to detect C4 immune adherence more C4 is required. With pure C4, rosette formation increases as EAC1 are treated with more than the limiting amount of C4 until a plateau value is obtained. However, when heat-inactivated serum is used as a C4 source, careful titration of the serum is required because of the presence of the C4b inactivator. The amount of C4 rosette formation obtained reaches a maximum level with a certain amount of serum, and then decreases sharply when only slightly more serum is added because of this inactivator. The maximal level of C4-dependent rosette formation when heat-inactivated serum is employed as a source of C4 is usually the same as the plateau value obtained when purified C4 is utilized, but occasionally this is not so. Thus, heat-inactivated serum from several individuals should be tested, and the one giving the best results should be stored in 0.5-ml volumes at −70°C. The amount of this serum found to produce a maximum level of C4 rosette formation is then used in all future preparations of optimally reactive EAC14. With several different heat-inactivated sera, this amount has been found to vary between 0.1 and 0.2 ml of heat-inactivated serum per 10^9 EAC1.

EAC14^{oxy}2 are produced from EAC14 by addition of 90 effective molecules of ^{oxy}C2 per EAC14 (see Section 2.6). Before addition of the ^{oxy}C2 source, it is necessary to add C1 (in a similar manner as when EAC1 is formed) to the EAC14 to restore that which comes off during EAC14 formation. Purified C2 (0.3–1.0 mg/ml) is oxidized just before use by addition of an equal volume of iodine stock solution (see Section 2.6) diluted approximately 1:500 with 0.09 M phosphate buffer, pH 6.0, incubation at room temperature for 5 min, and immediate cooling to 0°C. The exact amount of iodine required must be determined by treating samples of the C2 with various concentrations of iodine followed by tests to determine which amount produced the greatest enhancement of C2 activity (15). If the purified C2 is stored in low ionic strength pH 6.0 buffer with EDTA (14), then an appropriate amount of 5X Veronal buffer and Ca^{2+}–Mg^{2+} solution must be added to the ^{oxy}C2 to produce isotonicity and neutralize the EDTA. Either purified ^{oxy}C2 or I_2–KSCN-treated serum are incubated with the EAC14 for T_{max} at 32°C (see Section 2.6) and then immediately washed twice with ice-cold GVB. EAC14^{oxy}2 are stable for up to 1 week at 0°–2°C (15). Since I_2–KSCN treated serum may occasionally contain residual amounts of C4, EAC14^{oxy}2 formed from I_2–KSCN treated serum should be tested for lack of rosette formation with human E. If the EAC14^{oxy}2 form human E rosettes, then 25–50% less I_2–KSCN treated serum should be used in future preparations of EAC14^{oxy}2.

EAC14^{oxy}23b (EAC1-3b) are formed by addition of 30–70 µg of purified C3 to 10^9 EAC14^{oxy}2, followed by incubation at 37°C for 15 min and two washes with ice-cold GVB. Each batch of C3 should be titrated for amount required to produce EAC1-3b that detect a maximum number of CRL rosettes.

EAC1-3d are prepared from EAC1-3b by treatment with C4b-C3b INA for 1 hr at 37°C, followed by two washes with ice-cold GVB. Purified C4b-C3b INA should be titrated for inhibition of immune adherence (23) utilizing EAC1-3b containing the same amount of C3b used to detect a maximum number of CRL. EAC1-3b should be treated with eight times the amount of C4b-C3b INA required to produce 50% inhibition of immune adherence. When the modified serum reagent is used as a source of C4b-C3b INA it is important that C1 be removed from the complex. Thus the EAC1-3b must be first incubated for 90 min at 37°C with 0.04 GVBE, then washed once and resuspended at 2.5% in 0.04 GVBE. An equal volume of the serum reagent is then added and after 1 hr at 37°C, the EAC1-3d are washed once with ice-cold 0.04 GVBE and twice with ice-cold GVB.

3.3. Preparation of EAC^{mo}.

EAC14^{oxy}2^{hu}3b^{mo} (EAC1-3b^{mo}) are prepared from EAC14^{oxy}2^{hu} by addition of C5-deficient mouse serum diluted in GVB containing 1.5 mg/ml of suramin (GVB-S). Suramin inhibits the serum C4b-C3b INA (22) so that most, if not all, of the fixed C3 remains in the C3b form. At concentrations sufficient to inhibit C4b-C3b INA, suramin also completely inhibits C4 fixation, thus it is necessary to use EAC14^{oxy}2^{hu} rather than EA. At higher suramin concentrations, C3 fixation is also inhibited. Ten milliliters of EAC14^{oxy}2, suspended at 1% (v/v) in GVB-S, are mixed with 10 ml of C5-deficient mouse serum, that was previously diluted 1:5 in GVB-S and held at

37°C for 5 min just before use. After exactly 10 min at 37°C, the generated EAC1-3b^{mo} are diluted and washed once with ice-cold GVB-S and twice with ice-cold GVB.

EAC1-3d^{mo} are prepared by addition of C5-deficient mouse serum to EA, followed by treatment of the formed EAC with mouse serum diluted in EDTA. The second treatment assures complete cleavage of all cell-bound C4b and C3b by C4b-C3b INA. Ten milliliters of EA suspended at 2×10^8/ml in GVB are mixed with 10 ml of C5-deficient mouse serum diluted 1:2.5 in GVB, and incubated at 37°C for 45 min. After one wash with 0.04 GVBE, the EAC are resuspended in 10 ml of 0.04 GVBE and incubated at 37°C for 45 min. Next, the EAC are resuspended in 2 ml of 0.04 GVBE and mixed with 8 ml of C5-deficient mouse serum diluted 1:2 in 0.04 GVBE, and incubated at 37°C for 45 min. The EAC1-3d^{mo} are ready for use after one wash with ice-cold 0.04 GVBE and two washes with ice-cold GVB.

3.4. Testing EAC for Specificity and Potency. EAC14 are specific for immune adherence receptors, but may contain insufficient amounts of C4b to form rosettes with some cells with low numbers of receptors, particularly if the EAC14 were prepared with heat-inactivated serum. EAC14, EAC1-3b^{hu}, and EAC1-3b^{mo} should be tested for rosette formation with human E. E from different individuals vary greatly in the proportion of cells that form rosettes. Usually though, individual E donors will vary little from week to week and it is, therefore, advantageous to select one particular person (with the most reactive E) from the laboratory personnel as the E donor, since this allows comparison of new batches of EAC to those prepared in previous weeks. Also, a similar amount of cell-bound C4b or C3b is required to form a maximum number of rosettes with human E as with normal CRL. EAC14 which contain optimal amounts of C4b usually form only two-thirds as many human E rosettes as do optimal EAC1-3b. A small sample of the EAC14 from which the EAC1-3b were prepared should be put aside and tested later after the EAC1-3b are prepared. If these EAC14 (prepared with a small amount of C4) form no rosettes, then the rosettes formed with the EAC1-3b and the same indicator cells can be assumed to be C3b dependent.

Since EAC1-3b^{mo} are prepared with whole serum, it is difficult to quantitate the amount of C3 added and the amount of C3b subsequently bound. The proper ratio of suramin to serum is important. More suramin will inhibit C3 fixation, whereas less suramin will allow the serum C4b-C3b INA to cleave some C3b. If the EAC1-3b^{mo} produce as many human E rosettes as do the EAC1-3b^{hu} (prepared as described with purified C3), then they will detect all human CRL with immune adherence receptors and probably all mouse CRL with immune adherence receptors. However, even though it can be demonstrated that the EAC1-3b^{mo} probably contain optimal amounts of C3b^{mo}, there is at present no way to determining whether or not they also contain some small amount of C3d. Any small amount of C3d the EAC1-3b^{mo} may contain is probably insignificant, since with human CRL known to contain only C3d receptors, EAC1-3b^{mo} were found to form the same number of rosettes as did EAC1-3b^{hu} (prepared with purified C and therefore containing no C3d). Also, immature mouse neutrophils containing only C3d receptors were not rosetted by EAC1-3b^{mo} (7).

It is important that the EAC1-3d be tested for human E rosette formation. Since human E do not have C3d receptors. EAC1-3d specificity can be confirmed when they form less than 5% as many human E rosettes as do the EAC1-3b. The potency of the EAC1-3d is best tested by rosette formation with an established line of cultured human lymphoblastoid cells. Individual cell lines usually remain fairly constant from week to week in the proportion of cells that will form EAC1-3d rosettes. Ideally, a cell line should be used in which all the cells form EAC1-3d rosettes, but few cells, if any, form EAC14 rosettes. Many cell lines, including RAJI (24) have this characteristic. If the EAC1-3d^{mo} form more than 5% as many human E rosettes as the EAC1-3b, they must be retreated with C4b–C3b INA (or EDTA-mouse serum). If EAC1-3d^{hu} form too many rosettes with human E after a second treatment with C4b-C3b INA, it is possibly because they were prepared with too much C4. This can be confirmed by testing the EAC14^{oxy} 2 intermediate for human E rosette formation. The C4b contained on EAC1-3d^{hu} is completely resistant to the inactivator because it is complexed with oxidized C2 (21).

3.5. Rosette Assay for C Receptors. EAC, 0.1 ml, suspended at 0.5–1.0% (1 to 2×10^8/ml) is mixed with 0.1 ml of lymphocytes or human E suspended at 2 to 3×10^6/ml in 10×75 mm siliconized glass or plastic tubes. Any isotonic buffer (PBS, GVB, HBSS, etc.) may be used for the rosette assay. Sodium azide (0.02%) can be used to preserve EAC and has the additional benefit of inhibiting both sheep E-dependent rosettes with T cells (negligible at 37°C without azide) and receptor capping (particularly valuable in double-label assays for C receptor rosettes and surface immunoglobulin immunofluorescence). Continuous mixing for 5–20 min at 37°C on a rotator (see Section 2.13) at 40 rpm is essential for the cell–cell contact, which leads to rosette formation. With cells from some established lymphoid lines, more than 5 min of incubation with EAC1-3d will occasionally produce clumps of rosettes that are difficult to enumerate. With normal CRL, 20 min of incubation on the rotator is sufficient. A drop of the rosette suspension is then examined by phase-contrast microscopy utilizing a nail polish-sealed cover slip (or phase contrast hemocytometer) and a 70–100 × oil-immersion objective lens. With lymphocytes, 200–300 cells in random fields are counted as either rosetted (3 or more attached EAC) or not, and the percentage of CRL is calculated. With human E, a four-button counter is used and 200–300 human E in random fields are counted in four different categories: (a) unrosetted, 0 or 1 attached EAC; (b) rosetted with 2 attached EAC; (c) 3 attached EAC; or (d) 4 attached EAC. Human E with more than 4 attached EAC are rare. From the number of each type of rosette, the average number of EAC bound to 100 human E is calculated. This method of quantitating human E rosettes is more reproducible than calculating the percentage of rosettes, but is not practical for lymphocytes, since small CRL may contain up to 10 attached EAC.

3.6. Isolation of Lymphocytes. Human blood lymphocytes have been routinely isolated for CRL analysis by treatment of blood with carbonyl–iron followed by Ficoll–Hypaque centrifugation (2). If Ficoll–Hypaque alone is utilized, a considerably higher proportion of monocytes contaminate the lymphocyte preparation (25). Unfortunately, there is some recent preliminary evidence that carbonyl-iron may occasionally selectively deplete B cells from lymphocyte preparations (R. Winchester and G. Ross, unpublished observation). Since monocytes form rosettes with EAC that must be distinguished from CRL rosettes, contaminating monocytes should be labeled with latex. With mouse lymphocyte preparations, neutrophil and monocyte C receptor-dependent rosettes can be specifically inhibited by inclusion of 0.01 M EDTA in the CRL assay buffer (5).

Since even 5% undetected monocyte contamination can falsely increase the percentage of CRL, lymphocyte preparations should be routinely treated with latex to label monocytes. For this purpose, the lymphocytes are suspended in HBSS at 1×10^6/ml and 25 μl of 5% latex is added per 2×10^7 cells. After 45 min of gentle mixing at 37°C, the cells are washed 3 times at 200 g for 10 min and a sample of the cell suspension is examined for free latex. After each wash, it is necessary to resuspend the pellet rigorously in 1 ml with a vortex mixer. If free latex is observed, then the cells must be washed again. When the cells are resuspended after the final wash, care should be taken to break up clumps of monocytes (use a vortex mixer) which may contain trapped lymphocytes. Considerable caution must still be observed when counting CRL, since some monocytes do not phagocytize latex and some lymphocytes bind latex to their surface without ingesting it.

4. Interpretation

4.1. Human CRL. With normal blood lymphocytes, an average of 12% CRL (range 6–18%) has been demonstrated by several different investigators utilizing either EAC14, EAC1-3b, or EAC1-3d (1, 24, 26). Exact enumeration of CRL is complicated by several factors. First, neutrophils, erythrocytes, and especially monocytes that contaminate lymphocyte preparations may falsely increase CRL determinations. On the other hand, techniques that deplete phagocytic cells from lymphocyte preparations, such as nylon wool, plastic, glass, or carbonyl-iron adherence, have a variable tendency to also deplete CRL, especially those

CRL containing membrane-bound immunoglobulin (B cells). Finally, CRL are usually underestimated utilizing EAC made with whole serum (EAC1-3d). EAC1-3d usually detect only two-thirds as many normal blood CRL as do EAC1-3b. If normal blood lymphocytes are isolated by Ficoll–Hypaque centrifugation and the large number of contaminating monocytes are labeled with latex, 17% CRL (range 8–25%) are detected with EAC1-3b, and 12% CRL (range 6–18%) are detected with either EAC14 or EAC1-3d. Thus, 20–40% of normal blood CRL can only be detected with EAC1-3b. Since human C receptors react equally well with EAC prepared with either human C or mouse C, EAC1-3b^{mo} may be used to detect human CRL if purified human C3 is unavailable for preparation of EAC1-3b^{hu}. EAC1-3b probably detect the highest number of CRL with normal blood lymphocytes because of the ability of C3b to react with cells containing low numbers of both types of C receptors. EAC1-3b, however, do not react with CRL, having only weak C3d receptors. Such lymphocytes are rare in normal blood, but they characterize the lymphocytes from most patients with chronic lymphatic leukemia and make up 5–15% of normal tonsil lymphocytes (1). EAC14 react specifically with immune adherence receptors but may not detect as many cells with immune adherence receptors as do EAC1-3b. EAC1-3d can only be considered as specific for C3d receptors when they form <5% as many human E rosettes as do the EAC1-3b. Cells which form rosettes with EAC1-3b and EAC1-3d, but not with EAC14, have strong C3d receptors but no immune adherence receptors. Such cells characterize most established lymphoblastoid lines. Significant numbers of lymphocytes that form rosettes with EAC14 and EAC1-3b, but not with EAC1-3d, have been observed only in the blood from patients with Waldenström's macroglobulinemia (1). Such cells presumably have immune adherence receptors but lack C3d receptors.

4.2. Mouse CRL. As with human CRL, EAC1-3b^{mo} react with both types of C receptors, but do not react with CRL having only weak C3d receptors. In mouse spleen, EAC1-3b^{mo} detected slightly fewer CRL than did EAC1-3d^{mo}, but a mixture of EAC1-3b^{mo} and EAC1-3d^{mo} detected 10–15% more CRL than did EAC1-3d^{mo} alone. With mouse peripheral blood, EAC1-3b^{mo} and EAC1-3d^{mo} detected a similar number of CRL, with little or no increase in CRL detected when EAC1-3b^{mo} and EAC1-3d^{mo} were mixed. With various mouse strains, spleens contained 25–65% CRL, while blood contained 15–30% CRL. Mouse C receptors react poorly with EAC prepared with human C; EAC1-3d^{hu} detected less than 50% as many CRL as did EAC1-3d^{mo} (7).

REFERENCES

1. Ross, G. D., and Polley, M. J., *J. Exp. Med.* **141**, 1163 (1975).
2. Ross, G. D., Polley, M. J., Rabellino, E. M., and Grey, H. M., *J. Exp. Med.* **138**, 798 (1973).

3. Reynolds, H. Y., Atkinson, J. P., Newball, H. H., and Frank, M. M., *J. Immunol.* **114,** 1813 (1975).
4. Gupta, S., Ross, G. D., Good, R. A., and Siegal, F. P., *J. Allergy Clin. Immunol.* **57,** 189 (1976).
5. Bianco, C., Patrick, R., and Nussenzweig, V., *J. Exp. Med.* **132,** 702 (1970).
6. Dierich, M. P., Pellagrino, M. A., Ferrone, S., and Reisfeld, R. A., *J. Immunol.* **112,** 1766 (1974).
7. Ross, G. D., Rabellino, E. M., and Polley, M. J., *Fed. Proc., Fed. Am. Soc. Exp. Biol.* **35,** 254 (1976).
8. Griffin, F. M., Bianco, C., and Silverstein, S. C., *J. Exp. Med.* **141,** 1269 (1975).
9. Rabellino, E. M., and Metcalf, D., *J. Immunol.* **115,** 688 (1975).
10. Miller, G. W., Saluk, P. H., and Nussenzweig, V., *J. Exp. Med.* **138,** 495 (1973).
11. Theofilopoulos, A. N., Bokisch, V. A., and Dixon, F. J., *J. Exp. Med.* **139,** 696 (1974).
12. Cooper, N. R., and Müller-Eberhard, H. J., *Immunochemistry* **5,** 155 (1968).
13. Müller-Eberhard, H. J., and Biro, C. E., *J. Exp. Med.* **118,** 447 (1963).
14. Polley, M. J., and Müller-Eberhard, H. J., *J. Exp. Med.* **128,** 533 (1968).
15. Polley, M. J., and Müller-Eberhard, H. J., *J. Exp. Med.* **126,** 1013 (1967).
16. Polley, M. J., *J. Immunol.* **107,** 1493 (1971).
17. Dalmasso, A. P., and Müller-Eberhard, H. J., *J. Immunol.* **97,** 680 (1966).
18. Mayer, M. M., *in* "Experimental Immunochemistry" (by E. A. Kabat and M. M. Mayer), p. 184. Thomas, Springfield, Illinois, 1961.
19. Nilsson, U., and Müller-Eberhard, H. J., *J. Exp. Med.* **122,** 277 (1965).
20. Cinader, B., Dubiski, S., and Wardlaw, A. C., *J. Exp. Med.* **120,** 897 (1964).
21. Cooper, N. R., *J. Exp. Med.* **141,** 890 (1975).
22. Tamura, N., and Nelson, R. A., *J. Immunol.* **99,** 582 (1967).
23. Ruddy, S., Hunsicker, L. G., and Austen, K. F., *J. Immunol.* **108,** 657 (1972).
24. Bokisch, V. A., and Sobel, A. T., *J. Exp. Med.* **140,** 1336 (1974).
25. Zucker-Franklin, D., *J. Immunol.* **112,** 234 (1974).
26. Pincus, S., Bianco, C., and Nussenzweig, V., *Blood, J. Hematol.* **40,** 303 (1972).

7
_____

A Rosette Technique for Identification of
Human Lymphocytes with Fc Receptors

Stig S. Frøland and Finn Wisløff

1. Introduction

Surface receptors for the Fc portion of IgG molecules have been demonstrated on monocytes and granulocytes of human origin (1–3) and also on mouse lymphocytes (4, 5). Recently, similar binding sites for IgG both of homologous and heterologous origin have been demonstrated also on human lymphocytes by means of various test systems (6–10). In our laboratory we have been working with a rosette assay for human Fc receptor-bearing lymphocytes (EA-RFC), based on the ability of these cells to form rosettes with human indicator erythrocytes sensitized with human IgG (19). Studies with this rosette system have led us to conclude that EA-RFC, identified as described in the present paper, to a large extent represent lymphocytic cells different from T and B lymphocytes as demonstrated with conventional surface markers, and therefore possibly representing a third lymphocyte population (8, 9). This conclusion is compatible with recent results obtained by other workers (11, 12). Little is known about the biological importance to this "third lymphocyte population," which probably is heterogeneous, but it appears to contain the effector cells (the so-called K cells) in lymphocyte-mediated antibody-dependent cytotoxicity (13, 14) and also certain cells participating in lymphocyte cytotoxicity induced by unspecific mitogens (15). We feel that the rosette test for EA-RFC represents a useful and convenient marker system for cells belonging to this "third population" of lymphocytes, both in normal and pathological situations.

2. Materials

    2.1. Heparin, 5000 IU/ml (Novo, Copenhagen)
    2.2. Isopaque, 440 mg I/ml (Nyegaard & Co. A/S, Oslo)
    2.3. Ficoll (Pharmacia A/B, Uppsala)
    2.4. Hanks' balanced salt solution (Hanks' BSS, obtained from Grand Island Biological Company, Grand Island, New York).
    2.5. Medium 199 with Hanks' BSS (Grand Island Biological Company)

2.6. Pipettes, calibrated: 25 ml, 10 ml, 2 ml, 1 ml

2.7. Pasteur pipettes (Harshaw v.d. Hoorn, Utrecht)

2.8. Phosphate-buffered saline (PBS), pH 7.4

2.9. Bürker cell-counting chamber (hemocytometer).

2.10. Cell-counting pipette and staining fluid for counting leukocytes

2.11. Human O Rh+ ($R_1 R_2$) erythrocytes collected on acid-citrate-dextrose (ACD) and stored at $4°C$ for up to 3 weeks.

2.12. Anti-CD antiserum of Ripley type (16) kindly supplied by Dr. Marion Waller, Medical College of Virginia, Richmond, Virginia)

2.13. Microscope Dialux (Leitz, Wetslar)

3. Method

3.1. Separation of Lymphocytes. Venous blood (10 IU/ml of heparin) is drawn from healthy blood donors. The lymphocytes are separated by means of the Isopaque–Ficoll gradient centrifugation technique (17, 18). Instead of preparing the Isopaque–Ficoll mixture in the laboratory, one may use the equivalent commercial reagent Lymphoprep (Nyegaard & Co. A/S, Oslo). The mononuclear cells obtained are washed three times in Hanks' BSS and resuspended in Medium 199 at a concentration of 4×10^6/ml.

3.2. Preparation of Sensitized Indicator Erythrocytes. Human O Rh+ ($R_1 R_2$) erythrocytes are sensitized ("coated") with human IgG by incubating them with anti-CD antiserum (Ripley). Two drops (0.1 ml) of washed and packed erythrocytes are mixed with 1 drop (0.05 ml) of the Ripley antiserum and 8 drops (0.4 ml) of PBS and incubated for 1.5 hr at $37°C$. The cells are then washed 4 times in PBS and finally resuspended in PBS to give a 1% suspension. This cell suspension is either used on the day of preparation or after storage for at most 24 hr at $4°C$.

3.3. Preparation of Rosettes between Lymphocytes and Sensitized Indicator Erythrocytes. Of the 1% suspension of indicator erythrocytes, 0.25 ml is mixed with 0.25 ml of lymphocyte suspension (containing 1×10^6 lymphocytes). This cell mixture is centrifuged for 2 min at 200 g and left at room temperature for 15–30 min.

3.4. Qualitative and Quantitative Evaluation of EA-RFC. The cell pellet is resuspended gently with a long Pasteur-pipette, and a sample is placed in a conventional counting chamber (hemocytometer) of the Bürker type. The percentage of rosette-forming lymphocytes (EA-RFC) is determined by first counting the rosettes and then the lymphocytes (including those engaged in rosette formation). A rosette is defined as a lymphocytelike cell with five or more erythrocytes firmly bound to its surface.

Rosettes with the IgG-sensitized indicator erythrocytes may also be formed by some monocytes and granulocytes. Granulocytes are, however, unimportant for the results, since contamination of granulocytes is low in the cell suspension used (17, 18) and granulocyte rosettes are usually easy to identify. Somewhat greater difficulties may be caused by monocyte rosettes. With experience such rosettes may to a considerable extent be excluded, but it seems inevitable that a few rosette-forming monocytes are included in the EA-RFC count. However, this monocyte contribution seems insignificant, as demonstrated in the experiments where EA-RFC were counted before and after removal of adherent cells including monocytes by fractionation on nylon fiber columns (9). This has also been confirmed in experiments where stained smears of rosette preparations were examined.

Sometimes, a few small erythrocyte agglutinates with a superficial resemblance to EA rosettes are seen in rosette preparations, but with experience such agglutinates usually do not disturb counting.

4. Critical Comments

With the technique described, a mean of 15% positive lymphocytes (range 4–39%) is found in mononuclear cell suspensions obtained from venous blood by the Isopaque–Ficoll gradient centrifugation technique (9). We will emphasize that different anti-Rh isoantibodies vary widely in their suitability for the detection of human Fc-receptor-bearing lymphocytes (EA-RFC), which may at least partly explain the previous failure by some workers to detect such lymphocytes. The Ripley anti-CD antiserum, which is composed of IgG1 and IgG3 antibodies, with a minor admixture of IgG4 antibodies, seems particularly well suited for the EA-rosette test, but we have also discovered other anti-Rh isoantibodies of IgG1 or IgG3 subclass, which give numbers of EA-RFC approaching those of the Ripley antiserum (19). This is in agreement with findings by other workers (6). The high variability between different antisera with respect to their suitability in the rosette test for EA-RFC is not completely understood, but may in part reflect the density of IgG molecules achievable on the indicator erythrocytes. Preliminary studies in our laboratory suggest that the suitability of any particular anti-Rh antiserum is not correlated with a given IgG subclass or Gm type (19). The advantage of the Ripley anti-Rh antiserum in the rosette test compared to many other anti-Rh antisera is rather similar to previous observations on Fc receptors on granulocytes (3).

The receptors on EA-RFC responsible for rosette formation appear to have specificity only for IgG among the Ig classes, and about equal affinity for IgG1 and IgG3, with only weak binding capacity for IgG2 and IgG4 (19). The specificity for the Fc portion of the IgG molecule seems clear, and our data indicate that mainly the $C\lambda 2$ region is involved in the binding of IgG to EA-RFC (19). However, it is possible that also the $C\lambda 3$ region may participate in the binding of intact IgG molecules.

Human monocytes have previously been reported to form rosettes with IgG-sensitized indicator erythrocytes by means of rosette techniques resembling that used by us for lymphocytes (1, 2). As mentioned above, when care is taken to exclude monocyte rosettes, such rosettes apparently contribute insignificantly to the number of positive cells with the latter test. This was demonstrated by studies of EA-RFC before and after removal of adherent cells, including monocytes, by nylon fiber columns (9) and is also in agreement with recent findings by other workers (6). It seems, therefore, that not all monocytes necessarily form rosettes under the conditions employed by us, and that such rosettes may to a large extent be excluded by an experienced observer. An even higher degree of efficiency in identification of monocyte rosettes might probably be achieved by the simultaneous use of, for example, latex particle incubation or histochemical methods to demonstrate phagocytic cells, as well as cover-slip preparations where the identification of the central cell in rosettes is made more easily.

A series of experiments with various lymphocyte-fractionation techniques as well as studies of patients with pathological distribution of blood B and T lymphocytes have shown that the EA-RFC, detected with the technique described, largely represent lymphocytic cells lacking B and T lymphocyte characteristics as defined by conventional surface markers (8, 9). The EA rosette test is a convenient assay for this probably heterogeneous lymphocyte class provisionally termed by us "the third lymphocyte population." Among these cells are found the so-called K cells, i.e., the effector cells responsible for lymphocyte-mediated, antibody-dependent cytotoxicity *in vitro* (13, 14). It is possible that the K cells have Fc receptors with higher binding affinity for human IgG than the bulk of EA-RFC (20). By changing the concentration of IgG molecules on indicator erythrocytes, it is therefore possible that the EA rosette test may be made somewhat more specific for these lymphocytes. Cells within the EA-RFC category also participate in target-cell destruction *in vitro* mediated by lymphocytes upon activation by unspecific mitogens (15). Data supporting the existence of non-B, non-T lymphocytes in man have recently been reported from other laboratories (12, 21), but the origin and relationship of these cells to other cell types, particularly to the monocyte line, is at the present not clarified.

In addition to its use for the detection and quantitation of EA-RFC, including K cells, we have also used the EA-rosette phenomenon to deplete cell suspensions of these cells by subjecting the rosettes to gradient centrifugation over Isopaque–Ficoll (9, 14). This is an alternative to fractionation of lymphocyte suspensions on antigen–antibody-coated Degalan columns, which have also been used by us for the same purpose (9, 14).

A rosette test utilizing human indicator erythrocytes sensitized with rabbit IgG has previously been introduced by French workers claiming to detect IgG binding cells peculiar to rheumatoid arthritis (22). Our own studies have not confirmed the existence in patients with rheumatoid arthritis of any IgG-binding lymphocytic cells different from EA-RFC as also detected in normals (23).

Recently, the identification of human Fc receptor-bearing lymphocytes have been achieved by several workers using rosette assays different from that described by us both with respect to indicator erythrocytes and origin of IgG used for sensitization (10, 21, 24, 25). Also the binding of fluorescein-labeled IgG aggregates has been used for this purpose (7, 26). Results obtained with some of these techniques suggest that Fc receptors are found on many different lymphocyte populations, both B lymphocytes, certain T lymphocytes (activated?), as well as on non-B, non-T cells, previously termed "null cells." A major reason for these conflicting reports is probably that the particular method used to detect Fc-receptor-bearing cells is of the greatest importance for the results both with respect to number of positive cells and to the surface markers and possible origin. Thus, rosette tests can be designed using non human indicator erythrocytes, e.g., ox erythrocytes (10, 24) or sheep erythrocytes (25) sensitized with rabbit IgG antibodies, giving considerably higher proportions of positive lymphocytes than obtained with the presently described Ripley rosette test; this is due at least in part to a much higher B lymphocyte contribution to positive cells with the former assays. In these rosette assays, higher concentration of IgG molecules on indicator erythrocytes is probably achieved than with erythrocytes sensitized with anti-Rh isoantibodies, making it possible to detect lymphocytes with Fc receptors with weak binding affinity for IgG. The fact that different cell types have Fc receptors with unequal affinity for IgG has been clearly demonstrated in mouse (27). The concentration of IgG molecules on indicator erythrocytes appears, therefore, to be one of the most important parameters in any rosette assay, but other technical differences, including species origin of erythrocytes and IgG, also vary from laboratory to laboratory. It is therefore obvious that results reported with different rosette techniques are not necessarily comparable, explaining much of the present controversy concerning the characteristics and origin of human Fc receptor-bearing lymphocytes. With assays for Fc receptor-bearing cells depending on affinity for fluoresceinated IgG aggregates, results may be complicated even more by other phenomena than Fc receptor interaction with IgG—e.g., unspecific binding of large aggregates (26). It is imperative that any particular rosette test introduced and employed for the detection and quantitation of lymphocytes with Fc receptors be thoroughly standardized and characterized with respect to the lymphocyte populations it is claimed to detect. This can be achieved only through careful experiments with cell fractionation techniques, ideally supplemented with studies on cell suspensions with a pathological distribution of lymphocyte populations.

REFERENCES

1. Abramson, N., Gelfand, E. W., Jandl, J. H., and Rosen, F. S., *J. Exp. Med.* **132,** 1207 (1970).
2. Huber, H., and Fudenberg, H. H., *Int. Arch. Allergy Appl. Immunol.* **34,** 18 (1968).
3. Messner, R. P., and Jelinek, J., *J. Clin. Invest.* **49,** 2165 (1970).

4. Basten, A., Miller, J. F. A. P., Sprent, J., and Pye, J. A., *J. Exp. Med.* **135**, 610 (1972).
5. Paraskevas, F., Lee, S.-T., Orr, K. B., and Israels, L. G., *J. Immunol.* **108**, 1319 (1972).
6. Brain, P., and Marston, R. H., *Eur. J. Immunol.* **3**, 6 (1973).
7. Dickler, H. B., and Kunkel, H. G., *J. Exp. Med.* **136**, 191 (1972).
8. Frøland, S. S., and Natvig, J. B., *Transplant. Rev.* **16**, 114 (1973).
9. Frøland, S. S., Wisløff, F., and Michaelsen, T. E., *Int. Arch. Allergy Appl. Immunol.* **47**, 124 (1974).
10. Hallberg, T., Gurner, B. W., and Coombs, R. R. A., *Int. Arch. Allergy Appl. Immunol.* **44**, 500 (1973).
11. Grey, H. M., Anderson, C. L., Heusser, C. H., and Kurnick, J. T., *in* "Membrane Receptors of Lymphocytes" (N. Seligmann, J. L. Preud'homme, and F. M. Kourilsky, eds.), p. 185. North-Holland Publ., Amsterdam, 1975.
12. Lobo, P. I., Westervelt, F. B., and Horwitz, D. A., *J. Immunol.* **114**, 116 (1975).
13. Wisløff, F., and Frøland, S. S., *Scand. J. Immunol.* **2**, 151 (1973).
14. Wisløff, F., Frøland, S. S., and Michaelsen, T. E., *Int. Arch. Allergy Appl. Immunol.* **47**, 139 (1974).
15. Wisløff, F., Frøland, S. S., and Michaelsen, T. E., *Int. Arch. Allergy Appl. Immunol.* **47**, 488 (1974).
16. Waller, M., and Vaughan, J. H., *Proc. Soc. Exp. Biol. Med.* **92**, 198 (1965).
17. Böyum, A., *Scand. J. Clin. Lab. Invest.* **21**, 97 (1968).
18. Frøland, S. S., and Natvig, J. B., *Int. Arch. Allergy Appl. Immunol.* **39**, 121 (1970).
19. Frøland, S. S., Michaelsen, T. E., Wisløff, F., and Natvig, J. B., *Scand. J. Immunol.* **3**, 509 (1974).
20. Cordier, G., Samarut, C., Brochier, J., and Revillard, J. P., *Scand. J. Immunol.* **5**, 233 (1976).
21. Samarut, C., Brochier, J., and Revillard, J. P., *Scand. J. Immunol.* **5**, 221 (1976).
22. Bach, J.-F., Delrieu, F., and Delbarre, F., *Am. J. Med.* **49**, 213 (1970).
23. Frøland, S. S., Natvig, J. B., and Wisløff, F., *Rheumatology* **6**, 231 (1975).
24. Ferrarini, M., Moretta, L., Abrile, R., and Durante, M. L., *Eur. J. Immunol.* **5**, 70 (1975).
25. Tønder, O., Morse, P. A., and Humphrey, L. J., *J. Immunol.* **113**, 1162 (1974).
26. Frøland, S. S., Natvig, J. B., and Michaelsen, T. E., *Scand. J. Immunol.* **3**, 375 (1974).
27. Anderson, C. L., and Grey, H. M., *J. Exp. Med.* **139**, 1175 (1970).

8

Lymphocyte Binding of Heat-Aggregated and Antigen-Complexed Immunoglobulin

Robert D. Arbeit, Pierre A. Henkart, and Howard B. Dickler

1. Introduction

The surface membranes of certain lymphocytes bear sites which bind antigen-complexed or heat-aggregated Ig (1–3). Binding is dependent on an intact Fc portion of the Ig molecule and the binding site is therefore generally referred to as the Fc receptor (3–5). Although this term is both descriptive and convenient, it should be noted that the observed binding may involve several different membrane structures either on the same cell or on different subpopulations of lymphocytes. Furthermore, the actual role(s) of these binding sites in the immune response has not yet been fully defined.

Information about Fc receptors is largely derived from studies of lymphocyte binding of complexed Ig. The latter can be formed using specific antibody and soluble protein antigens. Such antigen–antibody complexes have been used on cell surfaces (1), in solution (3), in suspension (6), or immobilized on plastic surfaces (7). Alternatively, the antigen may be an erythrocyte which when coated with antibody forms a particulate complex (8). In addition, preparations of heat-aggregated Ig possess many of the properties of antigen–antibody complexes and appear to bind to the same membrane sites (5, 9, 10). The actual binding of the complexed Ig to the lymphocyte surface may be detected by a variety of methods including radioautography (1), direct or indirect fluorescence (2), or rosette formation (8). We will describe two methods in detail: (a) direct fluorescent detection of the binding of heat-aggregated human Ig; and (b) binding of soluble antigen–antibody complexes detected with indirect immunofluorescence. To date most studies have involved lymphocytes from human peripheral blood and murine lymphoid organs. Lymphocyte binding of antibody-coated erythrocytes will be discussed elsewhere in this volume.

Assays for Fc receptors are of value in a variety of investigations. Most directly, properties of the receptors for complexed Ig can be evaluated (4, 5). Further, Fc receptors are a useful marker in the characterization of normal lymphocyte subpopulations (11), cultured lymphoid cell lines (12), and abnormal human lymphoid cell populations [e.g., chronic lymphocytic leukemia (13), and hypogammaglobulinemia (14)].

Techniques are available to isolate the subpopulation(s) of lymphocytes which bear Fc receptors. These include the adherence of such cells to plastic surfaces coated with immobilized antigen—antibody complexes (7) and the use of the fluorescence-activated cell sorter (6).

An application of potential clinical importance derives from the observation that Fc receptors of normal murine splenic B lymphocytes are closely associated with alloantigens determined by the *I* (immune response gene) region of the *H-2* major histocompatibility complex (Ia antigens) (9). Thus, antibodies [and F(ab') fragments thereof] against Ia antigens specifically inhibit the binding of aggregated Ig to B lymphocytes, whereas alloantisera against antigens determined by the *K* and *D* regions of the *H-2* complex fail to inhibit binding. This relationship, along with tissue distribution, can be used as a correlative criterion for the detection of "Ia-like" antigens in an outbred species such as man, where, to date, there has been no definitive demonstration of an analogous immune response gene region. Thus, an anti-HLA alloantiserum has been shown to contain antibodies specific for B lymphocyte alloantigen(s). These antigens were distinct from HLA antigens and, unlike the latter, were closely associated with B lymphocyte Fc receptors (15). In the mouse, Ia antigens are stimulatory in the mixed lymphocyte reaction, and are associated with MHC-linked immune response genes. By analogy, the definition of human "Ia-like" antigens may be of significant clinical value in the study of transplantation genetics and of diseases possibly related to immune response genes. The assays for Fc receptors described here may provide a convenient means to this end.

2. Materials

2.1. Animals
Mice, C57BL/10 Sn(B10) (Jackson Laboratories, Bar Harbor, Maine)
Rabbits, outbred (NIH animal colony)

2.2. Reagents
Cohn fraction II human Ig (Miles Laboratories, Kankakee, Illinois)

FITC (fluorescein isothiocyanate) (Baltimore Biological Laboratories, Cockeysville, Maryland)

PBS (phosphate-buffered saline): 0.05 M PO_4, 0.15 M NaCl; pH 7.2 or 8.0, as indicated.

BSA (bovine serum albumin) (Miles Laboratories). For use in stock solutions—Cohn fraction V powder; for use in antigen preparation—BSA, crystallized (MW 68,000).

KLH (keyhole limpet hemocyanin) (Sigma Chemical Co., St. Louis, Missouri)

TNBS (trinitrobenzenesulfonic acid) (Sigma Chemical Co.). Referred to as TNP (trinitrophenyl) when covalently bound to a protein or cell as a haptenic group.

BSA–PBS: 2% BSA in PBS with 0.02% Na azide added; pH 7.2 or 8.0, as indicated.

DNP-lysine (ϵ-dinitrophenyl-L-lysine HCl) (Sigma Chemical Co.)

Sepharose 4B and Sephadex G200 (Pharmacia Fine Chemicals, Piscataway, New Jersey)

Fl-goat anti-rabbit IgG (fluorescein-conjugated IgG fraction of goat antiserum to rabbit IgG) (heavy and light chains) (Lot No. 7853, Cappel Laboratories, Downingtown, Pennsylvania)

2.3. Special Glassware

Dounce homogenizer (Kontes Glass Co., Vineland, New Jersey)

2.4. Microscope.

Leitz orthoplan (E. Leitz, Inc., Rockleigh, New Jersey). Equipped with a Ploem vertical illuminator, dc power source and HBO 100 W mercury arc lamp, Heine phase condenser and 90×1.32 NA apochromatic oil immersion objective, and a monocular head. The excitation filters for FITC were one BG38, two KP 490, and one K475. Dichroic mirror/suppression filters were TK510/K515. Owing to a variety of optical considerations, the above system appears to provide sensitivity equal to or greater than other equipment currently available.

3. Methods

3.1. Preparation of Fluorescein-Conjugated Heat-Aggregated Human Ig.

Cohn fraction II human Ig is dissolved in PBS, pH 7.2, with 10% (v/v) carbonate-bicarbonate buffer, 0.5 M, pH 9.0, and the pH is corrected to 9.0 with 10 N NaOH. The final concentration of Ig is 50 mg/ml. Fluorescein isothiocyanate (FITC) is added, and the preparation is stirred at 4°C for 18 hr followed by exhaustive dialysis with PBS, pH 7.2, to remove unconjugated FITC. Different batches of Cohn fraction II human Ig vary in the degree of conjugation obtained with a given quantity of FITC. Generally, preparations with absorption ratios (495 nm/280 nm) between 0.5 and 1.0 (obtained with 20–40 μg of FITC per milligram of protein) work well for subsequent cell surface immunofluorescence whereas those with absorption ratios less than 0.4 do not.

Aggregation is produced by heating the conjugated Ig in PBS, pH 7.2, at 62°–63°C for 20 min. The preparation is pelleted at 145,000 g for 1 hr at 4°C, and the supernatant is discarded. The pellet (20–25% of the original protein) is homogenized in PBS, pH 8.0, at 50 mg/ml in a 7-ml Dounce homogenizer, the pH is corrected to 8.3 with 0.1 N NaOH, and the aggregates are stored at 4°C until use. Freezing and thawing, lower protein concentrations, and lower pH all tend to precipitate the aggregates and are therefore avoided. Just prior to use the preparation is brought to 23°C and centrifuged at 600 g for 15 min at 23°C. This removes large, insoluble aggregates which cause clumping of cells in the assay. The aggregates are adjusted to appropriate concentrations (see below) with PBS, pH 8.0, 23°C.

3.2. Preparation of Affinity-Purified Rabbit IgG Anti-TNP. Rabbits are hyperimmunized with heavily substituted TNP–KLH prepared similarly to TNP–BSA (see below). The course of immunization and purification of antibody are followed by anti-TNP hemagglutination titers. Indicator cells are prepared by incubation of human erythrocytes (10% by volume) in 1.0 mM TNBS in PBS, pH 7.2, at 37°C for 15 min. The Ig is isolated from the antisera by precipitation with $(NH_4)_2SO_4$ and then affinity-purified on DNP-lysine-coupled Sepharose (16). The specific antibody is eluted from the column with 0.10 M acetic acid and neutralized immediately with Tris. The monomeric IgG is separated from IgM and aggregated IgG by gel filtration on Sephadex G-200. The IgG fraction is concentrated by vacuum dialysis (generally to 1 mg/ml), dialyzed against PBS, pH 7.2, aliquoted, and stored at −20°C. F(ab')$_2$ fragments are prepared by pepsin digestion and chromatography on G-200 (17). The F(ab')$_2$ preparations have a hemagglutination titer very similar to that of the intact antibody, but are unable to lyse TNP-red blood cells in the presence of complement and do not react with antirabbit Fc antibodies in Ouchterlony double diffusion.

3.3. Preparation of TNP$_{16}$ BSA. BSA (100 mg, 1.47 μmoles) is dissolved in 10 ml of 0.1 M borate buffer, pH 9.0, and to this is added 2.35 ml of 10 mM TNBS (23.5 μmoles) in PBS, pH 7.2. The solution is mixed well, incubated at 37°C for 1 hr, and then dialyzed overnight against PBS, pH 7.2. The degree of conjugation finally achieved is determined by spectroscopy.*

3.4. Preparation of TNP–Anti-TNP Complexes. A precipitin curve is used to establish the equivalence point for each batch of antigen and antibody. A fixed amount of antibody (e.g., 100 μl of 1 mg/ml) is mixed with various amounts of antigen (e.g., 0.3–30.0 μg) in a fixed volume (e.g., 200 μl). The mixture is incubated for 1 hr at 37°C and then overnight at 4°C. The precipitates are then washed 3 times with cold PBS pH 7.2 in a cold centrifuge at 600 $g \times$ 15 min, and finally resuspended in a constant volume of PBS. The protein precipitate is quantified by a Lowry determination. A typical equivalence point using TNP$_{16}$ BSA and affinity purified IgG is 10 μg antibody to 0.3 μg antigen. The ratio may vary with the degree of conjugation of the antigen and the particular

*The following spectroscopic constants are used: for TNP, ϵ_{360}=1.50× 10^4, ϵ_{280}=3.95× 10^5; for BSA, ϵ_{360}=0, ϵ_{280}=1.09× 10^5. The molar concentrations of TNP and BSA are calculated from the absorptions at 360 nm and 280 nm. That is [TNP] = A_{360}/1.50× 10^4 and [BSA] = $[A_{280} - (A_{360}/0.263)]$ (1.09× 10^5). The degree of conjugation is given by the ratio [TNP]/ [BSA].

preparation of antibody. Complexes are prepared fresh daily by mixing antigen and antibody at 4-fold antigen excess, which provides easily detectable and completely soluble complexes. Antigen and antibody are incubated at 23°C for at least 1 hr.

3.5. Preparation of Fl-Goat Anti-rabbit IgG. To remove any cross-reacting antibodies, the commercial Fl-goat antirabbit IgG is absorbed with an appropriate solid-phase immunoabsorbent: i.e., for use with mouse cells, Sepharose-coupled normal mouse ascites or mouse Ig; for use with human cells, Sepharose-coupled Cohn fraction II Ig. Subsequently, the reagent is titered against a fixed number of lymphocytes which have bound complexes (see below) to determine the maximum percentage of cells which can be stained (plateau value). Four times the concentration of conjugate required to reproduce the plateau value is used in subsequent tests (1:16 dilution). The reagent is routinely deaggregated by preparative ultracentrifugation immediately before use (5).

3.6. Preparation of Lymphocytes. Mononuclear cells from different species are isolated from peripheral blood or from single-cell suspensions of spleen, lymph node, or thymus by density centrifugation as described by Böyum (18) and washed 3 times with large volumes of PBS, pH 7.2. In the case of peripheral blood, monocytes (which constitute up to 30% of the mononuclear cells and which bear Fc receptors) are either removed by adherence to loosely packed nyion fiber columns or allowed to phagocytize polystyrene beads, or both (5). For use in the assays, the lymphocytes are suspended at 20×10^6/ml in BSA–PBS, pH 8.0 for aggregates, or pH 7.2 for antigen–antibody complexes. The Na azide minimizes shedding and/or movement of receptors, and the presence of protein improves reproducibility.

3.7. Lymphocyte Binding of Aggregated Ig. Lymphocytes and FITC-conjugated, heat-aggregated Ig (25 or 50 μl of each) are mixed and incubated at 23°C for 30 min. The cells are then washed 3 times with 10–20 volume excess of BSA–PBS and vigorously resuspended (to prevent clumping) in the same medium at the original concentration; wet mounts are prepared. Each lymphocyte preparation is tested with several concentrations of the aggregates to determine what concentration is necessary to obtain plateau values for the percentage of positive cells. This concentration (usually 1–8 mg/ml) varies, owing apparently to the number and avidity of aggregate-binding cells in any particular population and to the extent to which aggregates have been lost (secondary to insolubilization during storage). Binding of aggregates at pH 8.0 and 23°C produces a relatively uniform staining pattern, with small aggregates distributed over the entire cell surface. This is in contrast to the clumpy pattern of binding obtained at pH 7.2 and 4°C as first described (2). The clumpy pattern is apparently due to the formation of larger aggregates at lower temperature and pH.

3.8. Lymphocyte Binding of Antigen-Complexed Ig. Lymphocytes (25 μl) and complexes (100 μl) are mixed and incubated at 23°C for 30 min. Different concentrations of complexes are required to detect receptors on different subpopulations (see below). The cells are then washed 3 times with 10–20 volume excess of BSA–PBS pH 7.2 and resuspended in 25 μl. The working dilution of Fl-goat anti-rabbit IgG (25 μl) is added, and the cells are incubated at 4°C for 30 min. They are then washed 3 times and resuspended in 25 μl, and wet mounts are prepared. Under these conditions, the binding of complexes produces a relatively uniform punctate staining pattern, with small complexes distributed over the entire cell surface. There has been no difficulty with cell clumping over a wide range of concentrations of complexes.

3.9. Microscopy. Microscopic fields are read alternately under phase and fluorescent illumination for the percentage of fluorescent-positive lymphocytes. A cell showing 3 or more fluorescent spots is considered positive. Only cells that appeared to be lymphocytes by morphological criteria (and in the case of peripheral blood, cells that had neither phagocytized nor had adherent polystyrene beads) are counted. A minimum of 200 lymphocytes are counted per preparation.

4. Interpretation of Data and Critical Comments

4.1. Lymphocyte Subpopulations Bearing Fc Receptors. In the initial detection of murine lymphocyte Fc receptors with radiolabeled antigen–antibody complexes and short-term radioautography, Basten *et al.* (1) demonstrated in several cell populations that the Fc-receptor-bearing cells correlated very highly with B cells but not T cells. In the case of aggregated Ig, double-labeling experiments with mouse splenocytes showed that the Ig-staining (i.e., B cell) and the aggregate-binding populations are essentially overlapping (19). Studies with normal human peripheral blood lymphocytes similarly showed that the subpopulation that stains with polyvalent anti-Ig whole antibody is virtually identical to that which binds aggregated Ig (2). Further, only a small subpopulation (mean: 3.0%; range: 1–4%) binds aggregates and forms spontaneous sheep erythrocyte rosettes, generally accepted as a T cell marker (11). In normal members of all other species tested (i.e., monkey, rat, and guinea pig), there are also lymphocytes that show binding of aggregated human Ig and correspond in number to those detected by polyvalent anti-Ig (19). However, recent studies from several laboratories have provided evidence that among the normal human peripheral lymphocytes which stain with polyvalent anti-Ig whole antibody, there is a subpopulation whose Ig staining is due to the labile, secondary uptake of IgG—that is, these cells lack stable membrane Ig (IgM or IgD) (20, 21). These are probably the same cells described earlier by Frøland and Natvig (8). The exact relationship of these Fc receptor-positive, stable membrane Ig-negative, non-T peripheral lymphocytes to traditionally defined T and B cells and their role(s) in the immune system are not totally clear. Nevertheless, it can be inferred from the data (2, 20) that fluorescein-conjugated heat-aggregated human Ig detects the Fc receptors of these lymphocytes as well as those of true B lymphocytes.

Fc receptors have been demonstrated on a subpopulation of normal mouse T lymphocytes by techniques with increased sensitivity, such as long-term radio-autography (22, 23) and the fluorescence-activated cell sorter (6). Using indirect immunofluorescence to detect binding of soluble antigen–antibody complexes, we have observed Fc specific binding to approximately 10–20% of murine thymocytes and up to 80% of murine splenocytes (Fig. 1, Table 1). In titrating the amount of complexed antibody incubated with a constant number of cells in a constant volume, two plateaus were observed. On the plateau obtained with high concentrations (200–800 μg Ig/ml), the Fc receptors on both T and B cells were detected; on the lower concentration plateau (10–50 μg Ig/ml), the Fc receptors of only B cells were detected. The binding of complexes to splenic T cells was confirmed in a double-labeling experiment using anti-θ serum as a T cell marker (Table 2). Further evidence that increased sensitivity is required to detect the Fc receptors of normal T cells was provided by experiments which showed that the binding of aggregated Ig to murine T lymphocytes could be detected by indirect, but not by direct, fluorescent techniques (H. B. Dickler, unpublished observation).

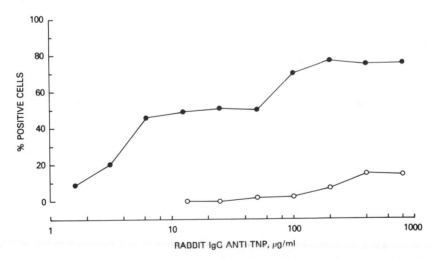

Fig. 1. Percentage of lymphocytes from spleen (●) or thymus (○) that bound various concentrations of TNP–BSA–anti-TNP complexes. The percentage of B lymphocytes as assessed by surface Ig staining was 50.0% in the spleen and <0.5% in the thymus. This experiment is representative of several that were performed.

TABLE 1

Indirect Fluorescent Detection of the Binding of
Antigen–Antibody Complexes to Murine
Lymphocytes: Dependence on the Fc Portion
of the Antibody

| | % Positive Cells | |
Preparation[a]	Expt. 1 spleen	Expt. 2 thymus
TNP–BSA–anti-TNP IgG	80.5	19.5
TNP–BSA–anti-TNP F(ab')$_2$	3.0	0.5

[a]The concentrations [1.4 mg/ml for IgG and 1.0
mg/ml for F(ab')$_2$] were chosen so as to be approximately equivalent in numbers of molecules. Binding
was detected with Fl-goat anti-rabbit IgG (see Section
3).

It is not completely clear why the Fc receptors of normal T cells are detected
only by methods of apparently greater sensitivity. There may be fewer Fc
receptors on T cells; they may have a lower affinity for complexed Ig; or they
may have significant affinity only for a particular subpopulation of complexed
Ig molecules.

The stimulation of T lymphocytes by alloantigens (22) or protein antigen (24)
has been shown to increase the size and ease of detection of the Fc receptor-
positive subpopulation. Further, antigen–antibody complexes inhibit the response of T cells to the mitrogen conconavalin A (25, 26). The Fc receptor-
positive T cell population appears to be primarily responsible for the response to
this mitogen (26), as well as for the generation of cytotoxic effector cells (27).
Such observations have led to the suggestion that those T cells with Fc receptors
have a particular role in the regulation of the immune responses (26).

4.2. The Specificity of the Fc Receptors. The binding of heat-aggregated
human Ig to human peripheral blood lymphocytes is quite stable and is not
dependent on complement, pH (6.0–8.2), temperature (4°, 23°, and 37°C),
protein content of the medium, or the divalent cations Ca^{2+} and Mg^{2+} (2). The
binding of noncomplexed Ig has not been detected by direct fluorescence or by
inhibition of aggregate binding (2, 5, 9). However, other studies using techniques
which may have been more sensitive have suggested that monomeric Ig may bind
in small quantities and/or with low affinity (1, 28). Lymphocytes do not bind
aggregates of human serum albumin, bovine serum albumin, or human trans-
ferrin (5). Aggregated Ig which lacks the Fc portion of the molecule, i.e.,
F(ab')$_2$, also does not bind (5). Similarly, the binding of antigen–antibody

TABLE 2
Double Labeling of Murine Splenic Lymphocytes[a] with Anti-θ and Antigen–Antibody Complexes

	Incubation No.			% Positive cells			
1	2	3	4	Only Rho[d]	Only Fl[d]	Both	Neither
Anti-theta[b]	Fl–goat anti-γG_2[b]	Medium	Medium	0	34.0	0	66.0
Medium	Medium	TNP–BSA rabbit anti-TNP[c]	Rho-goat anti-rabbit IgG	74.0	0	0	26.0
Anti-theta	Fl–goat anti-γG_2	TNP–BSA rabbit anti-TNP[c]	Rho-goat anti-rabbit IgG	57.0	16.0	16.5	10.5

[a] From a B10 mouse. Percentage of surface Ig positive lymphocytes was 51.0%.
[b] Anti-θ (AKR anti-C3H) and Fl–goat anti-γG_2 were a kind gift of Dr. Richard Asofsky, NIH.
[c] 400 μg/ml antibody.
[d] Fl, fluorescein isothiocyanate; Rho, tetramethylrhodamine isothiocyanate.

complexes is dependent on the presence of the appropriate antigen and antibody combination and on the presence of the Fc portion of the antibody (1, 3, 4, 6, 22) (Table 1). Finally, lymphocyte binding of aggregated Ig is inhibited by antigen–antibody complexes (but not by either antigen or antibody alone) and vice versa (5, 9, 10). Taken together these findings indicate that the binding is specifically dependent on an intact Fc portion of complexed Ig and that the same receptors bind heat-aggregated Ig and antigen–antibody complexes.

Studies with protein antigen–antibody complexes and aggregated Ig have suggested that Fc receptors have specificity for certain classes and subclasses of Ig. Murine B cells have been shown to bind IgG1 and IgG2b. IgM was bound less well, and no binding of IgA or IgG2a was observed (4). Normal mouse T cells bound IgG1 and IgG2b but not IgA (22). Human peripheral blood lymphocytes have been reported to bind all subclasses of complexed IgG as well as IgE, but not IgM, IgA, or IgD (28). Each of these studies is subject to limitations on the interpretation of the data, and further experiments are needed to clarify the question of class and subclass specificity.

In contrast, Fc receptors show relatively little species specificity. Thus, murine B-cell Fc receptors bind mouse, rabbit, and human Ig (1, 9, 10). There are conflicting data in the case of chicken Ig (1, 22). There is evidence that human peripheral lymphocytes bind human, monkey, and rabbit Ig, but not goat, sheep, or mouse Ig (5, 7). There are recent data that human peripheral lymphocytes with labile surface Ig will bind heat-aggregated guinea pig Ig, whereas those cells with stable membrane Ig (true B cells) will not (D. A. Horwitz, personal communication). The lymphocytes of several other species bind human Ig (19).

4.3. The Nature of Fc Receptors and Their Relationship to Other Surface Molecules. The Fc receptors of human peripheral blood lymphocytes were found to be pronase sensitive, which suggested that they were at least partially proteins (5). In addition, they were found to be distinct from endogenous membrane Ig, C3 receptors, and, in the mouse, from alloantigens determined by the K and D regions of the H-2 major histocompatibility complex [reviewed by Dickler (19)]. Recently, a glycoprotein (MW 65,000) that binds to aggregated Ig was isolated from murine B lymphocytes (29). Similarly, a factor that binds to Ig has been isolated from murine T lymphocytes (30). The relationship of these entities to Fc receptors remains to be definitively established.

Relationships between Fc receptors and certain other membrane molecules appear to exist. Thus, endogenous membrane Ig, when cross-linked by a ligand (anti-Ig), appears to associate with many, but not all, B cell Fc receptors as evidenced by cocapping (31, 32). It has been suggested that this association may have functional significance (31).

As mentioned earlier (see above), antibodies against Ia antigens, but not antibodies against other surface components, inhibit the binding of aggregated Ig to murine B lymphocytes. While this finding could have indicated that Fc receptors and Ia antigens were identical, other evidence suggests that at least some Ia antigens are distinct from Fc receptors (29, 32). Regardless of whether Ia antigens and Fc receptors are identical or separate but associated molecules, it has been suggested that this relationship is important in the regulation of the immune response (33).

4.4. Conclusions. In considering the relative advantages of the two methods described here, it should be noted that there is considerable experience with fluorescein-conjugated heat-aggregated human Ig indicating that under the conditions used it binds primarily to the Fc receptors of the B lymphocytes of several species. It is a direct assay involving only one readily prepared reagent. On the other hand, the aggregates tend to precipitate on storage, requiring frequent titration of the reagent for optimal binding and relatively frequent preparation of fresh aggregates. The use of antigen—antibody complexes requires the preparation of several specific reagents. However, these reagents are stable on storage and the formation of fresh complexes is highly reproducible. The system is, moreover, easily titrated for the detection of particular subpopulations of Fc receptor-bearing lymphocytes. Finally, the hapten-specific antibody can also be used to prepare complexes immobilized on plastic, a system that has proved to be useful in lymphocyte separation and in the study of the role of Fc receptor-bearing cells in mitogenesis.

In conclusion, it should be stressed that, whatever technique is used, it must be carefully characterized. The *sine qua non* is the formal demonstration of the Fc dependence of binding by a negative control using the $F(ab')_2$ from the same Ig preparation as that used in the assay. Further, it is important to titrate the system over a wide range of Ig concentrations and correlate the subpopulation(s) detected with other known lymphocyte markers.

REFERENCES

1. Basten, A., Miller, J. F. A. P., Sprent, J., and Pye, J., *J. Exp. Med.* **135**, 610 (1972).
2. Dickler, H. B., and Kunkel, H. G., *J. Exp. Med.* **136**, 191 (1972).
3. Paraskevas, F., Lee, S.-T., Orr, K. B., and Israels, L. G., *J. Immunol.* **108**, 1319 (1972).
4. Basten, A., Warner, N. L., and Mandel, T., *J. Exp. Med.* **135**, 627 (1972).
5. Dickler, H. B., *J. Exp. Med.* **140**, 508 (1974).
6. Stout, R. D., and Herzenberg, L. A., *J. Exp. Med.* **142**, 611 (1975).
7. Henkart, P. A., and Alexander, E. A., manuscript submitted for publication.
8. Frøland, S. S., and Natvig, J. B., *Transplant. Rev.* **16**, 114 (1973).
9. Dickler, H. B., and Sachs, D. H., *J. Exp. Med.* **140**, 779 (1974).
10. Basten, A., Miller, J. F. A. P., and Abraham, R., *J. Exp. Med.* **141**, 547 (1975).
11. Dickler, H. B., Adkinson, N. F., and Terry, W. D., *Nature (London)* **247**, 213 (1974).
12. Theofilopoulos, A. N., Dixon, F. J., and Bokisch, V. A., *J. Exp. Med.* **140**, 877 (1974).
13. Dickler, H. B., Siegal, F. P., Bentwich, Z. H., and Kunkel, H. G., *Clin. Exp. Immunol.* **14**, 97 (1973).
14. Dickler, H. B., Adkinson, N. F., Fisher, R. I., and Terry, W. D., *J. Clin. Invest.* **53**, 834 (1974).

15. Arbeit, R. D., Sachs, D. H., Amos, B. D., and Dickler, H. B., *J. Immunol.* **115**, 1173 (1975).
16. Robbins, J. B., Haimovitch, J., and Sela, M., *Immunochemistry* **4**, 11 (1967).
17. Nisonoff, A., Wissler, F. C., Lipman, L. N., and Woernley, D. L., *Arch. Biochem. Biophys.* **89**, 230 (1960).
18. Böyum, A., *Scand. J. Clin. Lab. Invest.* **21**, Suppl. 97, 77 (1968).
19. Dickler, H. B., *Scand. J. Immunol.* in press (1976).
20. Winchester, R. J., Fu, S. M., Hoffman, T., and Kunkel, H. G., *J. Immunol.* **114**, 1210 (1975).
21. Lobo, P., Wistervelt, F. B., and Horwitz, D. A., *J. Immunol.* **114**, 116 (1975).
22. Anderson, C. L., and Grey. H. M., *J. Exp. Med.* **139**, 1175 (1974).
23. Basten, A., Miller, J. F. A. P., Warner, N. L., Abraham, R., Chia, E., and Gamble, J., *J. Immunol.* **115**, 1159 (1975).
24. Van Boxel, J. A., and Rosenstreich, D. L., *J. Exp. Med.* **139**, 1002 (1974).
25. Ryan, J. L., Arbeit, R. A., Dickler, H. B., and Henkart, P. A., *J. Exp. Med.* **142**, 814 (1975).
26. Stout, R. D., and Herzenberg, L. A., *J. Exp. Med.* **142**, 1041 (1975).
27. Stout, R. D., Waksal, S. D., and Herzenberg, L. A., manuscript submitted for publication.
28. Lawrence, D. A., Weigle, W. O., and Spiegelberg, H. L., *J. Clin. Invest.* **55**, 368 (1975).
29. Rask, L., Klareskog, L., Ostberg, L., and Peterson, P. A., *Nature (London)* **257**, 231 (1975).
30. Fridman, W. H., and Golstein, P., *Cell Immunol.* **11**, 442 (1974).
31. Forni, L., and Pernis, B., *in* "Membrane Receptors of Lymphocytes" (M. Seligmann, J. L. Preud'homme, and F. M. Kourilsky, eds.), p. 193. North-Holland Publ., Amsterdam, 1975.
32. Abbas, A. K., and Unanue, E. R., *J. Immunol.* **115**, 1665 (1975).
33. Sachs, D. H., and Dickler, H. B., *Transplant. Rev.* **23**, 159 (1975).

9

Detection of Surface Immunoglobulins on Human Cells by Direct Immunofluorescence*

J. L. Preud'homme and S. Labaume

1. Introduction

The recent availability of various functional and antigenic lymphocyte surface markers has led to a large number of studies of human lymphocytes in health and disease. These studies, aiming at characterizing and categorizing B and T cells, have been undoubtedly rewarding and provided new insights into the pathogenesis of various diseases, as well as data useful for a better understanding of some basic aspects of the immune response (see 1–3). Surface immunoglobulins (S.Ig), as defined as readily demonstrable surface-membrane Ig that are actual products synthesized by the cells which carry them, occupy a prominent situation among the lymphocyte markers. Indeed, although a few immature B cells and some plasma cells may lack S.Ig, the presence of S.Ig constitutes the current operational definition of B cells and the other B and T markers have been considered in relation to S.Ig (4). In addition, when studied using mono-specific reagents to the various immunoglobulin (Ig) chains and eventually idio-typic antisera, S.Ig have the advantage of constituting a clonal marker in certain conditions. The study of S.Ig therefore resulted in the development of new concepts, such as those of homogeneous populations of proliferating monoclonal B cells and of maturation arrests at various steps of the differentiation pathway of the B cell line.

These considerations and the convenience of S.Ig detection by immunocyto-chemical methods, such as surface immunofluorescence (IF), explain the wide use of such techniques and their introduction into routine laboratory work. One may expect in the near future that only few patients affected with any kind of disease will escape enumeration of their blood B and T lymphocytes; and the literature already contains controversial results and some rather poor or bizarre data. There are indeed in S.Ig detection a number of causes of erroneous interpretation, and sufficient attention has not always been paid to the necessary

*This work was supported by INSERM (Grants Nos. 73.16.17 and 10.74.31.3), D.G.R.S.T. (Grant No. 71.7.3065), and CNRS (E.R.A. 239).

characteristics and controls of anti-Ig reagents (4, 5). We report here the methods used in our laboratory and emphasize the pitfalls we have encountered and the need for a critical evaluation of the results.

2. Materials

IF tests for the detection of plasma membrane molecules are based upon vital staining of living cells in suspension by properly controlled conjugates.

2.1. Anti-immunoglobulin Conjugates. Three main steps are involved in the preparation of anti-immunoglobulin reagents: selection and absorption of antisera, their conjugation to fluorochromes, and controls of their monospecificity.

Rabbits were immunized by normal polyclonal IgG obtained from pooled normal sera or commercial fraction II by diethylaminoethyl-cellulose chromatography (DEAE,Whatman Biochem. Ltd., Maidstone, Kent, United Kingdom), by myeloma proteins of the four main classes prepared by a combination of Pevikon (Pevikon C 870, Stockholm Superfosfat, Sweden) block electrophoresis (6), DEAE-cellulose chromatography and gel filtration, by heavy chains purified from normal IgG and monoclonal Ig or by κ and λ light chains prepared from urinary Bence-Jones proteins and from myeloma proteins.

Because we wanted conjugates usable at a low protein concentration and at a relatively low conjugation ratio, these antisera were carefully selected to obtain sera that reacted strongly with various determinants of S.Ig accessible to immunofluorescent staining. The carboxyterminal part of the Fc fragment of S.Ig is not accessible to conjugated antibodies (7–9). Anti-heavy-chain sera were hence tested by gel double-diffusion experiments with whole Ig and Ig chains and fragments in order to select sera reactive not only with the Fc fragment of heavy chain, but also with nonidiotypic determinants located on the Fd segment of Ig molecules or conformational determinants resulting from the association of one given heavy chain to light chains. The antisera to κ or λ light chains were studied to choose those that gave precipitation reactions as well with Bence-Jones proteins as with monoclonal IgG, IgA, and IgM of the same light-chain type. To obtain sera showing a reactivity as broad as possible within each given specificity, several sera of the same class or type specificity and obtained from rabbits immunized with different Ig molecules were pooled.

These pooled sera were made monospecific by adsorption of contaminant antibodies on the suitable antigens coupled to solid immunoadsorbents. We first used coupling of antigens to Sepharose 4B (10), then we preferred coupling to Sepharose 2B after activation with high concentrations of cyanogen bromide, according to Metzger (11), because of higher coupling capacity and antigenic efficiency: Sepharose (Pharmacia Fine Chemicals, Uppsala, Sweden) washed with distilled water was resuspended in an equal volume of water. After the pH was adjusted at 11 with 4 N NaOH, Sepharose was activated by the addition of

300 mg of settled Sepharose of cyanogen bromide per milliliter previously dissolved in distilled water. The pH was kept between 10 and 11 by adding 4 N NaOH, and the temperature below 30°C with ice. When the pH was stable or after the reaction had proceeded for 12–15 min, the activated Sepharose was rapidly washed (less than 90 sec) with ice-cold 0.1 N NaHCO$_3$ pH 8.5–8.7 (0.5–1 liter of bicarbonate for each 10 ml of Sepharose). The mixture of the antigen (5–10 mg/ml of Sepharose) and Sepharose in bicarbonate was incubated at 4°C for 16–18 hr with gentle stirring, then extensively washed with borate buffer (0.2 M borate, 0.15 M in NaCl pH 8.0) or phosphate-buffered saline (PBS:0.01 M sodium phosphate, 0.15 M in NaCl pH 7.2), then 0.5 N acetic acid and neutral buffer again. Eventual residual free sites on Sepharose were inactivated by 0.5 M ethanolamine in 0.1 M sodium bicarbonate buffer pH 9.0 (12).

In addition to the antigens that corresponded to the contaminant antibodies detected by Ouchterlony experiments, the immune sera were usually adsorbed on agammaglobulinemic serum and on Ig other than those that corresponded to the specificity of the sera. After specificity controls, the IgG fractions of these sera were purified by ammonium sulfate precipitation and DEAE-cellulose chromatography in 0.0175 M sodium phosphate buffer pH 7.5 with stepwise elution using the same buffer, successively without sodium chloride and 0.05 M and 0.1 M in NaCl. Highly purified IgG are necessary for vital IF to avoid nonspecific staining (which occurs with conjugated ammonium sulfate precipitates, for instance). As discussed in a later section, the use of whole IgG antibodies as anti-Ig reagents in surface IF may result in nonspecific staining due to binding to the strong-affinity IgG Fc receptor of certain cells, and it is safer to utilize F(ab')$_2$ fragments instead of whole IgG (13). We therefore use now F(ab')$_2$ fragments, prepared by hydrolysis with pepsin (14) followed by gel filtration on Sephadex G-200.

The IgG fractions of the antisera or their F(ab')$_2$ fragments were conjugated to fluorescein isothiocyanate (FITC) or tetramethylrhodamine isothiocyanate (TRITC). FITC conjugates are easily obtained by usual methods (15) whereas conjugation to TRITC is more difficult. However, TRITC conjugates are more valuable than FITC-coupled reagents for surface IF because of their much higher sensitivity and virtually negligible fading. The conjugation method we used was derived from those of Clark and Shepard (16) and Amante et al. (17) with modifications (18). We have chosen this procedure, rather expensive with fluorochrome, because it was the only one that regularly gave us a high yield (around 80%) in conjugates with the wanted conjugation ratio; however, other methods are satisfactory (17, 19). We had first to select a fairly soluble batch of TRITC. Several batches had to be checked before finding one satisfactory lot (Lot 1051345, Baltimore Biological Laboratories, Baltimore, Maryland). The IgG fractions of the immune sera, adjusted at a concentration of 10 mg/ml, were dialyzed for 4–6 hr against three changes of 0.05 M sodium carbonate–

bicarbonate buffer pH 9.5 and for 24 hr at 4°C with permanent stirring a volume of the same buffer equal to 10 times the volume of the IgG solution and containing 0.1 mg of TRITC per milliliter. After passage through a Sephadex G-50 column in 0.0175 M phosphate buffer pH 7.5, 0.05 M in NaCl (or extensive dialysis against this buffer), the conjugates were applied on DEAE-cellulose columns equilibrated in the same buffer. Stepwise elution was performed with increasing NaCl molarity (0.05, 0.1, 0.2, and 0.3 M) to select fractions with an optical density (OD) ratio between 2 and 3 ($OD_{280\ nm}$) $\times$ (protein)/$OD_{515\ nm}$ (TRITC). Their protein concentration was calculated according to the following formula (20).

$$\text{Protein (mg/ml)} = \frac{OD_{280\ nm} - 0.56\,(OD_{515\ nm})}{1.4}$$

These fractions were concentrated by negative pressure and dialyzed against PBS. Working dilutions of the conjugates were determined by dilution experiments with normal lymphocytes. In these experiments, a plateau was observed, then the percentage of positive cells decreased with increasing dilutions of the conjugates. A concentration 2 or 3 times higher than the last point of the plateau was chosen, usually 0.4–1 mg of IgG per milliliter. The specificity of these conjugates was carefully assessed, as will be described later. When contaminating antibodies were detected, further adsorptions on Sepharose-coupled antigens were performed.

The conjugates were made 0.2% in sodium azide (except for aliquots to be used for capping experiments, which were sterilized by membrane filtration) and stored frozen. In order to avoid nonspecific staining due to the presence of IgG aggregates, the conjugates were stored at protein concentrations greater than 5 mg/ml in small aliquots to be thawed only once. They were subjected to high speed centrifugation in a Beckman Microfuge centrifuge before every use. It is also recommended to ultracentrifuge them (150,000 g for 30 min) before storage (4).

2.2. Cells. Peripheral blood was obtained by defibrination on glass beads rather than by heparinization, because heparin may cause some degree of nonspecific staining. In addition, defibrination removes platelets that are stained by anti-Ig conjugates. Mononuclear cells were isolated by Ficoll–Triosil centrifugation (21, 22). The technical problems raised by this latter procedure are considered by Aiuti et al. (4). It must be stressed that Ficoll centrifugation removes most red cells and polymorphonuclear leukocytes whereas it leads to an enrichment in monocytes. In our experience, Ficoll preparations from normal bloods contained a mean of about 15% monocytes (23), but values as high as 50% or more are common in certain disease, such as immunodeficiency states. In marked hyperlymphocytosis (as in patients with chronic lymphocytic leukemia), a simple sedimentation led to reasonably pure lymphocyte suspensions: the mixture of 1 volume of 2.5% pig skin gelatin (Plasmagel, Roger Bellon, Paris, France) and 2 volumes of blood were allowed to sediment for 30 min at 37°C to obtain a supernatant free of red cells.

The same Plasmagel sedimentation procedure was used for the separation of nucleated bone marrow cells. Indeed, we were unable to separate marrow lymphoid cells from the other nucleated cells by Ficoll centrifugation. Lymph node or spleen cells were processed by gentle teasing of small fragments, followed by filtration through stainless steel gauze.

The cell suspensions were washed three times in Hanks' balanced salt solution that contained bovine serum albumin at 5 g/100 ml (Hanks'–BSA), and adjusted at a concentration of 10–20 X 10^6 cells/ml. Eagle's minimal essential medium (MEM) supplemented with 20% heat-inactivated fetal calf serum (FCS) was used instead of Hanks'–BSA when short-term culture experiments were performed.

3. Methods

3.1. Immunofluorescence Procedures. Surface immunoglobulins were detected by direct IF using monospecific sera to the four heavy-chain classes and the two light-chain types. Other experiments, such as double staining, are of interest in certain situations.

3.1.1. Usual Membrane Immunofluorescence. Surface staining was performed according to Pernis *et al.* (7) with minor modifications. A volume (0.05 ml) of cell suspension was incubated with the same volume of conjugate at the proper dilution for 30 min in an ice bath in the presence of 0.1% sodium azide (which did not need addition of azide since the conjugates contained 0.2% azide) to reduce pinocytosis and was washed 3 times at 4°C in 0.01 M phosphate buffer pH 7.2, 0.15 M in NaCl, that contained 5 g/100 ml bovine serum albumin (PBS–BSA). After the last washing, the cell pellet was resuspended in one drop of PBS–BSA. At that stage, the cells may be examined in suspension: one droplet is put on a slide, covered with a cover slip that is sealed with nail polish, and viewed immediately. However, we gave up this type of examination several years ago, and we systematically studied the stained cells after they were postfixed: one droplet of the cell suspension was spread on a slide using the bottom of a small test tube to form a small circle about 1 cm in diameter and let dry on the bench. (In our hands, this method was more satisfactory than the use of a cytocentrifuge.) The slides were fixed for 5 min in absolute ethanol, quickly washed in three changes of PBS, and mounted in buffered glycerol. This postfixation procedure increases the IF brightness. For instance, in several patients with chronic lymphocytic leukemia where the IF staining is often faint (24), lymphocytes, which apparently lacked S.Ig when examined in suspension, exhibited an obvious positivity for one heavy and one light chain when studied by this postfixation procedure. In addition, after the cover slips are sealed with nail polish, the slides may be kept at 4 °C for weeks or months for further examination. Using a different postfixation, the cells may be stained for endogenous peroxidase as described in Section 4.2. in order to identify monocytes. Postfixation may be also the first step of restaining for cytoplasmic Ig.

3.1.2. Double Labeling for Surface and Intracellular Ig. The simultaneous study of surface and intracellular Ig is often of interest and is easy to perform (25). After vital staining with a TRITC-coupled antiserum and ethanol postfixation, as described above, the slides were overlaid with a FITC conjugate (of the same or of another specificity), incubated for 30 min at room temperature in a moist chamber, washed in PBS, and mounted in buffered glycerol. Alternative illumination with filter combinations specific for each fluorochrome allows an easy comparison of Ig in and on the same cells.

3.1.3. Double Staining of S.Ig. Double labeling of surface molecules was performed by incubating the cells in the cold with a mixture of FITC and TRITC conjugates. Double labeling was also commonly performed in combination with antibody-induced redistribution. Indeed, a polar redistribution of human lymphocyte S.Ig (capping) is induced by anti-Ig antibodies at 37°C (26). The capping of one given surface determinant does not affect the surface distribution of independent molecules, which remains diffuse, and experiments that combine capping and double staining are very useful for studying molecular relationships between surface antigens (26, 27). The lymphocytes stained in the cold with a first conjugate in the absence of sodium azide were incubated for 45–60 min at 37°C to induce capping, then cooled down at 0°C, and labeled again in noncapping conditions with a second antiserum coupled to the opposite fluorochrome (26). Such experiments are often crucial when checking the specificity of conjugates (see below).

3.1.4. Indirect Staining. Indirect IF, more sensitive and less safe than direct staining, is definitely not recommended for S.Ig detection (4). We used sandwich techniques very seldom, mainly in some control experiments mentioned below and in the study of a few patients with lymphoproliferative diseases whose lymphocytes bore a monoclonal S.Ig in small amounts not detectable by direct staining. The second layer in these experiments was TRITC-conjugated sheep IgG anti-rabbit IgG. This reagent was adsorbed with human cells. It must be stressed that, at the level of sensitivity of membrane IF, these sheep antibodies to rabbit IgG strongly reacted with human Ig at the lymphocyte surface and had to be adsorbed with insolubilized normal human IgG.

3.1.5. Fluorescence Microscopy. Reflection illumination using an epiilluminator is highly preferable to the much less sensitive conventional transmission illumination system for membrane IF. We used a Leitz Orthoplan microscope equipped with an Osram HBO 200 mercury lamp, a Ploem's Opak-Fluor vertical illuminator (28), and filter combinations specific for each fluorochrome: for rhodamine, excitation filters 4 mm BG 38, 2 mm BG 36 and AL

546, dichroic mirror 580 nm, barrier filter K 550; for fluorescein, excitation filters 5 mm BG 12 and 2 mm BG 12, or 2 mm BG 12 and AL 470, dichroic mirror 495 nm and secondary filter K 495. More recently available filters and new vertical illuminators with easily interchangeable blocks containing complete sets of primary and secondary filters appear to be more convenient (29).

3.2. Demonstration of S.Ig Synthesis. The actual synthesis of S.Ig by the cells that carry them may be proved in IF experiments. The principle of such studies is to denude the cell surface of existing immunoglobulin molecules by exposing cells to proteolytic enzymes, such as trypsin (30, 31) or pronase (32), or to anti-Ig antibodies (since, after capping, S.Ig–anti-Ig complexes disappear from the cell surface owing to pinocytosis and shedding (31), then to incubate the cell *in vitro* long enough to allow S.Ig resynthesis to occur and to stain the regrown S.Ig, with proper controls. In our experience, the most effective system for removing S.Ig was the combination of trypsinization and capping as follows (31): The cells were stained at $0°C$ with the anti-Ig conjugates (which of course did not contain azide) and washed in the cold with MEM–20% FCS, the medium used throughout the experiment. After three washings, aliquots were examined by IF. The remaining cells were incubated for 30 min at $37°C$ in prewarmed culture medium where 2.5 mg/ml of twice-crystallized trypsin (Nutritional Biochemical Corp., Cleveland, Ohio) were added extemporaneously. This very high trypsin concentration was needed by the paradoxical presence of proteins from the calf serum in the medium. The reason for it is that, when trypsinizing leukemic cells, the cell survival was poor when FCS was not present in all steps. After three further washings, the cells were incubated at $37°C$ for 6–7 hr or overnight, preferably in a CO_2 incubator. The efficiency of the treatment with trypsin was controlled by IF examination of the cells after trypsinization and 1 hr later (with eventual restaining) and at the end of the incubation period. At that time, the cells were restained using the 6 anti-Ig conjugates. In the controls, and although the removal of S.Ig was effective, a small percentage of the cells showed some staining, probably owing to the attachment of Ig or fragments removed from the cell surface and complexed or aggregated. Such experiments yielded clear-cut results in the study of homogeneous populations of proliferating monoclonal B cells (24). However, the interpretation may be not as easy when dealing with relatively small percentages of heterogeneous polyclonal B cells diluted with T lymphocytes, as in normal subjects.

4. Critical Evaluation of S.Ig Detection

A critical examination of the data obtained by S.Ig vital staining is obviously required. Indeed S.Ig detection is reliable only if several pitfalls and possible errors are eliminated. Several problems must be considered to avoid erroneous interpretations: specificity of the reagents, identification of the IF-positive cells, nonspecific staining and labeling of exogenous Ig attached to, but not synthesized by, the cells.

4.1. Monospecificity of the Conjugates. This point is critical, and some unexpected published results are apparently due to a lack of monospecificity of the anti-Ig conjugates, which are not always properly controlled. The specificity of our antisera was assessed by the following experiments.

Before conjugation, specificity was checked by gel double-diffusion experiments for gross detection of important contaminants. When possible, the concentrations of these contaminating antibodies was assessed by semiquantitative experiments to estimate the amounts of Sepharose-coupled antigens needed for the adsorptions. To avoid conjugation of grossly impure sera, specificity was further checked after adsorption and prior to conjugation by Ouchterlony experiments in the best possible sensitivity conditions (thick gelose, large wells).

After conjugation, specificity controls were performed to detect two types of contaminating antibodies: antibodies reacting with surface antigens other than S.Ig, on the one hand, and antibodies directed against unwanted Ig determinants, on the other hand. Sera from immunized rabbits may contain antibodies that react with lymphocyte surface antigens, such as heterophilic antibodies. The presence in the conjugates of such antibodies detectable by vital staining may be ruled out by negative results of the staining of lymphocytes from immunodeficiency patients who lack circulating B lymphocytes [such as most patients with sex-linked infantile agammaglobulinemia (1)], of T lymphocytes purified from normal blood by filtration through nylon wool (33), and of Sezary cells (known to be of T cell origin) (1). Because we considered this type of control to be very important, we performed these experiments also by the more sensitive indirect staining method with the undiluted unconjugated sera and with an antirabbit IgG conjugate, as described above.

The specificity of the conjugates with respect to Ig chains was assessed by both cytoplasmic and membrane staining. Cytoplasmic IF provides a first necessary control and allows an estimation of the strength of the conjugates. Fixed smears of plasma cell-rich bone marrow cells from patients with myelomas and macroglobulinemias of known classes and types were used to test the conjugates. A panel of monoclonal plasma cells that synthesize the various Ig, including Bence–Jones proteins, is easy to constitute, because marrow smears can be kept (unfixed) frozen for cytoplasmic staining. For this purpose, marrow cells processed as described in Section 2.2 were smeared and air dried. The slides were individually wrapped in aluminum foil and stored at $-80°C$. When needed, the slides were unfrozen, fixed for 5 min in ethanol, rehydrated by washing in three changes of PBS, and incubated with the conjugate. The important point is, when getting the slides out of the freezer, to keep them wrapped while they thaw and to unwrap them only after they have reached the ambient temperature. If not, the atmospheric water vapor condenses on the slides and freezes, and the cells are destroyed by the ice crystals.

Specificity controls by cytoplasmic IF are not sufficient since surface IF is much more sensitive, probably because of the nonspecific background unavoidable in cytoplasmic staining (whereas, with proper conjugates, there is absolutely no background staining in surface IF, so that a very faint specific staining is easily detected). For instance, some of the sera we had used for cytoplasmic IF, and that appeared to be strictly monospecific at this level of sensitivity, revealed obvious contaminants when their specificity was checked by membrane IF. Control experiments by vital staining are therefore crucial. In a first set of controls, we took advantage of the homogeneous populations of lymphocytes bearing monoclonal S.Ig provided by lymphoproliferative diseases. Waldenström's macroglobulinemia represents a monoclonal proliferation of IgM carrying B lymphocytes with persistent differentiation (25), and bone marrow (where almost all lymphocytes belong to the proliferating clone) or blood (mean 50% of lymphocytes bear a monoclonal S.Ig marker) cells provide lymphocytes that carry IgM [and IgD (34)] with a single light chain. IgG- or IgA-bearing cells may be obtained from patients with pleomorphic lymphoid proliferation similar to macroglobulinemia but with serum monoclonal IgG or IgA, because lymphocytes from such patients bear the same Ig chains as the serum monoclonal component (24). Lymphocytes from chronic lymphocytic leukemia patients (which correspond in most instances to a monoclonal B cell proliferation) are also very useful when they have been previously characterized in terms of S.Ig or when the patient's serum contains a monoclonal Ig, because in most such cases the same Ig chains are found at the leukemic lymphocyte surface (24). Although the staining of these cells is often faint, plasma cells from myeloma or plasma cell leukemia patients are usable when they carry detectable monoclonal S.Ig (35). The study of several patients is necessary to test conjugate specificity against cells that bear S.Ig of each heavy-chain class and light-chain type. Purified Ig covalently coupled to Sepharose beads may also be used as substrate for microfluorometric evaluation of conjugate specificity (36).

Experiments that combine double staining and capping on normal and leukemic lymphocytes also represent a critical control. For instance, the finding that a conjugate stains at 0°C the caps induced by a first conjugate provides a strong argument for a cross-reactivity between the two sera. Such experiments are of utmost importance when testing specificity of antisera to μ and δ chains. Because these Ig are often present together but independent of each other on the same normal or leukemic B lymphocytes (37–41), it is crucial to demonstrate that the determinants identified by the anti-μ and anti-δ conjugates migrate independently during the antibody-induced redistribution process. The same kind of experiments may be applied to the comparison of anti-heavy- and anti-light-chain sera on normal lymphocytes, where one must find, in addition to cells with mixed stained caps, cells singly stained by each conjugate. Experiments of this type are also very useful for characterizing the cross-reactivity of impure sera in order to choose the Sepharose-coupled antigens appropriate for further adsorptions.

Following these procedures, we have studied the specificity of numerous conjugates from various commercial sources, in addition to that of our own antisera. With very few exceptions, we have virtually never found truly monospecific conjugates of commercial origin. Many of the commercial sera we have checked were even not specific at the level of sensitivity of cytoplasmic IF. We therefore strongly feel that most presently available commercial conjugates are not usable with confidence for S.Ig detection by membrane staining.

4.2. Identification of IF-Positive Cells. The occasional polymorphonuclear leukocytes that remain after Ficoll centrifugation are easily identified by their staining pattern of large patches, which contrasts with the homogeneously spotty pattern of lymphocytes and by phase microscopy. The homogeneous cytoplasmic staining of dead cells is easily recognized also. Conversely, monocytes represent an important source of potential errors. They bind serum IgG by their Fc receptor and therefore stain with conjugated antisera to γ, κ, and λ Ig chains. In addition, some monocytes are able to bind rabbit IgG used as reagents and react positively in IF tests, regardless of conjugate specificity.

Two approaches may be used to avoid erroneous interpretation due to monocytes: the use of cell suspensions free of monocytes or the identification of monocytic cells. None of the procedures used by us to remove monocytes [filtration through glass or nylon wool or through Sephadex G-10 (42) or incubation with iron carbonyl followed by Ficoll centrifugation (43)] was satisfactory, because they all produced a poor lymphocyte recovery and a selective loss of B cells. Therefore, in agreement with the recommendations of a WHO-sponsored group (4), we did not try to get rid of monocytes but kept separating blood lymphocytes by Ficoll centrifugation, and we tried to identify monocytic cells on the basis of criteria that were more objective than mere morphology under phase-contrast microscopy. Giemsa staining of IF slides cannot be used owing to a strong autofluorescence. We tried, therefore, to combine IF and cytochemical reactions. Esterase staining was employed first, but under UV illumination, it produced a diffuse cell staining that made the specific fluorescence barely visible. Moreover, some lymphocytes displayed some degree of esterase positivity. By contrast, peroxidase (POX) staining was found to be extremely useful (23).

The cells that had been incubated with the conjugates, washed, and smeared (see Section 3.1.1) were fixed for 3 min with an alcoholic solution of benzidine (0.25 g of benzidine + 0.5 g of sodium nitroprussiate per 100 ml of 96% ethanol). This fluid was discarded, then the slides were overlaid with a mixture of 1 volume of the same benzidine solution and 1 volume of a solution of hydrogen peroxide obtained by extemporaneous 1:500 dilution of a stock solution of 3% (11 volumes) H_2O_2 in distilled water, according to Hayhoe et al. (44). After a 5-min incubation, the slides were washed in phosphate buffer 1/15 M pH 7 and mounted in buffered glycerol. This procedure did not grossly affect the IF brightness of positive lymphocytes and allowed an easy identification of monocytes, since most of them (mean 93% of monocytes from Ficoll preparations from normal bloods) contained obvious POX grains when viewed in visible light (23). POX-negative monocytes appeared to be the most easily identifiable monocytes upon morphological criteria, and they accounted for only about 1% of the mononuclear cells obtained by Ficoll centrifugation of normal bloods. On the other hand, some monocytes showing a strong POX activity were hardly distinguishable from lymphocytes by phase-contrast microscopy. The occasional polymorphonuclears displayed a strong POX positivity. It must be emphasized that POX-positive lymphocytes were never found, as shown by Giemsa restaining after the enzymatic reaction.

Monocytes may be also identified by their phagocytic properties, mostly using latex beads (45, 46). In our hands, the cytochemical reaction provided a better identification since it allowed the recognition of more monocytes than did phagocytosis of latex particles, as revealed by Giemsa and POX staining after latex phagocytosis. In addition, latex particles may bind to the surface of some lymphocytes, and it may be difficult to distinguish the cells that have ingested the latex from those that have bound it. The latex method requires an incubation at 37°C for 30–60 min with the latex particles in 50% FCS containing medium (4) whereas POX staining takes less than 10 min. It is possible, however, that the combination of latex phagocytosis, prior to staining, and POX reaction after it, could lead to recognizing virtually all monocytes.

4.3. Nonspecific Staining. The major reason for nonspecific staining is the presence of aggregated IgG in the conjugates. Certain cells are indeed able to bind IgG aggregates, without strict species specificity. Aggregation of conjugated IgG may be due to a number of reasons, including hyperconjugation and hyperconcentration (we have observed that conjugates with a high conjugation ratio or used at very high concentration were responsible for nonspecific staining, probably because of the presence of aggregates), unpropitious storage conditions, and repeated freezing-thawing. These considerations have led to the procedures described above for the selection, preparation, and storage of the conjugates. In addition, it must be recalled that conjugates containing soluble immune complexes may stain any cell expressing an IgG Fc receptor. The removal of unwanted antibodies from the immune sera hence absolutely requires solid immunoadsorbents.

Another trivial but important reason for nonspecific staining is that, when the cells are damaged, they may bind all conjugates. We have observed such a nonspecific staining with cells whose processing was delayed, owing to transportation from another center, for instance. We therefore directly obtain in the laboratory the samples to be studied and process the cells as quickly as possible.

4.4. Detection of Exogenous Ig. The staining of exogenous Ig molecules attached to, but not synthesized by, the cells is the major pitfall in S.Ig detection. Practically, one must distinguish between the loose binding of normal IgG from the patients' serum to some cells with high-affinity Fc receptor and strong binding of Ig that react with the lymphocyte surface in an immunological reaction or that are complexed to their antigen.

The incidence of IgG-bearing cells in normal human blood has been for years a matter of controversy, since these cells were reported as being either the predominant or a minor population of B lymphocytes. It appears now to be clear that the incidence of IgG-bearing lymphocytes has been overestimated by many groups. The majority of cells that stain for IgG do not synthesize any Ig molecule, and they show positive IF because of the binding of serum IgG likely by a strong-affinity Fc receptor (13, 47). The bond is loose enough to be dissociated by a short incubation at $37°C$ (47). These IgG are not detected by $F(ab')_2$ fragments of anti-IgG antibodies, probably because the formation of immune complexes between whole anti-IgG antibodies and the small quantities of labile IgG loosely bound to the Fc receptor, leading to a strong attachment to this receptor, is necessary to prevent removal of these IgG during the washing subsequent to IF staining (13). The figures reported by our group for IgG-bearing cells were the lowest before the recent work of Winchester *et al.* using $F(ab')_2$ fragments (13), thus suggesting that we were not including most of the labile IgG-bearing cells in our counts, probably because we considered them as nonlymphocytic. Indeed, these cells appear to belong to a particular population of cells lacking true S.Ig and expressing an Fc receptor avid enough to be detected by the formation of EA rosettes with red cells coated with relatively small amounts of IgG ["third population" described by Frøland and Natvig (1)] (13, 48). These cells appear to show endogenous POX activity and are probably related to the monocytic line (49). However, it must be emphasized that lymphocytes that actually synthesize surface IgG do exist, although their incidence in normal blood is low.

In other situations, exogenous Ig is firmly bound to the cell surface. Circulating immune complexes from the patients' plasma may bind to Fc or complement receptors. This is a critical problem in autoimmune diseases, but circulating complexes are also found in a variety of pathological conditions, such as infectious and neoplastic diseases. It must be emphasized that the detection of Ig bound to Fc or C receptors, or of aggregate binding, is crucial in terms of S.Ig being a B cell marker. Indeed, the cells that express these receptors include the "third population" in addition to B lymphocytes, monocytes, and polymorphonuclears. Moreover, there is no doubt that many activated T cells (50–52) and a subpopulation of normal T cells (53) bear IgG Fc receptor. On the other hand, autoantibodies to lymphocyte surface determinants have recently been reported in several conditions, particularly autoimmune diseases and lymphoproliferative disorders (5). Such antibodies often show a T cell specificity, and their presence on the lymphocyte membrane may lead to erroneous conclusions. In addition, S.Ig on lymphocytes from patients affected with certain diseases may possess autoantibody activities, such as a rheumatoid factor activity (31). This anti-IgG activity of surface-bound IgM is not uncommon in B cell proliferations and should be considered in rheumatoid arthritis and related diseases. It results in a false polyclonal staining pattern due to *in vivo* binding of serum polyclonal IgG to the surface IgM.

It is therefore often crucial to prove that S.Ig detected at the lymphocyte surface are actually synthesized by the cells which carry them. This demonstration can be accomplished by studying S.Ig synthesized *in vitro,* either by restaining after culturing following stripping the S.Ig by anti-Ig antibodies and/or proteolytic enzymes (see Section 3.2.) or by biosynthesis experiments using radioactive amino acid incorporation (54). It should be stressed that surface staining showing an apparent restriction with respect to heavy-chain class and light-chain type do not provide in itself a sufficient argument for active production by the cells. Indeed, antibodies to the lymphocyte surface may be of restricted heterogeneity and mimic homogeneous S.Ig. This is the likely explanation for the finding of apparently monoclonal exogenous Ig on proliferating T lymphocytes (55). In addition, in several patients with B-type chronic lymphocytic leukemia, the cells bore a monoclonal surface IgM that was an actual cell product and IgG antibodies bound to the cell surface. Probably owing to steric hindrance, the determinants detectable by vital staining of fresh cells were restricted to the light chain of the monoclonal IgM and to the heavy chain of the IgG antibodies, thus resulting in a false appearance of homogeneous surface IgG (24).

Provided that S.Ig are detected by procedures that fulfill precise technical conditions similar to those described here, they represent by far the most reliable B cell marker. However, in the study of diseased individuals and in view of the pitfalls mentioned above and of the possibility for abnormal or malignant cells to express membrane properties different of those of normal lymphocytes, there is an absolute requirement for using several different B and T cell markers together with S.Ig detection.

REFERENCES

1. T and B lymphocytes in human. *Transplant. Rev.* **16** (1973).
2. Warner, N. L., *Adv. Immunol.* **19,** 67 (1974).
3. Preud'homme, J. L., and Seligmann, M., *Prog. Clin. Immunol.* **2,** 121 (1974).
4. Aiuti *et al.,* Report of a WHO sponsored Workshop. 1974. *Scand. J. Immunol.* **3,** 521 (1974). *Clin. Immunol. Immunopathol.* **3,** 584 (1975).

5. Preud'homme, J. L., and Seligmann, M., *Rheumatology* **6**, 178 (1975).
6. Congy, N., and Mihaesco, C., *Rev. Fr. Etud. Clin. Biol.* **6**, 608 (1967).
7. Pernis, B., Forni, L., and Amante, L., *J. Exp. Med.* **132**, 1001 (1970).
8. Frøland, S. S., and Natvig, J. B., *J. Exp. Med.* **139**, 1599 (1972).
9. Fu, S. M., and Kunkel, H. G., *J. Exp. Med.* **140**, 895 (1974).
10. Klein, M., *Rev. Eur. Etud. Clin. Biol.* **17**, 525 (1972).
11. Metzger, H., personal communication.
12. Capel, P. J. A., *J. Immunol. Methods* **5**, 165 (1974).
13. Winchester, R. J., Fu, S. M., Hoffman, T., and Kunkel, H. G., *J. Immunol.* **114**, 1210 (1975).
14. Nisonoff, A., Wissler, F. C., Lipmann, L. N., and Woernley, D. L., *Arch. Biochem. Biophys.* **89**, 230 (1960).
15. Hijmans, W. H., Schuit, H. R. E., and Klein, F., *Clin. Exp. Immunol.* **4**, 457 (1969).
16. Clark, H. F., and Shepard, C. C., *Virology* **20**, 242 (1963).
17. Amante, L., Ancona, A., and Forni, L., *J. Immunol. Methods* **1**, 289 (1972).
18. Preud'homme, J. L., and Labaume, S., *Ann. N. Y. Acad. Sci.* **254**, 254 (1975).
19. Brandtzaeg, P., *Ann. N. Y. Acad. Sci.* **254**, 35 (1975).
20. Cebra, J. J., and Goldstein, G., *J. Immunol.* **95**, 230 (1965).
21. Böyum, A., *Scand. J. Clin. Lab. Invest.* **21**, 77 (1968).
22. Thorsby, E., and Bratlie, A., *in* "Histocompatibility Testing" (P. Terasaki, ed.), p. 655. Munksgaard, Copenhagen, Denmark, 1970.
23. Preud'homme, J. L., and Flandrin, G., *J. Immunol.* **113**, 1650 (1974).
24. Preud'homme, J. L., and Seligmann, M., *Blood* **40**, 777 (1972).
25. Preud'homme, J. L., and Seligmann, M., *J. Clin. Invest.* **51**, 701 (1972).
26. Preud'homme, J. L., Neauport-Sautes, C., Piat, S., Silvestre, D., and Kourilsky, F. M., *Eur. J. Immunol.* **2**, 297 (1972).
27. Kourilsky, F. M., Silvestre, D., Neauport-Sautes, C., Loosfelt, Y., and Dausset, J., *Eur. J. Immunol.* **2**, 249 (1972).
28. Ploem, J. S., *Leitz-Mitt. Wiss. Technol.* **4**, 225 (1969).
29. Ploem, J. S., *Ann. N. Y. Acad. Sci.* **254**, 5 (1975).
30. Pernis, B., Ferrarini, M., Forni, L., and Amante, L., *Prog. Immunol.* **1**, 95 (1971).
31. Preud'homme, J. L., and Seligmann, M., *Proc. Natl. Acad. Sci. U.S.A.* **69**, 2132 (1972).
32. Jones, P. P., Cebra, J. J., and Herzenberg, L. A., *J. Immunol.* **11**, 1334 (1973).
33. Greaves, M. F., and Brown, G., *J. Immunol.* **112**, 420 (1974).
34. Pernis, B., Brouet, J. C., and Seligmann, M., *Eur. J. Immunol.* **4**, 776 (1974).
35. Preud'homme, J. L., Brouet, J. C., and Seligmann, M., *in* "Membrane Receptors of Lymphocytes" (M. Seligmann, J. L. Preud'homme, and F. M. Kourilsky, eds.), p. 417. North-Holland Publ., Amsterdam, 1975.
36. Knapp, W., Haaijman, J. J., Schuit, H. R. E., Radl, J., Van Den Berg, P., Ploem, J. S., and Hijmans, W., *Ann. N. Y. Acad. Sci.* **254**, 94 (1975).
37. Rowe, D. S., Hug, K., Forni, L., and Pernis, B., *J. Exp. Med.* **138**, 965 (1973).
38. Knapp, W., Bolhuis, R. L. H., Radl, J., and Hijmans, W., *J. Immunol.* **111**, 1295 (1973).
39. Kubo, R. T., Grey, H. M., and Pirofsky, B., *J. Immunol.* **112**, 1952 (1974).
40. Fu, S. M., Winchester, R. J., and Kunkel, H. G., *J. Exp. Med.* **139**, 451 (1974).
41. Preud'homme, J. L., Brouet, J. C., Clauvel, J. P., and Seligmann, M., *Scand. J. Immunol.* **3**, 853 (1974).
42. Wernet, P., and Kunkel, H. G., *J. Exp. Med.* **138**, 1021 (1973).
43. Tebbi, K., *Lancet* **1**, 1392 (1973).
44. Hayhoe, F. G., Quaglino, D., and Doll, R., *in* "The Cytology and Cytochemistry of Acute Leukemia: a Study of 140 Cases." Her Majesty's Stationery Office, London, England.

45. Cline, M. J., and Lehrer, R. I., *Blood* **32,** 423 (1968).
46. Zucker-Franklin, D., *J. Immunol.* **112,** 234 (1974).
47. Lobo, P. I., Westervelt, F. D., and Horwitz, D. A., *J. Immunol.* **114,** 116 (1975).
48. Kurnick, J. T., and Grey, H. M., *J. Immunol.* **115,** 305 (1975).
49. Hayward, A. R., and Greaves, M. F., *Scand. J. Immunol.* **4,** 563 (1975).
50. Fridman, W. H., and Golstein, P., *Cell Immunol.* **11,** 442 (1974).
51. Van Boxel, J. A., and Rosenstreich, D. L., *J. Exp. Med.* **139,** 1002 (1974).
52. Anderson, C. L., and Grey, H. M., *J. Exp. Med.* **139,** 1175 (1974).
53. Stout, R. D., and Herzenberg, L. A., *J. Exp. Med.* **142,** 611 (1975).
54. Nies, K. M., Oberlin, M. A., Brown, J. C., and Halpern, M. S., *J. Immunol.* **111,** 1236 (1973).
55. Brouet, J. C., and Prieur, A. M., *Clin. Immunol. Immunopathol.* **2,** 481 (1974).

Techniques of Surface Immunofluorescence Applied to the Analysis of the Lymphocyte

Robert J. Winchester

1. Introduction

The objectives of this chapter are to consider a number of the technical aspects of both direct and indirect fluorescent antibody analysis as they relate to studies of the lymphocyte surface. Because of the inherent sensitivity of surface immunofluorescence along with the presence of certain surface structures, such as the Fc receptor, there are major technical pitfalls of false-positive fluorescence that await the investigator. An awareness of these problems is stressed, and the methods utilize modifications to minimize interference from these hazards.

One of the most frequently performed measurements is the enumeration of B lymphocytes through detection of intrinsic surface membrane Ig. The procedures for this are contained in Section 3.2 on direct fluorescence. The methods for preparation of the reagents are also in that section.

The subject of indirect immunofluorescence is covered in Section 3.5 and includes the detection of autoreactive anti-lymphocyte antibodies as well as the broader use of the indirect method as a tool in the exploration of the lymphocyte surface primarily through the use of human antibodies with specificities for alloantigens. The subject of demonstrating B cell differentiation alloantigens is briefly covered.

2. Materials

2.1. Antigens and Immunogens. IgG, IgA, IgM, and IgD myeloma proteins isolated by methods such as preparative electrophoresis in Pevikon are the most suitable starting materials. Myeloma sera should be selected on the basis of ideally having a very high monoclonal band, over 30 mg/ml, and depression of normal IgG. Bands migrating in the β region are more likely to be contaminated with unwanted molecules and are less satisfactory as immunogens. Pooled IgG from several individuals or obtained as Cohn fraction II should be partially purified on a DEAE-cellulose column before use. F(ab')$_2$ fragments are prepared by pepsin digestion. Either the whole immunoglobulin or its fragment are useful both as immunogens in preparing a "polyvalent" reagent or in absorptions. $F(ab')_2$ fragments of IgG myelomas or light chains prepared by reduction and alkylation of the monoclonal band are distinctly preferable as immunogens for raising sera with K or L specificities. Bence-Jones proteins are particularly difficult to use as immunogens because of contaminants, among these β_2-microglobulin, which introduce many undesired specificities. Bence-Jones proteins are not suitable for certain absorptions because of small amounts of Ig fragments that could remove desired specificities. Sera from patients with severe hypogammaglobulinemia or selective absence of IgA are useful for absorptions.

2.2. Antisera. Rabbits are repetitively immunized according to conventional protocols and test bled until extremely strong antisera are produced. The strength of antisera are estimated most simply by capillary precipitin reactions using fraction II IgG at 10 mg/ml as the antigen. A dense flocculent precipitate forming at the interface within a few seconds indicates a sufficiently strong antiserum. A preliminary characterization of the specificity is carried out by Ouchterlony plate double diffusion against myeloma and Bence-Jones proteins.

2.3. Ig Isolation and Chromatography Equipment. One-liter stock solutions of the following are convenient to prepare and store as concentrates, the appropriate dilution being made before use:

> Sodium phosphate buffer, 0.5 M, pH 7.5
> Sodium chloride, 1.0 M
> Sodium carbonate-bicarbonate, 1.0 M, pH 9.6
> Sodium acetate, 1.0 M, pH 4.0
> Trizma base, 1.0 M

Saturated ammonium sulfate is prepared using distilled water and stored over an excess of ammonium sulfate crystals. DEAE-cellulose conveniently obtained as DE-52 (Whatman) is equilibrated with the phosphate buffer and stored. Other items include pepsin (Worthington Biochemical Corp.); 1 X 20 cm and 2 X 30 cm columns for ion-exchange chromatography; 23/32 Visking dialysis tubing; a flow-through cell for a spectrophotometer to facilitate the column procedures; a high-speed centrifuge for processing the salt precipitates. A fraction collector is not needed unless the G-150 gel filtration separation is undertaken. For the gel filtration procedure a 2.5 X 150 cm column of Sephadex G-150 equilibrated with 0.5 M sodium chloride, 0.1 M Tris HCl, pH 8.0, 0.01% sodium azide is operated by downward flow from a Marriotte bottle. For conjugation, tetramethylrhodamine isothiocyanate is obtained from Baltimore Biologic Laboratories. A Branson sonicator with a microtip adapter on the transducer probe is used to finely suspend the fluorochrome.

2.4. Cell Preparations. Mononuclear cells isolated from peripheral blood by Ficoll—Hypaque centrifugation contain monocytes that are often difficult to recognize by phase microscopy. One approach to this problem is to label the moncytes by latex. This incubation has the added advantage of permitting IgG molecules and autoreactive anti-lymphocyte antibodies to elute as described subsequently.

Adjust the mononuclear cell preparation to about 1×10^6 cells/ml in Hanks' balanced salt solution (HBSS). Add 1 drop (0.020 ml) of a 5% suspension of latex particles per $2 \pm 0.5 \times 10^7$ cells and incubate at 37°C for 45 min with occasional suspension. Wash three times with 30–40 ml of HBSS or phosphate-buffered saline–glucose (PBS–G) to eliminate excess latex. Monitor a drop of the suspended pellet to determine whether there are fewer than 1 free latex particle per 5–10 cells; if not, an additional wash is necessary. If monocytes are abundant, clumps of monocytes can form, incorporate other cells, and interfere with the analysis; they usually can be broken up by vortex mixing. Latex particles 1.1 μm in diameter are obtained from Dow Diagnostics as a 10% suspension. They are washed 5 times in PBS by centrifugation, (15,000 g, 10 min) and stored as a 5% suspension in PBS at 4°C. The particles are resuspended before use. The cells are suspended in phosphate-buffered physiologic saline, pH 7.4, containing 0.02% sodium azide and 10 mg of bovine serum per albumin per milliliter (PSB–BSA).

2.5. Materials for staining. These include microscope slides with frosted end, 22×22 mm cover slips, Pasteur pipettes; colorless, quick-drying nail polish. Colored polishes frequently contain fluorescent dyes that slowly stain the cell membrane. The use of a good grade of nail polish permits the slides to keep for several days without drying out. Round-bottom plastic tubes (Falcon), 10×75 mm, are used.

2.6. Fluorescence Microscopy. For cell-surface studies the microscope must perform near its design limits. A vertical (Ploem) incident illumination device is essential (1). A $60–100 \times$ oil or water immersion phase objective designed for fluorescence and with the greatest available numerical aperture should be selected. The ocular magnification should be no greater than $10 \times$. The enhanced brightness afforded by a monocular eye tube in the author's opinion more than offsets the inconvenience of its use. In general, all components should be chosen to give maximum illumination intensity and full transmission of cell fluorescence. The assistance of an experienced fluorescence microscopist in the selection of equipment and in ascertaining that its performance is up to the specifications is often a useful adjunct to the product literature and service features of the microscope suppliers. The author's laboratory uses the filter system described in Method 9.

2.7. Insolubilization of Antigen. Procedure for Insolubilization of Antigen on Sepharose Beads. This is given in Method 9.

3. Methods

3.1. Direct Immunofluoroescence *3.1.1. Selection of Specificities.* There are two approaches that can be taken to obtain a polyvalent screening reagent that detects all cells with surface Ig. One involves the preparation of separate reagents, each specific for one of the Ig classes and using a mixture of them as a pool. The other approach rests on detection of surface Ig primarily through K and L determinants and variable region antigens obtained by immunizing with whole pooled IgG or F(ab')$_2$ fragments. The relative merits of these two methods are discussed in Section 4.

3.1.2. Isolation of IgG. From 10 to 50 ml of antiserum are mixed with an equal volume of saturated ammonium sulfate, and the precipitate is harvested by centrifugation at 10,000 g for 10 min. The supernatant is poured off and discarded. The precipitate is dissolved in a minimum of distilled water and dialyzed against two changes of a buffer containing 0.05 M sodium chloride, 0.01 M sodium phosphate, pH 7.5, prepared by diluting the stock solutions with distilled water. The solution is passed over a 1 X 15 cm DEAE-cellulose column equilibrated with the same buffer, and only the "fall through" fraction is harvested. The solution is dialyzed against 0.1 M sodium acetate buffer, and the protein content is measured at 280 nM using 1.35 OD units/mg as the conversion factor. One milligram of pepsin per 100 mg of IgG are added, and the mixture is incubated at 37°C for 18 hr. The digest is neutralized by adding Trizma base. Depending on the available equipment and amount of antiserum, there is an alternative procedure for resolving the products of digestion.

3.1.3. Purification of F(ab')$_2$ Fragments (2). The simplest procedure involves dialysis against 0.05 M NaCl, 0.01 M sodium phosphate, pH 7.5, and passage over a 1 X 5 cm bed of DEAE-cellulose equilibrated with the same buffer, only the "fall through" is harvested and dialyzed against 0.15 M NaCl. Should the final protein content be below 5 mg/ml, the sample should be concentrated by salt precipitation as detailed in the next paragraph. This simple purification procedure relies on the fact that rabbit IgG is essentially completely digested to F(ab')$_2$ with virtually no F(ab') fragment or whole IgG detectable. The correctness of this assumption for the individual laboratory conditions and each serum should be verified.

In the case of species other than rabbit, such as sheep or goat, the pepsin digestion will have a lower yield of F(ab')$_2$ fragments and gel filtration through G-150 is essential. In the case of these latter species it has been recommended to perform the pepsin digestion in 0.2 M sodium acetate buffer, pH 4.5, for 15 hr to minimize production of F(ab') fragments (J. Haimovich, A. Cohen, and Z. Bentwich, personal communication). Gel filtration is also used for processing volumes of rabbit antiserum over 20 ml. It is clearly the preferable alternative if larger amounts of antiserum are available to offset the poorer recovery. Usually it is necessary to concentrate the digest prior to gel filtration in order to reduce its volume to under 10 ml. This is accomplished by adding ammonium sulfate crystals to at least half saturation, and after allowing the precipitate to flocculate, harvesting it by centrifugation, 10,000 g for 10 min. The pellet is dissolved in a small volume of distilled water and layered directly on the column. The F(ab')$_2$ fragments obtained from the column are concentrated in the same way and dialyzed against 0.1 M saline.

3.1.4. Fluorochrome Conjugation. The balance of opinion favors the use of rhodamine as superior to fluorescein for surface staining (3). The procedure used for the conjugation of the isothiocyanates of rhodamine or fluorescein are, however, essentially the same and are modified from the procedure of Amante *et al.* (4). Between 5 and 10 mg of tetramethylrhodamine isothiocyanate is weighed out with great accuracy and a suspension of exactly 1 mg/ml is prepared with 0.1 M sodium carbonate–bicarbonate buffer, pH 9.6. In a plastic tube the mixture is sonicated for 1–2 min at 50 W/cm^2, giving a finely divided suspension (2). The importance of this will be discussed in Section 4. The F(ab')$_2$ fragments are adjusted to a concentration of 5–15 mg/ml using the conversion coefficient at 280 nM of 1.35 OD unit/mg and are put in a small beaker gently stirred by a magnetic bar. The solution is rendered 0.1 M in sodium carbonate–bicarbonate buffer and a volume of the finely suspended tetramethylrhodamine isothiocyanate is added dropwise to give 0.030 mg of the fluorochrome per milligram of F(ab')$_2$ fragment. The mixture is stirred overnight at 4°C in the covered beaker.

A 2 × 25 cm bed of G-50 sephadex in 0.01 M phosphate buffer pH 7.5 and a DEAE-cellulose column 1 × 10 cm in the same buffer are prepared. The conjugation mixture is carefully layered on the gel bed and eluted slowly. Unconjugated dye and the buffer salts are separated and emerge as a second band after the conjugated proteins. The F(ab')$_2$ rhodamine conjugate peak is applied to the DEAE-cellulose column (5, 6). The fraction of conjugate that does not adhere in the initial 0.01 M phosphate buffer is not suitable for fluorescence work. The adsorbed conjugate is eluted by increasing concentrations of NaCl in a stepwise fashion. It is usually sufficient to use solutions of 0.01 M phosphate buffer containing 0.1 M, 0.125 M, and 0.15 M NaCl. Ratios of $OD_{280} - OD_{515}$ in the range of 1.3–2.0 are generally suitable. Conjugate fractions with ratios lower than 1.3 may have diminished antibody activity and can adhere to cells nonspecifically. Dilute eluates are concentrated by ammonium sulfate precipitation. The samples are dialyzed against PBS containing 0.02% sodium azide and are usually stored at 4°C with bovine serum albumin added to a concentration of 20 mg/ml.

3.2. Staining Procedure. The procedure used is essentially that of Pernis *et al.* (7) with minor modifications. In the case of the mononuclear cell layer from peripheral blood obtained by Ficoll–Hypaque centrifugation the monocytes are labeled by latex spherules as described in Section 2.4, and the suspension is adjusted to 2.5 × 10^7 cells per milliliter in PBS containing 0.2% sodium azide and 10 mg of BSA per milliliter. Cell suspension, 0.025 ml, is transferred to a 10 × 75-mm test tube. The staining is usually carried out at room temperature, although for special purposes 4° or 37°C are used as noted below; 0.025 ml of the antibody conjugate is added and mixed with the cells by forcibly rubbing the test-tube tip over the top of a wire test-tube rack. After a 30-min incubation 2 ml of **PBS-BSA** are added and the cells centrifuged. Any residual foam is aspirated and the supernatant wash is poured out in a smooth motion. The remaining droplet is blotted off with the tube inverted and the cells suspended. The cells are washed a total of three times in this manner. The remainder of the final wash is not poured off until immediately before making the slide; then the top of the tube is briefly pressed against a towel to dry it and the pellet is resuspended with several forcible strokes across a test-tube rack. A Pasteur pipette is quickly put in the tube and a column of 0.5–1.0 cm of cell suspension removed by capillary action and expressed on the slide by thumb pressure. The importance of these maneuvers is to achieve a cell density of 15–25 per oil immersion field. After 15–20 sec a cover glass is placed on the drop and pressed firmly down with the eraser of a pencil to flatten the cells. Such flattened preparations facilitate reading, particularly if the conjugate is irregularly distributed on the cell surface. The edges of the cover slip are sealed with a quick-drying high-quality colorless nail polish.

3.3. Slide Examination. The slides are examined with a high-resolution oil or water immersion objective of at least 60 X. Phase optics alternating with the incident fluorescent illumination are used to identify the cell type and perform the fluorescent analysis. Depending on the percentage of positive cells encountered, 200–500 cells are counted. Cells with homogeneous cytoplasmic staining due to early cell death are not counted. They are readily recognized by the absence of the circumferential ring of fluorescence and greater fluorescence intensity in the cell center.

Discrimination of lymphocytes from monocytes or the occasional granulocyte is an essential requirement and requires some practice. The majority of monocytes will have ingested latex particles, and these are seen to be clearly within the cytoplasm. However, a few other cells shown to be monocytes by specialized criteria fail to ingest latex. These may be recognized by an irregular profile of the cell membrane, granular cytoplasm, and an indistinct nuclear membrane. Occasionally one or a few latex particles can be found adhering to the surface membrane of a typical lymphocyte. These are not excluded from the lymphocyte population.

When applying statistics to the results it should be recalled that percentages are involved and that the distribution is not necessarily a normal one.

3.4. Specificity and Potency Testing. Arriving at the final state of having a fluorescent reagent that is both highly sensitive and of fully characterized specificity is perhaps the most difficult part of immunofluorescent microscopy. A general outline of the procedure is that first the strength of the newly conjugated reagent is assayed on normal mononuclear cells without absorption. After the reagent is absorbed, using the appropriate insolubilized antigens, the strength of the conjugate is again assayed and with the pattern of reaction and the aid of staining defined pathological cells the specificity of the conjugate is characterized as described below.

3.4.1. Absorbed Conjugate. The relative strength of the absorbed conjugate is determined by serial dilutions showing a maximal percentage of cells stained. To a series of tubes containing mononuclear cells with latex-labeled monocytes add 0.1 ml, 0.05 ml, 0.025 ml, and then 0.025 ml of 2-fold serially diluted conjugated antiserum up to a dilution of 1:16. The cells are stained and processed as described above. The number of lymphocytes positive in fluorescence are plotted versus the dilutions. The plateau percentage reflects the maximal number of positive cells bearing the Ig. As the amount of antiserum is reduced, only cells with the greatest abundance of mIg are stained, resulting in lower percentages. The reagent should be concentrated by ammonium sulfate precipitation to the extent that 0.025 ml contains sufficient antibodies to place the reaction on the plateau by a factor of at least two or preferably four.

The presence of Fc receptors on monocytes serves as a built in control for specific staining of the IgG adhering to the monocyte either through light or gamma heavy chain antigens or for nonspecific staining due to complexes or aggregates. Careful search for stained monocytes should be made particularly at the higher concentrations used in the plateau test.

3.4.2. Absorption. The $F(ab')_2$ fluorochrome conjugate is usually absorbed with well washed Sepharose beads to which antigens have been coupled following cyanogen bromide activation. The beads are washed and freed of buffer on a sintered-glass funnel and transferred to the $F(ab')_2$ conjugate for absorption. The reaction is performed at 37°C for 30 min, then the mixture is returned to the sintered funnel and with very gentle suction the conjugate is harvested without the production of foam. A few drops of BSA–PBS are used to wash the beads free of any remaining conjugate.

The quantity of beads needed is found empirically. There is considerable latitude in the amount of beads used, providing the antigens are completely free of any contaminant that would attenuate the intended major specificity of the reagent. The antigens required reflect the principal known undesired specificities detected in the whole unconjugated serum by double diffusion or other method. For example a mixture of DEAE-cellulose purified fraction II IgG and K chains would be used to absorb an anti-IgMK serum. If initially the whole antiserum gave additional uncharacterized precipitin reactions with whole human serum, hypogammaglobulinemic sera coupled to beads would also be used. Following the absorption, the reagents are tested as described in 3.4.1. Additional absorptions not indicated by the initial immunochemical characterization are sometimes necessary. With the vast majority of reagents prepared using myeloma proteins as immunogens, a single absorption step is all that is required. Occasionally with immunogens, such as fraction II IgG or Bence-Jones protein, dominant specificities were detected by surface fluorescence that defied removal without affecting the suitability of the reagent for recognizing the intended determinant. As discussed in Method 9, cocapping experiments are of particular use in defining the surface immunoglobulin specificities. No other immuno-chemical tests are performed, and it should be emphasized that fluorescent reagents shown to be specific only by techniques other than surface fluorescence have not been reliably characterized (8). In some circumstances, defined antigens coupled to Sepharose beads or to erythrocytes can be examined in the fluores-cent microscope and contribute greatly to the analysis of difficult samples (9). Another approach is to use lymphoid cell lines such a Daudi bearing IgMK but no IgG or IgD to define the specificity of the reagent. Characterized chronic lymphatic leukemic lymphocytes are particularly useful in this regard, since certain patients express only IgD molecules, and others only IgM molecules.

   3.4.3. Blocking. The central criterion of specificity is the absence of staining in a blocking experiment. This is performed by absorbing the fluorescent reagent with increasing amounts of a protein containing antigens for which the reagent has been rendered specific. There are some circumstances described in Section 4 where this test is not a sufficient guarantee of specificity.

   3.5. Indirect Immunofluorescence. There are two slightly different tech-niques for performing indirect immunofluroescence depending on whether the objective is the detection of autoreactive anti-lymphocyte antibodies or recogni-tion of iso- or heterospecific antibodies directed to cellular antigens. The reason for this is that the majority of autoreactive antibodies are of the IgM class and have a greatly increased avidity at 4°C whereas iso- and heteroantibodies are primarily of the IgG class and are warm reactive. Therefore, although the general procedures are similar, the conditions and the reagents differ.

   3.5.1. Detection of Autoreactive Anti-lymphocyte Antibodies. Lymphocytes are isolated in a conventional procedure and incubated at 37°C to ensure elution of antibodies as described in Section 4. The latex incubation period usually suffices for this although overnight incubation to allow shedding, might be necessary in some circumstances (10, 11). The cell suspensions are prepared as for direct fluorescence except that all procedures are carried out with the tubes in a melting-ice bath. In place of the fluorescent reagent, tubes containing 1 drop of autologous serum and control tubes with normal serum and no serum (BSA−PBS only) are prepared. The cells are added and incubated for 0.5 hr. They are then washed 4 times with ice-cold PBS−BSA using a refrigerated centrifuge. After the last wash, the wash is discarded, the tubes are blotted to remove any adherent solution, and the cell pellet is suspended by vigorous stroking. They are returned to the melting-ice bath and staining with F(ab′)₂ reagents carried out as described above except that all steps are carried out in the cold. The F(ab′)₂ reagents used should include an anti-IgM and an anti-IgG. In screening experi-ments these could be used as a mixture. Normal serum controls are included. Slides are prepared and promptly examined in the usual manner at room temperature. The air-dry method described in Method 9 is particularly useful here. The difference in percentage of positive cells between control and test serum reflects the presence of antilymphocyte antibodies on the cells.

3.5.2. Detection of Cryptoantigens. An example of the uncovering of a cryptoantigen is provided by experiments in which lymphocytes are digested with neuraminidase and then reincubated with autologous serum. Antibodies predominantly of IgM class are found in nearly all sera that react with determinants exposed by this digestion (12).

3.5.3. Detection of Alloantibodies and Lymphocyte Alloantigens. Alloantigens expressed on B lymphocytes but not T lymphocytes are detected through the use of pregnancy sera. The procedure is performed as described in Section 3.5.1 with the exception that all steps are carried out at room temperature in order to minimize nonspecific staining. In most instances the human alloantibodies are exclusively of the IgG class. Only the IgG-specific fluorochrome F(ab')$_2$ reagent is routinely used in these experiments. Backgrounds of nonspecific staining due to immune complex formation although low will vary according to the condition of the human alloserum. Two controls are included, PBS–BSA alone, and a normal serum processed in the same way as the human alloserum alone in the first stage followed by the anti-IgG reagent. If these two controls are widely divergent, fresh sera heat-inactivated at 56°C for 10 min should be run as additional controls.

3.5.4. Double Heteroantibody Systems in Indirect Immunofluorescence. The use of systems, such as rabbit antihuman lymphocyte antigen and sheep anti-rabbit, are extremely difficult. A major source of nonspecific reactivity are heteroantibodies in the first serum that are directed to antigens on the lymphocyte surface. Some of these are removed by absorbing with erythrocytes and agarose beads. Because of these and other subtleties of demonstrating specificity, this system is generally avoided by most workers unless there is no ready alternative. A preimmunization serum is a very important control to minimize uncertainties due to heteroantibodies.

3.5.5. Capping in Indirect Immunofluorescence. The nonimmunoglobulin antigens differ markedly in their ability to be redistributed on the surface of human lymphocytes. For most antigens there appears to be a "pro zone" type of phenomenon in which concentrations of reagents used for optimal staining fail to give adequate redistribution. Two-dimensional titrations of each reagent are performed, and the optimal redistribution is usually given with dilutions of 1:5 to 1:10.

4. Interpretation of Technical and Conceptual Problems in Immunofluorescence

4.1. Analysis of Some Technical Staining Problems in Surface Immunofluorescence.
Certain of the problems more frequently encountered in fluorescent antibody analysis of cell surfaces are grouped under the categories of either

insufficient staining or excessive staining. Table 1 summarizes these. Additional general information on this topic was the subject of a recent conference (13).

4.1.1. Insufficient Staining. This is most commonly due to difficulties with the amount or quality of the fluorochrome-conjugated antibodies. When a lower than anticipated percentage of cells with surface Ig staining is found, the plateau test should be repeated to determine whether an inadvertent absorption or dilution of the reagent occurred. Reagents stored at 4°C in the appropriate solution are stable for well over a year if insolubilized absorbing antigens have been used, and simple deterioration is usually not a problem.

4.1.1.1. Serum remaining in the medium in which the cells are suspended will block the added fluorescent reagent and prevent the staining of cells. This is particularly a problem in indirect fluorescence, where the critical efficiency of washing steps is constrained by the necessity of keeping the cells in the small test tube. It is well demonstrated that a few nanograms of Ig will block the staining and produce soluble complexes.

4.1.1.2. Serious contamination of a F(ab')$_2$ conjugate with Fab fragments will markedly alter the intensity of perceived fluorescence. Much of the sensitivity of surface fluorescence rests on the minute redistribution of the membrane components into "spots" or "speckles," and this redistribution does not occur with Fab reagents. Usually this is not a problem with digests of rabbit antibodies but can be encountered in sheep and goat reagents if improper pooling of column fractions was made. Fab fragments, however, are useful reagents in capping experiments (14).

4.1.1.3. The presence of a considerable proportion of hypoconjugated or unconjugated antibodies in the reagent results in competition with properly conjugated antibodies for the antigen on the cell surface. Elimination of poorly

TABLE 1

Analysis of Some Technical Problems in Immunofluorescence

Insufficient staining
    Inadequate quantity of antibody added
    Blocking of antibodies by residual serum
    Contamination by Fab fragments
    Hypoconjugated antibodies
    Instrument factors
Excessive staining (not removed in blocking experiments)
    Contaminant specificities
    Hyperconjugated protein
    Preexisting immune complexes or aggregates
Removed in blocking experiments
    Antigen antibody complexes formed during the staining procedure
    Failure to distinguish monocytes from lymphocytes
    Presence of interfering components, such as anti-lymphocyte antibodies

---

conjugated antibodies is achieved by rechromatography on DEAE-cellulose and elimination of fractions eluting with lower concentrations of sodium chloride. If problems of this nature are encountered a short continuous sodium chloride gradient may provide the clue to more appropriate fractionation.

4.1.1.4. Despite the availability of high-performance equipment from several sources, certain technical problems can frustrate the best efforts of an investigator. The exchange of a weak-staining preparation having a definite percentage of positive cells with another laboratory aids greatly in uncovering problems such as mislabeled filters or decentered optical components that prevent optimal fluorescence. The use of the defined antigen sphere technique (9) or equivalent approaches to achieving some degree of quantitative control over the amount of fluorescence are of particular relevance if problems of this nature are encountered.

4.1.2. Excessive Staining. This refers to the finding of a greater percentage of stained cells than are warranted. The analysis of this problem is aided by the performance of a blocking experiment in which a purified antigen, but preferably not the immunogen, is used to absorb selectively all antibodies having the intended specificity. It should be noted that there are some types of nonspecific staining that are removed in blocking experiments so that other adjunctive types of evidence may be required in particular situations (see 4.1.2.4).

4.1.2.1. Contaminant specificities can relate to persisting specificities for antigens on Ig molecules. An example would be persistant λ specificity in an antiserum raised against an IgD λ myeloma protein, so that the specificity is $\delta +$ λ where only δ was intended. Other contaminant specificities could be due to the presence of antibodies to determinants such as β_2-microglobulin or to other components of the lymphocyte membrane. Antisera raised to certain faster Bence-Jones proteins or to protein isolated from nondefibrinated plasma can have additional specificities reflecting β_2-microglobulin or bits of lymphocyte or platelet membrane inadvertently carried along in the isolation. Absorptions by hypogammaglobulinemic sera and very well washed human pooled erythrocytes are often helpful in this respect. They are of particular value in indirect fluorescence where the first antibody is from a species other than man. Intracellular staining is often of considerable utility in sorting out specificity problems of this variety (15).

4.1.2.2. Extremely hyperconjugated antibodies bind to the cell surface through charge–charge interactions because of their increased negative charge. Reagents eluted from DEAE-cellulose by concentrations of saline below 0.15 M usually do not present this problem. Rechromatography in 0.1 M NaCl, 0.01 M phosphate buffer, pH 7.5, or absorption with erythrocytes may correct this nonspecificity.

4.1.2.3. Preexisting immune complexes formed in absorption or aggregates of rabbit IgG conjugated with fluorochrome are taken up by the Fc receptor and simulate positive fluorescent staining (16). Ultracentrifugation of the reagents assists in decreasing this very major source of potential error. But the scrupulous use of solid-phase absorption and $F(ab')_2$ fluorescent reagents provides the best solution to this problem (2).

4.1.2.4. Another variety of nonspecific staining arises through the formation of immune complexes at the moment of fluorescent antibody addition to the cell suspension because of the presence of free molecules in solution bearing the antigen. For example, serum IgG, IgA, or IgM present in nanogram amounts forms complexes with the specific reagents that are then taken up by the Fc receptor. Blocking experiments remove the reagent specificity and provide an illusion of proof that the staining was specific. Staining of monocytes is often a clue that this variety of nonspecificity is a problem. $F(ab')_2$ reagents eliminate this problem except in the case of IgG, where if the antibodies are directed to the Fab end of the IgG it is possible to form an immune complex with enough of the Fc region of the human IgG exposed to be taken up on the Fc receptor. This event does not occur to an appreciable extent if antibody fragments with specificity for the IgG Fc region are present. In this latter case the Fc region on the human IgG is covered by antibody fragments themselves lacking Fc regions, resulting in immune complexes that do not adhere to the Fc receptor (2).

4.1.2.5. The failure to distinguish monocytes from lymphocytes in the case of staining with reagents specific for IgG or light chains will result in an overestimation of the number of positive cells. Method 9 provides several approaches to this problem.

4.1.2.6. Autoreactive anti-lymphocyte antibodies or other interfering substances can adhere to T as well as to B lymphocytes and confer false-positive staining, particularly since these antibodies are usually of the IgM class. Procedures involving elution at $37°C$ or shedding in overnight culture allow these antibodies to leave the lymphocyte surface (10, 11). Such antibodies are found in a number of malignant states as well as in the autoimmune diseases and some acute infections.

4.2. Conjugation of Antibody Fragments. While the introduction of the isothiocyanate moiety on the fluorochrome molecule has greatly improved the practicality of conjugation, a number of problems remain. These are particularly evident with the tetramethylrhodamine fluorochrome. Chief among these are difficult solubility and considerable batch-to-batch variability in being able to give any usable results. The marked superiority of rhodamine over fluorescein for surface fluorescence nevertheless justified the efforts to overcome these deficiencies in the reagent.

In our laboratory, the problem of solubility is largely overcome by sonicating the fluorochrome to yield a finely divided suspension prior to its addition to the protein. If the material is not finely divided, the yield of properly conjugated material is highly variable depending on batch-to-batch variations in the physical state of the fluorochrome.

Despite full solubilization, some batches of tetramethylrhodamine isothio-cyanate are useless for conjugation, perhaps because of hydrolysis of the iso-cyanate group. Each lot of fluorochrome should first be tried in a trial conjugation using purified rabbit or human fraction II IgG, to define the suitability of the chemical and discern whether there are any unusual propor-tions required to achieve a 70–80% yield of properly conjugated material. For additional comments on conjugation and its analysis, see Method 9.

4.3. Absorption. Perhaps the most difficult aspect of surface fluorescence is achieving specific reagents through appropriate absorptions. There are no firm guidelines to be followed since each antiserum presents its own challenge. The use of lymphoid cell lines permits the exchange among laboratories of standard cells with a defined variety of immunoglobulin expressed on the cell surface. We have found the Daudi line to be particularly useful since it bears a strong Fc receptor along with abundant IgMK. In general the specificities can be defined on peripheral blood with careful examination at each stage of absorption. Method 9 presents additional material on this subject.

4.4. Interpretation of Direct Surface Ig Staining. In normal peripheral blood, IgD and IgM constitute the major classes of cell-surface immunoglobulin. Ap-proximately two-thirds of the cells with either IgD or IgM express both simul-taneously on the same cell, and the remainder express a single class. This population of cells is usually detected by a mixture of reagents separately determined to be specific for IgD or IgM. The percentage of positive cells given by this mixture varies widely from 1 to 15 and rarely higher. Slightly higher levels are obtained with the complete polyvalent mixture specific for IgD, IgM, IgA plus IgD. Certain antisera raised against $F(ab')_2$ of pooled IgG give levels generally equivalent to the complete polyvalent mixture. It is not yet possible to be certain about the relative merits of detecting all surface immunoglobulin cells by polyvalent mixtures of class-specific reagents or alternatively by reagents specific for K and L determinants. In general, slightly higher levels are obtained by the latter reagents. This could reflect selective expression of light chains or a general superiority of detecting surface Ig through its most exposed regions. On the other hand, the use of reagents with primary specificity for the Fab portion of the molecule leaves open the possibility of forming immune complexes with portions of the Fc receptor uncovered that can be taken up on the Fc receptor. A resolution of this problem awaits further experiments.

In addition to their detection in the polyvalent mixture, IgG-bearing lympho-cytes are detected in an additional separate assay because of the difficulty sometimes experienced in the identification of a given cell as a lymphocyte in certain disease states. In normal individuals, usually 1% or less of typical small lymphocytes are stained by F(ab')$_2$ reagents specific for IgG. The staining is weaker than IgD, IgM, or IgA. The identity of larger cells that stain positively for IgG requires further study. Granulocytes and monocytes are variably stained by F(ab')$_2$ anti-IgG reagents; this most likely reflects the avidity of their Fc receptors for serum IgG. Nevertheless this staining greatly complicates the assay of IgG-positive lymphocytes.

IgA-bearing lymphocytes are usually detected at levels below 1% in normal peripheral blood. The morphology of the IgA-bearing cell is that of a small lymphocyte, and the staining is bright. Monocytes are not stained. Because of the low level of IgA-positive cells, they are assayed separately as well as being included in the polyvalent mixture. It is sometimes difficult to produce reagents specific for IgA unless sera of individuals with selective IgA absence is available for absorption.

4.5. General Problem of Fc Receptor Interference. In a number of situations where small amounts of the antigen are present in the solution about the cells, it is possible that immune complexes form with the staining reagent and are secondarily taken up by the Fc receptor. This has proved to be the case with an antiserum to α_2-macroglobulin, which in whole antibody form stained most B cells, yet in F(ab')$_2$ form failed to produce positive staining on any cell. Control experiments showing equivalent positive staining on insolubilized α_2-macroglobulin provided evidence that the antibody strengths of both preparations were satisfactory (S. Fu and J. Hurley, personal communication). In some instances this same mechanism appears to be operating in staining due to surface IgM, where much lower levels of stained cells were obtained with F(ab')$_2$ reagents.

4.6. B Cell Enumeration. Apart from the technical factors of measuring with minimum ambiguity the number of cells with surface Ig, there are several unresolved conceptual problems relating to the proper definition of a B cell in terms of surface markers. While the "classic" B cell has Fc receptors, complement receptors in addition to the surface Ig and fails to form rosettes with sheep erythrocytes, a sizable fraction of cells have some of these markers in unusual combinations. The "third population" of Fc receptor-positive Ig-negative lymphoid cells described by Frøland and Natvig (17) is an example of such an unusual population equal in number to "classic" B cells (2). While the remote possibility exists that monocytoid cells form a part of this population, this is not likely to account for the majority, and moreover some Fc receptor-positive cells lacking surface Ig have been shown to form E rosettes (2), a property not associated with monocytes.

Delineation of differentiation antigens, other than surface Ig, through allo- and heteroantisera now constitute a strong direction of investigation in this field, and it is hoped that these studies will resolve some of the questions of cell classification.

4.7. Autoreactive Anti-lymphocyte Antibodies. Fluorescent assays are a convenient method of detecting and characterizing these antibodies (10, 11). The fluorescent method gives results that are generally equivalent to those obtained in carefully performed cytotoxic assays carried out at 15°C. The nature of the target antigens is unknown, but a number of separate specificities exist, including those for determinants expressed solely on B cells or on T cells and those expressed on both B cells and T cells. The antibodies are predominantly of IgM class and secondarily of IgG class. There is little evidence for anti-lymphocyte antibodies of the IgD or IgA class in these patients. The antibodies vary in their reactivity at different temperatures. All show strongest reactivity at 4°C while a lesser proportion are demonstrable by incubation at 23° and 37° C. Evidence has been obtained that they participate in formation of cryoprecipitates with lymphocyte antigen.

Certain monoclonal cold agglutinins specific for either components of the Ii complex or Pr antigens cross-react strongly with molecules expressed on T or B lymphocytes (R. Winchester, unpublished observations).

In various lymphoproliferative malignancies, polyclonal as well as monoclonal, autoreactive anti-lymphocyte antibodies can be demonstrated; here also, they are sometimes associated with cryoprecipitation.

In contrast to these "pathologic" antibodies, all adults have various antibodies to cryptantigens on the lymphocyte surface, such as are exposed by neuraminidase digestion or other modification. These antibodies are of the IgM class, and their presence could under some experimental circumstances cause confusing fluorescence (12).

4.8. B Lymphocyte Alloantigens Demonstrable by Indirect Immunofluorescence. Evidence from several laboratories has come together to form a picture of a human B cell differentiation alloantigen system that is selectively expressed on all B cells and monocytes, but not the vast majority of T lymphocytes, erythrocytes, or platelets (18–20). Human allosera obtained from pregnant women or transplant recipients provide the reagents for study of this system by indirect immunofluorescence. There appear to be a set of several distinct molecules that characterize B lymphocytes. These are present on acute lymphatic leukemic lymphocytes that lack all other T or B cell markers (21). The same antigens are found on acute myelogenous leukemia blasts but not on mature polymorphonuclear leukocytes.

REFERENCES

1. Ploem, J. S., Z. Wiss. Mikrosk. **68**, 129 (1967).
2. Winchester, R. J., Fu, S. M., Hoffman, T., and Kunkel, H. G., J. Immunol. **114**, 1210 (1975).
3. Fauk, W. P., and Hijmans, W., Prog. Allergy **16**, 9 (1972).
4. Amante, L., Ancona, A., and Forni, L., J. Immunol. Methods **1**, 289 (1972).

5. Cebra, J. J., and Goldstein, G., *J. Immunol.* **95**, 230 (1965).
6. Brandtzaeg, P., *Scand. J. Immunol.* **2**, 273 (1973).
7. Pernis, B., Forni, L., and Amante, L., *J. Exp. Med.* **132**, 1001 (1970).
8. Seligmann, M., Preud'homme, J.-L., and Brouet, J.-C., *Transplant. Rev.* **16**, 85 (1973).
9. Knapp, W., Haaijamn, J. J., Schuit, H. R. E., Radl, J., van den Berg, P., Ploem, J. S., and Hijmans, W., *Immunofluorescence and Related Staining Techniques, 5th N. Y. Acad. Sci.* **254**, 94 (1975).
10. Winchester, R. J., Winfield, J. B., Siegal, F., Wernet, P., Bentwich, Z., and Kunkel, H. G., *J. Clin. Invest.* **54**, 1082 (1974).
11. Winfield, J. B., Winchester, R. J., Wernet, P., Fu, S. M., and Kunkel, H. G., *Arthritis Rheum.* **18**, 1 (1975).
12. Winchester, R. J., Fu, S. M., Winfield, J. B., and Kunkel, H. G., *J. Immunol.* **114**, 410 (1975).
13. Hijmans, W., and Schaeffer, M. (eds.), *Ann. N. Y. Acad. Sci.* **254**, 1–627 (1975).
14. Fu, S. M., Winchester, R. J., and Kunkel, H. G., *J. Immunol.* **114**, 250 (1975).
15. Hijmans, W., and Schaeffer, M., *Ann. N. Y. Acad. Sci.* **254**, 1 (1975).
16. Dickler, H. B., and Kunkel, H. G., *J. Exp. Med.* **136**, 191 (1972).
17. Frøland, S. S., and Natvig, J. B., *Transplant. Rev.* **16**, 114 (1973).
18. Winchester, R. J., Fu, S. M., Wernet, P., Kunkel, H. G., Dupont, B., and Jersild, C., *J. Exp. Med.* **141**, 924 (1975).
19. Mann, D. L., Abelson, L., Harris, S. D., and Amos, D. B., *J. Exp. Med.* **142**, 84 (1975).
20. van Rood, J. J., van Leeuwen, A., Keuning, J. J., and Termijtelen, O. O., *Transplant. Proc.* **7**, 31 (1975).
21. Fu, S. M., Winchester, R. J., and Kunkel, H. G., *J. Exp. Med.* **142**, 1334 (1975).

11

Assays for Epstein-Barr Virus (EBV) Receptors

Mikael Jondal

1. Introduction

The capacity to bind the Epstein-Barr virus (EBV) is a B lymphocyte characteristic and may be used as a B lymphocyte marker (1, 2). Recent evidence indicates that the EBV receptor is linked to the complement receptor complex (3); so far there is a complete correlation between the expression of C3d and EBV receptors although the actual binding sites do not appear to be identical (3). This correlation holds true only for *human cells of lymphoid origin;* i.e., no EBV receptors have been found on human monocytes or granulocytes or on mouse lymphocytes (3). This restriction of the EBV receptor to human lymphoid cells, in contrast to the wider distribution of complement receptors, indicates that the EBV receptor assay may be useful in the classification of human leukemias. However, as with most markers, exceptions from the general rule exist, thus Molt-4, a T cell line (4), has been found to express EBV as well as C3d receptors (1, 3).

Three different assays will be described. The first method consists of adsorption of virus that is secondarily visualized by direct membrane immunoflorescence (5). The second method is based on the fact that lytically infected, EBV-producing cells form rosettes with EBV receptor-positive cells (1). The third method allows quantitation, as it compares the capacity of different cells to adsorb virus by testing remaining viral activity in an antigen induction assay, in the nonadsorbed supernatant (6).

2. Material

2.1. For the Direct Membrane Immunofluorescence Method. *2.1.1. Preparation of EBV.* Two different producer cell lines may be used: P3HR-1, derived from a Burkitt's lymphoma patient (7) or B95-8, a marmoset-derived cell line producing virus of human origin (8). For viral production the cell lines are cultivated for 14 days at 33°C in RPMI 1640 medium supplemented with antibiotics and 2% fetal calf serum, the initial cell concentration being 2 ✕

10^5/ml. Subsequently cells and debris are removed by low speed centrifugation. B95-8 supernatants may be used unconcentrated whereas P3HR-1 supernatants should be concentrated by polyethylene glycol (PEG) (9); accordingly; solid, dry heat-sterilized NaCl (20 g/liter) is added to the supernatant and polyethylene glycol 6000 (AB Kebo, Stockholm, Sweden) as a 50% (w/v) sterile solution in 0.5 M NaCl to a final concentration of 8% PEG. The mixture is left for at least 1 hr at 4°C before the sedimentable phase is collected by centrifugation at 7000 g for 15 min in a Sorvall GS3 rotor. The virus pellets are resuspended in 1% of the initial volume.

2.1.2. Preparation of Antisera Directed against the EBV-Associated Membrane Antigen (MA). Sera containing antibodies against the MA antigen may be taken from patients with Burkitt's lymphoma or nasopharyngeal carcinoma (5, 10) or from certain normal individuals (2). The serum IgG fraction is conjugated to fluorescein isothiocyanate (FITC) or tetramethylrhodamine isothiocyanate (TRITC) by standard techniques (11).

2.2. For the Rosette Assay. *2.2.1. Isolation of EBV-Producing Cells.* For this purpose only the P3HR-1 cell line can be used. This line contains in general 1–5% EBV-producing cells, which may be isolated, or at least enriched, as they are less dense than the nonproducing cells, on a discontinuous two-step Ficoll–Isopaque gradient. Three milliliters of standard Ficoll–Iospaque (Ficoll, Pharmacia Fine Chemicals Ind., Uppsala, Sweden; Isopaque, Nyegaard & Cl., Oslo, Norway), with the same density, 1.077, as that used for lymphocyte isolation from whole blood (12), is loaded in a siliconized 15-ml tube and overlayered with 3 ml of Ficoll–Isopaque adjusted to density 1.042 with isotonic NaCl. P3HR-1 cells (5 ml; 4 × 10^6/ml) in buffer with 10% fetal calf serum is loaded on each gradient tube and centrifuged at 900 g for 20 min. The cells at the first interphase are harvested and washed twice.

2.3. For the EBV Adsorption Assay. *2.3.1. Preparation of EBV.* As described in Section 2.1.1.

2.3.2. Preparation of Antisera Directed against the EBV-Associated Early Antigen (EA). High-titered anti-EA sera are preferentially found among patients with Burkitt's lymphoma or nasopharyngeal carcinoma (5, 10). The serum IgG fraction is conjugated to FITC or TRITC by standard techniques (11).

3. Methods

3.1. Direct Membrane Immunofluorescence Method. Cells (0.5 × 10^6) are mixed with 1.0 ml of B95-8 supernatant or 1.0 ml of a dilution of the concentrated P3HR-1 supernatant (usually in the range of 1:5 to 1:40) for 1 hr at 4°C with shaking every 15 min. After two washes the cells and the medium-treated control cells are mixed with 50 μl of the conjugated anti-MA antiserum and incubated for 45 min at 4°C. The appropriate anti-MA titer should be found by analyzing a dilution series of the antiserum on EBV adsorbed and unadsorbed receptor-positive reference cells (Table 1). The test should be read soon after the last washing; positive cells appear stained in a ringlike, dotted fashion.

3.2. The Rosette Assay. To allow identification of the virus-producing cells these should be prestained with a FITC or TRITC conjugated anti-MA serum (see Section 2.1.2) for 30 min at 4°C. The producer cells will appear as strongly, ringlike stained. Of these cells, 10^5 are mixed with 2×10^6 of the cells under investigation in 100 μl of buffer (containing 5% fetal calf serum) and incubated at 4°C for 1 hr. Then the cells are gently shaken, mounted on a glass slide, and read in UV light. If the investigated cells have EBV receptors, they will bind to the MA-positive cells and *only to these cells*. The results may be recorded as (a) the percentage of MA-positive cells having adhering cells, or (b) the number of cells adhering to a fixed number of MA-positive cells.

TABLE 1

Lymphoid Cell Lines (B Cell Type) Used in Assays for
Epstein-Barr Virus (EBV) Receptors

Name of cell line	Characteristics and origin	Used for
P3HR-1	Derived from Burkitt's lymphoma (7)	Production of nontransforming EBV, EBV receptor-negative line
B95-8	Marmoset derived (8)	Production of transforming EBV, EBV receptor-negative line
RAJI	Derived from Burkitt's lymphoma (17, 18), a nonproducer cell line	EBV receptor-positive reference cell line
DAUDI	Derived from Burkitt's lymphoma (19), a low level-producer cell line.	EBV receptor-positive reference cell line
P3HR-1	See P3HR-1 above	Production of EBV-positive rosette-forming cells
RAJI	See RAJI above	EA induction assay
DAUDI	See DAUDI above	EA induction assay
BJAB	Derived from lymphoma, EBV-negative (20)	EBNA[a] induction assay
Ramos	Derived from lymphoma EBV negative (21)	EBNA[a] induction assay

[a]EBNA, Epstein-Barr virus nuclear antigen.

3.3. The Adsorption Assay. Fractions, 1.0 ml, of concentrated P3HR-1 supernatant (usually diluted 1:20 to 1:40) is mixed with a dilution series of the investigated cells, ranging from 10^7 to 10^5. The fractions are incubated for 2 hr at 4°C with continuous shaking; the cells are then spun down, and 0.5 ml of supernatant is harvested from each tube. The remaining EBV activity, in the supernatant, is then measured by the EA induction assay (5, 13): 0.5×10^6 RAJI cells are mixed with each 0.5-ml fraction and incubated for 1 hr at 37°C for superinfection to occur; the cells are then washed once and further incubated at 37°C for 48 hr under tissue-culture conditions. Finally, the cells are washed and smeared on glass slides. After air-drying, the slide is fixed in cold acetone: methanol (1:1) for 5 min, washed in buffer, and overlayered with 50 μl of a conjugated anti-EA serum for 30 min at room temperature in a humid chamber. After a final washing, a drop of glycerol:PBS (1:1) is used to cover the cells under a cover slip. B95-8 virus does not induce EA and can thus not be estimated by EA induction. A comparable assay for B95-8 virus is the EBV nuclear antigen (EBNA) induction assay in the EBV-negative cell lines, Ramos and BJAB (14, 15). However, this assay is technically more difficult.

4. Comments

The determination of EBV receptors is somewhat problematical as the virus does not exist in a purified form. The "EBV" preparations derived from supernatants of producer cell lines contain a variety of ill-defined proteins and cell-derived products. This may be less important, however, as the specificity in the direct membrane immunofluorescence method is determined not by the supernatant material, but by the conjugated anti-MA sera. Furthermore, it is most likely that a large proportion of the adsorbed and stained material consists of membrane fragments that contain the MA antigen known to cross-react with the outer surface of the virus particle (16).

The rosette assay was originally developed because the direct membrane immunofluorescence method, at that time, was too insensitive when applied to peripheral lymphocytes. Later it was found that the fluorescence test could be used also for peripheral lymphocytes if the conditions were optimized. The staining on these cells is weak, however. In general, the rosette assay is more difficult than the direct fluorescent test; for the sake of simplicity, the latter is thus to be preferred.

The adsorption method is important as it is the only method that measures binding of functional virus particles (6). Furthermore, it is seminquantitative as it allows comparison of the number of cell-bound virus particles between different receptor-positive cell types.

REFERENCES

1. Jondal, M., and Klein, G., *J. Exp. Med.* **138,** 1365 (1973).
2. Greaves, M. F., Brown, G., and Rickinson, A. B., *Clin. Immunol. Immunopathol.* **3,** 514 (1975).
3. Jondal, M., Klein, G., Oldstone, M. B. A., Bokisch, V., and Yefenof, E., *Scand. J. Immunol.* **5,** 401 (1976).
4. Minowada, J., Ohnuma, T., and Moore, G. E., *J. Natl. Cancer Inst.* **49,** 891 (1972).
5. Klein, G., Dombos, L., and Gothoskar, B., *Int. J. Cancer* **10,** 44 (1972).
6. Sairenji, T., and Hinuma, Y., *Gann* **64,** 583 (1973).
7. Hinuma, Y., and Grace, J. T., *Proc. Soc. Exp. Biol. Med.* **124,** 107 (1967).
8. Miller, G., and Lipmann, M., *Proc. Natl. Acad. Sci. U.S.A.* **70,** 190 (1973).
9. Adams, A., *J. Gen. Virol.* **20,** 391 (1973).
10. Klein, G., *in* "Oncogenesis and Herpesviruses" (G. de-Thè and H. zur Hausen, eds.), p. 293. IARC, Lyon 1974.
11. Weir, D. M. (ed.), "Handbook of Experimental Immunology," 2nd ed. Blackwell, Oxford, 1973.
12. Böyum, A. A., *Scand. J. Clin. Lab. Invest.* **21,** 51 (1968).
13. Klein, G., and Dombos, L., *Int. J. Cancer* **11,** 327 (1973).
14. Dölken, G., and Klein, G., *Virology* **70,** 210 (1976).
15. Reedman, B. M., and Klein, G., *Int. J. Cancer* **11,** 499 (1973).
16. Silvestre, D., Kourilsky, F. M., Klein, G., Yata, J., Neuport-Sautes, C., and Levy, J. P., *Int. J. Cancer* **49,** 891 (1971).
17. Epstein, M. A., Achong, B. G., Barr, Y. M., Zajac, B., Henle, G., and Henle, W., *J. Natl. Cancer Inst.* **37,** 547 (1966).
18. Pulvertaft, R. J. V., *J. Clin. Pathol.* **18,** 261 (1965).
19. Klein, G., Pearson, G., Nadkarni, J. S., Nadkarni, J. J., Klein, E., Henle, G., Henle, W., and Clifford, P., *J. Exp. Med.* **128,** 1011 (1968).
20. Menezes, J., Leibold, W., Klein, G., and Clements, G., *Biomedicine* **22,** 276 (1975).
21. Klein, G., Giovanelli, B., Westman, A., Stehlin, J., and Mumford, D., *Intervirology* **5,** 319 (1975).

12

Protein A from *Staphylococcus* as a Human Lymphocyte Mitogen*

A. Forsgren, A. Svedjelund, and Hans Wigzell

1. Introduction

Morphology and function complement each other in the characterization of a given cell type. Surface markers, such as the capacity to express and produce surface-attached immunoglobulin or the ability to bind sheep erythrocytes, have been found to be very useful characteristics of human B and T lymphocytes, respectively. With regard to functional markers, mitogens have found important applications in animal as well as in human research as markers of subpopulations of lymphocytes. In studies using human peripheral blood as a source for lymphocytes, there exists by now a relative abundance of substances such as phytohemagglutinin (PHA) and concanavalin A (Con A) with a seemingly selective capacity to trigger T lymphocytes into division (1–3). Other substances have been reported to trigger both T and subsequently B lymphocytes into increased DNA synthesis, perhaps the most frequently reported structure in this regard being pokeweed mitogen (PWM) (1, 3). It should be realized, however, that PWM as mostly used is a composite mixture of substances, and there exists no convincing evidence that purified B cells alone will be stimulated into mitosis by this mitogen(s) (3). There is thus a need for a specific B cell mitogen for human blood lymphocytes, and until recently only one such system was reported, that using anti-β_2-microglobulin antibodies as a B lymphocyte triggering agent (4). However, having to rely upon heterantisera, there is always a problem of standardization.

Very recently we have found that a bacterial substance obtainable in pure form, namely, protein A from the *Staphylcoccus aureus* (5, 6), can be used in a polymerized state as a selective mitogen for human peripheral blood B lymphocytes (7). No evidence has so far been obtained that T lymphocytes can respond to this structure, nor is there anything to suggest that they contribute in any measurable way to B lymphocyte activation. In the present article we will thus describe the optimal conditions for obtaining stimulation of DNA synthesis in human B cell-enriched population using this mitogen.

*This work was supported by grants from the Swedish Medical Research Council, the Swedish Cancer Society, and NIH Contract NOI-CB-43883.

2. Material and Methods

2.1. Bacterial Strains. *Staphylococcus aureus* Cowan I (with a high surface content of protein A) and Wood 46 (with esentially no protein A) were used (8). The bacteria were killed by incubation in 0.5% formaldehyde for 3 hr at room temperature followed by heat-killing at 80°C for 3 min.

2.2. Lymphocyte Separation Techniques. Human lymphocytes were obtained using whole blood in 10 IU/ml of heparin. The blood was diluted 1:2 in a balanced salt solution containing 40 mM EDTA and layered on a Ficoll–sodium metrizoate solution (Ficoll, Pharmacia, Uppsala, Sweden; sodium metrizoate, Nyegaard & Co., Oslo, Norway) using the concentrations prescribed by Böyum (9). The blood was centrifuged at 400 g for 25 min, and adherent cells were removed via carbonyl-iron and magnetism. The lymphocytes were then washed twice and finally resuspended in RPMI 1640 *without serum,* using 2 mM L-glutamine; 5 μl/liter 2-mercaptoethanol per 10 U/ml of penicillin and 10 μg/ml streptomycin. T lymphocytes were then prepared through removal over anti-Ig coated glass-bead columns (10; see also Method 18).

B lymphocytes were separated through depletion of cells forming rosettes with sheep erythrocytes, a good marker for human T lymphocytes (2). Rosette formation was carried out essentially as described (2; see also Method 17), using Ficoll–sodium metrizoate centrifugation.

2.3. Lymphocyte stimulation. Lymphocytes, 10^6 in 1-ml tissue culture tubes, were used throughout. Purified phytohemagglutinin (PHA, Wellcome) was used at a concentration of 1 μg per 10^6 cells. *Staphylococcus aureus* were added in varying numbers in volumes of 50 μl per milliliter of lymphocytes. Incubations were carried out at 37°C at 5% CO_2, adding 1 μCi of tritiated thymidine (0.2 mCi/μg, specific activity) to each culture 22 hr prior to termination.

3. Results

3.1. Lymphocyte Stimulation Experiments with *S. aureus*: Determination of Optimal Stimulating Numbers of Bacteria and Time of Incubation. In experiments establishing the optimal conditions for stimulation, it was found that maximal uptake of tritiated thymidine was obtained when adding Cowan I staphylococci to obtain a ratio of between 10 and 100 bacteria per lymphocyte. Using such numbers, stimulation of almost the same extent as that induced by PHA was found when terminating the cultures at day 3 of stimulation. Day 3 was also found to be optimal with regard to stimulation with protein A-positive bacteria, markedly lower stimulation being found at day 5 or 7. Cowan I always gave a significantly better stimulation then Wood 46, usually 4–10 times better (8).

3.2. Stimulation Experiments with Subpopulations of Lymphocytes. Control or B or T lymphocytes purified as described in Section 2 were used as responder cells when stimulating with Cowan I bacteria or PHA, harvesting at day 3. Figure

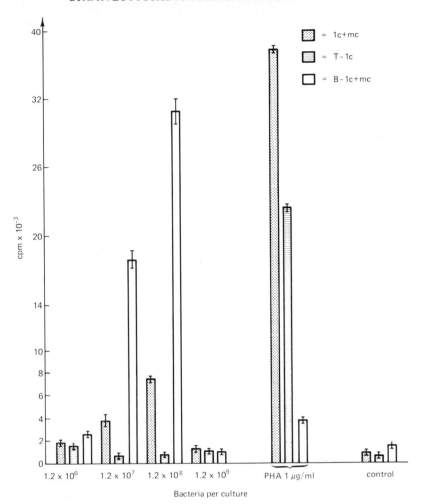

Fig. 1. Tritiated thymidine incorporation in human lymphocytes stimulated with phyto-hemagglutinin (PHA) or protein A-positive *Staphylococcus aureus,* strain Cowan I. lc+mc, Ficoll—Isopaque purified lymphocytes with monocytes. T-lc,T lymphocytes produced by sheep RBC rosetting. B-lc+mc,B lymphocytes enriched by depletion of sheep RBC rosetting lymphocytes, containing monocytes. Removal of monocytes has a marginal effect on DNA synthesis.

1 shows one representative experiment out of five. As shown in the figure, Cowan I bacteria significantly stimulated control lymphocytes to increased DNA synthesis, but the enriched B-lymphocyte population was by far the best-responding population of cells. Purified T cells, on the other hand, did not respond in a detectable manner to Cowan I staphylococci. Exactly opposite

results were obtained using PHA as mitogen. Here, control and T lymphocytes showed excellent responses whereas the B cell population displayed only very marginal increases. It would thus be fair to state that the Cowan I bacteria, in contrast to PHA, are excellent stimulators of cell division of human B lymphocyte-enriched, T lymphocyte-depleted populations.

4. Discusssion

Protein A of *Staphylococcus aureus* is known to display specific binding to the Fc region of IgG of the subclasses 1, 2, and 4 in the human (6). In the present system we know that protein A is a most relevant structure in the triggering of human B cell-enriched populations into DNA synthesis for the following reasons (7): (a) There exists a positive correlation between the amount of protein A expressed on the outer surface of the bacteria and their respective capacity to induce cell division. (b) $F(ab)_2$ anti-protein A antibodies will block the mitogenic activity. (c) Purified protein A polymerized via coupling to Sephadex or Sepharose beads will trigger as do the bacteria. (d) Monomeric protein A will tend to block the capacity of polymeric protein A to induce B cell division in a competitive manner.

It should be realized, however, that although we consider the present system to be a most promising one for the studies of activated human B cells, several questions remain as yet to be resolved at the theoretical level. First, we do not know whether the triggering is actually taking place via surface-bound IgG molecules, be they intrinsically produced or absorbed by cytophilic means. Also, the very good response as measured by DNA synthesis using B cell-enriched populations may or may not be produced by the low number of actual IgG-producing B cells present at time zero of stimulation. Finally, we do not know as yet whether the proliferation will lead to increased Ig synthesis in the blast cells.

Thus, several points remain to be established. However, the virtues of the present system are already obvious, as protein A can be produced in a biochemically pure form that would allow standardization of B cell activation.

REFERENCES

1. Greaves, M. F., and Janossy, G., *Transplant. Rev.* **11,** 87 (1972).
2. Jondal, M., Wigzell, H., and Aiuti, F., *Transplant. Rev.* **16,** 163 (1973).
3. Jondal, M., *Scand. J. Immunol.* **3,** 739 (1974).
4. Ringden, O., and Möller, E., *Scand. J. Immunol.* **4,** 171 (1975).
5. Forsgren, A., and Sjöquist, J., *J. Immunol.* **97,** 822 (1966).
6. Kronvall, G., and Williams, R. C., Jr., *J. Immunol.* **103,** 828 (1969).
7. Forsgren, A., Svedjelund, A., and Wigzell, H., *Eur. J. Immunol.* **6,** 207 (1976).
8. Forsgren, A., *Infect. Immun.* **2,** 672 (1972).
9. Böyum, A., *Scand. J. Clin. Lab. Invest.* **21,** Suppl. 97 (1968).
10. Wigzell, H., Sundqvist, K. G., and Yoshida, T. O., *Scand. J. Immunol.* **1,** 75 (1972).

Characterization and Enumeration of Lymphocyte Populations in Whole Human Peripheral Blood

M. B. Pepys

1. Introduction

There are serious drawbacks in many of the widely used methods for the characterization and enumeration of lymphocyte populations among cells isolated from either blood or lymphoid organs. These problems fall into three groups.

1.1. The data most likely to be of clinical significance in studies on peripheral blood are the true ratios and absolute concentrations of different circulating lymphocyte populations. However, it is not possible to derive this information from most previous work which has utilized mononuclear cells isolated from blood, since all the available procedures provide subtotal and variable yields. Brown and Greaves (1) have elegantly demonstrated that the ratio of T to B lymphocytes in a given cell suspension alters substantially with the yield during isolation. This obviously does not invalidate work in leukemias, where the point at issue is characterization of a large abnormal population, but it may be highly relevant to the study of other conditions, such as chronic inflammatory diseases, in many studies of which a moderate "depletion" of T cells has been reported (2). Various factors, such as alteration of the plasma protein profile, might cause sufficient reduction in the yield from a mononuclear cell separation procedure to cause an apparent loss of T cells. Brown and Greaves, who first clearly delineated this problem, overcame it by testing for lymphocyte surface markers in whole peripheral blood (1). The present method is a development of their approach.

1.2. Monocytes, as well as lymphocytes, bear C3 and Fc receptors, and they may bind immunoglobulin on their surface, where it is detected by immunofluorescence and other techniques (3) The identification of monocytes in either mononuclear cell isolates or whole blood is therefore essential for accurate enumeration of lymphocytes. Most workers have relied on criteria of size and phagocytic activity, but neither of these is completely satisfactory. When small size is used as the major criterion for identification of lymphocytes, and therefore exclusion of monocytes, the large and medium lymphocytes, which may constitute up to 10% of all lymphocytes in normals, will be excluded. Marking of phagocytic cells has other problems, particularly that only about 60% of monocytes will phagocytize at any one time (4). Endogenous myeloperoxidase is a better marker and identifies about 90% of monocytes (4), including the small cells which might be confused with lymphocytes, but there are some monocytes which lack peroxidase. Fortunately, most of these are large, distinctive cells, which are obviously not lymphocytes and can therefore be discounted.

1.3. A proportion of normal lymphocytes, including B cells, some T cells, and some cells which lack distinctive T or B characteristics, have the capacity to bind IgG both in a form that occurs in plasma and when it is the antibody in an immune complex. This is a serious potential cause of error in the detection of lymphocyte surface markers, especially immunoglobulin, by the use of labeled IgG antibodies (5–7). During the preparation and washing of blood or lymphocytes in the cold, IgG, and to a lesser extent IgA, from the plasma become associated with cells (5, 7). Labeled anti-immunoglobulin antibodies of IgG class form complexes with this cell-associated immunoglobulin, which then adhere via the Fc piece of the detecting antibody to lymphocyte surface $Fc(\gamma)$ receptors (6). This phenomenon can be overcome by washing cells at 37° or by applying a low pH shock before staining, both of which procedures seem to remove the cell-associated immunoglobulins (5, 7). Alternatively, use of the $F(ab)_2$ fragment of the detecting antibody (6) circumvents both this difficulty, and a further potential risk that any whole IgG antibody, irrespective of its specificity, might associate with cells in the cold and be detected there either by an intrinsic label or after application of a second-stage labeled reagent.

We have developed a method for immunofluorescent detection of lymphocyte surface markers in whole peripheral blood which overcomes many of the problems outlined above, and permits accurate enumeration of the proportions and absolute concentration of different circulating lymphocyte populations. The technique has been used mainly to study cell surface immunoglobulin, but it is applicable to other markers and should prove useful for routine clinical investigation.

2. Materials

2.1. Blood Samples. Venous blood from normal donors drawn into heparin is used for the whole-blood method, and a sample drawn into EDTA is sent for a routine blood count and 100-cell leukocyte differential.

2.2. Antisera and Other Immunological Reagents. Fluorescein isothiocyanate (FITC)-conjugated IgG fractions and their $F(ab)_2$ fragments from sheep and rabbit antisera specific for human immunoglobulins have been most extensively used. Preliminary work with FITC-aggregated IgG (for Fc receptors) and FITC–anti-lymphocyte antibodies (for T cells) has been undertaken.

2.3. Other materials and Reagents. Plastic tubes, 2.5-ml (LP3, Luckham Ltd., Sussex, England) are used for processing the blood. Diluent for washing cells is phosphate-buffered saline (PBS) pH 7.3 containing 0.2% bovine serum albumin (BSA, Sigma Chemical Co., St. Louis, Missouri) and 0.2% sodium azide (PBS/BSA/azide). Other reagents are: fetal calf serum (FCS) (GIBCO Biocult Ltd., Paisley, Scotland); 3,3-diaminobenzidine tetrahydrochloride (DAB, Sigma); methyl green (CI 42585, BDH Chemicals Ltd., Poole, England); glycerol/PBS (9:1) pH 7.2; and translucent nail enamel.

2.4. Microscopy. A Leitz Orthoplan microscope with incident illumination and water immersion fluorescence objectives is used, but any comparable instrument would suffice. The GG455 filter, which excludes the excitatory wavelength (420 nm) for the red fluorescence of methyl green, must be removed.

3. Method

3.1. Wash 0.25 ml of heparinized venous blood 3 times (200 g, 7 min, 4°C) with 1.2 ml of PBS/BSA/azide.

3.2. Incubate 25-μl volumes of washed blood on ice for 30 min with 25-μl volumes of optimal dilutions of fluorescein-conjugated reagents, then wash 3 times (200 g, 7 min, 4°C) with PBS/BSA/azide.

3.3. Reconstitute the cell pellet with 25 μl of FCS and make thin smears on clean glass microscope slides. Dry in air then fix with 95% ethanol/formaldehyde (9:1).

3.4. Wash fixed smears in PBS for 3 min in Coplin jar, then stain for peroxidase (9) as follows. Add 100 μl of fresh 1% H_2O_2 to 10 ml of a fresh 0.5% solution of DAB in Tris/HCl buffer, pH 7.6. Cover smears with this mixture for 7 min before rinsing in distilled water.

3.5. Counterstain for 6 min with 0.01% methyl green freshly diluted in PBS from a stock 0.1% solution in distilled water (10).

3.6. Wash smears for 1 min in PBS, then mount wet in glycerol/PBS; seal in with translucent nail enamel.

3.7. Examine each field under alternate bright and UV light. Lymphocytes are identified as peroxidase-negative mononuclear cells, and as many fluorescein-positive cells as possible, up to 35, are counted together with the negative cells seen in linear or battlement-pattern scanning of the slide. Occasional very large mononuclear cells, which clearly are not lymphocytes even though they lack intracellular peroxidase, are not counted.

3.8. Calculation of Results. Washing and staining blood as described here did not alter the total leukocyte count or the leukocyte differential, assessed after further staining with Giemsa–May–Grünwald. Furthermore, there was good correlation between the proportion of lymphocytes in the total leukocyte count and the proportion of peroxidase-negative leukocytes; in smears stained for peroxidase and counterstained with Giemsa—May—Grünwald, there were exceedingly few peroxidase negative cells which might have been monocytes. The absolute number of fluorescein-positive lymphocytes per microliter was therefore derived by multiplying the proportion of these cells by the absolute lymphocyte count.

4. Discussion

4.1. The identification of monocytes is critical, and it is essential to exclude cells with even a single brown granule or trace of staining. In contrast to the method of Preud'homme and Flandrin (4), we have found that the DAB technique leaves unstained almost no cells recognizable as monocytes by morphological criteria in Romanovsky stained smears (B. Bain, M. Druguet, and M. B. Pepys, unpublished).

4.2. The fluorescence of both fluorescein and methyl red are rather labile (24 hr) in these preparations, and it is essential that fresh PBS be used throughout, and fresh glycerol be used for mounting. The smears are, however, stable after fixation and can be kept in the dark and cold to be stained for peroxidase and counterstained immediately before counting.

4.3. The risks of sampling error in counting leukocytes in blood smears are well recognized. These are not readily soluble and can only be minimized by making good smears and counting thoroughly representative samples.

4.4. Some data obtained using antibodies to different immunoglobulins are shown in Table 1 (8). FITC-F(ab)$_2$ anti-whole Ig stains around 13% of lymphocytes, that is the same as the sum of cells stained by anti-IgM (or IgD), anti-IgA, and F(ab)$_2$ anti-IgG. We agree with Winchester et al. (6) that the lymphocytes stained by whole IgG polyvalent anti-immunoglobulin include both true B cells with intrinsic surface-membrane immunoglobulin and other cells with Fc receptors. Washing at 37°C before staining the blood reduces in parallel the number of lymphocytes stained by polyvalent anti-immunoglobulin and anti-IgG (Table 2). We have not yet applied F(ab)$_2$ anti-IgA for the detection of IgA-bearing cells, and it may be, in view of the observation that IgA as well as IgG can adhere to lymphoid cells (7), that our value of 2.2% overestimates the number of Bα cells.

The proportions of both B cells and Fc-receptor lymphocytes in and between individuals seem to be remarkably constant, though the absolute numbers vary with the lymphocyte count. Our values for B cells and for total lymphocytes stained by polyvalent anti-immunoglobulin are slightly greater than those obtained by Winchester et al. (6) and by Brown and Greaves (1) in their whole-blood method. A possible explanation is that these groups used small size as a

TABLE 1

Lymphocytes in Whole Blood Stained by Anti-immunoglobulin Antibodies

| | Positive cells | | | | |
| | Percentage | | Concentration | | |
Reagent	Mean ± SD	Range	Mean ± SD (No./μl)	Range	No. of individuals[a]
IgG anti-whole Ig	20.5 ± 1.0	18.7 – 22.2	380 ± 117	232 – 652	20
IgG anti-IgM	8.1 ± 2.3	4.5 – 12.4	142 ± 60	56 – 304	20
IgG anti-IgD	8.9 ± 2.2	5.2 – 13.3	212 ± 85	83 – 317	11
IgG anti-IgA	2.2 ± 1.6	0.8 – 4.0	41 ± 24	61 – 105	22
IgG anti-IgG	11.0 ± 1.6	7.7 – 12.8	195 ± 55	97 – 303	20
F(ab)$_2$ anti-IgG	2.3 ± 1.6	0.0 – 4.3	60 ± 47	6 – 128	7

[a]Each individual was tested once. Repeated testing of many individuals always gave very similar percentage results; the absolute values, however, varied with the absolute lymphocyte count at different times.

primary criterion for identification of lymphocytes and exclusion of monocytes. Since up to 10% of normal peripheral blood lymphocytes may be "large," these cells will have been excluded. The effect of strictly counting only small lymphocytes on results obtained with polyvalent anti-immunoglobulin is shown in Table 3, and the mean value of 15.7% is virtually the same as that of Brown and Greaves (1). It seems that a higher proportion of large than of small lymphocytes stain with anti-immunoglobulin.

4.6. The present method should be applicable to the study of any lymphocyte marker which can be detected by immunofluorescence. It should also permit accurate enumeration of circulating lymphocyte populations in disease.

TABLE 2

Effect of Washing Blood at 37°C before Immunofluorescent Staining

| | | Positive lymphocytees (%) | |
Donor	Reagent	Washed at 4°C	Washed at 37°C
1	IgG anti-whole Ig	20.3	14.2
	IgG anti-IgG	9.8	2.9
2	IgG anti-whole Ig	19.7	9.7
	IgG anti-IgG	11.6	3.8

TABLE 3
Small Lymphocytes Stainable by IgG Anti-whole Immunoglobulin Antibodies

Reagent	No. of individuals	Lymphocytes counted	Positive cells (%)	
			Mean ± SD	Range
Ig anti-whole Ig	7	All	19.4 ± 0.7	18.5 – 20.3
Ig anti-whole Ig	7	Small only	15.7 ± 1.7	12.5 – 17.7

ACKNOWLEDGMENTS

The present methods and results are the composite effort of several colleagues: Dr. Carla Sategna-Guidetti, D. D. Mirjah, A. C. Dash, Dr. M. H. Wansbrough-Jones, and Dr. M. Druguet. The advice of Dr. M. F. Greaves and Professor A. G. E. Pearse has been invaluable.

REFERENCES

1. Brown, G., and Greaves, M. F., *Scand. J. Immunol.* **3,** 161 (1974).
2. Editorial, *Brit. Med. J.* **2,** 1 (1975).
3. Aiuti, F., Cerottini, J.-C., Coombs, R. R. A., *et al., Scand. J. Immunol.* **3,** 521 (1974).
4. Preud'homme, J.-L., and Flandrin, G., *J. Immunol.* **113,** 1650 (1974).
5. Lobo, P. I., Westervelt, F. B., and Horwitz, D. A., *J. Immunol.* **114,** 116 (1975).
6. Winchester, R. J., Fu, S. M., Hoffman, T., and Kunkel, H. G., *J. Immunol.* **114,** 1210 (1975).
7. Kumagai, K., Abo, T., Sekizaka, T., and Sasaki, M., *J. Immunol.* **115,** 982 (1975).
8. Pepys, M. B., Sategna-Guidetti, C., Mirjah, D. D., Wansbrough-Jones, M. H., and Dash, A. C., *Clin Exp. Immunol.* in press.
9. Graham, R. C., and Karnovsky, M. J., *J. Histochem. Cytochem.* **14,** 291 (1966).
10. Schenk, E. A., and Churukian, C. J., *J. Histochem. Cytochem.* **22,** 962 (1974).

Detection of Specific Mononuclear Cell Receptors in Tissue Sections

Michael M. Frank, Elaine S. Jaffe, and Ira Green

1. Introduction

During the past several years, a variety of membrane receptors have been identified on the surface of bone marrow-derived (B) lymphocytes, thymus-derived (T) lymphocytes, and macrophages (1−7). Identification of the receptors on mononuclear cells in suspension has allowed these cells to be identified and distinguished from one another. As an extention of these techniques, it has been possible to identify a number of these receptors on cells in tissue section and, therefore, characterize the type of mononuclear cells in normal and diseased tissues (8−13).

There are a number of advantages in being able to identify mononuclear cells directly in tissue sections. Although a cellular suspension is easily prepared from peripheral blood and most lymphoid organs, any degree of fibrosis within the tissue may lead to difficulty in extracting some of the cells. An adequate cellular suspension is also difficult to obtain from nonlymphoid organs, such as the liver or breast, especially if the mononuclear cell infiltrate is sparse. Another advantage of tissue section techniques is that one can define the localization of cells within the same tissue and identify the physical interrelationships among different cells present. These considerations are of crucial importance in the study of malignant lymphoreticular infiltrates. For example, in many instances of malignant lymphoma, particularly nodular lymphoma, a lymph node may be only focally involved. It may be difficult to identify and characterize the malignant cells in suspension, although this is easily accomplished in tissue sections where one can observe binding of the indicator reagent to cells in the neoplastic nodules.

Similarly, topographical considerations are also important in the study of benign or reactive cellular infiltrates. For example, in a study of the lymphoid infiltrates associated with Sjögren's syndrome, it is desirable to characterize those cells surrounding the degenerate acinar cells of the salivary glands, since these mononuclear cells presumably are the ones mediating the damage.

This chapter reviews techniques used for the preparation of reagents and for the identification of receptors on mononuclear cells in tissue sections. We shall concentrate on the methods we have used to identify C3 and IgG Fc receptors, although other methods used for identification of mononuclear cells in tissue sections will be cited. Techniques for identifying T cells in tissue sections using E (unsensitized sheep erythrocyte) rosettes as a marker are considerably more difficult technically and in our hands have not lent themselves to routine use.

There are a number of generalizations that can be made. Indentification of these receptors in tissue sections is more difficult than identification of the same receptors on cells in suspensions. Presumably, only fragments of cell membrane exposing limited numbers of receptors are available for binding in the frozen sections, while considerably more membrane area is available for binding in suspensions. For this reason, in the frozen-section technique, the reagents used to identify receptors appear to be of critical importance. Reagents that are adequate for demonstrating receptors on cells in suspension may not be adequate for demonstrating the same receptors in tissue sections. In our studies, we have not used commercially available reagents for the preparation of the various cellular intermediates, but understand that it is more difficult to obtain adequate results with them.

2. Materials and Methods

2.1 Preparation of Boiled Sheep Erythrocyte Stromata and Immunization of Rabbits.   The technique employed follows closely that described by Mayer (14). One liter of sheep blood in acid–citrate–dextrose solution is filtered through glass wool to remove cell clumps. The cells are washed twice with saline with removal of the buffy coat, and the sedimented red cells are slowly added with constant stirring to 10 liters of ice-cold distilled water containing 4 ml of glacial acetic acid. The mixture is stored at $4°C$ until the stromata have settled, and the hemoglobin rich supernatant is removed. The stromata are washed with cold, 0.001 M acetate buffer in 500-ml bottles in a Sorvall centrifuge with the GS3 head until the supernatant fluid is relatively free of hemoglobin. Stromata are then washed free of acetate with cold saline and resuspended to a volume of about 300 ml. The material is transferred to an Erlenmeyer flask with a large stirring bar and heated in a boiling water bath for 1 hr with constant mixing. The boiled stromata are then brought to a concentration of 1 mg of N per milliliter (Kjeldahl), and Merthiolate is added to a final concentration of 1:10,000 (w/v). Rabbits are injected intravenously with this suspension in increasing doses, starting with 0.1 ml per injection and ending with about 2.0 ml per injection. In all, about 10 injections are given over 2.5 weeks, and the period between injections is never longer than 2 days. The rabbits are bled on days 4 and 5 following the last injection. Serum is removed from the clotted blood and used as a source of high-avidity IgM antibody. Although these sera also contain fairly large amounts of IgG antibody, the latter is not suitable for preparation of a reagent to identify the IgG Fc receptor, because the IgG antibody is not yet of sufficiently high avidity. The sera obtained at this step in preparation are screened by hemolytic antibody titration, and only those sera with titers higher than 25,000 U/ml are processed further (14). One may have to immunize a number of rabbits to achieve this goal. The IgM hemolysin prepared by this method is particularly useful in tissue-section techniques since it is of very high avidity. This is shown by the fact that it is virtually impossible to demonstrate transfer of the hemolytic antibody from sensitized to nonsensitized sheep erythrocytes in a mixture of the two cell types.

To prepare IgG antibody of high avidity which is satisfactory for demonstration of the Fc receptor, the same rabbits used to prepare IgM can be utilized after a rest period of 2–3 weeks or fresh rabbits can be used (15). The rabbits are immunized with 0.25 ml, in each foot pad, of the sheep erythrocyte stromata (1 mg of N per milliliter) emulsified in an equal volume of Freund's complete adjuvant. After several weeks, the animals receive another foot-pad injection of the same antigen emulsified in Freund's incomplete adjuvant, and 2–3 weeks later the rabbits are bled.

2.2. Preparation of IgG and IgM Fractions. For the purposes of these studies, it is of particular importance to prepare IgM antibody free of IgG contamination since IgM EAC prepared with contaminating IgG might bind to cells bearing either C3 or Fc receptors. On the other hand, contamination of IgG fractions with IgM will rarely cause problems, since no cells with heterologous IgM receptors have ever been detected in sections. We follow similar procedures for the preparation of both the IgG and IgM reagents. The appropriate antisera are mixed with ammonium sulfate to a final concentration of 5.4 M at $0°C$. The sedimented globulins are applied to a Sephadex G200 column equilibrated in Veronal-buffered saline. The crude IgG or IgM peak is collected, concentrated by negative pressure ultrafiltration (No. 100 Model, Schleicher and Schuell) and further purified by sedimentation in a linear 10–30% w/v sucrose gradient for 16 hr at 25,000 rpm in a Spinco Model L2 ultracentrifuge with a type 40 angle head rotor (16). Care is taken to exclude contaminants when collecting the 19 S and 7 S protein peaks by taking only the central part of each peak. The antibodies are stored at $4°C$ in the concentrated sucrose solutions of the gradients with added 1:2000 sodium azide until used, and are stable under these conditions for months to years. We do not freeze these preparations since we have observed the IgM to lose activity on freezing. Moreover, it may be useful to note that in our hands DEAE chromatography has not been useful in these preparations. In many sera, most of the anti-Forssman IgG does not appear in the fall-through fraction on DEAE, but rather is eluted with IgM-containing fractions.

2.3. Sensitization of Sheep Erythrocytes and Preparation of EAC. In preparing sensitized sheep erythrocytes (IgM EA and IgG EA) reagents, we have found it convenient to base the amount of antibody used on the results of a preliminary hemolytic titration assay. The method we use for doing this is as follows:

A volume of 0.5 ml of VBS (with 0.1% gelatin, 1 mM MgCl$_2$, and 0.15 mM CaCl$_2$) containing 5 × 10^8 sheep RBC per milliliter is mixed with 0.5 ml of VBS containing antibody over a broad range of antibody dilutions. The mixtures are incubated at 37°C for 30 min, and 2.25 ml of VBS are then added. The mixtures then receive 0.5 ml of a dilution of guinea pig serum that has been preabsorbed twice with sheep erythrocytes at 0.0°C. The concentration of guinea pig serum (usually 1:150–1:180) is chosen to produce partial lysis of the cell suspension at all antibody concentrations. The mixtures are incubated at 37°C for 1 hr. Appropriate controls consist of maximally sensitized erythrocytes incubated in the absence of complement and unsensitized cells incubated with the complement dilution. A typical dose–response curve is shown in Fig. 1. Note that with IgM antibody there is a broad flat portion of the lysis curve over a wide range of antibody concentrations, in which major changes in antibody concentrations make little change in the degree of hemolysis. This is the area of optimal sensitization. On the other hand, similar titrations with IgG antibody lead to the production of a much more steep curve with a clear area of prozone. Arrows on the diagram indicate those concentrations of IgG and IgM antibody that are used in preparing the RBC reagents used in these studies. At these levels of sensitization, the IgG does not agglutinate the erythrocytes. It should be noted that the IgG antibody preparations must be pretested on tissue sections before use in studies, because some preparations with the correct hemolytic characteristics

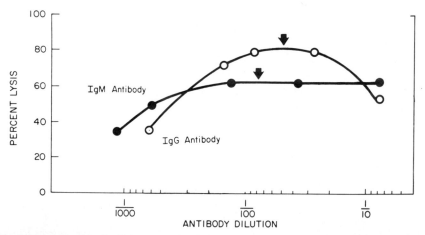

Fig. 1. Degree of lysis of sheep erythrocytes at 37°C in a mixture containing limiting amounts of guinea pig complement, as a function of IgG and IgM anti-Forssman antibody concentration.

still do not produce adequate tissue reagents. The reasons for this have not been carefully studied but may relate to antibody affinity.

For tissue-section studies, 1×10^9 washed sheep erythrocytes per milliliter (1:25 dilution in water reads OD 0.420 at 541 nm) in VBS is sensitized with an equal volume of antibody at the dilution chosen above. Because the antibody is highly avid, great care must be taken to see that the erythrocytes are uniformly sensitized. Antibody is always added to cells with the suspension being constantly mixed. It should be recognized that a vortex mixer may not be adequate to produce complete mixing of the solutions. We sensitize cell suspensions in an Erlenmeyer flask with constant swirling by hand.

After the IgG or IgM antibody is added to the cell suspensions, they are incubated at $30°C$ for 30 min to ensure adequate sensitization. The cells are washed and brought to a concentration of 5×10^8 cells/ml. Fresh mouse serum (C57B1 or AKR) as a source of complement is diluted 1:10 in ice cold VBS and added to an equal volume of IgM EA (5×10^8 cells per milliliter of VBS). The cell suspension is incubated at $37°C$ for 30 min, washed twice with cold VBS, and brought to a concentration of 1×10^8 cells/ml for use. Although there is no difficulty in storing the EA reagent for at least a week at $4°C$, we always add the complement on the day the cells are to be used. Moreover, we do not use frozen mouse serum as the complement source because there is a definite loss in hemolytic complement activity of the frozen serum (17).

Fresh serum from other species can be used as the complement source as well, but mouse serum is of particular value because it is only weakly lytic. Individual purified human and guinea pig complement components can be added sequentially to the sensitized cell suspensions, and these reagents can be used as well to characterize the fine specificity of complement receptor on particular cells; for example, receptors for both the C3b and C3d fragments of C3 have been identified, but the methods employed in preparing such reagents are beyond the scope of this review. [The reagents we use for these reactions are detailed elsewhere (18).]

2.4. Preparation of Tissue for Sections. Biopsy material should be obtained and processed for freezing as soon as possible after surgical removal, preferably within 1 hr. The use of autopsy material has been less satisfactory and to some extent depends upon the postmortem interval; although in some instances receptors have been intact and a satisfactory result is obtained, this is not always the case.

The tissue is maintained in cold sterile saline or tissue culture medium. A portion of this material can be processed as a cell suspension for correlation with frozen section results. To prepare the tissue for sectioning, a block no more than 3 mm in thickness is cut using a sharp blade. The other dimensions of the block are less crucial and can be as large as 2×2 cm. As a general rule, it is more difficult to cut frozen sections from a large block. The type of tissue may also determine the maximum dimensions of the block; for example, it is difficult to prepare frozen sections of adipose tissue.

The block is mounted and frozen on the specimen plate. The plate may be precooled on Dry Ice or in a cryostat. A small amount of embedding medium (O.C.T. Ames Co., Division of Miles Laboratories, Inc., Elkhart, Indiana) is placed on the plate as a base. The tissue block is placed on the plate, and additional embedding medium is added until the entire block is covered. The specimen mounted on the tissue plate should be frozen as rapidly as possible to minimize the formation of ice crystals. This can be accomplished by immersing the plate in 2-methylbutane to which Dry Ice has been added or liquid nitrogen. The specimen will be snap frozen within a few seconds.

2.5. Storage of Tissues. The frozen tissue can be cut and assayed immediately or the entire tissue block can be stored and saved for future use. For storage, the intact tissue block is wrapped in aluminum foil to prevent dehydration and stored at $-70°C$ or below. Short-term storage at $-20°C$ may be satisfactory for short periods. We have used tissue stored at $-70°C$ for up to 1 year and have obtained satisfactory results.

2.6. Rosette Assay. The frozen sections are cut and mounted on glass slides at the time the rosette assay is to be performed. The sections may be prepared 24 hr in advance, but storage of sections for more than 48 hr is not advised, and sections should never be refrozen. Cryostat sections are mounted on uncoated clean glass slides. If there is a problem with detachment of the sections during the washing procedure, gelatinized slides may be used, but this is usually not necessary if the sections are given adequate time to dry before the assay is performed. Air-drying at $20°C$ is adequate if the sections are prepared 24 hr in advance. If they are prepared on the day of the assay, they may be rapidly dried at $37°C$ for 45 min. The sections should be cut at a thickness of 6–8 μm. Thin sections give better histological detail but are more difficult to handle.

After adequate drying, the slides are layered with the indicator red cells at a concentration of 1×10^8/ml (Fig. 2). IgM EAC is used to detect cells bearing complement receptors. IgG EA is used to detect cells bearing receptors for cytophilic antibody, predominantly mononuclear phagocytes. IgM EA is a control reagent that should not bind to the sections and is used to ensure that adequate washing has occurred. The slides are incubated for 30 min at either $20°$ or $37°C$. If incubation is performed at $37°C$, a humid chamber should be used so that drying of the reagent on the sections does not occur. In contrast to Dukor *et al.* (8), we have found that $37°C$ may give preferable results with some tissues, especially lymph nodes; however, with other tissues, such as spleen, nonspecific adherence may occur at $37°C$.

After incubation, the slides are washed by immersion with gentle agitation in phosphate-buffered saline (PBS) in a large-mouthed vessel. Three washes are usually sufficient, but it is possible to tell by a rapid microscopic inspection if

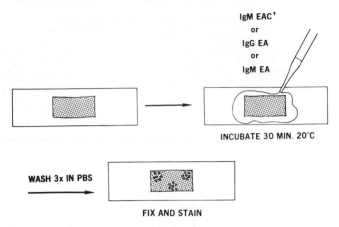

Fig. 2. Schematic for technique of layering reagent red cells on section for identification of cells bearing C3 receptors and IgG-Fc receptors in frozen tissue sections.

the washing is complete. After washing, the slides are immersed in fixative [either Perfix (Applied Bioscience, Fairfield, New Jersey) or 3% glutaraldehyde] for approximately 10 min. Fixatives commonly used for frozen sections, such as acid alcohol, are not suitable, as lysis of indicator red cells will occur. The fixed slides are stained with hematoxylin and eosin and viewed through a conventional microscope (Fig. 3). The stained sections can also be examined at low magnification through a dry-darkfield condenser. In this preparation, the adherent red cells appear as yellow-green refractile bodies against a dark background, and small numbers of adherent red cells can be easily identified (Fig. 4).

3. Interpretation of Data and Critical Comments

3.1. Detection of B Cells in Tissue Sections. The IgM EAC reagent was the first reagent used to detect lymphocytes bearing complement receptors in tissue section and still is widely employed for this purpose (8). Recently C3-coated gram-negative bacteria (fluorescein-labeled *Salmonella typhi*) have also been successfully used (19). The fact that these bacteria contain endotoxin allows them to fix complement from serum via activation of the alternative complement pathway in the absence of specific antibody. The use of the C3 receptor as a marker for B cells in sections is complicated by the fact that not all B cells may carry this receptor (20a) and, furthermore, a C3 receptor is also found on other cell types, such as monocytes and polymorphonuclear leukocytes (3, 20a, 31). Under ideal circumstances, therefore, positive identification of B cells in sections should also rest upon other criteria (see below). Our own experience suggests that the IgM EAC reagent binds best to B cells in follicles of lymph node and

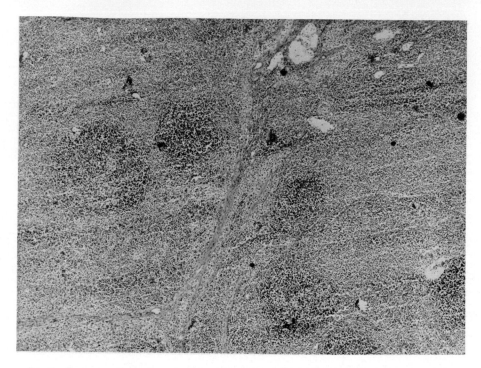

Fig. 3. Frozen section of normal lymph node layered with EAC. Reagent red cells adhere exclusively to lymphoid follicles. On the original section, areas of EAC adherence are easily visualized. (Hematoxylin and eosin; × 40.)

spleen. Other B-cell populations, for example those in the medulla of the lymph node, appear to lose this receptor as B cells mature into plasma cells. Most populations of macrophages in tissue section bind the EAC reagent poorly (20). However, in some lymphoid organs, such as the lymph node, tissue macrophages in the subcapsular areas also bind the IgM EAC reagent (12). Here, the use of both the IgM EAC reagent and the IgG EA reagent on serial sections is required because the latter reagent in tissue sections binds only to the Fc receptor of macrophages and does not bind to B cells. Thus, cells in a particular area of lymph node that bind both IgM EAC and IgG EA are classified as macrophages.

Another technique that has been used to detect B cells in sections is the use of anti-Ig sera to detect membrane bound Ig (21, 22). The use of this technique is complicated by several factors. First, since B cells, neutrophils, and macrophages have Fc receptors capable of capturing fluorescein-labeled intact IgG reagents, only $F(ab')_2$ fragments of the antibody should be employed (7). Of even greater theoretical difficulty is the fact that only a portion of the B cell membrane

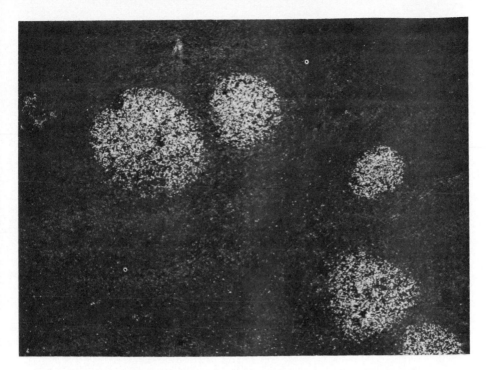

Fig. 4. Normal lymph node (same section as in Fig. 3) layered with EAC and viewed through a dry-darkfield condenser. Follicular localization of EAC is more readily apparent. × 40.

containing Ig is present in the section. Furthermore, each cell is bathed in interstitial fluid that contains Ig. Therefore, staining with an anti-Ig reagent may stain not only the small amount of Ig in the membrane, but also the Ig in the interstitium. Differentiating between these two localizations may not be simple. Gutman and Weissman, who have had some success with this technique in mice, caution that "the source and dilution of the fluorescein labeled anti-mouse Ig were chosen so as to minimize the fluorescence due to endogenous immunoglobulins in the tissue" (21). Unfortunately, the detailed methods involved in the "choosing process" were not mentioned. Several other authors have also used these anti-Ig techniques with success. However, in a recent paper describing the localization of B cells in human hepatic biopsies, many of the cells described in the captions as B cells actually had eccentric nuclei and abundant stained cytoplasm (23). These cells resembled mature plasma cells rather than B lymphocytes. Admittedly, the dividing line between a B cell and a plasma cell is somewhat arbitrary.

A more specific approach for the localization of B cells would be to use a heterologous anti-B cell serum. Such a highly specific B cell serum was prepared and used successfully by Goldschneider and McGregor to detect B cells in rat peripheral lymphoid tissue (24).

Since almost all B cells have Fc receptors, red cell reagents capable of binding to the receptors might also be expected to be useful (25, 26). However, IgG EA prepared as described in this chapter does not bind to Fc receptors on B lymphocytes in tissue sections. This reagent will nevertheless bind to B lymphocytes in suspension after centrifugation and incubation of the cell mixture (27). Moreover, Tønder has reported that if very large (agglutinating) amounts of IgG are used to coat the red cell and if gentle washing techniques are used, B cells as well as other cells may bind this reagent in tissue sections (28, 31a).

Husby (23) has reported the attempted use of an aggregated IgG reagent to detect Fc receptors of B cells in liver sections. He found, however, that macrophages and neutrophils bound this reagent, rendering interpretation of B-cell localization difficult. It would appear that since the affinity and number of these Fc receptors may be higher on mononuclear phagocytes and neutrophils than on B lymphocytes, these reagents will be difficult to use to detect B cells in sections.

Finally, in the mouse and human, antisera are now available that detect certain antigens (Ia) on cell surfaces coded for by genes of the major histocompatibility complex (29). The Ia antigens are not widely distributed on all tissues, but in fact are found in highest density on B lymphocytes (29, 30). Such anti-Ia sera might be useful for detecting B cells in tissue sections.

3.2. Detection of Macrophages in Tissue Sections. Peripheral blood monocytes have both the cytophilic receptor for the Fc portion of IgG as well as the complement receptor (7, 31). Tissue macrophages, derived from these cells, might be expected to have a similar array of receptors. The presence of the cytophilic receptor on macrophages in tissue sections is most commonly detected with an IgG EA reagent. As noted previously, when subagglutinating amounts of IgG antibody are used to sensitize the indicator RBC as in the present study, this reagent binds only to cytophilic receptor of the macrophage, not to the Fc receptor of the B lymphocytes. Although the receptor for C3 can also be utilized to detect monocytes in peripheral blood and alveolar macrophages (18), other macrophages appear operationally to lack the C3 receptor. That is, our own observations would indicate that the macrophages in the red pulp of the spleen, as well as macrophages present in some inflammatory sites, appear to have a quantitative or qualitative reduction in the numbers of C3 receptors (9, 20). This is shown by the lack of adherence of IgM EAC to macrophages in tissue sections, although these cells do bind IgG EA. Other macrophages, for example those in the subcapsular sinus of lymph nodes and the marginal zone of the spleen, do appear to have a C3 receptor. Monocytes and macrophages in other locations and in other states of maturity, such as in the bone marrow, brain, and macrophages scattered in inflammatory sites have not as yet been carefully studied for the presence and affinity of a receptor for C3.

One additional point can be made regarding the specificity of the C3 receptor. In cell suspensions, the C3 receptor of the mouse, guinea pig, and perhaps human macrophage seems to require the presence of divalent cations, whereas the C3 receptor of the B lymphocyte does not (6). Whether this distinction between the two types of C3 receptors also pertains to and may be useful in the study of B cells and monocytes in tissue sections has not been thoroughly investigated.

It should also be noted that cytochemical and histochemical methods have been traditionally used to detect lysosomal hydrolytic enzymes present in monocytes and macrophages (32). Such techniques provide perhaps the most accurate method for the identification of these cells and could conceivably be performed in tissue section in conjunction with the rosette technique described above.

3.3. Detection of T cells in Tissue Sections. In 1972, Silveira *et al.* (33) reported that T cell areas could be detected in human lymph nodes, spleen, and thymus by overlaying the tissue with E alone. The precise washing technique was not reported. The only other report that supports this claim is that of Tønder *et al.* (34). The latter incubated the E with tissue sections of lymph node and spleen in a special chamber in which the E adhering to the tissue were allowed to fall off the tissue by gravity. Under these conditions, bonds between the E and tissue of a much lower affinity might be expected to be detected. T cells diffusely located in a tissue were not detectable with this technique. Our own experience, as well as that of most other authors, is that, using ordinary washing techniques, we were unable to observe such binding of E to tissue sections known to contain T lymphocytes. This result is not unexpected since even in suspension the binding of E to living T cells is extremely weak.

T cells in tissue sections have to date been most successfully detected by using heterologous anti-T cell serum rendered specific by multiple absorption with a variety of different tissues. Weissman (22) and his collaborators have been successful using these techniques in the mouse, Talal *et al.* (35) with humans, and Goldschneider (24) reported success in the rat. Recently, Husby *et al.* (23) reported the use of heterologous anti-T cell sera to detect T cells in mononuclear cell infiltrates in liver diseases. These authors, using the same tissue, were unsuccessful in demonstrating E binding to the same sections.

Several other reagents which are candidates for use in tissue sections because of their reported affinity for T cells in suspension include a snail lectin and C-reactive protein (36, 37). Also in the mouse, special and more defined alloantisera directed to antigens found only on T cells deserve more attention. These would include anti-θ, anti-Ly, anti-G IX, and anti-TL (40a).

3.4. Future Directions. It is apparent from this brief chapter that a number of different techniques are now available for the detection of different types of mononuclear cells in tissue sections. Newer techniques are rapidly evolving, and indicator reagents of smaller size and higher degrees of specificity, allowing for identification of each individual mononuclear cell in a section, can be expected in the future. One of the chief aims of future studies will be to correlate the vast amount of information known about the activities and functions of various mononuclear cells *in vitro* with the function of these cells *in vivo*. It is hoped that such studies will some day allow for selective removal of mononuclear cells from biopsy specimens, the identification of the cell types, and the testing of the cells in a number of *in vitro* systems.

Another point that should receive considerable attention in the future is the fact that these receptors are not confined to the lymphocyte and mononuclear cell system but have recently been described on entirely different cell types. Thus, Tønder *et al.* (34) have described Fc receptors on malignant cells of epithelial origin as well as in normal placenta (38), and Staber *et al.* (39) have described E rosette formation between liver cells in suspension and also in sections of liver. Whether the receptor on liver cells bears any relationship to the receptor on T lymphocytes remains to be seen. Recently, Gelfand *et al.* (40) have described a receptor for C3b in the human renal glomerulus using tissue section techniques with IgM EAC. Shin *et al.* (41) have demonstrated that this receptor is on the epithelial cell of the glomerulus. It would seem likely that such a receptor would play an important role in the deposition and transport of complexes bearing C3 within the glomerulus. It appears that future studies of the localization and function of these membrane receptors should contribute greatly to our understanding of the pathophysiology of a good many human diseases.

REFERENCES

1. Shevach, E. M., Jaffe, E., and Green, I., *Tranplant. Rev.* **16**, 3 (1973).
2. Huber, H., Polley, M. J., Linscott, W. D., Fudenberg, H. H., and Müller-Eberhard, H. J., *Science* **162**, 1281 (1968).
3. LoBuglio, A. F., Cotran, R. S., and Jandl, J. H., *Science* **158**, 1582 (1967).
4. Lay, W. H., Mendes, N. F., Bianco, C., and Nussenzweig, V., *Nature (London)* **230**, 531 (1971).
5. Wybran, J., and Fudenberg, H. H., *Eur. J. Immunol.* **1**, 491 (1971).
6. Bianco, D., Patrick, R., and Nussenzweig, V., *J. Exp. Med.* **132**, 702 (1970).
7. Berken, B., and Benacerraf, B., *J. Exp. Med.* **123**, 119 (1966).
8. Dukor, P., Bianco, C., and Nussenzweig, V., *Proc. Natl. Acad. Sci. U.S.A.* **67**, 991 (1970).
9. Edelson, R. L., Smith, R. W., Frank, M. M., and Green, I., *J. Invest. Dermatol.* **61**, 82 (1973).
10. Chused, T. M., Hardin, J. A., Frank, M. M., and Green, I., *J. Immunol.* **112**, 641 (1974).

11. Jaffe, E. S., Shevach, E. M., Frank, M. M., Berard, C. W., and Green, I., *N. Engl. J. Med.* **290**, 813 (1974).
12. Green, I., Jaffe, E. S., Shevach, E. M., Edelson, R. L., Frank, M. M., and Berard, C. W., *in* "The Reticuloendothelial System" (J. Rebuck and C. Berard, eds.), p. 282. (The International Academy of Pathology, Monograph No. 16). Williams & Wilkins, Baltimore, Maryland, 1975.
13. Meijer, C. J. L. M., and Lindeman, J., *J. Immunol. Methods* **9**, 59 (1975).
14. M. M. Mayer, *in* "Experimental Immunochemistry" (by E. A. Kabat and M. M. Mayer), p. 133. Thomas, Springfield, Illinois. 1961.
15. Frank, M. M., and Gaither, T., *Immunology* **19**, 967 (1970).
16. Frank, M. M., and Humphrey, J. H., *J. Exp. Med.* **127**, 967 (1968).
17. Shin, H., personal communication.
18. Reynolds, H. Y., Atkinson, J. P., Newball, H. H., and Frank, M. M., *J. Immunol.* **114**, 1813 (1975).
19. Gelfand, J., Fauci, A., Green, I., and Frank, M. M., *J. Immunol.* **116**, 595 (1976).
20. Jaffe, E. S., Shevach, E. M., Frank, M. M., and Green, I., *Am. J. Med.* **57**, 108 (1974).
20a. Ross, G. D., Rabellino, E. M., Polley, M. J., and Grey, H. M., *J. Clin. Invest.* **52**, 377 (1973).
21. Gutman, G. A., and Weissman, I. L., *Immunology* **23**, 465 (1972).
22. Weissman, I. L., *Transplant. Rev.* **24**, 159 (1975).
23. Husby, G., Strickland, R. G., Caldwell, J. L., and Williams, R. C., *J. Clin. Invest.* **56**, 1198 (1975).
24. Goldschneider, I., and McGregor, D. D., *J. Exp. Med.* **138**, 1443 (1973).
25. Basten, A., Miller, J. F. A. P., Sprent, J., and Pye, J., *J. Exp. Med.* **135**, 610 (1972).
26. Dickler, H. B., and Kunkel, H. G., *J. Exp. Med.* **136**, 191 (1972).
27. Kedar, E., Ortiz de La dazuri, N., and Fahey, J. L., *J. Immunol.* **112**, 37 (1974).
28. Tønder, O., and Thunold, S., *Scand. J. Immunol.* **2**, 207 (1973).
29. Shreffler, D. C., and David, C. S., *Adv. Immunol.* **20**, 125 (1975).
30. Shevach, E., Rosenstreich, D. L., and Green, I., *Transplantation* **16**, 126 (1973).
31. Lay, W. H., and Nussenzweig, V., *J. Exp. Med.* **128**, 991 (1968).
31a. Thunold, S., Tønder, O., and Wiig, J. N., *Scand. J. Immunol.* **2**, 135 (1973).
32. Li, C. Y., Yam, L. T., and Crosby, W. H., *J. Histochem. Cytochem.* **20**, 1049 (1972).
33. Silveira, N. P. A., Mendes, N. F., and Tolnai, M. E. A., *J. Immunol.* **108**, 1456 (1972).
34. Tønder, O., Morse, P. A., and Humphrey, J., *J. Immunol.* **113**, 1162 (1974).
35. Talal, N., Sylvester, R. A., Daniels, T. E., Greenspan, J. S., and Williams, R. C., *J. Clin. Invest.* **53**, 180 (1974).
36. Hammerström, S., Hellström, V., Perlman, P., and Dillmer, M. L., *J. Exp. Med.* **130**, 1270 (1973).
37. Mortensen, R. F., Osmand, A. P., and Gewurz, H., *J. Exp. Med.* **141**, 821 (1975).
38. Matre, R., Tønder, O., and Endresen, C., *Scand. J. Immunol.* **4**, 741 (1975).
39. Staber, F. G., Fink, V., and Sack, W., *N. Engl. J. Med.* **291**, 795 (1974).
40. Gelfand, M. C., Frank, M. M., and Green, I., *J. Exp. Med.* **142**, 1029 (1975).
40a. Klein, J., "Biology of the Mouse Histocompatibility-2 Complex." Springer-Verlag, Berlin and New York, 1975.
41. Shin, H., Gelfand, M. C., Nagel, R., Cailo, J. R., Green, I., and Frank, M. M. Submitted for publication.

Purification of Human T Lymphocytes Using Nylon Fiber Columns

Melvyn F. Greaves, George Janossy, and Peter Curtis

1. Introduction

Since the "introduction" of glass bead filtration by Gavin and Rabinowitz, immunologists have extensively used adherence to solid surfaces as a means of removing relatively sticky cells, such as macrophages (reviewed in 1). In the presence of serum and at 37°C, macrophages and granulocytes will readily adhere to flat surfaces, beads, or fibers of glass, plastic, nylon, cotton, and polystyrene. It has, until relatively recently, been generally considered that lymphocytes were particularly nonadherent cells; however, all procedures used to remove macrophages also incur a loss of lymphocytes. This can in part be explained by temperature-independent mechanical effects (e.g., trapping), but it is now clear that lymphocytes cannot be considered as nonadherent. We have as yet no adequate chemical or biophysical interpretation of adherence and no means of calculating adherence capacity in absolute or quantitative terms. Given the appropriate conditions, virtually any cell will adhere to a solid surface. The time it takes to do so and the ease with which it can be displaced will vary considerably. It should be appreciated that adherence is at present only a comparative or relative quality of cells. In 1971, we reported studies on filtration through cotton wool of spleen cells from mice immunized against sheep red cells (2). These indicated an interesting rank order of adherence, namely: macrophages > plasma cells > antigen-binding (i.e., rosette forming) B cells > antigen-binding T cells.* The lymphoid cells removed by the column were immunologically activated cells and there was no clear selective adherence of cells with membrane phenotypes SmIg$^+$, θ^- (i.e., B) and SmIg$^-$, θ^+ (i.e., T). Shortman and colleagues have published rather similar results using glass bead columns (see Ref. 1). Julius *et al.* (3) reported later that B lymphocytes from

---

*Abbrevations: T, thymus derived (lymphocyte); B, "bursa equivalent" derived (lymphocyte); SmIg, surface membrane immunoglobulin; HuTLA, human T lymphocyte antigen(s); HuBLA, human B lymphocyte antigen(s); HuMA, human macrophage antigen(s); E, erythrocyte (rosette test); EAC, erythrocyte–antibody-complement complex; EBV, Epstein-Barr virus; SRBC, sheep red blood cells, PHA, phytohemagglutinin.

mouse tissues could be efficiently removed on columns of nylon wool enabling eluted populations to be obtained that were almost pure T (θ^+, SmIg$^-$) lymphocytes. Moreover, the purified T cells were viable and capable of expressing a variety of T cell functions *in vitro* and, after reinoculation, *in vivo* also.

We (4), and several other groups (5–7), have used nylon fiber columns as a routine method for preparing human T cell populations free of monocytes and B lymphocytes. In this report we present data relating to optimal conditions for separations. As with any method of physical separation, the criteria to be applied to determine the efficacy of the method should include: (a) the precise selectivity of the system, (b) the yield of desired cells, and (c) the functional capacity of purified cells.

2. Materials

2.1. Nylon fibers. These fibers were obtained from Travenol Laboratories (Thetford, United Kingdom, or Fenwal Laboratories, Morton Grove, Illinois). The trade name for the product is Fenwal Leukopak, and the fibers are dispatched as large polythene-contained filtration units. The loss of lymphocytes in using the whole unit is very high, and we routinely cut open the unit and use the nylon (after suitable preparation) to prepare small filtration columns (see below).

2.2. Cell Preparation. Cells are obtained from tonsils either by slicing and teasing with blunt forceps or by using an Ultra Turrax TP 10N homogenizer (Scientific Instruments Centre, London). The suspension is filtered first through a nylon strainer to remove large clumps and then through loosely packed glass wool columns at room temperature. The cells are then washed three times in Earle's saline (150–200 g, 10 min, at room temperature). Lymphocytes (and monocytes) were separated from defibrinated blood or heparinized blood using the Ficoll–Isopaque density centrifugation method of Böyum (8) i.e., $\psi = 1.077$ g/cm^3 centrifuged at 400 g for 40 min at 20°C. The resultant suspension has > 99% viability, and in our first series of experiments (9) consisted of over 88.3 ($\pm$ 1.6 SE) lymphocytes. The majority of the nonlymphoid cells are phagocytic monocytes. Yields obtained using this method have been variable over the three years of testing, but have usually been between 65 and 80% with blood from healthy adult donors.

2.3. Membrane Markers. A panel of membrane markers have been produced over the past three years at University College (reviewed in 10). Details of their production and selectivity are summarized in Table 1; specific points can be obtained from the references given [see also chapter on anti-T cell sera by Greaves and Janossy (Method 3)].

Antisera binding to cell surfaces was assessed using indirect immunofluorescence (with fluorescein-labeled goat antirabbit IgG) and either a Vickers M41

TABLE 1
Summary of Membrane Markers Used in Nylon Column Filtration Experiments

Marker	References		Reactive cells		
			T	B	Monocytes
1. Antisera					
i. Rabbit anti-human cerebrum (absorbed with CLL)	(9)	. −HuTLA$_1$	+	−	−
ii. Rabbit anti-monkey thymus^a (absorbed with CLL)	(11)	−HuTLA$_2$	+	−	−
iii. Rabbit anti-CLL (absorbed with thymus)		−HuBLA	−	+	−
iv. Rabbit anti-human Ig^b		−SmIg	−	+	(±)
v. Rabbit anti-human monocytes (absorbed with tonsils)	(12)	−HuMA	−	−	+
2. Rosette tests					
i. Sheep erythrocytes^c		E	+	−	−
ii. IgM plus complement-coated red cells^d		EAC	−	+	(±)
3. Heat-aggregated human IgG-FITC^e	(9)	AggIgG	± (few)	+	(±)

^{a}See Greaves and Janossy, this volume, Method 3.
^{b}See Preud'homme and La Baume, this volume, Method 9.
^{c}See Hoffman and Kunkel, this volume, Method 1.
^{d}See Ross and Polley, this volume, Method 6.
^{e}See Arbeit et al., this volume, Method 8.

Photoplan fluorescence microscope (HBO mercury lamp, incident illumination) or a Zeiss microscope with a IV/F epifluorescence condenser.

More recently, fluorescence has been evaluated using the fluorescence activated cell sorter (FACS, Becton Dickinson, Mountain View, California) (see results given by Greaves and Janossy in Method 3).

The EAC test was performed as described by Ross et al. (13). The E test was routinely performed by mixing 50 μl of lymphocytes (at 10^7/ml in Earle's saline) with 50 μl of SRBC-absorbed fetal calf serum and 100 μl of 2% sheep erythrocytes (< 2 weeks old).* This mixture is centrifuged at 200 g for 5–7 min

*In some experiments 20% SRBC were pretreated with neuraminidase (15 U/ml, 30 min, 37°C).

at 20°C (or room temperature) and left standing as a pellet on the bench for 60 min. The pellet is gently resuspended by tapping. The suspension is diluted 1X with cold Earle's saline and placed in a hemacytometer for evaluation.

Phagocytic cells were estimated by incubating 1 to 2 X 10^6 cells in 0.5 ml of Earle's saline plus 0.5 ml of fetal calf serum at 37°C for 45–60 min with 0.1 μm latex beads (Dowe-Latex, Serra, Feinbiochemica, Heidelberg).

2.4. Lymphocyte Culture and Stimulants. Lymphocytes were cultured in RPMI medium with fetal calf serum and antibiotics (14). Lectins used were purified phytohemagglutinin (PHA-p, Wellcome) or purified pokeweed [Pa-1 (ref. 15) given by Dr. M. J. Waxdal]. Synthesis of immunoglobulin was determined by radioimmunoassay (16).

3. Detailed Protocol of Nylon Fiber Filtration Method

3.1. Preparation of Fibers and Columns. Nylon fiber from Fenwal Leukopaks is washed in 0.2 N HCl for 2 hr, rinsed in distilled water, and allowed to dry; 300 mg or 600 mg of nylon are submerged in saline (in order to expel air bubbles) and pushed into a 5-ml polypropylene syringe (Plastipak, Becton Dickinson) up to either the 2.5 or 5.0 ml level, respectively. The syringe is rinsed through with at least 10 ml of Earle's saline containing 10% fetal calf serum. The syringe barrel column is sealed at the top with parafilm, and outflow is controlled by an attached polythene tubing and bunsen screw clip. Before lymphocytes are added, the columns were washed with 10% fetal calf serum in Earle's saline and incubated at 37°C for 25 min.

When columns need to be kept sterile, the fibers can be sterilized by autoclaving. They are then packed dry into the columns. Alternatively, fiber-packed glass syringe columns can be autoclaved.

3.2. Adsorption and Elution of Cells. Either 5 X 10^7 (300-mg column) or 1 X 10^8 (500-mg column) were added in 1 or 2 ml, respectively, of 10% fetal calf serum in Earle's saline, run carefully into the column, and incubated at 37°C for 30 min (in a warm room). To elute nonadherent cells, the column is flushed through with 10 ml of warm Earle's saline at approximately 1 drop/sec (or ~ 2 ml/min).

3.3. Marker Characteristics of Post- versus Precolumn Cells. Results from three independent series of experiments carried out over the past three years are given in Table 2. As shown, the purity of T cells in the eluted populations was generally 85–95% and could be improved up to 95% by recycling. Notice, however, that not only are 92–96% of the SmIg$^+$ B cells lost during filtration, but also a considerable number of T cells. We discuss below the possibility that T-cell subsets might be differentially adsorbed by the columns. There is some evidence that the few B cells in the nonadherent, eluted population may be a functional subset (see below). Platelets, granulocytes, and monocytes (in blood) are effectively removed by the columns. On a single occasion, we noticed that

TABLE 2
Yield and Purity of T Cells in Nylon Fiber-Filtered Suspensions

	No. of experiments	Unseparated (starting) population [% of E$^+$ (T) cells]	Filtered population		Yield (% of input)		
Tonsil			% E$^+$ (T) cells	% SmIg$^+$ cells	E$^+$ (T) cells	E$^-$ (non-T) cells	Total
Single cycle (A)	11[a]	46.1 ± 2.8	87.6 ± 2.2	5.0 ± 2.1	67.7	8.25	35.7 ± 3.0
Single cycle (B)	18[b]	55.0 ± 1.9	89.0 ± 2.1	NT[f]	44.8	6.77	27.7 ± 2.5
Single cycle (C)	27[b]	54.8 ± 1.6	94.0 ± 0.8	2.1 ± 0.3	49.0	3.78	28.5 ± 1.9
Double cycle	3[c]	55.0	95.0	0.4	26.6	1.5	14.7
6 g nylon fiber	2[d]	53.0	92.0	1.0	13.0	1.5	7.6
Blood							
Single cycle	4[e]	65.5	91.5	1–5	48.2	9.0	36.5

[a]Nylon fiber columns, 600 mg in 5-ml syringe loaded with 1 × 10^8 tonsil cells, as described.
[b]Columns, 300 mg in 5-ml syringe, loaded with 5 × 10^7 tonsil cells.
[c]As in b, except that eluted cells were made up to 5 × 10^7 concentration and loaded onto a second column. The analysis of cells eluted from the second column is shown.
[d]25 × 10^7 cells loaded onto a column made of 6 g of nylon fiber in a 20-ml syringe.
[e]Peripheral blood lymphocytes were separated on Ficoll–Isopaque, washed, and loaded onto 150-mg of nylon fiber.
[f]NT, not tested.

eosinophils were retained in the nonadherent eluted cell fraction. Notice also that besides the small number of $SmIg^+$ B cells in the eluates, there was also a population of E^-, $SmIg^-$ cells. When additional markers are used to characterize the eluted population, it is still difficult to draw any conclusions as to the nature of this small cell population (see Tables 3 and 4). Experiments described by Chess and Schlossman (see Method 19) suggest that this nonadherent population of "null" cells probably contains at least some cells that can synthesize and secrete immunoglobulin *in vitro* and others (or the same?) that can induce the lysis of appropriate antibody-coated cells.

3.4. Variables. The conditions described above have been found to be optimal after extensive testing of all variables. Yields of cells will be *decreased* if larger columns or more fibers are used—irrespective of cell number. Therefore for preparing large numbers of pure T cells use several columns in parallel. The columns, however, can be scaled down considerably. Column beds, 0.1 ml, in tuberculin syringes can be used to separate T cells from 0.5 to 3×10^6 cells (M. Greaves, unpublished observations).

Yields of cells will *increase* and B cell "contamination" will *increase* if (i) incubation time is less than 20 min (see Fig. 1); (ii) A fast elution rate is used or medium is forced through using the syringe plunger (see Fig. 2); (iii) B cells are not under optimal metabolic conditions (see below).

Solid surface or materials other than nylon appear to be less efficacious as judged by comparative experiments on mouse spleen cells (Table 5).

3.5. Some Requirements for Selection B-Cell Adhesion. Experiments summarized in Table 6 have indicated that selective adhesion of tonsil B to nylon

TABLE 3

Membrane Marker Analysis of Nylon Fiber Column-Filtered Cells

Marker[a]		Precolumn	Postcolumn	Reference
Anti-HuTLA$_1$	(4)	52.8 ± 1.9	95	(4)
Anti-HuTLA$_2$	(3)	45	92	Greaves and Janossy this volume, Method 3
Anti-HuBLA	(6)	44.5 ± 2.3	1.8	(4)
Anti-SmIg	(27)	43.2 ± 1.8	2.1±0.3	(4) and this paper
Anti-HuMA	(10)	0.2 – 1.5	<0.5	(12) and u.o.[b]
E	(27)	54.8 ± 1.6	94±0.8	(4) and this paper
AgglgG	(3)	43.1 ± 3.1	1.8	(4)
EAC	(5)	34.0 ± 2.3	0.2	(4)
EBV	(2)	44.0, 40.2	0.3. 1.1	(19)

[a]Numbers of observations in parentheses. Tonsil cells were used. HuTLA$_1$, anti-brain sera; HuTLA$_2$, anti-thymus sera.
[b]u.o., unpublished observations.

TABLE 4
Surface Marker Analysis of Nonadherent Tonsil Cells

	T cell markers		B cell markers			Anti-monocyte serum
	E⁺	anti-T	SmIg⁺	IgM⁺	IgG⁺	
Unseparated T+B	49	48	46	36	20	3
Purified B[a]	<1	3	71	51	30	2
Nylon column filtered (nonadherent)[b]	85	87	6	NT[d]	NT	1
Nonadherent T cells[c]	96	99.5	0.1	NT	NT	0
Nonadherent non-T cells	1	4	40	16	25	2

[a]B cells were purified by eliminating E⁺ T cells on a Ficoll–Triosil gradient. Neuraminidase-treated SRBC were used (SRBC-N).
[b]Nylon fiber, 600 mg in 5-ml syringe loaded with 1×10^8 cells.
[c]Cells eluted from nylon wool column were rosetted with SRBC-N. E⁺ cells (nonadherent T cells) were separated from E⁻ cells (nonadherent B + non-T cells) on a Ficoll–Triosil gradient. Nonadherent T cells were treated with $0.17\ M$ NH₄Cl for 10 min at 20°C and then passed through fetal calf serum.
[d]NT, not tested.

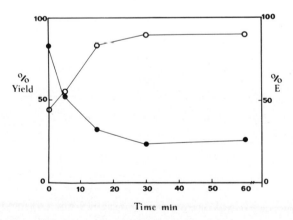

Fig. 1. Time requirement for selective B cell adhesion to nylon. ●———●, % yield; ○———○, % E rosettes. Tonsil lymphocytes, 25×10^6/150 mg of nylon, starting population 50.5% E⁺, 47.3% SmIg⁺. Series of individual identical columns were set up, and cells were harvested (on duplicate columns) after different periods of incubation at 37°C as shown.

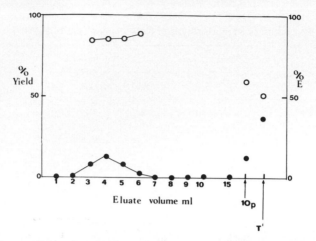

Fig. 2. Elution conditions for T cell purification through nylon. ●——●, % yield; ○——○, % E rosettes. Tonsil lymphocytes, $50 \times 10^6 / 300$ mg of nylon; starting population, 47% E^+. Eluted cells were collected in successive 1-ml aliquots, counted, and analyzed for E-rosetting cells. 10p: 10 ml forced through column under pressure; T: nylon removed from column and teased into medium. All columns were prewarmed to 37°C before the start of the experiments.

TABLE 5

Relative Efficiency of Different Adherence Columns for Removing B cells[a]

Column	Total yield	T (θ^+SmIg$^-$)	B (θ^-SmIg$^+$)	"Null" (E$^-$, SmIg$^-$)
1. Absorbent cotton wool				
175 mg	NT[c]	60.5	34.3	5.2
350 mg	20	51.5	31.0	17.5
2. Nylon fiber				
175 mg	NT	84.3	11.3	4.4
350 mg	11	83.2	7.8	9.0
3. Styrene copolymer benzene beads[b]				
5 ml	NT	74.8	18.3	6.9
10 ml	17	65.6	15.0	19.4

[a]Two experiments were pooled; 175-mg columns were used with CBA spleens and 350-mg columns with BDF, spleen cells. All three methods reduced phagocytic cells from $\sim 10\%$ to 0.2–1.0%. Pre-column, the suspensions were: CBA 55.7% SmIg$^+$ 33% θ^+, 11.3% "null," and 8% phagocytic; BDF$_1$ 52.5% SmIg$^+$, 31.5% θ^+, 16.5 "null," 9.5% phagocytic.
[b]Thompson et al. (20).
[c]NT, not tested.

TABLE 6
B Cells Require Active Metabolism, but No SmIg, for Their Adherence[a]

Treatment	Yield (%)	E⁺ cells in the effluent population (%)	E⁺ cells in precolumn population (%)
Positive controls			
Column temperature 37°,	22, 24	91, 89, 91, 93	
no inhibitors	26, 29		
Metabolic inhibitors[b]			
20°	28	81	
4°	50	63	
Azide, 0.2%, 37°	45	63	
0.02 M EDTA, 37°	51	66	
10 μg/ml cytochalasin B, 37°	64	68	
Removal of membrane-associated Ig[c]			49–61 (mean 57)
Positive control (NRS)	28	91	
Removal of SmIg (i)	27, 30	81, 85	
(ii)	24, 31	85, 89	
Incubation with anti-T cell serum[d]			
Positive control (NRS)	25, 27	89, 90	
Anti-T cell serum	24	91	

[a]Experiments were performed three times, and average values are given. 5× 10⁷ tonsil cells were loaded onto 300 mg of nylon fiber in a 5-ml syringe. The proportions of E⁺ and SmIg⁺ cells in the pre- and postcolumn suspensions were within the range shown in Table 2.

[b]Viability (pre- and postcolumn) was >90%. Inhibitors did not impair viability in these short-term experiments. In the effluent population the increase of yield and the decrease of % E⁺ cells corresponded to an increase of percentage of SmIg⁺ cells.

[c]Cells were treated with rabbit anti-human Ig (R-anti-Ig, 1:10 dilution) or normal rabbit serum (NRS, 1:10), for 60 min at 37°C. The removal of SmIg by R-anti-Ig was tested by staining cells with goat anti-rabbit Ig-FITC (G-anti-R Ig, 1:20, 4°C, 30 min). The residual SmIg⁺ cells were < 3%, whereas in NRS-treated samples 46% SmIg⁺ cells were seen.

[d]At the concentration of anti-T cell serum used (1:100, incubation for 30 min at 20°C) capping does not occur.

fibers is dependent upon temperature, azide inhibitable metabolic activity, and presence of calcium ions and it may involve microfilaments. In addition, the results are essentially unaffected by removing B-cell SmIg or by coating T cells with antibody to render them SmIg⁺ (Table 6). Notice that when little or no selective retention of B cells occurs, there is still a 50% cell loss distributed evenly in T and B populations. We assume that loss is most likely due to mechanical, physical trapping in the columns rather than temperature-independent adherence of both T and B subsets.

These observations correspond to what has previously been recorded with adherence of phagocytic cells but are in marked contrast to the temperature-independent adherence to glass beads of activated mouse lymphoid cells (1).

There is at present no explanation available for the differential adhesiveness of T and B lymphocytes. It presumably relates to some cell surface membrane property, possibly microfilament-regulated mobilization of appropriate membrane molecules or reactive groups. It might well be relevant in this respect that B cells on the whole appear to have more "spontaneous" microvilli and surface protrusions (and therefore a greater surface area) than T cells (16a). This is,

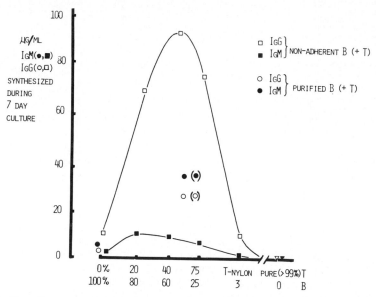

Fig. 3. Nonadherent B lymphocytes are T cell dependent and committed to synthesize predominantly IgG. Purified tonsil B cells were prepared by eliminating E$^+$ (T) cells on a Ficoll—Isopaque gradient. Nonadherent cells were from nylon column-filtered (T-cell enriched) populations. After E-rosetting followed by Ficoll—Isopaque separation, nonadherent T cells (> 99% E$^+$) were recovered from the pellet; these were treated with NH$_4$Cl to eliminate SRBC. Nonadherent B cells were from the interphase (see Table 4). B cells were mixed with pure T cells in varying proportions as shown. All cultures were set up at 1 × 10^6/ml cell concentration in flat-bottomed vials and stimulated for 7 days with 5 µg of Pa-1 [purified pokeweed mitogen (Ref. 21)]. The absolute amounts of IgM and IgG observed in the supernatants are shown. Results were confirmed by the cytological analysis (intracellular Ig staining) of stimulated cells. Symbols: □ ○, IgG; ■ ●, IgM; □ ■, nonadherent B (+ T) cells; ○ ●, "ordinary" purified B (+ T) cells. Symbols in parentheses show values observed in unseparated T + B tonsil cultures. In nonstimulated cultures < 3 µg/ml Ig was secreted. From Janossy et al. (22).

however, in itself a controversial observation. We are not aware of any convincing evidence for a relationship between adherence and either membrane viscosity or membrane lipid content, although these could well be relevant factors.

3.6. Functional Capacity of Column-Purified Lymphocytes. T cell-enriched populations eluted from nylon fiber columns have a high viability ($> 90\%$) and survive in culture for 4 or 7 days at the same rate as unfiltered cells. Their proliferative response to PHA lectin is superior to unfractionated cells on a cell-to-cell basis, which primarily reflects the enrichment in lectin-responsive cells (14).

A somewhat surprising functional characteristic of the eluted cells concerns the Ig biosynthetic capacity of the infrequent B cells. When unseparated tonsil cells are stimulated for 7 days with pokeweed mitogen, considerable quantities of both IgM and IgG are synthesized. This response is mostly T cell dependent as seen from the small levels of Ig biosynthesis in cultures of pokeweed-treated B cells (purified by E-rosette sedimentation). However, in the "pure-T" populations, the small residual fraction of B cells produce considerable quantities of Ig which is almost exclusively IgG (17). If the nylon fiber columns-purified T-enriched cells are further E-rosetted and separated on Ficoll–Isopaque, the pelleted fraction (containing $> 99\%$ E^+ cells), proliferates in response to purified pokeweed (preparation Pa-1) but does not biosynthesize Ig. This intriguing result could either reflect the existence of a relatively nonadherent IgG-committed (T dependent) B cell subset or perhaps be due to the loss of a particular B-regulator T cell subset on the column. This point was resolved by culturing the purified nonadherent $SmIg^+$ B cells (i.e., nylon filtered + E rosettes removed) and total $SmIg^+$ B cells (i.e., no nylon filtration but E rosettes removed) with varying numbers of purified E^+ T cells (i.e., nylon fiber filtered, pelleted E rosettes). The results show that the nonadherent B cell fraction appears to consist of an IgG-programmed subset and that the IgM-programmed B subset is lost on the column along with the bulk of B cells (Fig. 3).

4. Discussion

The nylon fiber column method as described appears to provide an inexpensive, simple and reproducible method for preparing reasonable quantities of T cell-enriched lymphocyte suspensions. With optimal conditions and recycling, 95% of the eluted cells have a T cell membrane phenotype. Between 5 and 15% of eluted cells, however, may be non-T cells; as discussed above, these are a mixture of IgG-programmed B cells plus a "null" cell population. Lymphocytes prepared by this method are functionally active in those tests that we have so far applied (i.e., proliferative response to lectins, helper activity in B cell Ig secretion).

One limitation of the method is its relatively poor yields (around 40–50% of T cells are lost). This compares reasonably well with T cell yields on some B cell immunoabsorbent columns (e.g., Degalan-anti-Ig) but is certainly inferior to what can be achieved on Sephadex-anti-Ig (see Method 19). This raises the serious question of whether T cell subsets, which certainly exist, could be differentially retained on the column. Experiments reported above indicated that, on recycling, the same porportion of T cells are lost. Also inhibition of selective B cell adherence by lowering temperatures in the presence of metabolic inhibitors or lack of Ca^{2+} resulted in an equal 50% loss of both T and B cells. We therefore have supposed that the T cell loss primarily reflects nonspecific physical or mechanical trapping in the column, and it is difficult to envisage how this could be selective for subsets. Nevertheless, this is still a real possibility and is reinforced by experiments in mice that have shown that IgG Fc receptor positive, θ^+, T cells in the mouse are adherent to nylon and their loss on "double cycle" filtration is accompanied by a simultaneous loss of the concanavalin A but *not* the PHA response (18, 19). Further tests are clearly necessary to determine the full functional repertory of nylon fiber column-purified human T cells.

Nylon fiber columns provide, therefore, a useful method for preparing human (and animal) T lymphocytes and are indeed used by many laboratories. The technique can form part of a strategy for a more extensive purification (see above and Method 19) or can provide T cells of sufficient purity for many functional tests *in vitro* and for assessing the specificity of membrane markers (see Method 3).

ACKNOWLEDGMENTS

This work was supported by the Imperial Cancer Research Fund and the Medical Research Council. The experiments described in this paper have been performed during the last three years at the University College, London, with the participation of G. Brown and R. Sutherland and at the Division of Immunology, Clinical Research Centre, Harrow, Middlesex, with the participation of Drs. A. Luquetti, E. Gomez de la Concha, and T. Platts-Mills.

REFERENCES

1. Shortman, K., *in* "Contemporary Topics in Molecular Immunology" (G. L. Ada, ed.), Vol. 3. Plenum, New York, 1975.
2. Hogg, N., and Greaves, M. F., *Immunology* 22, 959 (1971).
3. Julius, M. H., Simpson, E., and Herzenberg, L. A., *Eur. J. Immunol.* 3, 645 (1973).
4. Greaves, M. F., and Brown, G., *J. Immunol.* 112, 420 (1974).
5. Eisen, S. A., Wedner, H. J., and Parker, C. W., *Immunol. Commun.* 1, 571 (1972).
6. Fröland, S. S., Natvig, J. B., and Michaelsen, T. E., *Scand. J. Immunol.* 3, 375 (1974).
7. Chess, L., MacDermott, R. P., Sondel, P. M., and Schlossman, S. F., *in* "Progress in Immunology" (L. Brent and J. Holborow, eds.), Vol. 3, p. 125. North-Holland Publ., Amsterdam, 1974.
8. Böyum, A., *Scand. J. Clin. Lab. Invest.* 21, Suppl. 97.

9. Brown, G., and Greaves, M. F., *Eur. J. Immunol.* **4,** 302 (1974).
10. Greaves, M. F., *Prog. Haematol.* **9,** 255 (1975).
11. Greaves, M. F., and Brown, G., *Nature (London)* **246,** 116 (1973).
12. Greaves, M. F., Falk, J., and Falk, R., *Scand. J. Immunol.* **4,** 80 (1975).
13. Ross, G. D., Rabellino, E. M., Polley, M. J., and Grey, H. M., *J. Clin. Invest.* **52,** 377 (1973).
14. Greaves, M. F., Janossy, G., and Doenhoff, M. J., *J. Exp. Med.* **140,** 1 (1974).
15. Waxdal, M. J., *Biochemistry* **13,** 3671 (1974).
16. Platts-Mills, T. A. E., and Ishizaka, K., *J. Immunol.* **144,** 1058 (1975).
16a. Polliak, A., Lampen, N., Clarkson, B. D., deHarven, E., Bentwich, Z., Siegel, F. P., and Kunkel H. G., *J. Exp. Med.* **138,** 607 (1963).
17. Janossy, G., and Greaves, M. F., *Transplant. Rev.* **26,** 177 (1975).
18. Stout, R., and Herzenberg, L. A., personal communication, 1976.
19. Greaves, M. F., Brown, G., and Rickinson, A. B., *Clin. Immunol. Immunopathol.* **3,** 514 (1975).
20. Thompson, A. E. R., Bull, J. M., and Robinson, M. A., *Br. J. Haematol.* **12,** 433 (1966).
21. Janossy, G., Gomez de la Concha, E., Waxdal, M. J., and Platts-Mills, T., *Clin. Exp. Immunol.* in press.
22. Janossy, G., Gomez de la Concha, E., Luquetti, A., Waxdal, M. J., and Platts-Mills, T., submitted for publication.

Separation of Human Lymphocytes by E Rosette Sedimentation

S. M. Wahl, D. L. Rosenstreich, and J. J. Oppenheim

1. Introduction

Lymphocytes of man and other species consist of subpopulations of thymus-derived (T) and bone marrow-derived (B) cells. The T and B lymphocytes can be differentiated by specific cell membrane markers enabling the identification of unique functions for each subpopulation. These findings have provided new insights into the cellular basis of immunological events and thus into the pathogenesis of immunodeficiency and lymphoproliferative diseases. However, the identification of lymphocytes is still incomplete since some lymphoid cells have been shown to have no identifiable surface markers (null cells) and a small fraction to have both T and B cell markers (1). Nevertheless, since the majority of each population bear distinct cell surface characteristics, numerous methods have been devised to identify and quantitate these cells. The human T lymphocyte can be identified by specific surface antigens and by its ability to form spontaneous rosettes with unsensitized sheep erythrocytes (E) *in vitro* (2–4). In contrast, B lymphocytes with their unique surface membrane properties do not form rosettes with untreated sheep erythrocytes. This specificity of E rosette formation allows for identification and quantitation of the lymphocyte subpopulations present in lymphoid cell preparations. In addition to identification and enumeration of T cells, the phenomenon of spontaneous rosette formation also allows separation of T cells from B cells. Essentially the same procedure is used as for detection of E rosette-forming cells, except that larger quantities of cells are employed and separation is achieved by density centrifugation on Ficoll–Hypaque gradients. In contrast to many of the other techniques available for isolating subpopulations of T and B cells, this procedure allows for recovery of both the E-rosetted and non-E-rosetted populations from the same starting population of cells.

2. Materials

2.1. Isolation of Human Peripheral Blood Mononuclear Cells

2.1.1. Pharmaseal 50-ml plastic disposable syringes (American Hospital Supply, Washington, D. C.)

2.1.2. Butterfly—19 infusion set (Abbott Laboratories, Baltimore, Maryland)

2.1.3. Sodium heparin (1000 USP units/ml) (Eli Lilly & Co., Indianapolis, Indiana), stable at 4°C

2.1.4. Phosphate-buffered saline (PBS) (pH 7.2)

2.1.5. Ficoll 400,000 MW (Sigma, St. Louis, Missouri) diluted to 9% (v/v) in distilled H_2O.

2.1.6. Hypaque—M 90% (Winthrop Laboratories, New York), diluted to 33.9% with distilled H_2O

2.1.7. Screw-cap polystyrene tissue culture tubes, 16 × 150 mm (Falcon Plastics, Cockeysville, Maryland)

2.1.8. Conical polypropylene tubes, 50 ml (Falcon Plastics)

2.1.9. RPMI 1640 tissue culture media (Grand Island Biological Co., Grand Island, New York).

2.1.10. Penicillin—streptomycin (Flow Laboratories, Rockville, Maryland), 5000 IU/ml and 5000 μg/ml diluted to final concentration of 100 IU/ml and 100 μg/ml in media. Store at −20°C.

2.1.11. L-Glutamine, 200 mM (Grand Island Biological Co.), final concentration in media is 2 mmoles/ml. Store at −20°C.

2.2. Preparation of Sheep Red Blood Cells

2.2.1. Sheep red blood cells obtained under sterile conditions and added to an equivalent volume of Alsever's solution. Sheep cells should be stored at 4°C and be less than 2 weeks old.

2.2.2. Neuraminidase (*Vibrio cholerae*) (Behring Diagnostics, Somerville, New Jersey)

2.2.3. Saline: 0.85% NaCl

2.2.4. Ammonium chloride (NH_4Cl) lysing buffer (5)

2.3. Morphological Identification of Lymphocytes

2.3.1. Antihuman immunoglobulin (Ig) fluorescein-conjugated (IgG fraction) (Cappel Laboratories, Downington, Pennsylvania)

2.3.2. EACl-3b:sheep red blood cells (E) treated with antibody (A) and complement (Cl-3b) as described by Rapp and Borsos (6)

2.3.3. Esterase stain (7)

2.3.4. Polystyrene latex beads, 1.1 μm (Dow Chemical Co., Midland, Michigan)

2.3.5. Polypropylene tissue culture tube, 12 × 75 mm (Falcon Plastics)

2.3.6. Wright's stain

2.4. Functional Identification of Lymphocytes

2.4.1. Concanavalin A (Con A) (Calbiochem, Gaithersburg, Maryland)

2.4.2. Phytohemagglutinin (PHA) (Burroughs-Wellcome Co., Greenville, North Carolina)

2.4.3. [methyl-^{3}H] Thymidine (specific activity 6.0 Ci/mmole) (Schwarz/Mann, Orangeburg, New York)

2.4.4. Soda lima glass vials, 1 dram (Bellco Glass Inc., Vineland, New Jersey)

2.4.5. Microtiter trays (Falcon Microtest II, Falcon Plastics)

2.5. Equipment

2.5.1. 37°C water bath

2.5.2. 37°C water-jacketed CO_2 incubator (Thelco, Precision Scientific).

2.5.3. Ice-water bath

2.5.4. Refrigerated centrifuge

2.5.5. Skatron automatic cell harvester (Flow Laboratories, Rockville, Maryland)

2.5.6. Fluorescence microscope

2.5.7. Hemocytometer

3. Methodology

3.1. Isolation of Peripheral Blood Mononuclear Cells. Peripheral blood is drawn from adult donors into heparinized (100 units/ml) syringes and diluted 1:3 with sterile PBS. Mononuclear cells can be separated from erythrocytes and granulocytes on Ficoll–Hypaque gradients at room temperature (8). Ficoll–Hypaque (FH) is prepared by combining 2.4 parts of the 9% solution of Ficoll with 1 part of the diluted (33.9%) solution of Hypaque. Depending upon the total amount of blood being utilized, 12 ml of the diluted blood is layered on 3 ml of FH in 16 × 150 mm polystyrene tubes or, for larger amounts, 20–30 ml of diluted blood can be layered on 12 ml of FH in 50-ml polypropylene tubes. These tubes are centrifuged at 400 g for 40 min at 20°C. Better separation is obtained if the cells are not centrifuged in the cold. After centrifugation, the mixture of plasma and PBS is aspirated off to within approximately 1 inch from the cells at the FH interface and discarded. The cells are then aspirated along with about half of the FH. The mixture of cells, FH, and plasma obtained should be diluted about 4-fold with PBS and spun at 400 g. The supernatant fluid is discarded, then the pelleted cells can be pooled and washed 2–3 times with PBS before being suspended in tissue culture medium. These mononuclear cells (MNL) consist of approximately 70–80% lymphocytes, the remaining cells being monocytes. One can generally expect a yield of 2 × 10⁶ MNL from each milliliter of blood initially obtained.

3.2. Preparation of Sheep Erythrocytes (E). Two milliliters of sheep blood suspended in an equivalent volume of Alsever's solution are placed in a 50-ml centrifuge tube, diluted to 50 ml with PBS, and centrifuged (400 g) for 10 min. After gently decanting the fluid, the pelleted E are resuspended in PBS and washed twice more. Packed E, 1 ml suspended in 10 ml of PBS (roughly equivalent to 2 × 10⁹ E/ml), are then incubated with 4.0 units of neuraminidase (*vibrio cholerae*) at 37°C for 1 hr to enhance binding to the T lymphocytes (9).

The neuraminidase-treated E are washed 3 times in PBS and suspended in RPMI 1640 medium at approximately 1×10^9/ml.

3.3. Rosetting and Fractionating Procedure. Five milliliters of the neuraminidase-treated E are added to an equivalent volume of the leukocyte suspension containing a total of 50 to 100×10^6 MNL (a ratio of E to MNL of 50:1). These volumes can be decreased or expanded depending upon the number of cells being separated. The cells are mixed and then incubated for 15 min at 37°C. A slow spin (200 g) for 5 min gently pellets the E with the MNL, and the tubes are then carefully placed in an ice-water bath so as not to disturb the pellets for 60 min. After the incubation, the cells are very gently pipetted to resuspend the cells without dissociating the rosettes. This cell suspension is layered onto 10 ml of cold FH (4°C) in 50-ml tubes or onto 3 ml of FH in 16 × 150 mm tubes and centrifuged for 30 min at 4°C (400 g). The centrifuge should be accelerated gradually for best results. The non-rosette-forming cells (Fig. 1) found at the interface are collected by aspirating off the media and half of the FH, diluting this cell suspension 1:3 with medium and centrifuging at 525 g for 15 min. The cell pellets can be pooled and washed twice more before being subjected to a second rosetting. The pellet at the bottom of the FH gradient (Fig. 1) contains lymphocytes that have formed rosettes with E and free E. If these cells are warmed to 37°C, the rosettes will dissociate and the E can be lysed with NH_4Cl lysing buffer at 4°C for 10 min. After 2–3 washings these cells, which are predominantly T lymphocytes, can be suspended at 1×10^6/ml in RPMI 1640 tissue culture medium containing glutamine and antibiotics.

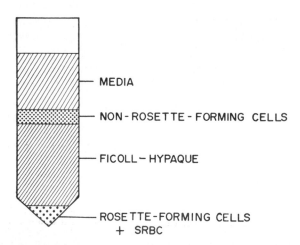

Fig. 1. Schematic representation of E-rosette sedimentation on Ficoll–Hypaque gradients after centrifugation (30 min, 400 g, 4°C). The non-rosette-forming cells (B enriched) float on the surface of the Ficoll–Hypaque while the E rosetted cells (T enriched) settle to the bottom of the Ficoll–Hypaque along with the free sheep red blood cells (SRBC).

Those cells that did not rosette during the first rosetting procedure and are enriched in B cells can be further enriched for B cells by a second rosetting with E as described above. The cells are then washed 3 times and suspended at 1 × 10^6/ml in RPMI 1640. Those rosetted cells below the FH after this second sedimentation are discarded since they are not as enriched in T lymphocytes as those obtained after the first rosetting.

3.4. Characterization of Surface Receptors of Lymphocyte Subpopulations. Lymphocytes, 5 × 10^6 unseparated, nonrosetting (B-enriched) or rosetted (T-enriched), are pelleted by centrifugation at 400 g for 5 min in a 12 × 75 mm plastic tube, suspended in 1 drop of medium containing 10 mM sodium azide, and 0.1 ml of fluorescein-conjugated anti-human Ig is added. The antiserum is ultracentrifuged at 100,000 g for 60 min to remove aggregates prior to use. The tubes are incubated at 4°C for 30 min (10) during which time the tubes should be agitated every 5–10 min. After 2–3 washes with cold medium containing 2% fetal calf serum, 2 drops of the cell suspension are placed on glass slides under cover slips sealed with petroleum jelly. Fluorescein-positive cells are quantitated using a fluorescence microscope alternating bright-field illumination and ultraviolet light observations of the same field. Slides should be maintained at 4°C until examined.

A second method of identifying the cells involves rosetting of the B lymphocytes with EACl-3b. The lymphocyte (1 × 10^6) subpopulations are incubated with the prepared EACl-3b (20 × 10^6) in 1.0 ml of RPMI 1640 at 37°C for 30 min with intermittent agitation. The cells are gently placed onto a hemocytometer, and the percentage of lymphocytes forming EAC rosettes consisting of 3 or more red cells is quantitated.

Phagocytic monocytes in the preparation can be identified by the ingestion of polystyrene latex particles. Cells, 1 × 10^6, are incubated with a 1:1000 dilution of latex beads in media containing 5% FCS for 30 min at 37°C, washed twice with PBS, and then gently smeared on a slide, air dried, ethanol fixed, and stained with Wright's stain. The percentage of cells ingesting latex can then be quantitated. Additionally, monocytes can be detected by a specific esterase stain (7).

3.5. Functional Properties of Lymphocyte Subpopulations. The lymphocyte subpopulations can be assessed functionally by their response to certain mitogens that appear to be relatively specific for B or T cells. Human peripheral blood T cells, but not purified B cells, are activated by PHA and Con A to proliferate and produce mediators. By utilizing this specificity, one can determine how pure the separated cell populations are. One milliliter of serum-free RPMI 1640 with 0.5% human plasma containing 1 × 10^6 cells is cultured in a 1-dram vial with PHA or Con A for 48–72 hr. Proliferation can be assessed by the degree of thymidine uptake as described in Method 54 (11). Mediator production, in particular the presence of chemotactic factor, can be determined by harvesting the supernatants from these cultures after 24–48 hr of incubation and measuring the chemotactic activity for monocytes by the method of Snyderman (12).

4. Interpretation of Data and Critical Comments

Table 1 summarizes the results of a representative experiment involving fractionation of subpopulations of human peripheral blood mononuclear cells by the E-rosette sedimentation method. The number of T and B lymphocytes was determined before and after separation using fluorescent staining with anti-human immunoglobulin and C3 receptors detected by EAC rosetting as markers for B lymphocytes (13, 14). Unseparated populations of peripheral blood mononuclear cells contained approximately 15% immunoglobulin-positive cells. After a single rosetting procedure, the T-enriched population (E rosette-forming cells) was almost completely depleted of Ig-positive cells while the non-rosette-forming cells contained an increased proportion of Ig-positive cells. Comparable values were obtained using EACl-3b as a B cell marker. After a repetition of the rosetting technique with those cells that did not rosette the first time, the percentage of cells in the non-rosette-forming population was increased to about 60% Ig or complement receptor positive. However, the E-rosette-forming cells also contain greater numbers of Ig-positive cells after this second sedimentation. These Ig-positive cells may in part be accounted for by dead cells that sediment,

TABLE 1

Morphological Identification of Lymphocytes Separated by E Rosette Sedimentation

	Percent of cells positive for		
Cell population	Surface Ig	C3 Receptor	Phagocytosis
Mononuclear cells	15.0 ± 2.0^a	18.3 ± 0.88^b	36.0 ± 1.15^c
First E rosette sedimentation			
E rosettes	3.7 ± 0.33	4.3 ± 0.67	2.3 ± 0.88
Non-E-rosettes	30.0 ± 1.2	44.7 ± 2.4	19.5 ± 4.5
Second E rosette sedimentation			
E rosettes	15.6 ± 1.7	9.7 ± 1.8	9.0 ± 1
Non-E-rosettes	62.0 ± 0.88	$57 \quad \pm 4.9$	19.0 ± 1

[a]Cells from the Ficoll–Hypaque isolated, nonseparated mononuclear cells or at various stages of purification were assessed for the presence of surface Ig by fluorescent staining with anti-Ig as described in Methods.
[b]Lymphocytes bearing C3 receptors were identified by the formation of rosettes with EACl-3b (> 3 EACl-3b per lymphocyte).
[c]Ingestion of latex beads as described in Methods served as a marker for phagocytic cells.

TABLE 2
Mitogenic Response of Lymphocytes Separated by E Rosette Sedimentation

Cells	Mitogenic response $(E/C)^a$	
	PHA	Con A
Mononuclear cells (FH)	73.6	69.7
T lymphocytes (E rosettes)	151.8	33.8
B lymphocytes (nonrosetted cells)	7.2	5.6

^{a}Unseparated mononuclear cells, T-enriched or B-enriched populations were cultured at 1×10^6 cells/ml in medium containing 0.5% heat inactivated AB + plasma. After 68 hr, the cells were pulsed with 1 μCi ^{3}H-thymidine per milliliter for 4 hr and then harvested. Counts per minute per culture were determined, and the data are expressed as stimulated/control.

or may be cells bearing both T and B cell markers (1). Alternatively, alteration of their membrane properties may occur during this treatment. Therefore these cells are routinely discarded and not added to the T cell-enriched population.

That the cells which do not rosette after two exposures to E are not all Ig positive is of some concern, but a consistent finding. By means of functional criteria (Table 2) the proliferative response to the T cell mitogens, PHA and Con A, is substantially eliminated in these B cell-enriched populations. Since the response to these mitogens is decreased 90–95% of nonseparated controls, the Ig-negative cells do not appear to be functional T lymphocytes. A portion of these Ig- and C3b-receptor-negative cells may be null cells which can constitute up to 13% of peripheral blood mononuclear cells (1) and would be enhanced in numbers in these preparations of nonrosetting cells. Moreover, Lobo *et al.* (15) have identified a population of C3-negative, Fc-positive, human B cells that have labile surface Ig and thus would not be detected by staining with fluorescein-conjugated anti-Ig at 37°C or by EAC1-3b. Additionally, monocytes do not appear to bind E under the conditions of this assay (2) and would therefore be found with the nonrosetting cells.

Pretreatment of the E with neuraminidase stabilizes the rosettes (9) enabling them to remain intact during the separation procedure. Although it is believed to unmask receptor sites, the neuraminidase treatment may also stabilize the rosettes by reducing the surface charge of the cells creating a more effective interaction between E and T cell (16) or by removing sialic acid residues in the vicinity of rosette receptors (17). Whatever the mechanism, the rosettes are not as fragile as with untreated E, thereby facilitating handling and increasing purity in separation.

This method for isolating B cells is preferable to other commonly employed methods, such as immunoadsorbent columns or EAC rosetting, for a number of reasons. This negative separation technique avoids interaction of immunoglobulins or complement components with surface receptors leading to aggregation, capping or cross-linking of the receptors which may actually activate the B cells (18). Moreover, by cell surface markers and proliferative criteria greater purification is achieved and the T cells appear to be quite homogenous. As seen in Table 2, the T lymphocytes show enhanced reactivity to the T cell mitogen PHA (> 100% increase) as compared to the unseparated cells. Conversely, the B-enriched populations had a 90–95% decreased mitogenic response to both the T cell mitogens, PHA and Con A, indicative of the reduction in numbers of functionally reactive T cells. Unfortunately, unlike in the mouse and guinea pig, B cell mitogens, such as endotoxin, which provide a functional test for purity are not yet available for human cells.

In contrast to the relative mitogenic specificity achievable by utilizing this E-rosette-sedimentation method for separating T and B cells, the method is not adequate for assessing mediator production by these subpopulations. It is evident in Table 3 that the mononuclear cells separated on Ficoll–Hypaque gradients produce significant levels of monocyte (MNL) chemotactic factor (CTX) in the absence of additional stimulation. A similar finding is evident in the supernatants of nonstimulated B cell-enriched populations in which chemotactic activity is as high as in the supernatants of mitogen-stimulated cultures. Since the T cells do not spontaneously release MNL CTX under these same conditions, it appears that the separation on FH is directly stimulatory to B lymphocytes. Because of the spontaneous lymphokine synthesis triggered under these conditions by human peripheral blood cells, it is difficult to assess the activation of these cells by additional B cell stimulants.

TABLE 3

Mediator Production by Lymphocytes Separated by E Rosette Sedimentation

Cells	Chemotactic activity		
	PHA	Con A	Nonstimulated
Mononuclear cells[a]	188 ± 15^{b}	197 ± 18	159 ± 12
T lymphocytes (E rosettes)	127 ± 2	61 ± 9	12 ± 1
B lymphocytes (nonrosetted cells)	211 ± 25	197 ± 21	226 ± 7

[a]Unseparated mononuclear cells, T-enriched or B-enriched populations were cultured at 1×10^6 cells/ml for 48 hr. The cell-free supernatants were then assayed in triplicate for chemotactic activity for monocytes in modified Boyden chambers.
[b]Chemotactic activity is represented as the mean number of migrated cells per oil immersion field for triplicate samples ± 1 SE.

Thus E-rosette sedimentation as a method for separation of T and B cells in human peripheral blood has certain drawbacks. The entire procedure is time consuming, requiring several hours for the incubations and centrifugation. Furthermore, one sporadically obtains inexplicable low yields of the T and B-enriched cells. While the T-enriched populations are by surface marker studies and by functional criteria a fairly homogeneous population, the B-enriched lymphocytes are less so. By surface markers the B lymphocytes are not homogeneous although they do not proliferate in response to T cell mitogens. Additionally, these cells appear to be triggered by the separation procedure to spontaneously release lymphokines. This finding of activation of the B lymphocytes by procedures used in their isolation is frequently encountered. While exposure to FH does not activate B cells in other species, such as the guinea pig (18), it is a consistent finding in human peripheral blood cells in this laboratory and has been reported by others (19).

In summary, this technique of E rosetting for separating T and B cells does have certain advantages. Both T and B lymphocyte-enriched cells can be recovered from the same initial population of cells. The T-enriched populations are homogeneous both by surface marker and functional criteria. They respond to T cell mitogens by proliferating and by producing lymphokines. Since the rosettes can be dissociated and the red cells lysed, the T cells can be freed of any interference with their surface receptors. Additionally, the non-rosette-forming cells that are B cell-enriched demonstrate significantly enhanced functional purity as determined by proliferative assays. Since this technique involves a negative separation of the B cells, no molecules have bound to their Fc, Ig, and C3 receptors that might interfere with subsequent binding, making this population of cells useful for further studies. Moreover, this technique can be successfully applied to separating T and B cell populations in animal models utilizing red cells of the appropriate species (Table 4) as reported by numerous

TABLE 4

Erythrocyte Species Requirement for Spontaneous Rosette Formation
by T Lymphocytes

Source of T lymphocytes	Source of erythrocytes			
	Sheep	Rhesus monkey	Rabbit	Human
Human	+	+		
Guinea pig			+	
Mouse	+			
South African baboon	+			
Vervet monkey	+			
Dog				+

investigators. Such separation procedures will enable further definition of the roles of T and B lymphocytes in immune phenomena.

REFERENCES

1. Dickler, H. B., Adkinson, N. F., Jr., and Terry, W. D., *Nature (London)* **247**, 213 (1974).
2. Jondal, G., Holm, G., and Wigzell, H., *J. Exp. Med.* **136**, 207 (1972).
3. Wybran, J., Carr, M. C., and Fudenburg, H. H., *J. Clin. Invest.* **51**, 2537 (1972).
4. Greaves, M. F., and Brown, G., *J. Immunol.* **112**, 420 (1974).
5. Roos, D., and Loos, J. A., *Biochim. Biophys. Acta.* **222**, 565 (1970).
6. Rapp, H. J., and Borsos, T., (eds.), "Molecular Basis of Complement Action," p. 75. Appleton, New York, 1970.
7. Lake, B. D., *J. Clin. Pathol.* **24**, 617 (1971).
8. Böyum, A., *Scand. J. Clin. Lab. Invest.* **21**, 31 (1968).
9. Weiner, M. S., Bianco, C., and Nussenzweig, V., *Blood* **42**, 939 (1973).
10. Van Boxel, J. A., and Rosenstreich, D., *J. Exp. Med.* **139**, 1002 (1974).
11. Oppenheim, J. J., and Rosenstreich, D. L., this volume, Method 54.
12. Snyderman, R., and Pike, M., this volume, Method 62.
13. Lay, W. H., and Nussenzweig, V., *J. Exp. Med.* **128**, 991 (1968).
14. Möller, G. (ed.), *Transplant. Rev.* **16** (1973).
15. Lobo, P., Westervelt, F. B., and Horowitz, D. A., *J. Immunol.* **144**, 116 (1975).
16. Galili, U., and Schlesinger, *J. Immunol.* **112**, 1628 (1974).
17. Lohrmann, H., and Novikovs, L., *Clin. Immunol. Immunopathol.* **3**, 99 (1974).
18. Wahl, S. M., Iverson, G. M., and Oppenheim, J. J., *J. Exp. Med.* **140**, 1631 (1974).
19. Arvilommi, H., and Räsänen, L., *Nature (London)* **257**, 144 (1975).

Isolation of Human T Lymphocytes from Tumor Tissues by SRBC Rosette Sedimentation

Mikael Jondal

1. Introduction

If the cell-mediated immune system is influencing tumor growth after macroscopic tumor development, reactive lymphocytes may be present at the tumor site. Lymphoid infiltration has long been regarded as a favorable prognostic sign (1).

It will here be described how human T lymphocytes can be detected, enumerated, and fractionated from tumor tissues by taking advantage of the affinity between human T lymphocytes and sheep red blood cells (SRBC) (2). In this context it is important to realize that activated T cells retain SRBC receptors and display an even increased capacity to bind SRBC (3, 4). There is some evidence that the SRBC receptor is localized near a T cell-specific antigen associated with T cell recognition (5–7).

2. Material

2.1. For SRBC Rosette Formation
SRBC
Fetal calf serum, heat-inactivated
RPMI 1640 medium

2.2. Additional Material for SRBC-Rosette Sedimentation
Ficoll (Pharmacia Fine Chemicals Inc., Uppsala, Sweden)
Isopaque (Nyegaard & Co., Oslo, Norway)
Tubes, 50-ml (Falcon Plastics, Oxnard, California)

3. Method

3.1. Preparation of Tumor Tissue. A single-cell suspension should be prepared from the tumor tissue, adapting the procedure to each particular tumor. No enzymes that affect SRBC receptors may be used (trypsin, phospholipase A, etc.). Large tissue pieces and debris are allowed to settle by 1 *g* sedimentation.

The supernatant is harvested and centrifugated on a one-step standard. Ficoll–Isopaque gradient, used (8) to remove dead cells: 20 ml of tumor-cell suspension (2×10^6 cells/ml), in RPMI 1640 medium with 10% fetal calf serum, is layered on 15 ml of cold Ficoll–Isopaque in a 50-ml tube and spun at 850 g for 15 min. The cells at the interphase are harvested and washed twice and resuspended in undiluted fetal calf serum at a cell concentration of 2×10^6/ml.

3.2. Rosette Formation. Washed SRBC (100 μl, packed) is added to 20 ml of tumor cell suspension (see Section 3.1). The cell suspension is mixed and pelleted by centrifugation at 700 g for 3 min and incubated for 5 min at 37°C and for an additional hour at 4°C. Thereafter the cells are *gently* resuspended, still at 4°C, and a small sample is taken to analyze the number of small and large (larger than 12 μm) rosette-forming T cells.

3.3. Fractionation of SRBC Rosettes. Each 20-ml fraction of the "rosetted" cell suspension is immediately layered on 15 ml of cold Ficoll–Isopaque and centrifugated as described in Section 3.1. The handling of the cells and the centrifugation should be done at 4°C. After centrifugation the tumor cells will be at the interphase, and the rosette-forming T cells in the pellet. When the interphase cells are harvested care should be taken to remove all cells and fluid above the pellet. Then 5 ml of Tris-buffered 0.83% NH_4Cl is added to the pellet to lyse the SRBC. After lysis the tube is immediately filled with buffer, and the T cells are washed twice. The purity of the T cell population usually ranges between 60 and 80%.

4. Comments

Treatment of SRBC with 2-aminoethylisothiouronium (AET) (9) or with neuraminidase (10) may be used to stabilize the SRBC rosettes and to facilitate the fractionation procedure. In certain situations, however, such treatments may cause rosette formation between treated SRBC and non-T cells or nonlymphoid cells. This must be checked for each individual tumor.

In this laboratory successful fractionation of immunocompetent T cells has so far been achieved from two different tumors: from the circulation of patients with chronic lymphatic leukemia (which had a very high number of malignant cells in the differential count) (11) and from biopsy cells derived from Burkitt's lymphoma (12). In the latter case the isolated T cells appeared to be selectively cytotoxic for the autologous tumor cells.

REFERENCES

1. Black, M. M., *Prog. Clin. Cancer* **26** (1965).
2. Möller, G. (ed.), *Transplant. Rev.* **16** (1973).
3. Jondal, M., *Scand. J. Immunol.* **3**, 793 (1974).
4. Owen, F. L., and Fanger, M. W., *J. Immunol.* **115**, 765 (1975).

5. Owen, F. L., and Fanger, M. W., *J. Immunol.* **113,** 1128 (1974).
6. Owen, F. L., and Fanger, M. W., *J. Immunol.* **113,** 1138 (1974).
7. Wortis, H. H., Cooper, A. G., and Brown, M. C., *Nature (London)* **243,** 106 (1973).
8. Böyum, A. A., *Scand. J. Clin. Lab. Invest.* **21,** 51 (1968).
9. Kaplan, M. E., and Clark, C., *J. Immunol. Methods* **5,** 131 (1974).
10. Bentwick, Z., Douglas, S. D., Skutelsky, E., and Kunkel, H., *J. Exp. Med.* **137,** 1532 (1973).
11. Blomgren, H., Jondal, M., and Johansson, B., *Acta Rad. Ther. Phys. Biol.* **15,** 23 (1976).
12. Jondal, M., Svedmyr, E., Klein, E., and Singh, S., *Nature (London)* **255,** 405 (1975).

Enrichment or Depletion of Surface-Immunoglobulin-Coated Cells Using Anti-immunoglobulin Antibodies and Glass or Plastic Bead Columns

Hans Wigzell

1. Introduction

Affinity chromatography of cells, first introduced to remove specific antigen-binding cells (1), is one of several approaches to deplete or enrich for a given cell type in a population. Additional structures besides antigen-binding receptors have since been included in such selection procedures, and it is now possible via bead column separation procedures to fractionate cells according to a variety of surface markers including Fc receptors for Ig (2), receptors for activated complement components (2, 3), Ig molecules (4, 5), or surface antigens (4, 6). Solid-phase sorbents for cellular fractionation have included a variety of material, but bead columns have been the dominating approach in these systems. A variety of bead materials have also been used to achieve efficient cell separation including glass, plastic (1–4), cross-linked dextrans, agarose, or acrylamide (5, 7). The different materials have varying vices and virtues, with nonspecific retention of cells matched against efficiency of selective retention as the two dominating factors to be considered. In the present description, beads of glass or poly-methacrylic plastic will be discussed as to their use when packed into columns to function as selective cellular sorbents.

2. Materials

2.1. Columns. Virtually any column will do, provided the filter pore size in the bottom allows passage of the cells to be fractionated. Most nylon and sintered-glass membranes are suitable and cause only minor retention of cells on their own. When using other kinds of material to provide a "membrane" in the bottom, e.g., of a Pasteur pipette, cotton wool or glass fibers in tiny quantities can be used. However, these materials, especially cotton wool, have sometimes quite high capacity on their own to remove cells from a passing population, and this removal is sometimes highly selective (8). If commercial columns are used, bottom membranes should be changed (or removed and thoroughly washed) after 10–20 passages of cells to maintain proper pore sizes and keep the low retaining behavior of the membrane. If sterile work is to be done with the cells, glass columns are preferred by us for reasons of ease of sterilization (70% ethanol overnight), a treatment that many plastic columns will not endure.

2.2. Beads. For separation of cells of lymphoid type, beads with a mean diameter of around 200 μm would seem optimal for providing surface contact between cells and beads while still allowing the majority of the cells to pass through according to simple "size filtration." Smaller beads can be used but should not go below 150 μm, as for most bead material mechanical retention of cells according to size will then start to become a major factor. Also, when using beads of smaller size, variation of bead sizes within the population must be minimized, as this would tend to decrease still further the "average" pore size between the beads and increase the degree of mechanical retention. Beads with sizes well above 1 mm have been used in affinity chromatography of cells, but flow rates must then be extremely slow or cells must be allowed to sit in the column for appreciable periods of time (30 min or more) in order to allow contact between beads and cells.

Glass beads, 200–225 μm (obtained from 3M Company under the name Super-Brite Glass Beads or from Ballotini, Barnsley, Yorkshire, England) have been used by us extensively and found to be highly suitable for the present procedures. When freshly obtained as well as before each labeling procedure, the glass beads should be acid cleaned to allow optimal coating with subsequent material. Beads to be cleaned are put in an Erlenmeyer bottle or beaker in a suction hood, mixed with a 1:1 mixture of concentrated HCl and HNO_3, and left for 15 min. Subsequently, the beads are washed with sterile 0.9% NaCl until the pH of the washing fluid is that of the original saline solution. The beads are now ready for coating.

Polymethacrylic plastic beads in a similar size as the above-mentioned glass beads can be obtained commercially from Degussa Wolfgang AG, Hanau am Main, West Germany under the trade name Degalan V26 (1). Certain batches of the Degalan require decantation in sterile saline to remove minor granules, which would otherwise tend to clog the bead column and remove cells because of poor "pore size" geometry. Degalan beads upon arrival can normally be considered to be sterile and are ready for use without acid cleaning. The Degalan beads are in a price range that allows many users to throw away the beads after usage, but the beads can be reused after acid cleaning at room temperature using 1 M HCl for 1 hr.

After the incubation with anti-Ig antiserum the columns should be washed with three void volumes of saline or tissue culture medium (the same medium in which the cells to be passed), and they are now ready for use, as the anti-Ig serum also has provided the column beads with the necessary "lubrication."

2.3. Cells. With anti-Ig columns, it is most common to use such bead columns to remove lymphoid cells with their own, actively synthesized Ig as the target antigen on the cell surface. However, the Ig on the cells to be separated can also be passively acquired either, most likely, by cytophilic antibodies or by the coating of surface antigens by antibodies. It should in this context be realized that anti-Ig columns can be used to selectively remove Ig-positive nonlymphoid cells. The bead size is important if the cells to be separated are larger than the mean free pore size between the beads. With anti-Ig coated columns we normally use lymphoid cells, whether from blood, spleen, lymph nodes, or thymus. Such cells are brought into single-cell suspension by pressing the organs through stainless steel mesh screens using routine procedures, followed by repeated, careful sucking up and down in Pasteur pipettes to further increase the yield of single cells. Clumps of cells are removed by allowing them to stand in tubes for 2 min followed by decanting and centrifugation of the cells at 250 g for 4 min. The washing is repeated once, and the cells are then adjusted to 5 X 10^7 cells/ml or less. It is necessary in order to achieve efficient separation that the concentration of the cells to be fractionated not exceed the 5 X 10^7/ml level, most likely because steric hindrance causes mechanical disturbances during filtration. When the cells are waiting for column fractionation they should be kept at 4°C in suspended form (pelleted cells tend to display increased clumping upon resuspension if not resuspended soon after centrifugation, especially if a sizable proportion of the cells are dead).

The media used for suspending the cells should fulfill two minimum requirements; they should keep the cells in satisfactory condition and they should not contain Ig molecules of the same species as the cells, as these would then abolish the capacity of the anti-Ig column to remove the Ig-positive cells. The medium we use most frequently when, for example, separating mouse, human, or rat lymphocytes is PBS according to Dulbecco (9) with 5% fetal calf serum. Keeping the cells at 4°C before fractionation is not obligatory but should be done unless the subsequent cellular assays demand otherwise, as storage at 4°C decreases the possibility of detachment of Ig molecules from the surface of the cells.

3. Methods

3.1. Coating of Beads: General Principle. Most proteins can be shown to bind comparatively firmly to glass or plastic beads (when ready for coating as described above), but the exact forces involved are still unknown (1). Whatever the exact mechanism, the binding is frequently of a strength comparable to that obtained via covalent coupling procedures yielding beads coated with, e.g., albumin molecules, which can subsequently be used as specific immunosorbents for the binding and elution of anti-BSA antibodies. It is wise, however, to establish the coupling conditions for any new protein previously not tried, using the present bead material to ensure the relative strength of the binding to the beads. Binding of the protein to the beads is normally carried out at isotonic conditions using neutral pH (or the pH to be used subsequently) and a protein concentration of around 1 mg/ml or more (1). With most proteins 1 mg/ml will saturate the bead surfaces, but occasional proteins might require higher concentrations. That saturation has been obtained can be assessed by the admixing of radioactively labeled protein to the protein to be coupled to and look for plateau levels of radiolabel attached in relation to added protein concentration. Using proteins in the molecular size range of 50,000, a density of molecules of the order of $10^4/\mu m^2$ is reached, indicating a virtually completely covered surface if random distribution of molecules is assumed. The density of protein molecules adsorbed would seem to be somewhat higher using Degalan beads as compared to glass beads, but no significant behavior in the specific capacity of the two bead types due to this difference has been noted. Use of radioactively labeled material when coating bead columns can also be used in the search for any possible detachment of material from the bead surfaces after labeling.

Actual labeling of beads can be carried out using uncoated beads either already packed in the column to be subsequently used or in an Erlenmeyer bottle of suitable size. Beads are in isotonic saline at neutral pH, and the protein (or other suitable macromolecules) to be attached is added in the same saline solution at 1 mg/ml concentrations (or above) when labeling in columns. If labeling is carried out in bottles, protein concentrations high enough to ensure a 1 mg/ml concentration should be used when finally mixed with the beads. Labeling can be carried out either rapidly, allowing coating at 45°C for 30 min to be followed by at least another 30 min at 4°C or, more often, by labeling via incubation overnight at 4°C. Larger batches of beads in protein solutions can be kept at 4°C for prolonged periods of time using sodium azide at 0.01% as a preservative.

Washing away of unattached protein is then carried out in columns, pouring the beads from the bottles or using the already packed, labeled bead columns for washing straight away. When pouring the beads into the columns, it is wise to already have some saline in the column to ensure that no trapping of air in the bottom of the columns occurs during packing. The washing of beads in the column is then carried out using at least twice the void volume of the bead column fluid to pass through, making sure that in the initial addition of washing fluid the protein-containing fluid going into the column does not mix at the top with the added washing saline solution.

After two void volumes have been washed through the column (three void volumes added), the effluent fluid from the bottom of the column is normally not contaminated in any detectable manner with soluble protein (1). With most proteins, however, the bead column is still not ready for use, as addition of cells to filter through the columns at this stage would lead to very high losses of cells that stick for "nonspecific" reasons to the beads. Thus, an additional incubation with isotonic saline containing at least 5% serum (any serum that would not interfere with the actual test would do; we normally use fetal calf serum) for 60 min at 4°C is advisable. Such an additional incubation procedure will "lubricate" the columns so as to allow a more specific retention of passing cells with affinity for the protein used as first coating agent. We assume the lubrication step to involve coating of the beads with additional serum material, maybe of lipoprotein nature, making the surface of the beads less sticky for passing cells. No investigation as to what is actually occurring at this step has, however, been carried out. After the "lubrication" labeling, the bead columns can be used straight away for removal of cells via affinity chromatography.

3.2. Coating of Beads: Preparation of Columns for Removal of Ig-Positive Cells. The underlying principle for specific removal and, under certain circumstances, enrichment of cells with immunoglobulin (Ig) molecules on their outer surface is the use of bead columns coated with antibodies against Ig molecules of the species providing the cells to be fractionated (4–6). This can be achieved using various variations of bead material, anti-immunoglobulin reagents, etc. We shall here deal only with such anti-Ig columns using as the underlying principle glass or Degalan beads coated with Ig molecules and on top of this anti-Ig antibodies in excess (4). Alternatively, we shall describe methods where the latter antibodies are used in excess to cover the Ig-positive cells, subsequently passed through Ig-coated bead columns and thereby removed. The use of excess anti-Ig antibodies will in principle in both cases leave one (in case of IgG antibodies) antigen-binding site free for combination with the second solid phase (the Ig-positive cells in the first case, the Ig-coated beads in the second case). The advantage of the present approach lies in its very high capacity with regard to cell numbers, its ease of preparation, and the high efficiency of removing of virtually all Ig-positive cells. The disadvantages of the technique reside in the relatively high capacity for nonspecific retention of the present beads with regard to "sticky" cells. With regard to enrichment of Ig-positive cells by elution from the anti-Ig columns of the present kind, the degree of enrichment is poor (4) unless preruns are made over normal serum-coated columns. In the latter case, mechanical elution of cells retained by anti-Ig column techniques of the present kind can yield preparations of close to 100% purity (6).

Standard procedures for making anti-Ig columns in our laboratory are as follows: Acid-cleaned glass beads or Degalan beads are incubated with immunoglobulin of the species providing the cells to be fractionated. We normally prepare our immunoglobulin from normal serum by ammonium sulfate precipitation (choosing the optimal concentrations of ammonium sulfate according to the species providing the serum). In most mammalian systems a 45% ammonium sulfate solution at pH 7 is adequate to bring down immunoglobulin in a purity adequate for the column coating. Normally, saturated ammonium sulfate solution is added to the serum at 4°C to make the ammonium sulfate concentration 45%. The precipitate formed after 30 min is centrifuged and washed twice with 45% ammonium sulfate solution with centrifugations, and is then dissolved to original serum volume using isotonic saline. Although containing high salt concentrations this solution can now be used for coating the beads (after reading in the spectrophotometer at 2800 Å to test that the protein concentration will be adequate, see Section 3.1), but we normally dialyze overnight against isotonic saline, pH 7.4, to remove the ammonium sulfate. With most mammalian sera, such ammonium sulfate precipitation procedures will yield, when reconstituted back to original serum volume protein, solutions with a concentration of between 5 and sometimes more than 10 mg of immunoglobulin per milliliter. During labeling of beads use concentrations of immunoglobulins in the fluid of at least 1 mg/ml. After coating, the beads (see Section 3.1) are transferred into a suitable column (unless labeled already in the relevant column). For most experiments we use Pharmacia columns 1.5 × 30 cm, but most commercial columns will do (see Section 2.1). The bead columns are then washed with at least three void volumes of saline and again incubated, this time with anti-Ig serum, and usually labeling for 60 min at 4°C or at room temperature. We generally use anti-Ig sera of polyvalent nature, directed against both heavy chains of most Ig classes as well as against light chains (4). The amount of anti-Ig antibodies in the sera used in our department do usually exceed 1 mg/ml in undiluted serum and is used at dilution 1:3 during column labeling.

An easy test to determine whether an anti-Ig serum contains enough anti-Ig antibodies involves the use of small precipitin tubes to which are added equal volumes of the antiserum, carefully overlaid by a solution of 1 mg/ml in isotonic saline of IgG molecules of the relevant species. Clear-cut precipitation should occur between the two reagents within 1–2 min. We have found no evidence that any particular species of animals are better than others in providing suitable anti-Ig antibodies for the present test, and in our department we usually use rabbit or sheep anti-Ig sera produced by ourselves for these assays.

3.3. Cell Separation. Columns with beads labeled with anti-Ig antibodies and washed should not be moved from cold to warm (e.g., from 4°C to 20°C) environments, as bubbles might form that could seriously impede the subsequent cellular passage. Column separation should be carried out at 4°C if shedding from the cells of the relevant affinity structure is anticipated, otherwise at room temperature or at 37°C. For our own purposes, when using fractionation of lymphocytes from normal, nonimmune donors, we usually carry out the separations at room temperature. The columns should be placed on a solid support with as little vibration as possible (e.g., not with table centrifuges on the same laboratory table).

Cells to be filtered at a maximum concentration per milliliter of 5×10^7 cells are now overlaid on the top of the column, using a maximum of 5×10^6 cells per milliliter of total beads, e.g., to a bead column of 50 ml do not normally exceed 250×10^6 cells added as this will start to oversaturate the capacity of the columns. Start the flow rate of the column using an adjustable controller at the bottom of the column and set the speed of the column flow in such a way that the cells will move through the columns at around 1 cm/min and never above 2 cm/min. Start collecting cells in fractions somewhat before the known void volume and continue collecting until there are no visible cells coming out from the columns. The columns function both as absolute retaining devices but will also allow a certain fraction of the specifically binding cells to sneak through, and these cells will come preferentially in the later fractions (10). Be prepared to add more medium when the top surface of the cell suspension is entering the upper bead surface in order to avoid any unintentional stop in the flow of the cells through the bead columns. If viability of the cells to be separated is low clogging of the columns may occur, as visible by decreased flow rate and eventual halt. This is normally easily cured by the introduction of a pipette into the top of the column, stirring the top bead layer as this is the place where the clogging does occur. It is mostly adequate to do this mild stirring once in case of signs of decreased flow rates.

The passed cells can now be washed and used for further analysis. Detailed descriptions as to percentage of nonspecific retentions, efficiency of specific retention, and variations as to recovery of the bound cells can be obtained from several articles (1, 2, 4, 6). The bound cells using the present kind of bead material can, however, be eluted using mechanical means yielding some 85% viable, functionally intact cells. The recovery is simply carried out by opening the bottom of the bead columns after cellular passage, allowing the beads to fall into a beaker with medium, make 2 or 3 swirling movements of the beaker, and collect the supernatant. If variations as to separations are included, such eluted cells can be recovered in close to 100% purity, e.g., with regard to specific immune reactivity against a given antigen (6).

A modification of the present technique when removing Ig-positive cells is to use only Ig-coated bead columns. Cells are incubated with excess anti-Ig, followed by one wash. Such cells, if carrying proper Ig surface markers, will now be coated with anti-Ig antibodies with one antigen-binding site free (if IgG antibodies), making these cells stick to the Ig-coated beads during fractionation. This modification is especially useful when expensive reagents are used, as only minimal amounts of anti-Ig antibodies are needed in comparison to the conventional anti-Ig column technique.

4. Discussion

The underlying principle behind the use of the present bead columns to function as selective absorbing agents for a subfraction of the passing cells probably resides at two levels. The glass or plastic beads have by themselves the capacity to bind cells in a "nonspecific" manner, and, in order as far as possible to eliminate this characteristic, one must precoat the beads with serum proteins as well as run the columns at a minimal flow rate. Otherwise, too high a fraction of the passing cells will stick to the beads because of these nonselective forces. However, these cell-binding activities of the present bead materials are probably responsible for the extreme efficiency with which these columns normally function. The forces making the specific fractionation of, e.g., Ig-positive cells possible using the present system are thus 2-fold: a specific but weak force that will retard the flow rate of the Ig-positive cells through the column. This decreased flow rate in itself will then greatly enhance the possibility that the cell will be bound to the beads via the nonspecific forces (10). In agreement with this is the finding that only mechanical elution procedures have been useful to recover specifically bound cells using the present bead material. Controlled coating procedures and flow rates are thus essential to make these columns optimal for selective retention of subgroups of cells.

Use of double-layer techniques to obtain efficient anti-Ig columns also have vices and virtues. By this approach it is possible by simple means to get an extremely high density of specific anti-Ig antibody molecules, admittedly only with some 50% of their antigen-binding sites free to interact with the passing Ig-positive cells. Straightforward coupling of Ig from unpurified anti-Ig antisera to the beads will yield columns of significantly inferior capacity to remove Ig-positive cells. Problems as to simultaneous removal of cells with Fc receptors for IgG being enhanced by the use of double layers of IgG (or Ig) molecules are real (11). However, such factors may also help to explain the high efficiency of the present columns in removing surface Ig-positive, Fc-receptor-bearing B lymphocytes. It should also be realized that removal of Ig-positive cells without removal of Fc-receptor-bearing cells would require either the use of F(ab)-anti-Ig-coated bead columns or anti-Ig antibodies produced in a species of animal whose Ig shows no binding to the Fc receptors of the cells to be fractionated (e.g., fowl antimouse Ig in the fractionation of mouse Ig-positive cells).

ACKNOWLEDGMENTS

Development of the techniques presented herein were made possible by support from the Swedish Cancer Society and by NIH contract NCI-CB-33859.

REFERENCES

1. Wigzell, H., and Andersson, B., *J. Exp. Med.* **129**, 23 (1969).
2. Jondal, M., Wigzell, H., and Aiuti, F., *Transplant. Rev.* **16**, 163 (1973).
3. Wigzell, H., Huber, C., and Schirrmacher, V., *Haematologia* **6**, 369 (1972).
4. Wigzell, H., Sundqvist, K. G., and Yoshida, T. O., *Scand. J. Immunol.* **1**, 75 (1972).
5. Chess, L., MacDermott, R. P., Sondel, P. M., and Schlossman, S. F., *Prog. Immunol.* **3**, 125 (1974).
6. Binz, H., and Wigzell, H., *J. Exp. Med.* **142**, 1231 (1975).

7. Truffa-Bachi, P., and Wofsy, L., *Proc. Nat. Acad. Sci. U.S.A.* **66**, 685 (1970).
8. Wigzell, H., *Cold Spring Harbor Symp. Quant. Biol.* **32**, 507 (1967).
9. Dulbecco, R., *J. Exp. Med.* **99**, 167 (1954).
10. Wigzell, H., and Andersson, B., *Annu. Rev. Microbiol.* **25**, 291 (1971).
11. Perlmann, P., Wigzell, H., Golstein, P., Lamon, E. W., Larsson, A., O'Toole, C., Perlmann, H., and Svedmyr, E. A. J., *Adv. Biosci.* **12**, 71 (1973).

19

Anti-immunoglobulin Columns and the Separation of T, B, and Null Cells*

Leonard Chess and Stuart F. Schlossman

1. Introduction

The specific fractionation of lymphocytes according to their affinity for various antibody-containing immunoabsorbents has permitted the isolation of both depleted and enriched populations of immunologically competent cells. While many of the published techniques allow for depletion of specific cells, only a few allow for their enrichment. Perhaps more important, even fewer permit quantitative recovery of the separated populations of cells (1–6). We shall describe in detail methods used in our laboratory for the fractionation of human T, B, and null cells utilizing Sephadex anti-immunoglobulin columns to prepare cell populations that are either enriched or depleted of lymphocytes with readily detectable surface immunoglobulins and the subsequent fractionation of the immunoglobulin-negative population into an E-rosette-positive and E-rosette-negative population (7, 8). Sephadex anti-Fab columns retain B cells by virtue of their surface immunoglobulins, whereas non-immunoglobulin-bearing cells are not retained. Immunoglobulin-positive cells retained by the column can be quantitatively recovered by elution with free immunoglobulin that competes with the B cell for the anti-Fab or, under special circumstances, by dextranase digestion of the insoluble immunoabsorbent. After separation of the human lymphocytes into immunoglobulin-negative and immunoglobulin-positive populations, the rosette depletion technique allows for further subfractionation of the immunoglobulin-negative population. T cells alone form spontaneous rosettes with sheep erythrocytes, whereas B cells, null cells, and to a certain extent monocytes form rosettes only when the sheep cells are coated with antibody or antibody and complement (EAC rosettes). The immunoglobulin-negative population is allowed to react with sheep cells, and the more dense sheep cell coated lymphocytes are separated from the nonrosetted lymphocytes by sedimentation through Ficoll–Hypaque. The nonrosetting cells are isolated at the interface.

*Supported by contracts CB-53881 and CB-43964 and Grant AI-12069 from the National Institutes of Health, Bethesda, Maryland.

Both immunoabsorbent column fractionation and rosetting techniques allow for the isolation of three distinct surface membrane populations of human lymphocytes: a T cell population that is Ig negative and E positive, a B cell population that is Ig positive and E negative, and a null cell population that is both Ig negative and E negative. Functional properties of surface characteristics of these isolated populations have been described in detail elsewhere (8–13).

The Sephadex anti-Fab immunoabsorbent technique described above is not restricted to the purification of T, B, and null cells, but also allows specific depletion and recovery of subsets of cells defined by specific antibody. For example, a subset of null cells that is extremely active in antibody-dependent cell-mediated cytotoxicity develops with time surface immunoglobulins and, more important, the capacity to secrete immunoglobulins *in vitro* (14, 15). This subset of cells reacts with rabbit antibody prepared against a human B cell complex, p23,30, whereas T cells are totally unreactive (16). Null cells treated with rabbit anti-p23,30 can be depleted by passage through a goat anti-rabbit Fc column and can be eluted specifically as above by rabbit immunoglobulin, which saturates the goat anti-rabbit column. This approach, plus the capacity to recover specifically adherent cells on antigen columns by dextranase digestion, provides additional versatility for Sephadex affinity chromatography of immunologically competent cells.

2. Materials

2.1. Solutions, Chemicals, and Reagents
2.1.1. Human γ-globulin (Miles-Pentex, Kankakee, Illinois)
2.1.2. Crystallized pepsin (Miles-Pentex, Kankakee, Illinois)
2.1.3. Sodium acetate, 0.1 M, pH 4.5
2.1.4. Sodium sulfate
2.1.5. Phosphate-buffered saline (PBS), pH 7.4
2.1.6. Complete Freund's adjuvant (CFA) (Difco Laboratory, Detroit, Michigan)
2.1.7. Cyanogen bromide (Eastman Kodak, Co., Rochester, New York)
2.1.8. Glycine buffer, 0.1 M, pH 2.5
2.1.9. Phosphate buffer, 2 M, pH 8.0
2.1.10. Sepharose 4-B (Pharmacia Fine Chemicals, Uppsala, Sweden)
2.1.11. Sephadex G-200 (Pharmacia Fine Chemicals, Uppsala, Sweden)
2.1.12. Medium 199 (GIBCO, Grand Island, New York)
2.1.13. Penicillin–streptomycin solution (GIBCO, Grand Island, New York)
2.1.14. EDTA, 2.5 mM
2.1.15. Fetal calf serum (Microbiological Associates, Bethesda, Maryland)
2.1.16. Hanks' balanced salt solution (HBBS) (Microbiologic Associates, Bethesda, Maryland)

2.1.17. Ficoll (Pharmacia Fine Chemicals, Uppsala, Sweden)

2.1.18. Hypaque (Sigma Chemical Co., St. Louis, Missouri)

2.1.19. Sheep erythrocytes (Microbiological Associates, Bethesda, Maryland)

2.1.20. EAC cells (Cordis Laboratories, Miami, Florida)

2.2. Special Equipment

2.2.1. Light microscope

2.2.2. Fluorescence microscope

2.2.3. Refrigerated centrifuges

2.2.4. Disposable syringes

2.2.5. Plastic stopcocks

2.2.6. Polyethylene sintered disks (Bell Art Products, Benwalk, New Jersey)

2.2.7. Glass columns (1 X 40 cm)

2.2.8. Spectrophotometer

2.2.9. pH meter

2.3. Animals. Rabbits and animal care facilities

3. Methods of Cellular Immunoabsorbent Chromatography

3.1. Preparation of Rabbit Anti-(Fab)$_2$ Sera

3.1.1. To obtain human (Fab)$_2$ fragments, 500 mg of human γ-globulin are dissolved in a 0.1 M sodium acetate buffer at pH 4.5 containing 5 mg of pepsin, and the mixture is incubated at 37°C for 20 hr. The digested γ-globulin solution is then adjusted to pH 8.0, and 50 ml of Na$_2$SO$_4$ (25 g/100 ml) is added dropwise.

3.1.2. The white precipitate containing (Fab)$_2$ is dissolved in water and dialyzed against 0.1 M sodium acetate and then PBS and brought to a concentration of 5 mg/ml in PBS. Undigested material can be removed by passage through a G-150 column. The excluded first peak contains undigested γ-globulin, whereas the second peak is (Fab)$_2$.

3.2. Purification of Rabbit Anti-(Fab)$_2$ Sera

3.2.1. Sepharose 4-B, 30 ml, is activated with cyanogen bromide (20 ml of 50 mg/ml solution) for 12 min, maintaining the pH at 11.0 with 1 N NaOH.

3.2.2. The activated Sepharose is washed in borate-buffered saline (pH 8.3), and 200 mg of human γ-globulin are added for 18 hr at 4°C.

3.2.3. The conjugated Sepharose is washed with PBS exhaustively and packed in a glass column.

3.2.4. Rabbit anti-(Fab)$_2$ serum, 100 ml, is passed through 10 ml of packed human γ-globulin-conjugated Sepharose.

3.2.5. The retained anti-(Fab)$_2$ antibody is then eluted from the column with 0.1 M glycine-HCl buffer (pH 2.5) and collected in 2 M phosphate buffer (pH 8.0).

3.2.6. The purified antibody is then dialyzed against PBS, concentrated to approximately 10 mg/ml, and stored at $-70°$C.

3.3. Preparation of Sephadex G-200 Anti-(Fab)$_2$ Immunoabsorbent Columns

3.3.1. Sephadex G-200, 60 ml, is sieved to achieve uniform bead size (88–120 μm), activated with 100 mg of cyanogen bromide, maintaining the pH at 10.2 with 1 N NaOH, for 10 min.

3.3.2. Proper activation should result in a 20–30% loss in volume.

3.3.3. The activated Sephadex G-200 is washed with borate-buffered saline (pH 8.3), and 20 mg of purified anti-(Fab)$_2$ are added for 4 hr at room temperature without mechanical stirring. Stir occasionally with a glass rod so as not to fracture the beads.

3.3.4. The resulting Sephadex G-200 anti-(Fab)$_2$ conjugate is washed with PBS over a sintered-glass funnel without suction.

3.3.5. Disposable syringes (12 ml) are fitted with polyethylene disks and packed with 8–10 ml of the anti-(Fab)$_2$ conjugated Sephadex.

3.3.6. The columns are washed with medium 199 containing 5% fetal calf serum, 2.5 mM EDTA, and 1% penicillin–streptomycin. At this point the columns are ready for cell fractionation.

3.4. Cell Preparation and Fractionation

3.4.1. The mononuclear cells from either whole peripheral blood or other peripheral lymphoid tissues should be isolated and purified by Ficoll–Hypaque centrifugation, to remove RBC granulocytes and debris. The cells are then washed 3 times in medium 199 containing 5% fetal calf serum and made monocyte-deficient using the iron carbonyl technique (6). One should avoid depletion of monocytes using nylon wool columns, since these columns will also selectively deplete B cells. The resulting highly purified lymphocyte populations, which should contain more than 98% lymphocytes, is then brought to a concentration of 10 to 20 $\times$ 10^6 per milliliter in media containing 5% FCS and 2.5 mM EDTA (starting media) before application to Sephadex antihuman Fab columns.

3.4.2. Lymphocyte suspension, 5–10 ml, is applied to each 8-ml column at room temperature, and eluates are collected by stepwise elution with 15-ml aliquots of starting media at a flow rate of approximately 0.3–0.5 ml/min. Elution with starting medium is continued until the effluent is virtually cell free.

3.4.3. The retained cells are eluted by competitive inhibition using two 15-ml aliquots of media containing 10 mg of human γ-globulin per milliliter. During the elution of bound cells the column can be gently mixed by simply drawing the column material up and down in a Pasteur pipette.

3.4.4. The recovered cell populations are then washed 3–4 times in medium 199 containing fetal calf serum before analysis of surface characteristics or before other investigations are carried out in cell culture. All cells passing directly through the column are surface immunoglobulin negative, whereas more than 98% of the cells eluted with human Ig stain with fluoresceinated anti-$(Fab)_2$ reagents. Greater than 90% of all cells applied to the immunoabsorbent columns are routinely recovered.

4. Comments on Cellular Immunoabsorbent Chromatography

4.1.1. Sephadex G-200 serves as an excellent filter for lymphocytes since cells are not nonspecifically retained. This property allows for "total" cell recovery.

4.1.2. The anti-$(Fab)_2$ must be purified and tested for antibody activity prior to conjugation to Sephadex G-200. Use of anti-$(Fab)_2$ serum without purification of the antibody is not advised.

4.1.3. Once prepared, anti-$(Fab)_2$-conjugated Sephadex can be stored in sodium azide at 4°C for as long as 3 months and maintain its activity.

4.1.4. The Ig-negative fraction isolated from anti-$(Fab)_2$ immunoabsorbent columns is composed predominantly of T cells but is heterogeneous in that there exists an Ig-negative, E-rosette-negative subset (null cell) within this population (see below).

4.1.5. The Ig-positive fraction is routinely more than 98% B cells by surface markers and functional properties.

4.1.6. Residual monocytes, not removed by the iron carbonyl technique, are found distributed in both the Ig-negative and Ig-positive populations and can be removed by nylon wool for special studies.

5. Use of Rosetting Techniques to Further Fractionate Human Lymphocyte Subpopulations

5.1. Isolation of the E-Rosette-Negative, Ig-Negative Subset from the Nonimmunoglobulin Bearing Population

5.1.1. Sheep RBC (E cells) are washed 3 times in Hanks' balanced salt solution (HBSS) and made up to a final concentration of 5% cells in HBBS.

5.1.2. Nonimmunoglobulin-bearing lymphocytes isolated from the immunoabsorbent column above, are washed 3 times in HBSS and brought to a concentration of 15×10^6 cells/ml.

5.1.3. Equal volumes of the washed nonimmunoglobulin lymphocytes are mixed with the 5% suspension of E cells, spun for 5 min at 250 g, and placed at room temperature for 1–2 hr.

5.1.4. The E-rosetted cells are then gently resuspended, layered over Ficoll–Hypaque, and spun at 400 g for 40 min at 20°C. The interface containing the nonrosetted cells is then aspirated and washed 3 times in medium 199 with 5%

fetal calf serum. The recovered lymphocyte population is surface-Ig negative and E-rosette-negative and represents a population of null cells.

5.2. Isolation of the E-Rosette-Positive (T Cell) Subset from the Nonimmunoglobulin Population

5.2.1. Sheep RBC coated with antibody and complement (EAC cells) are washed 3 times in HBSS and brought to a 5% concentration.

5.2.2. Equal volumes of EAC cells and HBSS washed nonimmunoglobulin bearing lymphocytes are gently mixed, incubated for 0.5 hr at 37°C, and centrifuged at 250 g for 5 min.

5.2.3. The EAC rosettes are then gently resuspended, layered over Ficoll–Hypaque and spun at 400 g at 37°C for 40 min. The non-EAC rosetting lymphocytes recovered from the interface are washed 3 times in medium 199 with 5% FCS. This population of cells is E-rosette positive and surface-Ig negative and represents a highly purified T-cell population.

6. Comments on Rosetting Techniques

6.1.1. Fresh E and EAC cells ($<$ 1 week old) are required for optimum separation to be achieved.

6.1.2. The temperature requirements outlined above are crucial for adequate cell separation.

6.1.3. With both the E and the EAC depletion techniques one routinely has a 20–40% cell loss. This makes use of these techniques for the separation of whole lymphocytes into T and B cell populations subject to the criticism that unique subpopulations may be lost.

6.1.4. Utilizing rosette depletion techniques alone, one requires two depletions before highly purified populations are obtained.

7. Depletion of Subsets of Cells on a Goat Anti-rabbit Fab Cellular Immunoabsorbent

7.1.1. Goat anti-rabbit Fab (G/R Fab) is prepared as described above for rabbit anti-human Fab. The G/R Fab is purified on a rabbit IgG Sepharose column and then passed through a human Ig-Sepharose column to remove cross-reacting antibodies. The purified, absorbed G/R Fab is covalently linked to Sephadex G-200 (Section 3.3).

7.1.2. The G/R Fab cellular immunoabsorbents are used to deplete human lymphocyte subpopulations that have specific rabbit antibody bound to their surface (piggy-back experiments).

7.1.3. With rabbit antisera to a specific null cell subset (anti-p23,30) the null cell can be depleted from the T + null cell population (Ig negative) by reaction with rabbit antisera and removal on G/R Fab columns. Similar studies can be performed with rabbit antisera to T cell and B cell subsets.

7.1.4. 60 × 10^6 cells (T + null) are incubated with either heat-inactivated normal rabbit serum (dilution 1:20) or rabbit anti-p23,30 (1:20 dilution) for 1 hr at room temperature. Cells are then washed 4 times in starting medium (see Section 3.4) and applied to G/R Fab columns using a flow rate of 0.5 ml/min as described in Section 3.4. Control cells incubated in the presence of NRS and then washed were not retained (17).

7.1.5. Effluent cells (nonretained) can be studied as the depleted population. Depleted (retained cells) can be recovered by competitive inhibition using 15-ml aliquots of medium containing 10 mg of rabbit γ-globulin per milliliter.

With all cell separation techniques it is extremely important to characterize each isolated population not only by surface marker criteria, but also by functional studies.

REFERENCES

1. Geha, R. S., Rosen, F. S., and Merler, E. J., *J. Clin. Invest.* **52,** 1726 (1973).
2. Eisen, S. A., Wedner, H. J., and Porter, C. W., *Immunol. Commun.* **1,** 571 (1972).
3. Zeiller, K., Pascher, G., and Hannig, K., *Prep. Biochem.* **2,** 21 (1972).
4. Mendes, N. F., Tolnai, M. E. A., Silveira, N. P. A., Gilbertsen, R. B., and Metzgar, R. S. *J. Immunol.* **111,** 860 (1973).
5. Wigzell, H., *Prog. Immunol.* **1,** 1105 (1971).
6. Wofsy, L., Kimura, J., and Truffa-Bachi, P. J., *J. Immunol.* **107,** 725 (1971).
7. Schlossman, S. F., and Hudson, L., *J. Immunol.* **110,** 313 (1973).
8. Chess, L., MacDermott, R. P., and Schlossman, S. F., *J. Immunol.* **113,** 1113 (1974).
9. Chess, L., MacDermott, R. P., Sondel, P. M., and Schlossman, S. F., *Prog. Immunol.*, 2nd Int-Congr. Vol. 3, p. 125, 1974.
10. Rocklin, R. E., MacDermott, R. P., Chess, L., Schlossman, S. F., and David, J. F. *J. Exp. Med.* **140,** 1303 (1974).
11. Sondel, P. M., Chess, L., MacDermott, P., and Schlossman, S. F., *J. Immunol.* **114,** 982 (1975).
12. MacDermott, R. P., Chess, L., and Schlossman, S. F., *Clin. Immunol. Immunopathol.* **4,** 415 (1975).
13. Chess, L., Rocklin, R. E., MacDermott, R. P., David, J. R., and Schlossman, S. F., *J. Immunol.* **115,** 315 (1975).
14. Brier, A. M., Chess, L., and Schlossman, S. F., *J. Clin. Invest.* **56,** 1580 (1975).
15. Chess, L., Levine, H., MacDermott, R. P., and Schlossman, S. F., *J. Immunol.* **115,** 1483 (1975).
16. Schlossman, S. F., Chess, L., Humphreys, R. E., and Strominger, J. L., *Proc. Nat. Acad. Sci. U.S.A.* **73,** 1288 (1976).
17. Chess, L., Evans, R., Humphreys, R. E., Strominger, J. L., and Schlossman, S. F., *J. Exp. Med.* **144,** 113 (1976).

Spontaneous Lymphocyte-Mediated Cytotoxicity (SLMC) *in Vitro*: Assay for, and Removal of, the Effector Cell

Mikael Jondal

1. Introduction

Lymphocyte-mediated cytotoxicity is one important *in vitro* parameter for cell-mediated immunity (1). For cytotoxicity testing it would be ideal to isolate both lymphocytes and target cells from the same individual; this is, however, seldom feasible, as the target cells in most situations are difficult to obtain. Many investigators have thus used allogeneic target cells, of a corresponding histological origin, grown as continuous cell lines (2). However, it has recently been clearly demonstrated that lymphocytes from normal donors, used as the base-line control, mediate a considerable cytotoxicity against established cell lines (3–5). This activity is a property of a small subpopulation of peripheral lymphocytes bearing complement (C) and Fc receptors and is called Spontaneous Lymphocyte-Mediated Cytotoxicity (SLMC) (4). SLMC may reflect a surveillance mechanism *in vivo* although no evidence in support of this has so far been presented. SLMC is anyhow important in two respects: (a) it creates a background "noise" in cytotoxicity test; and (b) it can be used as a functional marker for Fc/C receptor-bearing lymphocytes.

This paper deals with SLMC, measured by ^{51}Cr release, as a functional test and reports a method for removal of the effector cells.

2. Material

2.1. For the SLMC Test

RPMI 1640 medium
Antibiotics
Fetal calf serum
V-shaped microplates (Linbro, New Haven, Connecticut)
$Na_2{}^{51}CrO_4$
Target cells (see below)
Isolated peripheral lymphocytes (adherent cells should be removed)
Micropipette for 50–100 μl volumes

Holder for centrifugation of microplates (Damon/IEC Division, Catalogue No. 442, only for International centrifuges)

2.2. Additional Material for Rosette Sedimentation of Fc/C Receptor Lymphocytes (CRL)

Sheep red blood cells (SRBC)
Rabbit anti-SRBC
A-strain mouse serum (as complement source)
Ficoll (Pharmacia Fine Chemicals Inc., Uppsala, Sweden)
Isopaque (Nyegaard & Co., Oslo, Norway)

3. Methods

3.1. The ^{51}Cr Release SLMC Assay *3.1.1. Selection of Target Cells for SLMC.* All cell lines tested so far have been found susceptible, to varying degrees, to SLMC when tested for a 17-hr incubation period (4). The cytotoxicity against most lines starts at 1 hr and proceeds in a linear fashion during overnight incubation (Fig. 1). T-cell lines are in general more rapidly and completely killed (Fig. 1). One cell line, K-562, derived from chronic myelocytic leukemia (6) is exceptionally useful as a target in SLMC testing, as it is killed very rapidly and displays a low spontaneous release (1% per hour) (4). Xenogeneic target cells (mouse derived) may also be used (5). It is advised that SLMC be tested against a selected panel of cell lines.

3.1.2. Labeling of Target Cells. About 5×10^6 cells (or less) in 200 μl of

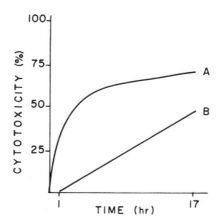

Fig. 1. Kinetics of spontaneous lymphocyte-mediated cytotoxicity against different groups of cells. Group A includes T-cell lines and the K-562 cell line. Group B includes B cell lines and most nonlymphoid cell lines.

HEPES-buffered medium with 5% fetal calf serum is mixed with 200 μl of ^{51}Cr and incubated for 1 hr at 37°C with occasional shaking. After three washes the cell concentration is adjusted to 0.2 × 10^6/ml.

3.1.3. The SLMC Test. It is recommended that only the central part of the microplate be used, i.e., between the vertical lines 3 and 10, as the cell mixtures in the periphery do not pellet in a central position during centrifugation. Target cells, 50 μl (=10^4), are added in duplicate wells and mixed with 100 μl of lymphocytes, with a lymphocyte:target cell ratio ranging between 50:1 and 1:1. The plate is centrifuged at 700 g for 5 min and then incubated under tissue-culture conditions. Duration of incubation has to be determined in relation to the particular target cells used; a 5–10-hr period is usually suitable. At the end of the incubation period, 100 μl of supernatant are harvested from each well, including wells containing only target cells (for spontaneous release); 100 μl of resuspended target cells are taken as the maximum value. Cytotoxicity is estimated according to the standard formula:

$$\frac{\text{test cpm} - \text{spontaneous release cpm}}{\text{maximum cpm} - \text{spontaneous release cpm}} \times 100$$

3.2. Removal of the Effector Cell by Rosette Sedimentation. One part washed SRBC (4%) is mixed with one part rabbit anti-SRBC and shaken for 1 hr at room temperature. The antiserum should be hyperimmune, consist primarily of IgG antibodies, and be used at a concentration that allows the highest number of antibodies bound to the SRBC without causing agglutination. EAC cells prepared with IgM anti-SRBC are not suitable for depletion of SLMC effector cells; this may be explained either by the fact that EAC(IgM) are less efficient in this particular fractionation procedure or by the fact that some effector cells express mostly Fc receptors and few (or no) C3 receptors. After two washes one part of antibody-treated SRBC (4%) is mixed with one part of 1:2 diluted fresh A-strain serum and incubated for 30 min at 37°C. After two washes the erythrocyte–antibody–complement (EAC) cells are mixed with the lymphocytes in 3 ml of medium, with a total of 6 × 10^6 lymphocytes, in siliconized 15-ml tubes. The ratio of EAC cells to lymphocytes should be 5:1; this is important because a greater number of EAC cells will result in a poor recovery of lymphocytes. The recovery under the present conditions is 25%. The cell mixture is then pelleted and incubated for 30 min at 37°C; the cells are then gently resuspended, and the percentage of rosettes is calculated. The cell suspension is then mixed with 0.3 ml of fetal calf serum and layered on 3 ml of cold standard Ficoll–Isopaque (7) and centrifuged at 850 g for 15 min. The cells at the interphase are depleted in effector cells and should be harvested and washed twice.

4. Comments

The importance of SLMC in the study of specific cell-mediated immunity has been clearly demonstrated in patients with infectious mononucleosis (8). During the acute phase of the disease the patients generate killer cells in the circulation that are specific for Epstein—Barr virus-transformed lymphoid cell lines. Such effector cells can be clearly demonstrated only if the nonspecific killer cells are removed. When these findings were applied to a model system in the rat, similar results were obtained (9); i.e., unspecific killer cells with Fc/C receptors had to be removed to pick up the specific *in vitro* cytotoxicity which correlated with the *in vivo* situation.

As far as human peripheral lymphocytes go, it should be remembered that the population also includes the K cells, although no evidence exists that SLMC should be similar to K-cell killing—in fact this is most unlikely.

Other fractionation procedures than rosette sedimentation may be used to minimize SLMC; these include anti-Ig columns, nylon wool columns, or treatment with Tris-buffered 0.83% NH_4Cl. However, none of these procedures are as efficient as rosette sedimentation.

REFERENCES

1. Bloom, B. R., Landy, M., and Lawrence, H. S., *Cell Immunol.* **6**, 331 (1973).
2. Perlmann, P., and Holm, G., *Adv. Immunol.* **11**, 117 (1969).
3. Takasugi, M., Mikey, M. R., and Terasaki, P. I., *Cancer Res.* **33**, 2898 (1973).
4. Jondal, M., and Pross, H., *Int. J. Cancer* **15**, 596 (1975).
5. Pross, H., and Jondal, M., *Clin. Exp. Immunol.* **21**, 226 (1975).
6. Lozzio, C. B., and Lozzio, B. B., *J. Natl. Cancer Inst.* **50**, 535 (1973).
7. Böyum, A. A., *Scand. J. Clin. Lab. Invest.* **21**, 51 (1968).
8. Svedmyr, E., and Jondal, M., *Proc. Natl. Acad. Sci. U.S.A.* **72**, 1622 (1975).
9. Cornain, S., Carnaud, C., Silverman, D., Klein, E., and Rajewsky, M. F., *Int. J. Cancer* **16**, 301 (1975).

Buoyant Density Separation of Lymphocyte Populations by Continuous Albumin Gradient Analysis and Simple Albumin Density Cuts

Ken Shortman

1. Introduction

The buoyant density of a cell, determined by centrifugation to equilibrium in a density gradient, reflects its average chemical composition, including its relative water content. As a physical parameter it is independent of cell size although the larger, activated or immature lymphocyte forms tend to be of light density, and the mature, compact small lymphocytes tend to be dense (1–5). This is not an absolute role, and many exceptions have been documented (3, 4). At neutral (not acid) pH, dense red cells are separated from lighter white cells (6–8). Extensive separation of mononuclear cells from the denser granulocytic elements of blood is also readily obtained (9). The procedure is not effective for separating T from B lymphocytes since two populations overlap extensively both in mice and man (4, 5, 9, 10). However, it is a powerful tool for isolating distinct subsets and stages of differentiation within each lineage (4, 5, 10–13). Density separation is also a useful technique for the separation of hemopoietic stem cells and precursor cells, and for distinguishing normal from leukemic stem cell forms in human blood (9, 14, 15).

Density separation of lymphocytes on continuous albumin gradients can be used as a precise, high-resolution analytical tool, as well as a preparative procedure, with 70–100% recovery of viable, immunologically active cells. Buoyant density is a highly reproducible parameter for characterizing a given cell type ($\pm$ 0.0003 g/cm^3) (16), a point first made by Leif and Vinograd (17). However, precision of this order demands close control over the pH, the temperature, the ion composition, and the osmolarity of the density gradient medium, since the physical properties of the cells are partially a function of the environment. High resolution in albumin gradients demands avoidance of cell aggregation, tube wall effects, streaming, and turbulence. Low pH albumin is chosen to minimize cell association while maintaining viability (16). The method of dispersing cells into the gradient and the centrifugal force used also reduce aggregation, wall effects, and streaming (1, 16). A simple but very accurate density estimation procedure, applicable to small samples of each fraction, is used to determine the exact density range sampled by each fraction, so a true density distribution profile can be calculated. The full analytical procedure of necessity is relatively lengthy and demanding.

A simpler density separation method is useful where a full density distribution analysis of a population is not required. Discontinuous gradients are often used for this purpose. An alternative procedure, which is simple and fast but conserves the efficiency, resolution, and accuracy of the analytical procedure, is presented in this chapter. A single 10-min centrifugation is used to divide a population into cells lighter and denser than a given value; if necessary a second-stage separation can produce 3 or 4 fractions. The density cut procedure has been used for separating damaged from viable cells (18), and as a clinical diagnostic test distinguishing leukemic from normal macrophage-granulocyte progenitor cells (15).

2. Materials

2.1. Salt Solutions. These are isoosmotic with human serum (269 milliosmolar absolute osmolarity compared to a mannitol standard, equivalent to 0.147 M NaCl). For use with mouse cells all concentrations are increased proportionally to give 308 milliosmolar, equivalent to 0.168 M NaCl and isoosmotic with mouse serum (19).

2.1.1. Buffered Balanced Salt Solution. The solution is prepared by mixing the following isoosmotic solutions: NaCl, 0.147 M, 121 volumes; KCl, 0.147 M, 4 volumes; CaCl$_2$ 0.098 M, 3 volumes; MgSO$_4$, 0.147 M, 1 volume; isoosmotic potassium phosphate buffer pH 7.2, 2 volumes; isoosmotic HEPES buffer, pH 7.2, 6 volumes. Isoosmotic potassium phosphate buffer is prepared by mixing 0.147 M KH$_2$PO$_4$ and 0.098 K$_2$HPO$_4$ to give pH 7.2 on 50-fold dilution of a small sample. Isoosmotic HEPES buffer is prepared by mixing 0.294 M N-2-hydroxyethylpiperazine-N-2-ethanesulfonic acid (HEPES, Calbiochem) with 0.294 M NaOH to give pH 7.2 on 50-fold dilution of a small sample. Stock solutions can be prepared and stored 5-fold concentrated. The medium is sterilized by Millipore filtration.

2.1.2. Unbuffered Balanced Salt Solution. This is prepared by mixing the following isoosmotic solutions: NaCl, 0.147 M, 121 volumes; KCl 0.147 M, 4 volumes; CaCl$_2$, 0.098 M, 3 volumes; MgSO$_4$ 0.147 M, 1 volume; KH$_2$PO$_4$, 0.147 M, 1 volume. The stock solutions can be prepared and stored 10-fold concentrated. The medium is sterilized by Millipore filtration.

2.2. Albumin *2.2.1. Preliminary Treatment.* Bovine plasma albumin, fraction V powder (Armour), a nonneutralized preparation, is used. Salt contaminants as well as absorbed water must be removed before use, as follows. The powder (100–300 g) is dissolved in water (4°C) to make a 15–20% solution and dialyzed for 2 days (4°C) against 4 changes of 10–20 volumes of precooled deionized water containing a few drops of chloroform. Thorough and frequent mixing of the internal contents of the dialysis bag (leave an air bubble to facilitate mixing), as well as stirring the external solution, is essential. After dialysis, the albumin solution is filtered (Millipore, 0.45 μm with prefilter), then freeze-dried. To remove residual water, the powder is further dried for 1–2 days over P_2O_5 in a vacuum desiccator.

2.2.2. Albumin Medium, Isoosmotic, pH 5.1. A 35% (w/w) stock solution is first prepared. Dry, dialyzed albumin powder, 100 g, is dissolved in 181 ml of "human osmolarity" unbuffered balanced salt solution and 5 ml of water (the latter to compensate for the slight osmotic pressure of the albumin itself). If working with mouse cells at mouse osmolarity, the ratio is 182 ml of unbuffered balanced salt solution and 4 ml of H_2O. To effect solution (at $4°C$) the albumin powder is layered above all but 50 ml of the liquid in a conical flask sealed with Parafilm to prevent evaporation. The mixture is shaken at low speed in a wrist-action shaker for a few hours, then mixed using a magnetic stirring bar and a powerful motor. The last 50 ml of liquid is added in two stages to the top of the solution, to dissolve residual albumin. Solution takes about 2 days, at $4°C$. The light and dense media for generating continuous gradients [generally 17% (w/w), ~ $1.055/cm^3$ and 29% (w/w), ~ $1.090 g/cm^3$, respectively, for wide range gradients] are prepared by diluting the stock by weight in unbuffered balanced salt solution. All albumin media are stored frozen in firmly sealed polythene bottles. Before use, thorough thawing (at $30°–37°C$) and extensive mixing is essential. If required, small quantities of the media are sterilized before use by passage through Millipore filters (0.45 μm with prefilter, using a Swinney filter holder and syringe pressure). The media are kept cold before use, and frozen immediately after use, to prevent bacterial growth.

2.2.3. Albumin Standards for Density Determination. For use as standards in the nonaqueous density-determination procedure, albumin media of density around 1.06, 1.07, 1.08, and 1.09 g/cm^3 are prepared and colored with a few drops of concentrated methyl violet solution. Absolute densities of the standards at $4°C$ are determined to five places by direct weighing in the cold, using 25-ml weighing bottles previously calibrated with water. Samples, 5 ml, of the standards are sealed in glass ampoules for long-term storage and kept frozen. Each 1–2 months an ampoule is opened, and the standard is dispensed into small, tightly stoppered plastic tubes, and frozen. A fresh tube is thawed at $30°–37°C$ for each week's work, with care to ensure thorough mixing.

2.3. Nonaqueous Solutions for Density Estimation. Light (usually 1.05 g/cm^3) and dense (usually 1.10 g/cm^3) mixtures of bromobenzene (AR, density 1.52 g/cm^3) and petroleum spirit (AR, boiling range $80°–100°C$, density 0.64 g/cm^3) are prepared in 5-liter lots, and stored at $4°C$ in tightly sealed bottles.

2.4. Albumin Gradient Generation Apparatus. The system used for generating linear albumin gradients is illustrated in Fig. 1. The acrylic mixing chamber

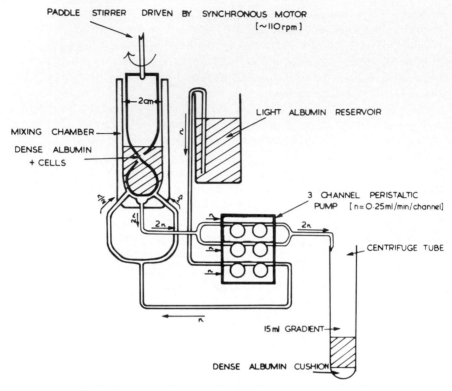

Fig. 1. Apparatus for generating continuous albumin gradients.

with stainless steel entry and exit tubes, and the acrylic paddle, are built in a workshop. The additional items required are a synchronous motor for constant-speed stirring and a peristaltic pump (a unit with at least 3 channels, and producing minimum pulsing is required, e.g., a Perpex 3-channel stack unit, Werner Meyer, Lucerne, or LKB). For sterile work the tubes and chambers are first washed with chlorhexidine, followed by a rinse with sterile saline or sterile H_2O. The chamber is dried with alcohol and drained before use.

2.5. Centrifuge. A refrigerated centrifuge with a swing-out head, capable of 4000 g and having relatively slow acceleration and deceleration, is required. A Sorvall RC2-B with an HB-40 rotor is recommended, provided a switch and simple circuitry permitting slow acceleration are installed. The tubes used are 15 ml, polyallomer thin-wall Sorvall tubes, fitted with an acrylic cap to prevent evaporation. The tube may be sterilized with chlorhexidine, washed with sterile water then alcohol, and drained dry.

2.6. Fraction-Collection Apparatus. The system used for collecting fractions from continuous albumin gradients is illustrated in Fig. 2. The tube-holder is conveniently made from a clear acrylic. The exit cap, and all tubing in contact with bromobenzene, are nylon or Teflon, since bromobenzene will dissolve certain plastics, including peristaltic pump tubing. A low viscosity, dense silicone oil may be an alternative solution for displacing the gradient. The peristaltic pump is the same unit used for gradient generation, and it may be convenient to employ several channels in parallel to obtain adequate speed. A stopwatch is required. The exit tube may be sterilized with chlorhexidine, as for the mixing chamber of the gradient generator.

2.7. Apparatus for Density Estimation in Nonaqueous Gradients. The apparatus required is illustrated in Fig. 3. The open mixing chambers are of glass, the mixing paddle is a spiral of stainless steel wire, and tubing and valve are of nylon or Teflon or other plastic not affected by the organic solvents. The burette tube and the outer water jacket are of glass. Boxes of disposable, narrow-bore Pasteur pipettes are required.

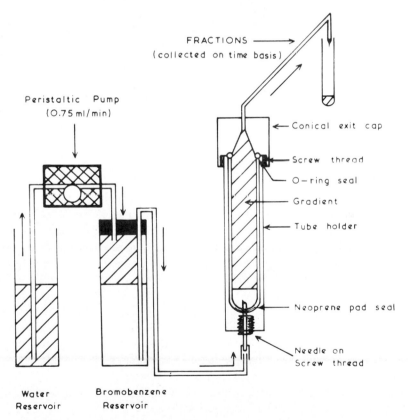

Fig. 2. Apparatus for collecting fractions from continuous albumin gradients.

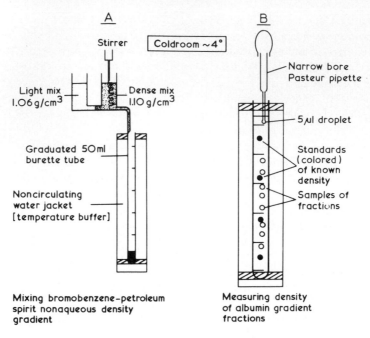

Fig. 3. Technique for measuring the density of small samples of albumin gradient fractions.

3. Methods

3.1. Continuous Gradient Separation and Analysis *3.1.1. Cell Suspension.* The gradient can accommodate up to 10^9 cells, but for good resolution the load should be less than 5×10^8 cells. The cell suspension is prepared in a suitable cold, pH 7.2 buffered, balanced salt solution, containing, if desired, 10% fetal calf serum. Tissue culture medium requiring CO_2 buffering should be avoided, since it becomes alkaline. The suspension medium should be the same osmolarity as the gradient medium. Removal of damaged cells and debris from the suspension improves the resolution and increases the allowable cell load; however, their presence can often be tolerated because most damaged cells sediment out of the gradient and appear in the pellet. It is important to avoid methods of eliminating damaged cells or nonlymphoid cells which cause marked lymphocyte losses and preselect the population to be analyzed. Many popular techniques do this. Damaged cell removal procedures which do not cause selective lymphocyte losses are available (1, 2, 18, 20). Before separation, a known sample (usually 5%) of the original suspension is reserved for later analysis with the fractions, to allow complete balance sheets and recovery estimations.

3.1.2. Gradient Generation. A typical wide-range gradient would run from around 1.055–1.09 g/cm^3 (human osmolarity medium), equivalent to 17–29% w/w albumin. Narrower-range gradients, restricted to the region of interest, give better resolution (3, 16). The generation system is shown in Fig. 1. It is operated in a cold room. For sterile work the whole apparatus is enclosed in a hood. The mixing chamber and lines are first washed through by pumping through a small quantity of dense albumin. The light-density albumin reservoir is filled and the light-density line pumped full almost to the mixing chamber entry port. The cells are spun to a pellet (400 *g*, 7 min), the supernatant is removed, and the pellet is directly dispersed in about 4 ml of the dense albumin medium, using a vortex mixer. The cells and dense albumin are transferred to the mixing chamber, and further dense albumin solution added to a final volume of 7.5 ml. Stirring is commenced, at 110 rpm, the direction of paddle rotation generating a downward, rather than upward, screw action thrust on the liquid. The peristaltic pump (0.25 ml/min per channel) is then activated, using two channels in parallel for the cells and albumin mixture exit, and one channel for the light albumin entry. The mixture is run down the side of the centrifuge tube from the top. This produces a linear gradient with cells well dispersed, but mainly concentrated toward the bottom of the tube. Pumping is continued until the chamber is empty and bubbles just begin to enter the 15-ml centrifuge tube. The apparatus should be rinsed soon after use.

3.1.3. Centrifugation. The centrifuge tube is capped to prevent evaporation, then centrifuged at 4000 *g* for 30 min at 0°–4°C using a swing-out head. Both the early stage of acceleration and the terminal stages of deceleration should be slow, to prevent swirling in the tube.

3.1.4. Fraction Collection. The technique used is illustrated in Fig. 2. Collection is done in a cold room, using a hood if sterile conditions are required. The tube is placed in a holder with a conical exit cap at the top and a needle on a screw thread at the base. A hole is pierced in the tube, and a drop of dense albumin is allowed to flow out, to displace air. The prefilled line carrying bromobenzene is then connected, and the bromobenzene is pumped in underneath the albumin to slowly (0.75 ml/min) displace the gradient upward out the conical exit. The bromobenzene is pumped indirectly, by displacing it from a reservoir with water. The water is pumped directly by the peristaltic unit. Fractions, 15–30, are collected on a time basis, using a stopwatch, and switching off the peristaltic pump to change fraction tubes. After the last fraction is collected the bromobenzene may be replaced in the reservoir by reversing the pump. The tube holder and lines in contact with the albumin should be rinsed soon after use.

3.1.5. Density Estimation. The set-up for measuring the density of microdroplets of each fraction is illustrated in Fig. 3. All operations are in a cold room. A continuous, linear nonaqueous gradient, wider in density range than the albumin gradient, is generated from the mixtures of bromobenzene and petroleum spirit. This gradient is conveniently made the day before, and the tube sealed with a stopper to prevent evaporation. Colored albumin solution standards of known density are thawed, thoroughly mixed, and left to stand several hours before use (sealed to prevent evaporation). Each fraction is briefly mixed and allowed to stand for 10 min to allow air bubbles to rise. Droplets (~5 μl) of each fraction in turn, and of the density standards, are then placed in the nonaqueous gradient, starting with the most dense. Using a separate narrow-bore Pasteur pipette for each fraction, a small sample is withdrawn from the center of the tube, with care to avoid minute air bubbles. The bulb of the Pasteur pipette is only compressed slightly, so there is no tendency for the sample to rise too high into the tube. After wiping the outside of the Pasteur pipette, a small droplet is expressed from the tip just below the meniscus of nonaqueous gradient. Lifting the pipette up through the meniscus releases the droplet, which then sinks to the region of its buoyant density. All droplets should be close to the same size. At 15–30 min after all samples are applied, the position of the fractions and standards is read off the burette scale.

3.1.6. Recovery of Cells from Fractions. After removal of samples for density estimation, each fraction is diluted 10-fold with buffered balanced salt solution, with thorough mixing, and centrifuged (400 g, 10 min) to recover the cells as a pellet. The cells from each fraction are then made to a fixed volume of suspension, and samples are withdrawn for a total cell count (Coulter counter with appropriate threshold set) and for other assays.

3.1.7. Expression of Results. The average density of each fraction is calculated from the burette readings, using the known standards to provide a calibration line. The value of each fraction is known from the collection time. A plot of density against cumulative fraction volume is made to determine the shape of the gradient. This also allows an estimation of the density at the beginning and end of each fraction, and of the density range or density increment that each fraction represents. The total number of cells in each fraction is calculated. In like manner the *total* activity or *total* number of cells of any particular type in each fraction is calculated. If the assay involves some form of per cell estimation (such as results of a culture of a fixed number of cells) or relative proportion of a given cell type (such as a differential count on smeared and stained cells), this must be multiplied by the total cell count to give the absolute number of cells or activity units per fraction. The total cells or total activity per fraction is then divided by the density increment covered by each fraction, and this is plotted against density to give the true density distribution profile. Such calculations are conveniently handled by a computer program.

3.2. Simplified Density Cut. The procedure for separating cells above and below a given density value is summarized in Fig. 4. All procedures are at

DENSITY CUT TECHNIQUE

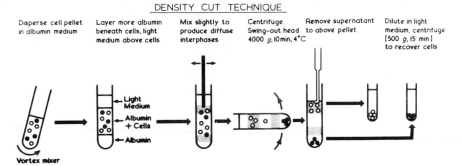

Fig. 4. Simple density cut procedure for selecting cells above and below a given density.

$0°-4°C$. Up to 5×10^8 cells can be handled in a single tube. The cells are spun to a pellet (400 g, 7 min), the supernatant is carefully removed, and 5 ml of albumin of the appropriate density are added. The cells are immediately dispersed, using a Vortex mixer. The trace of supernatant left in the cell pellet usually makes the average density of the suspension a little less than the albumin medium itself. A further 4 ml of the albumin is then layered below the cells in albumin, and 4 ml of some lighter medium is layered above, using a Pasteur pipette. The two interphase zones are then deliberately disturbed to produce a more diffuse zone or gradient region by gently mixing with a rod or Pasteur pipette. The tube is then centrifuged at 4000 g for 10–15 min, using a swing-out head. The supernatant, including the cell bands, the two interphase zones, and all layers down to a few millimeters above the cell pellet, is removed, using a bent Pasteur pipette. The supernatant is diluted 10-fold with buffered balanced salt solution. The pellet is suspended in buffered balanced salt solution. Cells in the two fractions are then recovered by centrifugation (400 g, 10 min). If further fractionation is required, the pellet may be directly suspended in the dense albumin for the next cut, without prior washing.

4. Interpretation of Data and Critical Comments

4.1. Osmolarity of Media. A high degree of reproducibility is possible only if osmolarity is carefully controlled, and steps like eliminating salts from the albumin powder are essential. Under these conditions the gradient is isoosmotic throughout. Other media, such as Ficoll, directly affect the osmolarity of salt solutions and make generation of isoosmotic gradients difficult (19). Note that the osmolarity of different species differs significantly (19). Mouse (and other rodent) cells may be separated at human osmolarity, but somewhat better results are obtainable if the gradient medium and salt solution are the same osmolarity as the serum of the species studied.

4.2. pH of Media. Under the conditions given, albumin buffers the medium at pH 5.1, close to its isoelectric point. At this pH lymphocytes survive well, maintain "normal" physical properties, and, most important, aggregation is markedly reduced. However erythrocytes and certain types of damaged cells swell at this acid pH. Neutral pH albumin may be employed, to separate these elements from viable lymphocytes (1, 2, 6–8, 18). In this case the osmotic contribution of the sodium ion added to produce a neutral albumin salt must be considered, and in addition the allowable cell load must be reduced owing to the increased aggregation effects.

4.3. Other Gradient Materials. A similar approach can be taken using other materials, such as Ficoll, to generate a density gradient. However, Ficoll, at neutral pH, causes extensive cell aggregation, and at high concentrations markedly alters the osmolarity of the basic salt solution.

4.4. Resolution. The degree of resolution is limited by the number of fractions taken, the width of the gradient, the cell load, and cell-to-cell association effects. For maximum resolution, the cell load should be reduced and the gradient restricted to a relatively narrow range around the region of interest (1–3, 16).

4.5. Density Estimations. The density estimation technique is fast, precise, and uses only small samples of each fraction. However, it does require a steady hand and some practice at producing small droplets of uniform size free of minute air bubbles. Care is required in handling the volatile organic solvents. The high accuracy of density estimation is required, not only to estimate the density of each fraction, but also to estimate the density increment or density range covered by each fraction, and so correct for deviations from linearity. If reasonably linear gradients can be generated, if fewer fractions are taken and high analytic precision is not required, a simple procedure such as refractive index measurements may suffice.

4.6. Expression of Results. The aim of the analytical procedure is to characterize a cell type or cell population by its density distribution, and the method of expression of results should be in accordance with this aim. Presentation of results on an "activity per cell" or "percent cells of a given type" basis provides important relative enrichment data, but does not characterize the absolute properties of the population under study. This requires calculation of the total response or total number of cells per fraction. A second point is that presentation of results on the basis of cells per fraction plotted against fraction number or mean fraction density will be misleading if the gradient is not strictly linear. With nonlinear gradients cells concentrate in fractions from the steep regions and are depleted in fractions from the flat regions. This can produce quite artificial "peaks," such as those deliberately created in discontinuous gradients. Strictly linear gradients are difficult to obtain, owing both to the limitations of the pumping system, and to the redistribution of cells within the gradient if the cell load is high. Reexpression of data as cells per density increment plotted against density overcomes such artifacts and reduces the data to true density distribution profiles.

4.7. Recoveries. Recoveries of viable cells and biological activity from the gradient is normally high (70–100%). This aspect should be monitored with a balance sheet approach, assaying a sample of the original suspension, and if a problem arises, a back-mix of samples from each fraction. Loss of apparent activity can be an index of cell interaction, with separation of the required interacting cells into different fractions.

4.8. Density-Cut Procedure. The appropriate albumin concentration and density for separating particular types of cells could be determined by trial and error. However, the method will be most useful if a careful density distribution analysis of the cell population has first been performed. The optimum density for maximum separation can then be read off directly from the distribution profiles.

REFERENCES

1. Shortman, K., *Annu. Rev. Biophys. Bioeng.* **1**, 93 (1972).
2. Shortman, K., *Contemp. Top. Mol. Immunol.* **3**, 161 (1974).
3. Shortman, K., *J. Cell. Physiol.* **77**, 319 (1971).
4. Shortman, K., von Boehmer, H., Lipp, J., and Hopper, K., *Transplant. Rev.* **25**, 163 (1975).
5. Shortman, K., Fidler, J. M., Schlegel, R. A., Nossal, G. J. V., Howard, M., Lipp, J., and von Boehmer, H., *Contemp. Top. Immunbiol.* **5**, in press.
6. Legge, D., and Shortman, K., *Br. J. Haematol.* **14**, 323 (1968).
7. Shortman, K., and Seligman, K., *J. Cell. Biol.* **42**, 783 (1969).
8. Williams, N., and Shortman, K., *Aust. J. Exp. Biol. Med. Sci.* **50**, 133 (1972).
9. Williams, N., Moore, M. A. S., Shortman, K., Condon, L., Pike, B. and Nossal, G. J. V., *Aust. J. Exp. Biol. Med. Sci.* **52**, 491 (1974).
10. Shortman, K., Cerottini, J.-C., and Brunner, K. T., *Eur. J. Immunol.* **2**, 313 (1972).
11. Kraft, N., and Shortman, K., *J. Cell Biol.* **52**, 438 (1972).
12. Shortman, K., Brunner, K. T., and Cerottini, J.-C., *J. Exp. Med.* **135**, 1375 (1972).
13. Roberts, I. M., Whittingham, S., and Mackay, I. R., *Clin. Exp. Immunol.* **19**, 251 (1975).
14. Moore, M. A. S., Williams, N., and Metcalf, D., *J. Cell. Physiol.* **79**, 283 (1972).
15. Moore, M. A. S., Williams, N., and Metcalf, D., *J. Natl. Cancer Inst.* **50**, 603 (1973).
16. Shortman, K., *Aust. J. Exp. Biol. Med. Sci.* **46**, 375 (1968).
17. Leif, R. C., and Vinograd, J., *Proc. Natl. Acad. Sci. U.S.A.* **51**, 520 (1964).
18. Shortman, K., Williams, N., and Adams, P., *J. Immunol. Methods* **1**, 273 (1972).
19. Williams, N., Kraft, N., and Shortman, K., *Immunology* **22**, 885 (1972).
20. von Boehmer, H., and Shortman, K., *J. Immunol. Methods* **2**, 293 (1973).

Separation of Human Peripheral Blood Lymphocytes by Sedimentation in Density Gradients of Bovine Serum Albumin (BSA)

E. Merler

Morphological analysis of human lymphocytes with the light microscope reveals a marked heterogeneity in size. It was, therefore, the obvious course to attempt to separate these variously sized cells in a gradient of changing density. Glycerol and sucrose, suitable for separating polymers of varying molecular weight, interfere with the structural integrity of the cell membrane. The use of a high-molecular-weight substance to form the gradient overcomes this difficulty: bovine serum albumin, readily available and highly soluble in dilute salt solution, has the necessary prerequisites for this purpose.

Principally, two methods have been used for separating lymphocytes in bovine serum albumin. One is described by Raidt, Mishell, and Dutton (1) and the other by Dicke, Tridente, and van Bekkum (2). It is a modification of the latter that will be described here.

1. Materials and Equipment

1.1. Buffers
1.1.1. Tris buffer, adjusted to pH 7.2 with HCl is filtered through a 0.22 μm Millipore filter into a sterile 1000-ml flask.
1.1.2. Phosphate-buffered saline: 0.15 M NaCl, 0.0076 M Na$_2$H PO$_4$, and 0.0024 M Na$_2$HPO$_4$ adjusted to between pH 7.1 and 7.3 with concentrated HCl. The solution is filtered through a 0.22 μm Millipore filter into a sterile 1000-ml flask.

1.2. Preparation of Stock BSA Solution of 35% Concentration
1.2.1. To 190 ml of Tris buffer in a sterile, covered 600-ml beaker, add slowly 100 g of powdered BSA (Sigma Chemical Co., N.A. 4503 Albumin bovine, fraction V).
1.2.2. Allow to stand at 4°C without stirring for 2–3 days.
1.2.3. Run through a 1.2 μm Millipore filter fitted with a prefilter pad.
1.2.4. Measure the pH of the solution and adjust to pH 5.1–5.3 with 0.1 M HCl. Equilibrate overnight.

1.2.5. Adjust to 35% concentration (w/v) using a reading of refractive index of 1.4036 at 20°C (Abbe refractometer).

1.2.6. Measure the osmolarity of a 1 + 1 dilution of the BSA with water.

1.2.7. Adjust the osmolarity of the stock solution to 360 mOsm/liter with solid NaCl by the formula:

$$\text{Volume BSA (liter)} \times \frac{(360 - \text{observed osmolarity})}{100} = \text{mOsm NaCl to be added}$$

where 2.922 g of NaCl = 100 mOsm/liter.

1.2.8. Filter through a sterile 0.45 μm Millipore filter and store in sterile 100-ml bottles.

1.2.9. Culture the contents of each bottle onto plates of blood agar.

1.3. Preparation of Lymphocytes

1.3.1. Peripheral blood to which preservative-free heparin has been added (100 units/4 ml of blood) is mixed with 6% dextran (Macrodex 70,000, Pharmacia) in saline (5 volumes of blood and 1 volume of dextran).

1.3.2. After sedimentation of the red cells for 1 hr at 37°C, the leukocyte-rich plasma is centrifuged (600 g) at 4°C for 10 min.

1.3.3. Cells suspended in medium 199 supplemented with 10% AB⁺ serum (complete medium), are adsorbed on glass beads (Potters Ind., Carlstadt, New Jersey, screen 35–40) contained in a jacketed glass column (50 X 3 cm) maintained at 37°C. Cells obtained from 450 ml of blood are added to a column that has been filled with 30 cm of glass beads. For smaller volumes of blood, proportional volumes of glass beads are used.

1.3.4. Leukocytes are suspended in an appropriate volume of complete medium, so that they can be totally adsorbed on the column bed. For this purpose, approximately 50 ml of a suspension of cells is added to a column of glass beads of 30 cm in height.

1.3.5. After 30 min, cells are eluted from the column with 1.5 to 2 volumes of complete medium.

1.3.6. Store in Medium 199.

1.4. Fractionation of Lymphocytes on Gradients of BSA

1.4.1. Prepare dilutions of the stock 35% BSA solution according to the tabulation on p. 281.

1.4.2. Layer in plastic tubes of 16 X 125 mm, 1 ml volumes of the different concentrations of BSA, starting at the bottom of the tube with a solution consisting of 35% BSA and continuing in 2% decrements to 19%. Keep the albumin cold and do not allow the layers to mix.

1.4.3. Suspend the cells in 17% BSA and carefully layer the suspension over the gradient.

1.4.4. Spin the tubes at 900 g (max) at 5°–10°C for 40 min.

Albumin concentration (%)	35% Albumin (ml)	PBS (ml)
35	3.5	0
33	3.3	0.2
31	3.1	0.4
29	2.9	0.6
27	2.7	0.8
25	2.5	1.0
23	2.3	1.2
21	2.1	1.4
19	1.9	1.6
17	1.7	1.8

1.4.5. Remove the cells at the interface of each layer into a separate tube, centrifuge, and wash twice with Hanks' balanced salt solution.

1.4.6. Count the cells in each layer and plot the numbers on graph paper.

2. Comments

2.1. Cell Suspensions. While the described procedure applies to peripheral blood lymphocytes, cells from the thymus, lymph nodes, bone marrow, spleen, and tonsil have been fractionated repeatedly and with good success. Recovery of cells should be nearly quantitative.

2.2. Distribution of Cells in the Gradient. The profile of the gradient is quite complex. Not only does the concentration of BSA change, but the pH and osmolarity change as well. A pH of the stock BSA in excess of 5.3 results in poor fractionation of the subpopulation of cells. Osmolarity changes in excess of 10 mOsm affect the separation adversely. In general, larger cells are found at the top of the gradient and smaller cells in the lower fractions. Layers 1–3 contain macrophages (if present) and blastlike precursor cells (3). *In vitro,* these cells can mature into T cells. When first separated from the gradient, they are reactive with EAC3 but not with E. They represent 3–5% of the total lymphocyte population.

Layers 4–6 contain primarily T cells (4). Sixty percent of these cells form spontaneous rosettes with E and exhibit *in vitro* reactivity to phytohemagglutinin, concanavalin A, antigens, allogeneic cells, etc. If the percentage of spontaneous E rosettes falls to 40% or less, the separation must be considered atypical. No more than 3–10% of these cells should form rosettes with EAC3;

20–30% can be considered "null" with respect to E and EAC3 and are probably "activated" cells. Red cells will start to appear in layer 5. Of peripheral blood lymphocytes, 60–70% appear in layer 4–6.

Cells in layer 7–9 are primarily B cells. Over 80% form rosettes with EAC3. Generally, there are no "null" cells in this area of the gradient, and less than 7% E reactive cells. Red cells will usually stop at layer 7. Monocytes are distributed between layers 5 and 8. Cells in this area of the gradient are the nonactivated precursors of antibody-forming cells. Damaged cells, i.e., cells that stain with Trypan blue, are found as a pellet at the bottom of the gradient. Of peripheral blood lymphocytes, 10–20% appear in layers 7–9.

REFERENCES

1. D. J. Raidt, R. J. Mishell, and R. W. Dutton, *J. Exp. Med.* **128,** 681 (1968).
2. K. A. Dicke, G. Tridente, and D. W. van Bekkum, *Transplantation* **8,** 422 (1968).
3. Gatien, J. A., Schneeberger, E., and Merler, E., *Eur. J. Immunol.* **5,** 312 (1975).
4. Geha, R. S., and Merler, E., *Eur. J. Immunol.* **4,** 193 (1974).

23

Separation of Cells by Velocity Sedimentation*[†]

Richard G. Miller

1. Introduction

In many problems in cell biology it would be useful to fractionate a complex population of viable cells into component subpopulations differing in function. Since cell function is often correlated with physical parameters, such as cell size, useful separations can often be obtained by fractionating on the basis of such parameters. The procedure could be used preparatively to obtain a purified subpopulation for further experiments or, analytically, to study directly the properties of a particular subpopulation under varying conditions. The analogy with biochemistry, in which various physically based techniques such as centrifugation and electrophoresis are used both preparatively and analytically, is obvious.

This article will be restricted to separation of cells by velocity sedimentation in the earth's gravitational field, but it is worthwhile to consider briefly other separation methods. If one limits oneself to physical methods for which the basis of the separation is reasonably well understood and which, at least potentially, can be applied analytically, five methods stand out: sedimentation, equilibrium density-gradient centrifugation, countercurrent distribution, electrophoresis, and electronic sorting. The first four methods have been concisely reviewed by Shortman (1, 2). They are all bulk processes in that they separate a population of cells into subpopulations essentially at one time in contrast to electronic sorting, which analyzes and separates cells one at a time, usually on the basis of fluorescent markers (see, e.g., 3).

Sedimentation and density separation are not completely independent procedures. Sedimentation separates cells primarily on the basis of size, rather than density. However, cell density is roughly inversely proportional to cell size, since

*This work was supported by the National Cancer Institute of Canada and the Medical Research Council (Grant MT-3017).
†This article is a revised and updated version of an article that appeared in "New Techniques in Biophysics and Cell Biology", (R. Pain and B. Smith, eds.), Vol. 1. Wiley, New York, 1973.

the nucleus of a cell is much more dense than the cytoplasm and larger cells tend to have a smaller nucleus-to-cytoplasm ratio. None the less, there are significant exceptions to this relationship; e.g., cytoplasmic granules such as are found in granulocytes, can markedly increase cytoplasmic density. Thus, sedimentation and density separation can often be complementary.

The physical bases of countercurrent and electrophoretic separation are not completely understood, but it appears that they may both be separating on the basis of the same cellular parameter, surface charge density (1, 2). In any case, either should be complementary to both sedimentation and density separation.

2. Theory

Consider a sphere (volume V, radius r, density ρ) falling through a viscous medium under the action of the earth's gravitational field. The net gravitational force on the particle is given by $(\rho - \rho')gV$, where ρ' is the density of the viscous medium and g is the acceleration due to gravity (980 cm/sec^2). The net gravitational force is opposed by a viscous drag force set up in opposition to the motion of the particle. For a sphere, the drag force is given by $6\pi\eta rv$ (Stokes' law) where η is the coefficient of viscosity and v is the velocity of the sedimenting particle. An equilibrium state is soon reached in which the net gravitational force is exactly balanced by the viscous drag force and the particle falls at a constant velocity, its terminal velocity, s. Equating the two forces, one finds that s is given by Eq. (1):

$$s = \frac{2(\rho - \rho')gr^2}{9\eta} \tag{1}$$

Under physiological conditions, the vast majority of mammalian cells have radii varying from 2.5 to 10 μm, and densities varying from 1.05 to 1.10 g/cm^3. If they are falling through an aqueous medium with a density of 1.0 g/cm^3, one can see that size variations can give rise to about a 16-fold variation in terminal velocity whereas density variations give rise to only about a 2-fold variation in terminal velocity. Thus, variations in s will primarily be due to variations in size.

Cells are seldom perfectly spherical and some, such as erythrocytes, are not even approximately so. However, the above expression still holds true (4) with an error of less than 10% for both prolate and oblate spheroids with axial ratios $a/b<3$ providing that one takes r to be that of an equivalent sphere, i.e., $r = (3V/4\pi)^{1/3}$. Thus, independent of shape, we have

$$s \cong \frac{g\,(\rho - \rho')\,V^{2/3}}{(16^2\pi^2)^{1/3}\eta} \tag{2}$$

The above expressions assume the cell to be moving at terminal velocity and, for typical cells under typical conditions, the time required to reach this speed is, at most, a few microseconds.

If one knew the density and volume of a cell, one should, in principle, be able to calculate its s value directly from Eq. (1). This has been verified experimentally for sheep erythrocytes (4), antibody-producing cells (5), and mouse L cells (6). Under conditions representative of actual experimental conditions used for separating cells by sedimentation, $\rho' = 1.01$ g/cm^3 and $\eta = 1.567$ centipoise (water at 4°C). Thus, we have

$$s = 5.0\,(\rho - 1.01)\,r^2 \tag{3}$$

in which s is in mm/hr, ρ in g/cm^3, and r in μ. A typical nucleated cell has a density of 1.06 g/cm^3, for which this expression becomes $s = r^2/4$.

3. Methods

The objective is to form a thin layer of cell suspension on top of a fluid column, let the cells sediment under the influence of gravity for an appropriate length of time, and collect fractions containing cells that have moved different distances. The cells should be as little affected as possible by the procedure. In particular, they should preserve their viability. Any changes resulting from metabolic activity should be greatly reduced by lowering the temperature. For this reason, we have usually performed separations in a cold room at 4°C, although we have also obtained satisfactory results at room temperature. The fluid column in which the cells sediment should be a buffered isotonic saline such as PBS (Dulbecco's phosphate-buffered saline). Any further additives should not affect the cells.

The following sections describe two closely related practical systems for meeting the above objectives and discuss their limitations.

3.1. **Apparatus.** The fluid column as described will be unstable to convection and mechanical jarring. Stability can be maintained by introducing a shallow density gradient into the fluid column. The choice of gradient material is important. It should have sufficiently high molecular weight so as not to create an appreciable tonicity gradient, and it should also be nontoxic to cells. Materials such as fetal calf serum, bovine serum albumin (BSA) (Cohn fraction 5), or Ficoll have proved to be satisfactory. Materials such as sucrose are not satisfactory on the basis of both tonicity and toxicity problems.

The gradient is made as shallow as possible, with ρ' as low as possible to ensure that separation is on the basis of differences in sedimentation rate rather than differences in density. A typical gradient might vary from 0 to 2% BSA in PBS which covers the density range 1.0074 to 1.0113 g/cm^3. The equivalent serum gradient would be 0 to 30% serum in PBS.

The next problem is the formation of a cell layer on top of the gradient. The first method described for doing this is the "staflo" system of Mel (7). The system is rather complicated, and it is difficult to get as good resolution as with

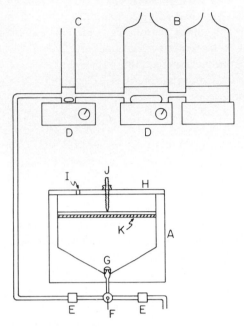

Fig. 1. The "staput" sedimentation chamber: A, sedimentation chamber; B, gradient maker; C, intermediate vessel; D, magnetic stirrers; E, flow-rate regulators; F, three-way valve; G, flow baffle; H, chamber lid; I, vent hole in chamber lid; J, screw; K, cell band shortly after loading is completed.

the simpler systems described below. The apparatus of Fig. 1 evolved from attempts to set up the "staflo" system (4). It is very similar to apparatus described by Peterson and Evans (8).

The apparatus of Fig. 1 ("staput") has three main parts: the sedimentation chamber (A), the gradient maker (B), and a small intermediate vessel (C). The sedimentation chamber should be transparent, as it is a big advantage to be able to see cell bands during the separation process. We have used sedimentation chambers made of Lucite, polycarbonate, or glass. The last two may be steam sterilized. The angle in the cone of the sedimentation chamber is nominally 30°, but this is not critical and cone angles as low as 15° to the horizontal appear to be satisfactory. All tubing interconnections are made using silicone tubing (Silastic, Dow Corning) because of the very low tendency for cells to stick to silicone rubber.

Cells are loaded into the chamber through (C) and are lifted into their starting position (indicated by K in Fig. 1) by the gradient (loaded via gravity) introduced through the gradient maker (B). The small stainless steel baffle (G) at the bottom of the chamber is used to deflect incoming fluid during the loading procedure. Without this baffle it is very difficult to load a gradient without mixing. Figure 2 gives details of the baffle and inlet construction for a chamber 12 cm in internal diameter. Returning to Fig. 1, the chamber has a lid (H), which serves to keep out dust. The screw (J) mounted in the lid has a sharpened point. This enables one reproducibly to fill the chamber to the same volume by stopping the filling process when the screw tip just touches the rising gradient. E represents a two-way needle valve, and F a three-way tap. After the cells have sedimented for an appropriate length of time, fractions are collected through the bottom of the chamber. The apparatus of Peterson and Evans (8) differs from that of Fig. 1 in that it has a second cone mounted on top of the chamber and fractions are collected by displacing the chamber contents upward through the upper cone using a dense sucrose gradient.

If the concentration of cells in the starting band exceeds a certain critical limit, a phenomenon called "streaming" takes place, and useful separations cannot be achieved. The highest concentration at which streaming does not take place (the "streaming limit") is characteristic of the cells being sedimented. For cells having

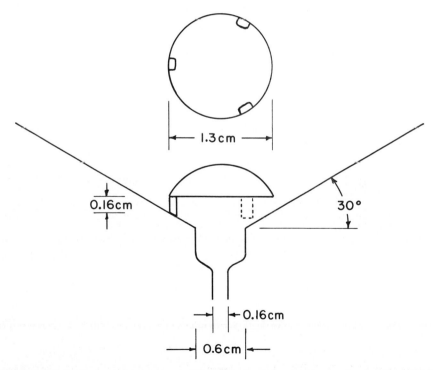

Fig. 2. Detail of chamber inlet and flow baffle for apparatus of Fig. 1 using a sedimentation chamber 12 cm in diameter.

a volume of about 100 μm^3, the streaming limit is about 5×10^6 cells/ml. Thus, for a given chamber, the maximum cell load is determined by the streaming limit and the maximum allowable thickness of the starting band for the resolution desired. (See the next section for a detailed discussion of both streaming and resolution.) To process more cells, one must use a chamber of larger diameter. We have successfully used chambers ranging in diameter from 11 to 39 cm. Chamber size is more conveniently designated by volume in cubic centimeters per millimeter of length in the cylindrical part of the chamber, since this is the parameter required to determine resolution and calculate sedimentation velocities. Call this the chamber constant a. Then the chamber diameter range of 11 to 39 cm corresponds to a values of 9.5 to 119 cm^3/mm.

One problem was encountered with the 39-cm diameter chamber: The total volume of gradient in this chamber is about 20 liters so that to collect fractions in a reasonable length of time we have used rather high drain rates (up to 400 ml/min). At these drain rates, swirling occurred similar to that seen in a draining bathtub. This problem was solved by attaching to the chamber lid a vane that splits the chamber into two sections almost to the bottom. This problem did not occur for a chamber 24 cm in diameter. A complete cell-separating apparatus, made of glass, with chamber diameters of approximately 11, 17, or 25 cm is available commercially from O. H. Johns Scientific, Toronto, Canada.

The detailed protocol we use for performing a separation in a chamber 12 cm in diameter ($a = 11.4$ cm^3/mm) is as follows.

3.1.1. Set up apparatus in coldroom as in Fig. 1. We use gradient bottles and an intermediate vessel with internal diameter of 7 and 2.2 cm, respectively.

3.1.2. Prepare at least 300 ml each of 1 and 2% BSA in PBS. Bring to a temperature of 4°C.

3.1.3. Fill all the connecting tubing (made of silicone rubber) of the apparatus on the chamber side of (C) with PBS, making sure to get rid of all air bubbles.

3.1.4. Center the flow baffle (G) inside the cone of the sedimentation chamber. It is important that this be centered carefully.

3.1.5. Clamp the lines between all three gradient chambers. Load 300 ml of 1% BSA into the left-hand bottle of (B) and 300 ml of 2% BSA into the right-hand bottle.

3.1.6. Load top layer (30 ml of saline) into the sedimentation chamber through the intermediate vessel (C). Note that the total volume of the top layer will be whatever fluid is put in (C) plus the volume of the tubing between (C) and the sedimentation chamber (typically less than 5 ml). Check that the flow baffle is still correctly centered. The function of this top layer is to prevent disturbance of the cell band by erratic movements of the rising fluid meniscus as the chamber is filling.

3.1.7. Load cells in 20 ml of 0.2% BSA in PBS through (C). The cell concentration must be below the streaming limit for the cells being loaded. Clamp the line the instant the buffer chamber empties.

3.1.8. Rinse the buffer chamber twice with 0.2% BSA in PBS. Use a 50-ml syringe and a piece of tubing to do this. Check that no air bubbles entered the lines during the rinse.

3.1.9. Fill (C) with the buffer gradient (0.35% BSA in saline) to the level of the fluid in the gradient bottles. Adjust the needle valve for a flow rate of 2–3 ml/min. Turn on magnetic stirrers.

3.1.10. Remove all clamps and record time (t_1); the gradient will load itself. It will rise rapidly from 0.35 to 1.0% BSA and slowly thereafter to 2.0% BSA. The reasons for using a gradient of this shape are described in the next section. Once the cells have been lifted off the bottom, the flow rate can be increased. Continuously adjust by eye to a rate just below that at which the cell band is disturbed. Small disturbances will settle out. Loading should be as rapid as possible (10–15 min). The time elapsed between loading cells and starting the gradient should also be as short as possible (4–8 min).

3.1.11. Record time cell band reaches top of cone (t_2).

3.1.12. After an appropriate sedimentation time (4 hr are usually adequate), start unloading the chamber through the bottom at a rate of about 30 ml/min. Record time (t_3). Discard the cone volume.

3.1.13. Collect remainder of gradient in equal-sized fractions (e.g., 15 ml). Record time first fraction started (t_4) and last fraction finished (t_5). Also record number and volume of last fraction.

Occasionally, one wishes to separate very large or very sticky cells. There is a reasonable probability that some of these will sediment onto or, in passing, stick to the cone during the loading procedure. These cells may either be permanently lost, or even worse, come off randomly during the draining procedure and contaminate all fractions. To avoid these possibilities, it is desirable to have a procedure in which cells can be layered on top of a preformed gradient. A system for doing this is shown in Fig. 3, which also illustrates the operating procedure.

The sedimentation chamber ("muffin") is a completely closed cylinder with entrance ports on opposite sides of the top and bottom, as depicted. The chamber is mounted between two stands and is free to rotate about axis A which is perpendicular to the plane determined by the entrance ports. To load, the chamber is first rotated to an angle of approximately 30° with respect to the horizontal and filled with saline. Next, a linear gradient (e.g., 1–2% BSA) is introduced through the bottom port. The gradient displaces the saline already in the chamber through the top port. Next, cells (in 0.5% BSA, for example) are

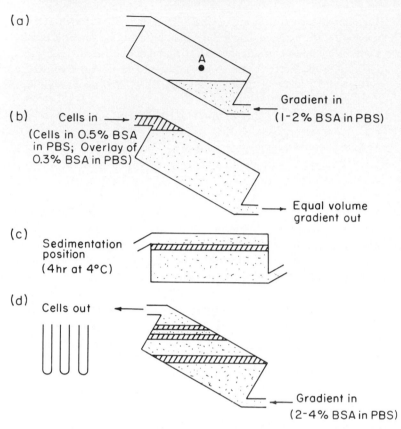

Fig. 3. Operating procedure for "muffin" sedimentation chamber. (a) The chamber is tilted to approximately 30° from the horizontal about axis A and a gradient is introduced through the lower port. (b) The cells and overlay are introduced through the upper port. (c) The chamber is carefully rotated to horizontal for cell sedimentation. (d) The chamber is again rotated to 30° from the horizontal, and fractions are collected by displacing the chamber contents through either the upper or lower port with an appropriate gradient (collection through the upper port is illustrated).

loaded through the top port followed by, if desired, an overlay (e.g., 0.3% BSA). Then the chamber is slowly and smoothly rotated to a horizontal position and left in this position for the duration of the sedimentation time (e.g., 4 hr). It may seem surprising that one can rotate the chamber in this way without complete disruption of the gradient. However, even mild density gradients are remarkably stable and all fluid appears to preserve its relative position during the rotation providing this is performed without jerking. To drain the chamber, one first rotates it back to its original position. It can then be unloaded through either the top or bottom. This is best done by displacing the contents with an appropriate gradient, e.g., 0.3–0% BSA for displacement through the bottom.

We have successfully used Lucite chambers of this design with a diameter of 14 cm and a depth of either 3.8 or 8 cm and a glass chamber of this design with diameter 13 cm and depth 8 cm. Problems were experienced with a much larger chamber, 39 cm in diameter and 13 cm deep, in that it was difficult to rotate it by hand sufficiently smoothly to prevent disturbance of the gradient during rotation although some kind of mechanical device could almost certainly be used to avoid this problem.

We have built a special version of this chamber 30 cm in diameter and only 1.8 cm deep for one particular job. The problem was to separate rosettes (lymphoid cells coated with heterologous erythrocytes) from a suspension of single cells. Most of the rosettes were expected to sediment at rates exceeding 1 cm/hr whereas most of the single cells were expected to sediment at rates less than 4 mm/hr. It was possible to get good separation between the two cell classes using cell loads in excess of 10^9 cells in times as short as 45 min (9). This is a preparative application of cell separation, whereas most of the other applications considered in this chapter are analytical in nature.

3.2. Streaming, Resolution and Cell-Load Limitations. The major limitation to separation of cells by velocity sedimentation is the phenomenon of streaming. This occurs if the cell concentration (cells/ml) in the cell band loaded into the chamber exceeds a certain number, called the streaming limit. Shortly after loading, large numbers of filaments ("streamers") a few millimeters long can be seen hanging down from the cell band. When viewed from above, the cell band has a mottled appearance. Streaming does not appear to be a cell-aggregation phenomenon because, when streaming is set up in a small cuvette and viewed with a microscope, all cells in streamers appear to be single and to move relatively independently of one another.

Streaming is probably due to some kind of density inversion phenomenon taking place at the interface between the cell band and the gradient. Tulp and Bont (10) reasoned that adding a small quantity of viscous material to the cell band to make its viscosity slightly greater than that of the underlying gradient would prevent accumulation of cells at the interface and thus would prevent any such inversion phenomenon. Using this procedure, we have not been able to increase the streaming limit. Streaming can, however, be considerably reduced by introducing a "rounding off" of the sharp edge of the gradient immediately below the band of cells. This is called a buffered-step gradient and is illustrated in Fig. 4. For sheep erythrocytes, the streaming limit using the sheer-step gradient is 5×10^6/ml. The streaming limit increases to about 1.5×10^7/ml when a buffered-step gradient is used (4).

Buffered-step gradients of a wide shape range can be generated by appropriate choice of the areas of the two bottles in a two-bottle gradient generating system.

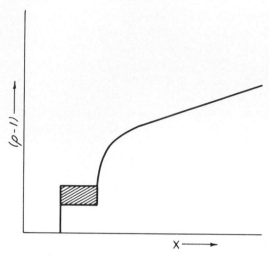

Fig. 4. Density distribution for attenuated step gradient immediately after loading. The part contributed by the cells is shown hatched.

Let the gradient be taken from bottle 1, which has area A_1 and contains material of density ρ_1; bottle 2 has area A_2 and contains materials of density ρ_2. Then

$$\rho(x) = \rho_2 - (\rho_2 - \rho_1)(1 - x/x_0)A_2/A_1 \tag{4}$$

where x is distance measured from the top of the gradient and x_0 is the depth of the gradient when the bottles are empty.

Both sheer-step and buffered-step gradients can be generated with the apparatus of Fig. 1. The gradient bottles of (B) are filled to the desired level with 1% and 2% BSA in PBS. For a sheer-step gradient, cells (in 0.2% BSA in PBS) are loaded into the sedimentation chamber via (C) which is then rinsed out with saline and used as a subsidiary mixing vessel for the 1–2% BSA gradient from (B). For a buffered-step gradient, the cells are loaded as above and chamber (C) is again rinsed, but this time filled to the same level as the bottles of (B) with 0.35% BSA in PBS. When flow resumes, a gradient similar to that in Fig. 4 will be generated. The precise details of the shape of the buffered-step gradient do not seem to be important; the increase in the streaming limit appears to be about the same whether the gradient is sharply or gradually rounded off.

The streaming limit varies with the cells being sedimented. All tests made to date are consistent with the streaming limit being inversely proportional to V, the average cell volume. Thus, large cells have a lower streaming limit than small cells.

The maximum cell load that can be separated on a given chamber is determined by the resolution desired and the streaming limit. What is the intrinsic resolution of the system; i.e., at what point do further reductions in the width of the starting band yield no significant improvement in resolution? This is a more difficult question.

Consider a population of cells, all of which have the same density and volume. Load these as a very thin band and measure the sedimentation profile after different sedimentation times. Then one can define the intrinsic resolution of the system as δs where δs is the full width at half height of the sedimentation profile. In various experiments (see, e.g., Fig. 5) approximating this situation using both cells and plastic beads, it has been found that $\delta s/s$ is a constant, independent of both s and the sedimentation time (for time ranges of 3–6 hr), having the value of 0.18. (This corresponds to an intrinsic coefficient of variation for the sedimentation distribution of 0.076.) This intrinsic dispersion is disturbingly large, much larger than one would expect on the basis of diffusion alone, and we have been unable to find a satisfactory explanation for it.

To get the optimum resolution while processing the maximum number of cells possible for a cell population with an s value of 5 mm/hr and a sedimentation time of 4 hr proceed as follows. The width of the band in the sedimentation chamber resulting from the intrinsic dispersion after 4 hr of sedimentation will be $4 \times 5 \times 0.18 = 3.6$ mm. Assuming that the intrinsic dispersion in the separation and the loss of resolution resulting from a starting band of finite width are independent (which, experimentally, seems approximately true), the sedimentation profile of the 5 mm/hr cell would be only $\sqrt{2} \times 3.6$ mm wide if the starting band were also 3.6 mm wide. Clearly, using the above assumption about how to add dispersive factors, there is little point in making the starting band much narrower than about 1.8 mm.

Suppose, in the above example, one wished to process 3×10^8 cells and that the streaming limit for this population is 10^7 cells/ml. The cells can be loaded in no less than 30 ml. To get a starting band 1.8 mm wide implies a chamber constant, a, of $30/1.8 = 16.7$ cm^3/mm corresponding to a chamber 14.6 cm in diameter.

3.3. Preparation of Cell Suspensions. The method used for preparation of cell suspensions is critical to the success of any cell-separation experiment because of the posssibility of generating artifacts from dead cells, cellular debris, or cellular aggregates. Our experience has been largely limited to cell suspensions of lymphoid or myeloid origin from mice. For a solid organ, such as thymus or spleen, the procedure we have found to be the best is as follows: Place the organ in the middle of a saucer-shaped wire screen (60 mesh) and cut it into several hundred pieces with sharp scissors. Rub the pieces through the screen with a glass pestle, keeping the screen center in buffered saline containing 0.2% BSA. Put this initial suspension into a tube and allow the large aggregates to settle out for 3–5 min and discard. Next, wash by centrifugation at a force not exceeding 250 g for the minimum time required to pellet all cells. This step gets rid of much of the cellular debris. Rewash if necessary. The wash medium should contain some protein (e.g., 0.2% BSA) to prevent cell loss and, if a glass centrifuge tube is used, it should be siliconized to avoid specific loss of adherent cells. After discarding the wash supernatant, resuspend the pellet in the solution to be used for cell loading in the sedimentation chamber.

More recently, we have been using the FCS wash procedure of Shortman, Williams, and Adams (11) which gives almost complete removal of debris and some additional removal of aggregates. After allowing large aggregates to settle out, as above, the cell suspension is gently layered over a few milliliters of FCS in a plastic or siliconized glass tube. Within 10–15 min, many of the remaining aggregates will settle into the FCS. Next, the overlay is removed with a Pasteur pipette and gently layered into a second tube containing a few milliliters (2–3 cm deep) of FCS. The cells are spun through the FCS at a force not exceeding 250 g for the minimum time required to pellet all of them. The pellet is then resuspended in the solution to be used for cell loading in the sedimentation chamber, as described above.

Next, the cell suspension is filtered through a capillary array filter (Mosaic Fabrications, Sturbridge, Massachusetts) to break up cell doublets and other small aggregates. We have used a capillary array filter 1 inch in diameter and 0.1 inch thick with a pore size of 37 μm. The cell suspension is taken up into a syringe and forced through the filter under slight positive pressure such that the shear force generated as the cells passed through the filter is sufficient to break up doublets, but not sufficient to shear the cells themselves. Next, the cell suspension is counted and diluted to the desired concentration for loading. The resulting suspension is more than 90% viable by either fluorescein diacetate (12) or trypan blue (13) viability tests and contains less than 1% cell aggregates (often much less).

Cell suspensions with similar viability can be made from spleen or thymus by enzymatic digestion using, for example, trypsin. We have not used such methods for fear of altering the chemical and biological properties of the cells. Meistrich (14), in studies of mouse sperm-cell differentiations, has shown that if a cell suspension prepared mechanically from mouse seminiferous tubules is treated with trypsin (0.25%, w/v) and deoxyribonuclease (20 μg/ml) at room temperature for a short period of time (less than 3 min) all nonviable cells are destroyed with no apparent loss of viable cells (as measured by trypan blue uptake). The same procedure appears to work for suspensions of lymphoid and myeloid cells but, again, this procedure undoubtedly alters the biological properties of the cells.

3.4. Counting and Size Analysis. In a typical cell-separation experiment it is necessary to determine the cell concentration in many fractions and therefore some kind of automated cell counter is called for. The best currently available is an electronic cell detector of the Coulter type (15). The heart of this instrument is a small aperture, typically about 100 μm in diameter, which is mounted in a glass tube and immersed in saline containing the cells to be counted. Electrodes are mounted on either side of the aperture, and electrical current flows from one electrode to the other through the aperture. To count cells, a known volume of fluid is sucked through the aperture. Each time a cell goes through the aperture, it increases the electrical resistance of the aperture and a pulse is generated, which can be amplified and counted in appropriate electronics. This instrument allows very rapid determination of cell concentration per fraction. Unless very carefully cleaned beforehand (e.g., by using the FCS wash procedure described in the preceding section), accurate counts of cell suspensions prepared from solid tissues are difficult to obtain in the cell counter because of the debris included in the suspension. However, in a sedimentation separation, the debris is largely left behind by the sedimenting cells, and this problem does not occur. Cell suspensions initially at 4°C appear to produce clogging of the aperture if they are warmed to room temperature before counting.

Using the Coulter counter, it is possible to get much more information than just the cell concentration. The magnitude of the signal produced by a cell traversing the aperture is proportional, over a restricted but useful range (16), to the volume of the cell detected. One can get a direct measure of the volume distribution of the cells in the sample by connecting the Coulter counter to a pulse-height analyzer. This instrument analyzes each incident pulse and adds the count to one of a set of serially arranged memory locations ("channels") according to the size of the pulse. At the completion of a run, the memory can be displayed visually or printed out to produce a graph of pulse number versus pulse size, i.e., cell number versus cell volume.

The rise time of the signal produced by a cell traversing an aperture will be determined, among other things, by aperture length. Commercial apertures tend to be so short (<100 μm) that the rise time is too short to be handled with fidelity by readily designable electronics. This problem can be overcome by making one's own apertures using ruby watch jewels 200 μm long. These can be obtained very cheaply from Erismann-Schinz, S. A., La Neuveville, Switzerland. The jewels should be directly fused to a soft-glass tube having a coefficient of thermal expansion close to but slightly greater than that of the watch jewel.

The electronics of most commercial cell counters of the Coulter type is such as to produce some distortion of the recorded volume spectrum (17), but these problems can be overcome by appropriate redesign of the circuitry (18). Some further distortion and dispersion of the volume spectrum is inherent in the nature of the events taking place in the detection aperture but, although very complex, these processes are largely understood (19, 20) and do not detract from the usefulness of the method. The coefficient of variation of the volume distribution measured for a uniform population of particles of volume 100 μm^3 detected in an aperture 100 μm in diameter and 200 μm long is about 0.1. Volume dispersions greater than this are due to true dispersion in the sample itself.

If one wishes to measure absolute volumes with the volume spectrometer outlined above, it is necessary to have some good volume standards in the cell-volume region being investigated. We have found the most satisfactory volume standards to be plastic beads (styrene divinylbenzene copolymer beads, 6–14 μm, Dow Chemical). Uniform beads in the volume range of cells cannot be obtained commercially. However, the Dow beads can be fractionated by velocity sedimentation using the techniques described in this article to give a large number of samples, each of quite uniform volume. The problem remains of how to measure the volume of the beads in each fraction. Ideally, one would like an accuracy of about 5%. This would require a diameter measurement accuracy of 5/3%, not obtainable by optical measurement because of diffraction problems. Electron microscopy is difficult because spherical aberration makes it almost impossible to make measurements at this level of precision even if the beads are put on a grid of known spacing at the time of the photograph. A solution to the problem is to calculate the absolute volume of the bead standard from the bead density as measured on a sucrose density gradient and the bead sedimentation velocity as measured by the methods described in this article. Alternatively the number of spheres in a volume containing a known weight of particles of known density can be counted. Absolute accuracies of 5% can be obtained.

3.5. Calculation of s Values. Homogeneous populations of cells can be characterized by their s value (sedimentation velocity in mm/hr) providing that all separations are related to a standard set of conditions. The standard conditions we have adopted are a temperature of 4°C and a gradient in which the average density in the region through which the cells sediment is very close to 1.010 g/cm^3. Under these conditions, absolute s values can be measured with a precision of 5%.

In calculating s values from experimental data, the distance a cell sediments is inferred from the volume of fluid through which it falls. To do this accurately, some conventions and corrections that are not altogether obvious are required. Consider a separation done in the apparatus of Fig. 1. i.e., the cells have been both loaded and drained through the bottom of a conical chamber. On draining, one cone volume of fluid is discarded and the rest of the chamber contents are collected as fractions of equal volume, v. Number the fractions in the order of collection, the last fraction having number N_f and volume V_f.

Define the $s = 0$ point as the middle of the input cell band. Treating fraction number as a continuous variable, the corresponding position, in terms of fraction number, is given by Eq. (5).

$$N(s = 0) = N_f - \frac{(V_0 + \frac{1}{2}V_{cb} - V_f)}{v} - \frac{1}{2} \tag{5}$$

where V_0 is the total volume of fluid above the cell band and V_{cb} is the volume of the cell band. The final subtraction of $\frac{1}{2}$ is necessary when one treats N as a continuous variable: A particular fraction, when collected, extends from $N-1$ to N on a continuous scale, but we wish to consider integer values of N, and the s value associated with them, as representing the average properties of the cells in the fraction having that N value.

Both loading and unloading of the chamber take finite time, during which the cells will sediment. When a cell sediments while in the cone, the volume of fluid fallen through per unit distance fallen is smaller than while in the cylindrical region. Thus, if one calculates the s value solely on the basis of the volume of the fluid fallen through, one will underestimate the s value. This is most easily allowed for by correcting the time the cells spend in the cone during loading and unloading by an appropriate factor. If the volume flow rate is constant and the cells start precisely at the apex of the cone, one can show that the actual time the cells spend in the cone during loading and unloading should be reduced by 40%. Using this correction factor and also allowing for the fact that cells in the last fraction collected sediment for a longer time than the cells in the first fraction collected, the s value (in mm/hr) for fraction N is given by Eq. (6).

$$s(N) = \frac{(N_f - N - \frac{1}{2})v - (V_0 + \frac{1}{2}V_{cb} - V_f)}{a[(t_4 - t_1) - 0.4(t_4 + t_2 - t_3 - t_1) + N(t_5 - t_4)/N_f]} \qquad (6)$$

where the times t_1 to t_5 (all in hours) are, respectively, the times at which loading started (t_1), the cells reach the top of the cone (t_2), draining started (t_3), first fraction started (t_4), and last fraction finished (t_5), a is the chamber constant, i.e., the milliliters of fluid per millimeter of length in the cylindrical region of the chamber. If one uses a chamber in which the cells are unloaded through a second conical region on top of the chamber (8), and if one loads the chamber to the bottom of the upper cone for sedimentation and collects all the chamber contents, the above expression takes on a slightly different form [Eq. (7)].

$$s(N) = \frac{(N - \frac{1}{2})v - (V_o + \frac{1}{2}V_{cb})}{a[(t_4 - t_1) - 0.4(t_4 + t_2 - t_3 - t_1) + N(t_5 - t_4)/N_f]} \qquad (7)$$

Equations (6) and (7) are still not exact because of variations in the loading rate and the finite thickness of the cell band, but they should be correct to within 1–2% if the cells spend less than 10% of the total sedimentation time in the conical portion of the chamber.

Calculation of accurate s values for the sedimentation chamber of Fig. 3 is much more difficult because a simple analytic expression for the cone correction factor cannot be obtained. Assuming the chamber to be unloaded from the top, and its entire contents to be collected

$$s(N) = \frac{(N - \frac{1}{2})v - (V_o + \frac{1}{2}V_{cb})}{a[(t_2 - t_1) + fN(t_3 - t_2)/N_f]} \qquad (8)$$

where t_1 is the time the cells are loaded and the chamber is rotated to the sedimentation position, t_2 the time the chamber is rotated back and the first fraction started, t_3 the time the last fraction, N_f, is finished, and f an undetermined constant, which should be approximately equal to l/D, l and D being chamber depth and diameter, respectively.

In establishing standard conditions for sedimentation, temperature control is of critical importance. From the sedimentation [Eq. (1)] it is seen that s is inversely proportional to the coefficient of viscosity. The viscosity of the BSA in PBS solutions used does not differ appreciably from water. The most viscous material used, 2% BSA in PBS, has a viscosity only about 2% greater than that of distilled water. However, the viscosity of water decreases 36% between 4° and 20°C, the rate of change being greatest near 4°C. It has been verified experimentally (4) that the s value for sheep erythrocytes increases accordingly.

4. Applications

This section describes some representative sedimentation experiments chosen to illustrate artifacts and limitations of the method, relative merits of measuring activity or enrichment profiles for cell types of interest, and some applications of biological interest.

Figure 5 shows the results of an experiment in which mouse bone marrow was sedimented and one fraction from the separation run a second time under identical conditions in an attempt to determine the ultimate resolution of the system. The starting bands were 1 mm thick, the sedimentation times were 4 hr, and the sedimentation chamber was of the type shown in Fig. 3 ("muffin").

Reproducible sedimentation profiles can be obtained over more than a 100-fold variation in cell concentration. Therefore, the results have been plotted on a logarithmic scale. The peaks in the total cell count profile in the regions of $s = 2$, 3, and 5 mm/hr are primarily mature red cells, lymphoid cells, and granuloid cells, respectively. However, some of the remaining profile is artifact.

Cell counts performed with the electronic cell detector indicate a peak at $s = 0.2$ mm/hr. Counts performed visually with a microscope indicate almost no cells in this region. This peak corresponds to cell debris. It is almost completely absent when the FCS wash procedure described in Section 3.3 is used. The shoulder in the profile in the region of $s = 7$ is also mostly artifact. It arises from cell doublets (primarily granulocyte doublets) present in the initial cell suspension, as shown by the doublet profile in the figure, which was determined by microscopic examination of the fractions. Theoretically [Eq. (2)], a doublet formed between two spheres of the same volume should sediment $2^{2/3}$ times as fast as the single spheres themselves. This has been verified experimentally using plastic spheres of known volume. The shoulder in the nucleated cell profile in the $s = 2$ region appears to consist almost entirely of nonviable cells (mostly lymphocytes) as determined by the fluorescein diacetate viability test. The

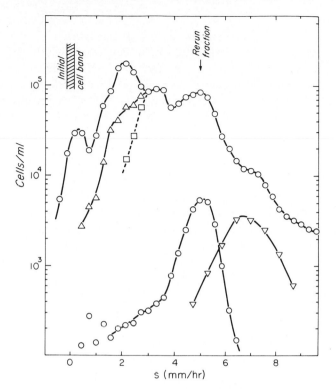

Fig. 5. Sedimentation profile of mouse bone marrow cells. One fraction from the separation (indicated by the arrow) was run a second time under identical conditions. ○, Total cells/ml as measured in an electronic cell detector for the initial separation (upper curve) and the rerun fraction (lower curve); △, nucleated cells/ml as measured visually with a microscope (where different from total cell count) in the initial separation; □, viable cells/ml as measured visually using FDA viability test (where different from total cell count) in the initial separation; ▽, doublets/ml as measured visually (mainly granulocyte doublets) in the initial separation.

magnitude of this peak increases with increasing harshness of the procedures used to prepare the cell suspension.

The s values of the various peaks in the profile are reproducible to an accuracy of at least 5% from one run to another, provided the separation conditions, particularly temperature, are maintained constant. Thus, for the conditions used (defined earlier), mouse red cells have a modal s value of 2.0 ± 0.1 mm/hr.

The mean s value of the rerun fraction is within 1% of its initial value. This indicates that the sedimentation properties of the cells do not change throughout the separation procedure. However, the rerun peak is very broad $[(\delta s/s) =$

0.20; see Section 3.2], broader than can be explained on the basis of diffusion or the finite widths of the starting bands. Similar results ($\delta s/s \geqslant 0.18$) are obtained if one repeats the experiment with Dow beads, which clearly cannot change in any way during the two separations. Thus, the broad width of the rerun peak must be taken as a measure of the intrinsic resolution of the system. Any measurement (e.g., a functional assay for cells of a particular type) that leads to a sedimentation profile with a width less than this limit must be viewed with suspicion.

Consider, next, an experiment in which the sedimentation profile of a particular subclass of cells is determined using an assay of cell function. The cells investigated were mouse spleen antibody-forming cells (AFC) making IgG antibody against sheep erythrocytes. These were obtained 4 days after a second immunization of the mouse with sheep erythrocytes. A single-cell suspension was made from mouse spleen and fractionated by sedimentation. Each fraction was assayed for its content of IgG AFC using the Jerne plaque assay [for details, see (5)].

Figure 6 shows the results of one such experiment. The starting band was 1.7 mm thick, sedimentation time was 3.5 hr, and the sedimentation chamber was of the type shown in Fig. 1. Nucleated and total cell count profiles are similar to those in Fig. 5 except that spleen contains far fewer granuloid cells than bone marrow so that there is not a peak in the $s = 5$ mm/hr region. However, there is a pronounced red cell peak at 2.0 mm/hr, and a lymphocyte peak at 3.1 mm/hr. Similarly, there is a debris peak at $s = 0.3$ mm/hr and a peak of nonviable nucleated cells (mostly lymphocytes) in the $s = 2$ mm/hr region.

The AFC content of each fraction was measured and is expressed on the figure both as an activity profile (AFC/ml) and as an enrichment profile (AFC/nucleated cell). Maximum activity is found around $s = 4.4$ mm/hr; maximum enrichment is found in two peaks at higher s values.

Calculation of the recovery of the cell of interest is very simple with an activity profile. Thus, in Fig. 6, one merely adds up the number of AFC/ml in each fraction (i.e., the values plotted), multiplies by the fraction volume, and compares the result with the total number of AFC loaded. For the experiment in Fig. 6, the recovery was 90%.

If one is using an assay that depends upon cell function for a response to occur, it is essential to have complete knowledge of the dose-response curve (the ideal being linearity) and to know that it is independent of relative enrichment or depletion of other cell types present in the unfractionated tissue. It was verified that the Jerne plaque assay, under the conditions used for the experiment of Fig. 6, had a linear dose–response curve independent of the number of AFC plated, total number of cells plated, or relative enrichment and depletion of particular cell types. Given all this, it is simple to construct either activity or enrichment profiles. However, very few functional assays have all these proper-

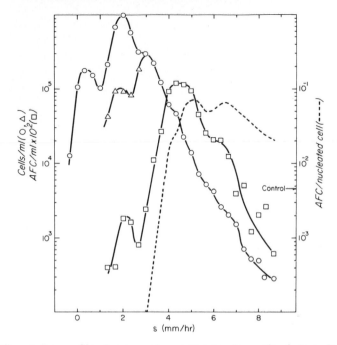

Fig. 6. Sedimentation profile of mouse spleen cells taken from mice 4 days after a second immunization with sheep erythrocytes. ○, Total cells/ml; △, nucleated cells/ml (when different from the total cell count); □, antibody-forming cells (AFC)/ml. The dashed line is antibody-forming cells per nucleated cell referred to right-hand axis, on which the control value is indicated.

ties, and to get meaningful profiles it may be necessary to measure dose–response curves on individual fractions. By doing this, it is sometimes possible to get meaningful activity and enrichment profiles even using a nonlinear functional assay.

The experiment in Fig. 6 has been repeated more than ten times. Although the modal sedimentation velocity of the IgG AFC was the same (4.4 ± 0.2 mm/hr) in all experiments, the peak was always much broader than that routinely obtained with other types of cells such as red cells or lymphocytes, and the shape tended to vary from one experiment to the next. An explanation for the broadness of the peak can be found from the fact that AFC are a population of dividing cells. If a cell has a volume $2V_o$ just before mitosis, then its daughters just after mitosis will have volumes V_o. In a randomly dividing population, if N_o cells are entering mitosis, then $2N_o$ cells should be leaving mitosis (see Fig. 7a, top). If one assumes that the density of a cell is independent of position in the cell cycle, then [from Eq. (2)] when the volume doubles, the sedimentation rate should

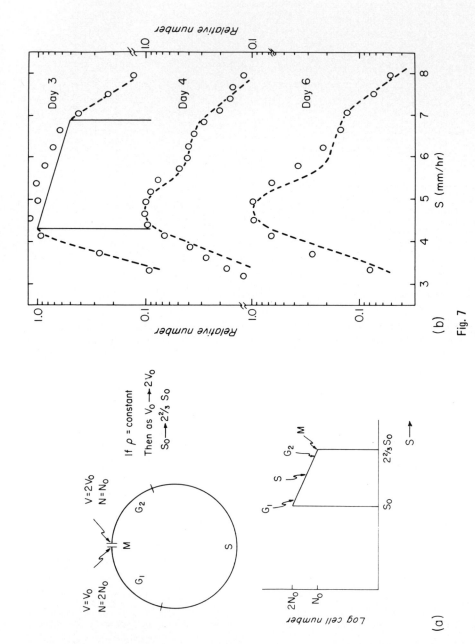

Fig. 7

increase by $2^{2/3}$. Such a population of cells should have sedimentation profile resembling that shown in Fig. 7b (bottom).

Thus, the variability in shape of the IgG AFC profile of Fig. 6 can be explained by noting that 4 days after immunization, the time at which the profile was measured, corresponds to the time of maximum number of IgG AFC. One might expect cell division to stop at about this time. However, if one compares the IgG AFC profiles 3 days and 6 days after immunization, then the AFC should be mostly in or out of cell cycle, respectively (see Fig. 7b). The day 3 profile fits the theoretical distribution rather well. The day 6 profile suggests that, when a cell stops dividing, it does so with a volume close to that of a cell just leaving mitosis. The variability seen on day 4 can be explained as a variable composite population of dividing and nondividing cells. Note that this model for the sedimentation distribution of AFC was based entirely on an analysis of the activity profile. Such an analysis is almost impossible starting from the enrichment profile, since it is determined by the distribution of other (irrelevant) cells as well as that of the AFC.

The definitive test of the cell-cycle model just outlined would be to demonstrate directly that different parts of the profile are in different parts of the cell cycle by scoring for, e.g., mitotic AFC and AFC undergoing DNA synthesis. This direct experiment is difficult because AFC are a minority population in the fractions collected. Thus, in Fig. 6, the most purified fraction is only about 8% AFC (corresponding to an 18-fold enrichment over unfractionated cells), and the most purified fractions obtained in any experiments were still only 28% AFC. [The highest enrichment over control in the series was 110-fold and was not correlated with purification (5)].

A direct test of the model is most simply made by investigating a homogeneous population of cells, all of which are in cycle. To this end, the sedimentation profile of mouse L cells, in asynchronous exponential growth in suspension culture, was investigated (6). The sedimentation profile from one experiment is shown in Fig. 8. The peak at $s \sim 4.5$ corresponds to cell fragments and the profile beyond $s = 18$ is largely clumps and polyploid cells. The limits of the theoretical sedimentation distribution, assuming no density variation through the cell cycle

---

Fig. 7. Relationship of cell growth and division cycle to sedimentation profile. (a) Above: Cell cycle model. M represents the period during which the cell is in mitosis, S the period when the cell is replicating its DNA, and G_1 and G_2 the two intervening periods. Below: Theoretical sedimentation profile for a homogeneous population of cells all in completely asynchronous exponential growth and having cell density independent of position in the cell cycle. (b) IgG antibody-forming cell activity profile measured 3 days, 4 days, and 6 days after a second immunization with sheep erythrocytes. The solid line on the day 3 profile is the theoretical curve shown in (a). The dashed line in all three curves represents the theoretical curve broadened by the known finite resolution of the sedimentation equation and includes a progressively increasing noncycling component on days 4 and 6.

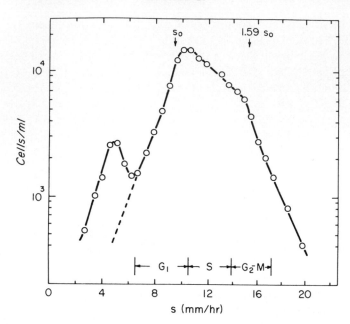

Fig. 8. Sedimentation profile of mouse L cells in asynchronous exponential growth. The dashed line extrapolates the true cell distribution into the region of cell debris.

and perfect resolution for the sedimentation separation, are indicated on the figure by arrows. The cells were pulse labeled with ^{3}H-thymidine before separation, and the fractions were scored for percent labeled cells and percent mitosis after fractionation. By defining S phase to be the region of the distribution in which the percentage of ^{3}H-labeled thymidine cells exceeds the asynchronous control and by excluding the outermost 4% of the cell-concentration distribution as being clumps and polyploid cells at large s, and debris at small s, one can establish the boundaries of G_1, S, and G_2-M, as shown on the figure. The percentage of cells found in each phase in this manner is in excellent agreement with the values found by other methods (6).

From Eq. (2), one can see that if all cells have the same density, then $s = kV^{2/3}$, or $\log s = k' + \frac{2}{3} \log V$ so that a plot of $\log s$ versus $\log V$ would have a slope of $\frac{2}{3}$. Volume distributions were obtained for the L cell fractions using the volume spectrometer described earlier. A plot of $\log s$ versus $\log V_o$, where V_o is the modal volume of the volume distribution obtained for each fraction, does indeed fit a straight line with slope of about $\frac{2}{3}$ (6). However, this plot fails to utilize much of the information contained in the volume distributions. The latter vary in shape as well as modal volume, and this shape variation appears to reflect real properties of the cells being analyzed. This information can all be represented on a contour map in which cell sedimentation velocity and volume are the independent variables and contours of equal cell number are plotted as illustrated in Fig. 9.

Figure 10 shows such a contour map or "fingerprint" for mouse L cells in exponential growth. The contours of equal cell number represent 2-fold changes in cell concentration. Thus, contour 10 represents 2^{10} cells per milliliter per s interval per V interval. The data points give modal volume as a function of s and can be fitted reasonably well with a straight line parallel to the slanted lines shown, which are contours of equal density calculated from Eq. (2). From the figure, the mean density of the cells is about 1.048 g/cm^3, not significantly different from the density of 1.051 g/cm^3 (6) measured on a continuous Ficoll density gradient (21), and density is approximately independent of position in the cell cycle. However, some very small cells appear to have an anomalously high density, and some very large cells appear to have an anomalously low density. Fingerprints of more complex cell suspensions show much more complicated structure and may give information difficult to obtain in any other way. In particular, such fingerprints may be useful in distinguishing between various myeloproliferative disorders of human bone marrow (22).

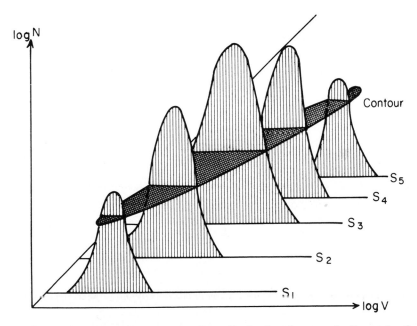

Fig. 9. Schematic representation of the volume distributions for several adjacent fractions from a velocity sedimentation separation indicating how the data are to be combined to form a contour map ("fingerprint") as in Fig. 10.

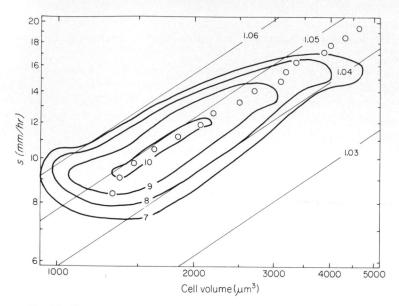

Fig. 10. Fingerprint of mouse L cells in asynchronous exponential growth.

The basic procedures outlined in this chapter have been successfully applied in studies of the cerebellum, pituitary gland, lung, liver, hemopoietic system, sperm development, and various tumor systems as well as cellular immunology. Our cell separation studies of B and T lymphocyte differentiation have been recently reviewed (23).

REFERENCES

1. Shortman, K., *Annu. Rev. Biophys. Bioeng.* **1**, 93 (1972).
2. Shortman, K., *Contemp. Top. Mol. Immunol.* **3**, 161 (1974).
3. Bonner, W. A., Hulett, H. R., Sweet, R. G., and Herzenberg, L. A., *Rev. Sci. Instrum.* **43**, 404 (1972).
4. Miller, R. G., and Phillips, R. A., *J. Cell. Physiol.* **73**, 191 (1969).
5. Phillips, R. A., and Miller, R. G., *Cell Tissue Kinet.* **3**, 263 (1970).
6. MacDonald, H. R., and Miller, R. G., *Biophys. J.* **10**, 834 (1970).
7. Mel, H. C., *Nature (London)* **200**, 423 (1963).
8. Peterson, E. A., and Evans, W. H., *Nature (London)* **214**, 824 (1967).
9. Edwards, G. E., Miller, R. G., and Phillips, R. A., *J. Immunol.* **105**, 719 (1970).
10. Tulp, A., and Bont, W. S., *Anal. Biochem.* **67**, 11 (1975).
11. Shortman, K., Williams, N., and Adams, P., *J. Immunol. Meth.* **1**, 273 (1972).
12. Rotman, B., and Papermaster, B. W., *Proc. Natl. Acad. Sci. U.S.A.* **55**, 134 (1966).
13. Pappenheimer, A. M., *J. Exp. Med.* **25**, 633 (1917).
14. Meistrich, M. L., *J. Cell. Physiol.* **80**, 299 (1972).
15. Coulter, W. H., U.S. Patent, 2,656,508 (1953).
16. Kubitschek, H. E., *Research* **13**, 128 (1960).

17. Harvey, R. J., *in* "Methods in Cell Physiology" (D. M. Prescott, ed.), Vol. III, p. 1. Academic Press, New York. (1968).
18. Taylor, W. B., *Med. Biol. Eng.* 8, 281 (1970).
19. Grover, N. B., Naaman, J., Ben-Sasson, S., and Dolijanski, F., *Biophys. J.* 9, 1398 (1969).
20. Miller, R. G., and Wuest, L. J., *Ser. Haematol.* 2, 128 (1972).
21. Gorczynski, R. M., Miller, R. G., and Phillips, R. A., *Immunology* 19, 817 (1970).
22. Moon, R., Phillips, R. A., and Miller, R. G., *Ser. Haematol.* 2, 163 (1972).
23. Miller, R. G., Gorczynski, R. M., Lafleur, L., MacDonald, H. R., and Phillips, R. A., *Transplant. Rev.* 25, 59 (1975).

Charge Fractionation of Lymphoid Cells*

P. Häyry, S. Nordling, and L. C. Andersson

1. Introduction

Mammalian cells in a physiological milieu carry a net negative surface charge. The charge density of different cell types varies to some extent. Accordingly, the differently charged cells have different anodic mobilities in an electrical field.

The first methods for the measurement of the electrophoretic mobility (and electrical surface charge density) of individual cells were based on the microscopic analysis of the mobilities of cells in an electric field. These methods have been discussed at length by, e.g., Brinton and Lauffer (1) and in a book edited by Ambrose (2). A major breakthrough in *preparative* fractionation of cells possessing different surface charges was the development of the "continuous deflection electrophoresis principle" (3). This field has been pioneered by Hannig and his collaborators (4).

Free-flow electrophoresis has proved to be a useful and reproducible method for the fractionation of the major lymphocyte subpopulations, both resting and activated T and B lymphocytes in all rodent species investigated (mouse, rat, guinea pig). Although a difference in the electrophoretic mobility of human T and B cells has been observed in analytical cell electrophoresis, the charge difference is not big enough to allow their preparative fractionation (5). In the mouse, newly formed and long-lived T cells have somewhat different electrophoretic mobilities, although present equipment does not permit their preparative fractionation either (5).

Cell electrophoresis can also be combined with other physical methods of cell fractionation, e.g., with density fractionation or 1 g velocity sedimentation.

---

*Abbreviations used: B, thymus-independent lymphocyte; CLM, cell-mediated lysis (after priming in MLC); E-RFC, cells forming rosettes with normal erythrocytes; EAC–RFC, cells forming rosettes with antibody and complement-coated erythrocytes; GVH, graft vs host (reaction); HMC, high-mobility (T) cells in electrophoresis; LMC, low-mobility (B) cells in electrophoresis; LPS, *Escherichia coli* lipopolysaccharide; MEM, Eagle's minimal essential medium; MLC, mixed lymphocyte culture (reaction); PFC, plaque-forming cell; PHA, phytohemagglutinin-M; RFC, rosette-forming cell; T, thymus-dependent lymphocyte.

The main advantages of the electrophoretic method are that no immunological manipulation of the cells is required and that (in contrast to, e.g., affinity column chromatography) all fractionated populations are directly recovered. Preparative cell electophoresis carries a reasonable capacity and enables fractionation of up to 60×10^6 cells/hr. The major disadvantages are the high basic cost of the equipment and the laborious sterilization procedure required for aseptical fractionation of cells. Furthermore, preparative fractionation of diverse subclasses of lymphoid cells is presently limited to the fractionation of the major subpopulations. Thus, selective preparation of small populations of lymphoid cells (e.g., cells carrying a given idiotypic receptor specificity) has not been accomplished.

Hannig (4) has given a detailed technical description of the most commonly used preparative free-flow electrophoretic device, Desaga FF4 (Desaga GmbH, Heidelberg). At least the following groups have also reported results on preparative charge-fractionation of lymphoid cells: Hannig and collaborators (6) and von Boehmer, Shortman, and Nossal (7). For their technical procedures the reader is referred to the original articles.

2. Materials

2.1. Equipment. Figure 1 shows the working principle of the Free Flow Electrophoresis Model FF4 (Desaga GmbH, Heidelberg, Germany). The main part of the device developed by Hannig used in our laboratory is a vertical separation chamber. The chamber consists of two glass plates 0.5 mm apart. The chamber is 50 cm high and 12 cm wide and has 92 outlet tubes at its lower end. The electrode chambers are located on both sides of the separation chamber. They are separated from the separation chamber by ion-exchange membranes.

A buffer solution of low ionic strength and physiological pH is continuously introduced to the upper rim of the separation chamber, and it flows vertically in a laminar fashion at a right angle to the electrical field. The cells suspended in the buffer are continuously injected into the separation chamber through a hole in the front glass by a peristaltic pump. The cells migrate sideways toward the anode owing to their negative net charge density and downward in the buffer stream owing to the velocity of the laminar buffer flow and are collected through the outlet tubes at the lower end of the separation chamber. The deflection is directly proportional to the surface charge density of the cell and to the strength of the electrical field, and in theory is inversely proportional to the streaming velocity of the buffer and to the square root of the ionic strength of the buffer. The last condition does not hold for very low ionic strengths, i.e., in the millimolar regions, because of adsorption and other phenomena.

Thus a higher electrical field strength gives a broader separation. For the separation of lymphocytes we have used a field strength of 100 V/cm and a

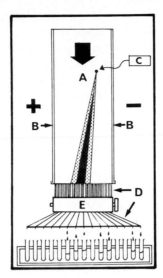

Fig. 1. Principle of the Desaga FF4 Free Flow Electrophoresis apparatus. A, separation chamber; B, electrode chambers; C, cell suspension and the site of injection; D, outlet tubes and fraction collector; E, 92-channel peristaltic pump that regulates the flow rate of the electrophoresis buffer. For details see Hannig (4).

current of 100 mA. These values are close to the upper limit of this equipment because, despite the low ionic strength of the electrophoresis buffer, there is considerable generation of heat. With a higher field strength, and consequently current, the capacity of the cooling system (Peltier elements attached to the back plate of the separation chamber in the FF4) is exceeded.

The vertical streaming velocity of the electrophoresis buffer should be kept low to keep the cells long in the electric field, but velocities of less than about 10 cm/min result in turbulences in the chamber. A homogeneous electrical field is essential for the linear flow of the particles to be separated. This is achieved by removing electrolysis products generated around the electrodes by a rapid, continuous flow of the electrode buffer through the electrode chambers.

2.2. Electrophoresis Buffer. The electrophoresis buffer used for fractionation of living cells must be isoosmolar and the pH within physiological limits. The correct osmolarity cannot be attained with salts alone, as the conductivity would be too high. The osmolarity is therefore made up by adding substances that do not themselves contribute to the conductivity, i.e., do not dissociate. Sucrose, glucose, and glycine are usually used for this purpose. For fractionation of lymphoid cells we have used a buffer developed by Hannig (4): 0.04 M potassium acetate, 0.015 M triethanolamine, 0.24 M glycine, pH 7.35, made isotonic with 0.011 M glucose and 0.03 M sucrose.

2.3. Electrode Buffer. The electrode compartment is completely separated from the main chambers by ion-exchange membranes. Thus the electrode buffer does not have to be isoosmolar. It must have a good buffer capacity because the electrolysis products tend to alter the pH. An electrode buffer suitable for our purposes is, e.g., 0.075 M triethanolamine and 4 mM potassium acetate in water.

2.4. Sterilization of the Device. The electrophoresis buffer with its high sugar content is an excellent culture medium for bacteria and especially for fungi. When the separated cells are used for *in vitro* experiments the conditions must be aseptic. Sterilization of the separation chamber can be performed with 1% formaldehyde or 0.2% chlorodioxide (left in the chamber overnight) followed by rinsing with several (3–5) liters of sterile water. The electrode chambers can be sterilized similarly with 1% formaldehyde followed by rinsing with water.

For details on the construction of the apparatus and its use, we refer to the original publications of Hannig and collaborators (4, 6).

3. Methods

3.1. Preparation of Cells. This is exemplified in the mouse; for preparation of cells of other species the method must be modified accordingly. The *thymus, spleen,* and *lymph nodes* are teased apart in 5% fetal calf serum containing Eagle's minimal essential medium (MEM) at +4°C on ice. The cell clumps are removed by sedimentation or by filtration through a loose cotton wool plug. Phagocytic cells are removed by incubation 100 $\times$ 10^6 cells in 10 ml of fetal calf serum containing MEM with 3 mg of carbonyl iron (GAF, Svenska Ab, Stockholm, Sweden) at 37°C for 30 min and by immersing a magnet bar into the cell suspension. Alternatively, the cell suspension is incubated in the same medium on glass for two 30-min periods at 37°C, and nonadherent cells are decanted for use. The red cells are lysed by suspending a cell button containing up to 100 $\times$ 10^6 cells in 0.83% ammonium chloride for 10 min at 4°C. This treatment results in reasonably well purified ($>$ 95%) populations of lymphoid cells from the thymus and the lymph nodes; the spleen cell population is still contaminated by approximately 20% of nonphagocytic precursor cells. Highly purified ($>$ 95%) small mouse spleen lymphocytes are obtained by 1 g velocity sedimentation and by removal of the large-sized precursor cells by the procedure (5).

Blood white cells are obtained by sedimentation of heparinized mouse blood with an equal volume of Plasmagel (Roger Bellon, Neuilly, France) for 15 min at 37°C. The white cells are recovered from the top layer and the remaining red cells are lysed by ammonium chloride. The bulk of granulocytes is removed by iron powder plus magnetic treatment as above. These procedures result in a population containing more than 90% blood lymphocytes.

3.2. Transfer of Cells to the Electrophoresis Buffer. For electrophoresis the cells are transferred into the electrophoresis buffer. This buffer tends to make cells stick together. This can be prevented to a great extent by using a step-by-step transfer. After one wash in cold serum-free medium, the cells are resuspended in the medium and mixed with an equal volume of cold buffer. After centrifugation in cold (90 g for 8 min), the pellet is resuspended in cold buffer. Clumps are removed by filtration through a loose cotton wool plug. After an additional wash with the buffer, the cell concentration is adjusted to a maximum of 20 $\times$ 10^6 cells/ml, and the electrophoretic separation is performed. All operations should be done rapidly at temperatures below 5°C.

3.3. Electrophoresis Procedure. The cell suspension of a maximum of 20 $\times$ 10^6 cells/hr is injected into the electrophoresis chamber at a flow rate of 3 ml/min at the most. With a vertical chamber electrolyte flow of 280 ml/hr, each cell remains in the electrical field for about 300 sec. The fractions are collected into test tubes immersed in ice. One milliliter of MEM containing 20% fetal calf serum in the collecting tubes minimizes cell damage. The procedure allows the fractionation of up to 60 $\times$ 10^6 cells per hour with a viability exceeding 95% of the fractionated cells as judged by trypan blue exclusion.

3.4. Data Processing. Rodent lymphocytes separate into two main peaks with some overlap. For preparative purposes it is sufficient to discard the overlapping fractions. For analytical purposes it is necessary to resolve the distribution patterns. If it is assumed that the populations have Gaussian distribution the semigraphical resolution methods developed by Bhattacharya (8) can be used (because computer programs are not readily available). In most cases this method gives a fairly good resolution into two main peaks, but leaves "tails," especially in the the anodic end. When one of the populations is small, $<$5 to 10% of total, the method is less satisfactory.

4. Examples of Charge Fractionation of Lymphoid Cells

4.1. Fractionation of Mouse T and B Lymphocytes in Resting State. When *spleen, lymph node,* or *blood* lymphocytes from nonimmunized mice are fractionated in free-flow electrophoresis, two populations of cells with different mobilities can be distinguished: a population with low electrophoretic mobility (LMC) and a population with high electrophoretic mobility (HMC) (Fig. 2). The peak fractions are located 4 or 5 tubes apart. Since the electrophoretic mobilities of nonlymphocytic hematopoietic cells overlap with the mobilities of lymphocytes, biphasic Gaussian-type distribution patterns of spleen cells can be obtained only when highly purified (e.g., by 1 g velocity sedimentation) small lymphocytes are used for fractionation (Fig. 2).

The distribution pattern of purified *bone marrow* lymphocytes and thymus cells is monophasic. The majority of the thymus cells have an electrophoretic mobility only slightly higher than that of the lymph node and spleen LMC. In the thymus there is also a smaller (5–10%) cell population located in the HMC

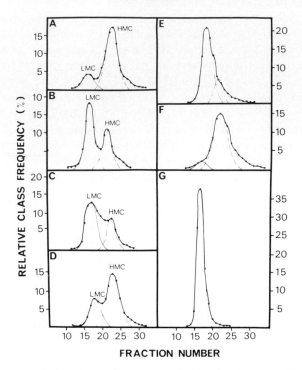

Fig. 2. Mouse: separation profiles of lymphocytes. (A) Lymph node cells (CBA). (B) Spleen lymphocytes (purified by 1 g velocity sedimentation; CBA). (C) Spleen cells (about 80% of which were lymphocytes) purified by iron powder plus magnetic treatment (random-bred mouse). (D) Blood lymphocytes (phagocytic cells removed with iron powder plus magnet; random-bred mouse). (E) Thymus cells (C3H). (F) Thymus cells (C3H) 2 days after injection of hydrocortisone. (G) Bone marrow lymphocytes (purified by 1 g velocity sedimentation; CBA). The curves have been resolved into Gaussian distributions by a semigraphical method.

area. Two days after injection of 2.5 mg of hydrocortisone acetate, there are mainly HMC thymus cells left, a finding which indicates that HMC thymus cells are more "mature" medullary type of cells (Fig. 2).

The fractionated spleen and lymph node cells have been characterized by the following procedures (Table 1). The results unequivocally demonstrate that the HMC fractions contain the T cells and the LMC fractions the B cells. To obtain reasonably "pure" (> 95%) T and B cells for experimentation, the intermediary fractions containing overlapping populations of T and B cells must be discarded.

4.2. Fractionation of T and B Lymphocytes of Other Species in Their Resting State. Preparative fractionation of spleen, blood, and lymph node T and B

TABLE 1
Characterization of Electrophoretically Separated Mouse Lymphocytes

Test	Source of cells	Result LMC	Result HMC
Cytotoxic effect of anti-θ + C′	CBA spleen, lymph node	−	+
Cytotoxic effect of anti-MBLA + C′	CBA spleen, lymph node	+	−
Complement receptor bearing cells (EAC-RFC)	CBA spleen, lymph node	+	−
Presence of surface Ig (FITC-anti-Ig positive cells)	CBA spleen	+	−
Adherence in anti-Ig column	CBA spleen, lymph node	+	−
Response to PHA *in vitro*	CBA spleen, blood	−	+
Response to LPS *in vitro*	CBA spleen	+	−
Ability to mount GVH reaction	CBA spleen to newborn (CBAxA)F$_1$ mice i.v.	−	+

lymphocytes has first been achieved in the rat (9). Lymphocytes from guinea pig blood and lymph nodes can also be separated into two different populations with T cells in the HMC population and the B cells in the LMC population (10). Electrophoresis of guinea pig spleen lymphocytes results in one single peak that contains both T and B cells (10). Whether this reflects the presence of different subpopulations of T cells in guinea pig spleen and lymph nodes is not known. Preparative fractionation of the T and B lymphocytes of subhuman primates has been reported by Seiler *et al.* (11). In our experience, preparative fractionation of human blood, tonsillar, and spleen lymphocytes by our equipment is not possible, but the T and B cells distribute in one (though broad) peak in largely overlapping populations (5).

4.3. Fractionation of Newly Formed and Long-Lived Mouse T Lymphocytes.

There is a small though definite difference in the surface charge densities of newly formed vs. long-lived resting mouse spleen and lymph node T cells. Thus, if a mouse is labeled *in vivo* with ^{3}H-thymidine and the spleen and lymph node cells are passed through an Ig-anti-Ig-coated column prior to the electrophoresis procedure, the labeled T cells distribute in slower moving (T) fractions than do the nonlabeled T cells (5). Noteworthy, however, is that the differences in the net negative surface charge densities are not great enough to enable preparative fractionation of the populations.

4.4. Electrophoretic Distribution of Immune Lymphocytes. It is noteworthy that the electrophoretic mobility of lymphocytes—especially that of B cells—may alter after being triggered to an immune response. When CBA mice are injected i.p. with 5×10^8 sheep erythrocytes and the electrophoretic distribution of the anti-sheep erythrocyte antibody-producing spleen cells, determined by modified Cunningham PFC assay, is compared to that of resting B cells, an increased electrophoretic mobility is observed. As shown in Fig. 3, the direct 19 S PFC have a higher anodal mobility than the cells carrying abundant surface Ig (resting B cells). The indirect (7 S) PFC showed a further increased mobility, and distribute in the area between the HMC and LMC of resting spleen and also

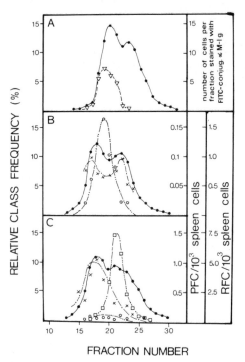

Fig. 3. Localization of mouse cells containing surface immunoglobulin, SRBC rosette-forming cells, and direct and indirect PFC in the electrophoresis profile in resting state and after immunization with SRBC. (A) Cells giving positive staining with FITC-conjugated anti-mouse-Ig (△———△). (B and C) cells forming rosettes (x — · —x) and giving direct (o — ·· —o) and indirect (□ — ·· —□) plaques with SRBC at 4 (B) and 12 (C) days after intraperitoneal immunization with 8×10^6 SRBC.

overlap with the HMC. These findings demonstrate an increased electrophoretic mobility of the B lymphocytes along their course of antigen-induced differentiation toward the plasma cell. This should be kept in mind when electrophoretic separation of immune spleen cells is attempted.

The effect of immunization on the electrokinetic behavior of the T cells is negligible. When CBA mice are given a single i.p. injection of allogeneic cells, the killer (T) cells (as determined by ^{51}Cr release assay against relevant target cells) are always located within the HMC. Thus there is no demonstrable change in the net surface charge density in activated T cells, at least when tested in the direct cytotoxicity assay.

The electrophoretic mobility of T killer cells recovered from day 6 one-way mixed lymphocyte culture has also been tested. The MLC-activated killer cells are located in the HMC fractions.

4.5. Localization of the "K" Cells in the Electrophoresis Profile. The "K" cells—lymphoid and nonlymphoid cells able to lyse antibody-coated target cells—constitute heterogeneous population of cells with one common denominator, receptor to Fc-part of IgG. In the chicken red cell–anti-chicken red cell system the spleen killer cells distribute in the intermediary fractions between the T and B peaks of nonimmune mouse spleen cells (12).

4.6. Comments. Rodent lymphocytes separating in electrophoresis into the high-mobility (HMC) and the low-mobility (LMC) populations represent highly purified populations of T and B lymphocytes. When the overlapping fractions are omitted, the contamination of B cells among the HMC and of T cells among the LMC is always less than 5%. Although preparative fractionation of the T and B lymphocytes of subhuman primates has also been reported, in our experience this has not been achieved in man. The free-flow electrophoresis can also distinguish between newly formed and long-lived T cells in the mouse, though preparative fractionation is not possible in this respect, either.

The main advantages of the electrophoretic fractionation method are that no (immunological) manipulation of the cells to be fractionated is necessary and that all fractionated populations are directly recovered. The major drawbacks are the high cost of the equipment and the rather complicated technical procedure required for its operation.

REFERENCES

1. Brinton, C. C., and Lauffer, M. A., in "Electrophoresis, Theory, Methods and Applications" (M. Bier, ed.), p. 427. Academic Press, New York, 1959.
2. Ambrose, E. J. (ed.), "Cell Electrophoresis," p. 204. Churchill, London, 1965.
3. Svensson, H., and Brattsten, I., Ark. Kemi 1:401 (1949).
4. Hannig, K., Methods Microbiol. 5B,513 (1971).
5. Häyry, P., Andersson, L. C., Gahmberg, C., Roberts, P., Ranki, A., and Nordling, S., Isr. J. Med. Sci. 11, 1299 (1975).
6. Hannig, K., Techniques Biochem. Biophys. Morphol. 1,191 (1972).

7. von Boehmer, H., Shortman, K., and Nossal, G. J. V., *J. Cell. Physiol.* **83,** 231 (1974).
8. Bhattacharya, C. G., *Biometrics* **23,** 115 (1967).
9. Zeiller, K., Hannig, K., and Pascher, G., *Hoppe-Seyler's Z. Physiol. Chem.* **352,** 1168 (1971).
10. Andersson, L. C., Nordling, S., and Häyry, P., *J. Immunol.* **114,** 1226 (1975).
11. Seiler, F. R., Johanssen, R., Sedlacek, H. H., and Zeiller, K., *Transplant. Proc.* **6,** 173 (1974).
12. Wigzell, H., and Häyry, P., *Curr. Top. Microbiol. Immunol.* **67,** 1 (1974).

Application of the Virus Plaque Assay to Studies of Human Lymphocytes

Simon Sutcliffe, Anna Kadish, Gerald Stoner, and Barry R. Bloom

1. Introduction

Understanding of cellular immunology has been greatly enhanced by the study of lymphocyte populations *in vitro*. In the case of cell-mediated immunity, most *in vitro* studies have been concerned with problems at the qualitative or phenomenological level. In contrast, the Jerne plaque assay for antibody-forming cells has permitted detailed exploration of antibody formation at a more quantitative level.

In hopes of contributing to the more precise study of cell-mediated immunity, we have developed a virus plaque assay (VPA) for enumerating activated lymphocytes. The experimental basis for the assay derives from the observations of many laboratories that resting lymphocytes are incapable of permitting replication of a wide variety of RNA and DNA viruses, and that, upon activation by mitogens or antigens, they rapidly acquire the ability to produce infectious virus (reviewed in 1–3). In the virus plaque assay, lymphocytes are cultured for various periods of time in the presence or in the absence of antigen or mitogen, and then aliquots of cells are removed and tested for their ability to produce virus, generally vesicular stomatitis virus (VSV). By the use of an infectious centers technique (1, 4), the activated infected lymphocytes are plated in agar above a monolayer of indicator cells for the virus, so that it is possible to count individual virus-producing lymphocytes (virus plaque-forming cells or V-PFC). In the method described, the indicator cell for detecting virus is L cells, which can be grown in suspension culture and plated to make indicator monolayer for the assay.

In any lymphoid population studied, there is a background of virus-producing cells comprised generally of macrophages and some lymphocytes activated either *in vivo* or by the culture conditions *in vitro*. When lymph node cells from tuberculin-sensitive guinea pigs were stimulated with purified protein derivative of tuberculin (PPD) in culture, the maximum number of V-PFC above background capable of replication VSV was found to be approximately 20 per 10^3 cells (1). In cultures of human peripheral blood lymphocytes from tuberculin-positive donors, the increase in V-PFC above background was approximately 5 per 10^3 cells (4). In these studies it was observed that the increase in V-PFC was a linear function of time of stimulation and that development of some V-PFC was not affected by inhibitors of DNA synthesis or mitosis (4), suggesting the existence of an antigen-sensitive, nondividing cell. Classical-type kinetic studies indicated in the case of stimulation of antigen-sensitive lymphocytes that inter-action of two cells was required for the production of one virus-producing cell (5).

The nature of the cell type measured by the virus plaque assay has been investigated at two levels. When continuous lymphoblastoid cell lines were examined for V-PFC, it was found that mouse and human T-cell lines were permissive for replication of VSV, polio virus and NDV, while most B-cell lines were much less able to produce virus (6, 7). In studies of primary mouse spleen cultures activated with mitogens, concanavalin A (Con A), phytohemagglutinin (PHA), and pokeweed mitogen (PWM) induced high levels of V-PFC while lipopolysaccharide (LPS) failed to stimulate virus production (8). Essentially all virus-producing cells were eliminated by treatment with anti-Thy 1 serum plus complement either prior to stimulation or prior to plating after stimulation.

The precise molecular event in stimulated lymphocytes governing their ability to replicate virus remains unclear. In comparisons of permissive and nonpermis-sive lymphoblastoid cell lines, it was found that cells of both types could be infected and synthesize viral mRNA and viral proteins; however, only the permissive lines were seen to contain virion RNA. These results suggest that VSV was able to infect even nonpermissive cells, but that such cells could not support a complete virus replicative cycle (9, 10). Recent studies on primary human and mouse lymphocytes indicate that resting lymphocytes can be infected with VSV, but that the infection remains latent until the cells are activated at a later time (11).

In summary, the virus-plaque assay offers the potential of estimating the number of activated T lymphocytes in a cell population. However, while improved conditions for its application to human lymphoid cell populations are presented here, a number of important questions, namely, its selectivity for activated human T rather than B lymphocytes, its efficiency in detecting activated T cells, its possible selectivity for only a subpopulation of activated cells, will require further study.

2. Materials

2.1. Plasticware
2.1.1. Test tube, 12 × 75 mm (Falcon 2054)
2.1.2. Conical centrifuge tube, 50 ml (Falcon 2070)
2.1.3. Petri dish, 60 × 15 mm (Falcon 3002)
2.1.4. Syringe, 50 ml

2.2. Glassware

2.2.1. Long-tip pipettes, 1 ml (one for each plate)

2.2.2. Regular-tip pipettes, 1 ml (one for each plate)

2.2.3. Spinner flasks, 500-ml (Bellco glass)

2.2.4. 10 ml pipettes (one for 5–6 plates)

2.2.5. Glass beads (3 mm diameter) in sterile 125 ml Erlenmeyer flask

2.3. Needles

2.3.1. No. 18 or No. 19, thin walled

2.3.2. Disposable, lumbar puncture (for underlaying Ficoll–Hypaque)

2.4. Media and Sera

2.4.1. 1X Eagle's minimal essential medium (MEM) with 100 U of penicillin and 100 μg of streptomycin per milliliter, and 2 mM glutamine added freshly (GIBCO No. 109)

2.4.2. 2 X MEM as above

2.4.3. Joklik-modified Eagle's MEM for spinner cultures (GIBCO)

2.4.4. Phosphate-buffered saline (PBS), pH 7.2

2.4.5. Hanks' balanced salt solution containing penicillin, streptomycin (GIBCO)

2.4.6. Fetal calf serum, heat inactivated and Millipore-filtered before use (Rehcis Chemical Co., Chicago, Lot No. 24910)

2.4.7. Medium 1640 with added penicillin, streptomycin, and glutamine (GIBCO)

2.5. Solutions

2.5.1. Ficoll–Hypaque solution, specific gravity 1.077

2.5.2. PBS, pH 7.2

2.5.3. Neutral red solution, 15 mg/100 ml in PBS–Hanks' (1:1) prepared freshly, or 4% formol–saline, pH 7.2 and crystal violet (1 g in 200 ml of methanol + 800 ml of H_2O)

2.5.4. Ammonium chloride, 0.83%, in H_2O

2.5.5. Trypan blue solution, 0.2% in PBS

2.6. Mitogens and Antigens

Con A (Miles Laboratories)

PHA-P (Difco)

PWM (GIBCO)

PPD Stock, 1.25 mg/ml in Tris-saline, pH 7.2 (Ministry of Agriculture, Weybridge, England)

Streptokinase–streptodornase (SK-SD) 1000 U/ml in PBS (Lederle)

2.7. Virus and Anti-viral Antibody

2.7.1. Vesicular stomatitis virus, stock 2 X 10^9 to 5 X 10^9 PFU/ml stored at −70°C. Prepared as in Section 3.

2.7.2. Anti-VSV guinea pig serum, heat inactivated (titer, 1:10,000). Prepared by immunizing guinea pigs with 0.5 ml of 1:10–1:100 dilution of

VSV stock (10^7 to 10^8 PFU) emulsified in 0.5 ml of complete Freund's adjuvant in footpads and nuchal muscles. Bleedings are made at 3–6 weeks.

2.8. Indicator Cells for Virus

L-929 cells carried in spinner culture in 6% FCS–Joklik modified spinner MEM; carried at a density of 3 × 10^5 cells/ml; doubling time, approximately 24 hr

3. Procedures

3.1. Preparation of Human Lymphocytes

3.1.1. Defibrination Blood (40–60 ml) is drawn into sterile syringe (containing no anticoagulant) and immediately expressed into a 125-ml Erlenmeyer flask containing sterile glass beads (approximately 12 beads/50 ml of blood). The beads are swirled gently for 5–10 min until a clot forms.

3.1.2. The defibrinated blood is drawn into a sterile 50-ml syringe using a lumbar puncture needle, and diluted 1:1 with PBS in 50-ml conical centrifuge tubes.

3.1.3. Ficoll–Hypaque Sedimentation. Using a lumbar puncture needle, 10 ml of Ficoll–Hypaque (density 1.077) solution is carefully layered under the diluted blood in each tube. The tubes are centrifuged at 300 g for 40 min at room temperature.

3.1.4. The monocyte–lymphocyte-rich layer is carefully aspirated with a Pasteur pipette, transferred to a 50-ml centrifuge tube, diluted with Hanks' BSS, and washed three times.

3.2. Lymphocyte Cultures

3.2.1. Lymphocytes are cultured in 12 × 75 mm test tubes, at a density of 1.5 × 10^6 to 2.0 × 10^6 cells per tube in 2 ml of 5% FCS-RPMI 1640 at 37°C in an atmosphere of 7% CO_2 in air. Duplicate or triplicate tubes are set up with each antigen or mitogen.

3.2.2. For mitogen-stimulated V-PFC, cultures are stimulated with 10 μg of Con A or 5 μg of PHA-P per milliliter and harvested at 72 hr.

3.2.3. For antigens, lymphocytes are cultured with 5 μg of PPD or 100 U of SK-SD per milliliter and harvested at 4–6 days.

3.3. Preparation of Indicator L Cell Monolayers.

The L cells used to detect virus production by individual lymphocytes can be plated as monolayers either the same day as the assay or 1 day in advance. The required cells are harvested from the spinner cultures, centrifuged, and resuspended in 6% FCS–MEM. When monolayers are prepared on the day of assay, the L cells are plated at a concentration of 3.5 × 10^6 to 4.0 × 10^6 per 4 ml of 6% FCS–MEM in each 60-mm petri dish to be used. When prepared 1 day in advance, 2.0 × 10^6 cells are plated in 4.0 ml in each petri dish. The plates are incubated at 37°C in 7%

CO_2 in humidified air until use (at least 3 hr when monolayers are prepared on the same day as the experiment). In general, the assay is performed on 3 log dilutions (1:1, 1:10, 1:100 of the lymphocyte suspension) of an infected lymphocyte culture, each in duplicate, so that for each experimental sample there will be 6 plates.

3.4. Agar-Containing Medium for Virus Plaque Assay. Each plate will receive 2.5 ml of agar medium, but ample allowance should be made for extra agar-containing medium. The final concentration is 1% agar in MEM containing 6% FCS with 100 U of penicillin per milliliter + streptomycin + 200 mM glutamine.

3.4.1. To prepare the agar medium, two separate solutions are prepared. To an amount of 2X MEM equal to half of the final desired agar-medium solution is added FCS, penicillin, streptomycin, and glutamine to yield the final desired concentrations. This soluation is kept in a 44°–46°C water bath until use.

3.4.2. An amount of agar needed to bring the final concentration of agar medium mixture to 1% is dissolved in distilled water. The amount of distilled water is that required to bring the final mixture to the desired volume when mixed with the 2X MEM containing antibiotics + FCS. The agar–water solution is autoclaved and then allowed to cool in a 44°–46°C water bath.

3.4.3. The warm 2X MEM is mixed with the agar solution just prior to plating.

3.5. Preparation of Vesicular Stomatitis Virus (VSV). The preparation of virus is critical to obtaining optimal results in the virus plaque assay. VSV exists in several forms, the principal ones being infectious particles (B particles) and defective particles (T particles). The latter are smaller, nonreplicating particles capable in many systems of blocking infectivity of infectious particles. Therefore the method of viral preparation must ensure a high yield of infectious particles with minimal contamination by defective T particles, which could interfere in the assay. There are two conditions that have assured us of highly infectious virus with minimal contamination with defective particles in a great many preparations. The first is that chicken embryo fibroblasts rather than L cells or HeLa cells be used for the preparation of stock virus, since considerably higher yields are obtained. The second is that the multiplicity of infection, i.e., the number of viruses used to infect the fibroblasts, be relatively low. The value chosen is a multiplicity of infection (MOI) of 0.5–1, that is, approximately 1 PFU/cell. Under these conditions stock titers of 2×10^9 to 4×10^9 PFU/ml are routinely obtained, with essentially no significant contamination by defective interfering particles.

To produce virus, chicken embryo fibroblasts are obtained from 9-day-old chicken embryos. The embryos are removed by sterile means from the egg, decapitated, and eviscerated. The remaining tissue is minced into fine pieces with scissors in 25 ml of PBS, transferred to a 250-ml flask and magnetically stirred for 5 min. After allowing the tissue to settle, the supernatant is discarded. Then 30 ml of 0.25% trypsin is added to the tissue and again magnetically stirred for approximately 20–30 min. The tissue is allowed to settle out; the supernatant is harvested and chilled on ice, and fetal calf serum is added to a 10% concentration to stop further trypsin digestion. The remaining tissue fragments are once again suspended in 0.25% trypsin, and the cycle is repeated two more times as described. The supernatants are pooled, filtered through sterile gauze to remove large particles, and centrifuged at 250 g for 10 min; the sedimented cells are resuspended in culture medium (Eagle's MEM + 6% FCS) and counted. For small batches, the cells are adjusted to a concentration of 1.5×10^6 viable cells/ml and distributed in 5-ml volumes into 60-ml plastic petri dishes. The yield is approximately 6×10^7 cells from each embryo. For larger preparations, 2×10^8 to 5×10^8 cells are added to roller bottles in 100-ml volumes of medium. The cells are allowed to adhere at the lowest possible speed of rotation, and the cultures are maintained until a monolayer is formed. The cells can either be infected at that point, or trypsinized again to produce 3–4 roller bottles of secondary chicken embryo fibroblast cultures to increase the yield of virus. Approximately 5×10^7 PFU of virus are added in a volume of 12 ml and allowed to adsorb with slow rotation in serum-free medium for a 2-hr period. Then approximately 50 ml of medium are added to the bottles, and they are cultured overnight.

The virus replication in the fibroblasts causes virtually complete lysis of the monolayers and release of infectious viruses into the supernatants. At 16–20 hr the bottles or plates are shaken vigorously, and the cell debris is removed by centrifugation at 2000 rpm for 15 minutes. We have found it convenient to add 10% dimethyl sulfoxide (DMSO) to the supernatants before aliquoting into 0.5- or 1-ml volumes and freezing and storing at $-70°C$. Titers of virus are prepared by making serial 10-fold dilutions of virus, and plating 0.2 ml on monolayers of L cells for a 2-hr period with occasional rocking to spread the virus evenly over the plates. Then 2 ml of 1% warm agar containing 6% FCS-MEM as described below for the virus plaque assay is added and allowed to cool. Plaques are counted at 24 or 48 hr and corrected for dilution to give the titer of stock virus.

3.6. Virus Plaque Assay *3.6.1. Infection with VSV.* The cultures are washed once in MEM supplemented with 6% FCS, antibiotics, and glutamine. All but 0.2 ml of supernate is removed and 0.02 ml of VSV (2×10^9 PFU/ml, approximate multiplicity 20:1) is added. The cells are resuspended, "gassed" with CO_2 and incubated 2 hr at 37°C, with periodic shaking.

3.6.2. Addition of Anti-VSV. 3–4 ml of MEM are added to each tube. The tubes are centrifuged for 10 min at 200 g. The supernatant is removed as completely as possible. 0.02 ml of guinea pig anti-VSV serum (1:10 dilution of stock, sufficient to neutralize the entire virus input) is added to each pellet, followed by 0.5 ml MEM. The tubes are "gassed" with CO_2 and placed at 4°C for 1 hr to neutralize free virus.

3.6.3. Washing.   Three to four milliliters of MEM are added to each tube. The tubes are centrifuged 10 min at 200 *g* and the supernatants removed. Repeat three times. The cells are then resuspended in 2 ml MEM.

3.6.4. Viable Cell Count.   One-tenth milliliter of cells are mixed with 0.1 ml of Trypan blue, and a viable cell count is done and recorded for each tube. This can be done before or after plating.

3.6.5. Plating.   Six plates are prepared for each culture, with duplicate plates for each of 3 log dilutions. Prior to plating, a dilution (1:10) tube containing 5.4 ml MEM is made for each culture.

Medium is removed from L cell monolayers. With a 1 ml long tip pipette 1 ml of cell suspension is drawn up. Two-tenths milliliter is dispersed on to each of 2 L cell plates. The remaining 0.6 ml of cell suspension is added to the appropriate dilution tube. The plates are gently shaken to disperse evenly the infected lymphocytes over the L cell monolayer.

To overlay with agar, 1 ml of warm agar–medium solution is drawn into 1 ml (short tip) pipette, and delivered on to each plate. The solution is then redrawn into the pipette to mix lymphocytes with agar–medium and redelivered on to the plate. Plates are then gently shaken to disperse agar evenly and are allowed to cool on a flat surface. After 5 min an additional 1.5 ml agar–medium overlay is added and the plates are allowed to cool. Similarly, 0.2 ml from each 1:10 dilution tube are dispensed into duplicate plates for 1:10 dilutions, and 0.02 ml for 1:100 dilutions and overlayed with agar–medium.

Plates are incubated in a humid 7% CO_2 incubator at 37°C for 24–48 hr until clear plaques are visible. (Culture times vary with humidity, L cells, etc., and must be established for each laboratory.)

3.6.6. Staining of Plates.   For counting plaques, plates are fixed in formol saline (10% formaldehyde in saline) and stained with crystal violet after removal of the agar. After formalin fixation, staining and counting may be postponed to a later time.

Alternatively vital staining with neutral red may be done; 1.5 ml of fresh neutral red (15 mg/100 ml PBS-MEM, 1:1) are added to each plate and the plates are incubated 2–3 hr in a humidified 7% CO_2 incubator at 37°C. When neutral red is used, counts must be made the same day.

3.6.7. Calculations.   The number of plaques per plate is recorded. Results are expressed as virus plaque-forming cells (V-PFC) per 10^3 viable cells plated.

Example: When 0.2 ml of undiluted cell suspension is plated

$$\text{V-PFC/plate} \times 5 = \text{V-PFC/ml plated}$$

$$(\text{V-PFC/ml})/(\text{viable count/ml} \times 10^{-3}) = \text{V-PFC/}10^3 \text{ cells plated}$$

Appropriate corrections are made for calculations for dilution plates.

4. Critical comments

4.1. The method of preparation of human peripheral blood lymphocytes for use in this assay is critical. After an extensive series of experiments comparing different cell separation techniques, it appears that defibrination followed by Ficoll–Hypaque purification is the most effective (Table 1). Cells prepared by Ficoll–Hypaque sedimentation of heparinized blood yield high backgrounds of V-PFC in unstimulated cultures, and such high background may obscure low numbers of V-PFC in antigen-stimulated cultures. While the background-producing cells could be largely removed on nylon columns, under the conditions used, such columns often removed a portion of Con A and antigen-responding V-PFC. The majority of background-producing cells in lymphoid populations appear to be of two types: monocytes or macrophages, and lymphocytes activated *in vivo* or by culture conditions. Defibrination alone reduces the background without significantly altering the proportions of E or EAC rosetting cells, yet the reason for the efficiency of so simple a procedure remains unknown.

Sedimentation of defibrinated blood through dextran or gelatin provides cells adequate for use in the virus plaque assay, but this method results in high numbers of contaminating polymorphonuclear leukocytes and red blood cells, many of which die in culture. Lysis of erythrocytes with ammonium chloride does not affect the V-PFC response to antigens or mitogens.

While defibrination followed by Ficoll–Hypaque appears to be the optimal procedure for reproducibly preparing human blood lymphocytes it must be pointed out that a number of other conditions, such as duration of infection and antigen dose, remain to be optimized.

4.2. In the mouse it has been demonstrated that marked increases in V-PFC result from stimulation with Con A or PHA, but not with LPS. Further, treatment of normal spleen cells with anti-Thy 1 serum and complement either at day 0 or after stimulation but before infection with VSV, eliminates the V-PFC. These results suggest that in the mouse there is selectivity for activated T lymphocytes, but not for activated B lymphocytes (8).

We have considerably fewer data on the nature of the V-PFC in human blood or tonsils. T cells purified by passage of cells through nylon columns or positively selected by E-rosetting are markedly stimulated by PHA and Con A to produce V-PFC. The numbers of such V-PFC range from 5 to 50 per 10^3 cells. Populations of cells depleted of T cells by two cycles of E-rosetting are considerably less responsive to PHA, Con A, or even PWM, and stimulation is generally 10-fold less than with T cells. It has been difficult to ascertain whether the stimulation of a small number of non-T cells reflects the ability of B cells or a subpopulation of non-T cells to produce VSV, or represents the cloning out of a small number of contaminating T cells. Recent studies using staphylococci

studies on synchronized lymphoblastoid lines indicate that infectivity is highly dependent on cell cycle such that infection must occur in the G_1 phase in order for plaques to be optimally produced. By optimizing the time and multiplicity of infection, a truer index of the number of activated T cells may be achieved.

A second possibility is that the virus plaque assay measures only a subpopulation of activated T cells. In studies of primary mixed lymphocyte cultures (MLC) in the mouse, the increase in V-PFC parallels incorporation of ^{3}H-thymidine, both are stimulated by I-region differences and both are inhibited by cytosine arabinoside (Ara C), an inhibitor of DNA synthesis. Preinfection of resting spleen cells with VSV eliminates the proliferative response following later stimulation in MLC (11). These results suggest that the proliferating (Ly 1) cells can be detected by the VPA in an MLC. Preliminary experiments using murine spleen cells obtained from mice immunized against major histocompatibility antigens and "boosted" *in vitro* for 48 hr indicate a parallelism between killer T-cell activity and V-PFC, which persist even in the presence of cytosine arabinoside, which blocks DNA synthesis and T cell proliferation. Both

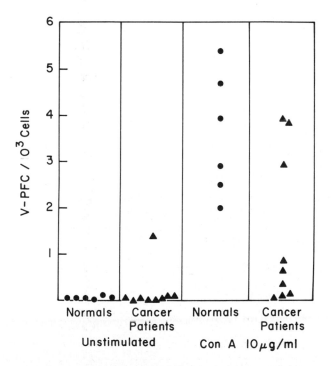

Fig. 1. Virus plaque-forming cells (V-PFC) following concanavalin A (Con A) stimulation of nylon wool-purified lymphocytes from cancer patients and normal donors

TABLE 3
Incorporation of ^{3}H-Thymidine and Virus Plaque Assay in a Normal and a Cancer Patient[a]

Assay	Normal control	Cancer patient
Virus plaque assay (VPA)	V-PFC/10^3 cells[b]	
Unstimulated	0.069	1.400
Con A stimulated	5.371	0.820
Lymphocyte transformation	^{3}H-Thymidine incorporation (cpm)	
Unstimulated	115	1,051
Con A stimulated	38,035	39,582

[a]Lymphocytes were prepared by defibrination followed by nylon column purification as in Fig. 1. VPA was performed and ^{3}H-thymidine incorporation was measured on aliquots of the same culture at 72 hr.
[b]V-PFC, virus plaque-forming cells.

functions are destroyed by treatment with anti-Ly 2,3 serum + C, suggesting that the VPA may measure activated killer T cells as well.

4.4. Preliminary studies using the virus plaque assay in a group of human cancer patients and normals appear to show a markedly decreased production of V-PFC stimulated by Con A in the cancer patients as compared to normal individuals (Fig. 1).

It is noteworthy that in these experiments there was often little correlation between results of the virus plaque assay and the incorporation of tritiated thymidine done on the same cultures. A representative experiment is illustrated in Table 3. This is consistent with the possibility the two assays may be measuring different subpopulations or functional sets of lymphocytes. The significance of the abnormal Con A response in the cancer patients as measured in the VPA remains to be established.

REFERENCES

1. Bloom, B. R., Jimenez, L., and Marcus, P. I., *J. Exp. Med.* **132,** 16 (1970).
2. Wheelock, E. F., and Toy, S. T., *Adv. Immunol.* **16,** 123 (1973).
3. Woodruff, J. F., and Woodruff, J. J., *Prog. Med. Virol.* **19,** 120 (1975).
4. Jimenez, L., Bloom, B. R., Blume, M. R., and Oettgen, H. F., *J. Exp. Med.* **133,** 740 (1971).
5. Jimenez, L., and Bloom, B. R., *Cell Immunol.* **3,** 175 (1972).
6. Bloom, B. R., Stoner, G., Fischetti, V., Nowakowski, M., Muschel, R., and Rubinstein, A., *Prog. Immunol. II* **3,** 133 (1974).

7. Nowakowski, M., Bloom, B. R., and Feldman, J. R., *J. Exp. Med.* **137**, 1042 (1973).
8. Kano, S., Bloom, B. R., and Howe, M. L., *Proc. Natl. Acad. Sci. U.S.A.* **70**, 2299 (1973).
9. Nowakowski, M., Bloom, B. R., Ehrenfeld, E., and Summers, D. F., *J. Virol.* **12**, 1272 (1973).
10. Bloom, B. R., Nowakowski, M., and Kano, S., *in* "Mechanisms of Viral Disease" (W. S. Robinson and C. F. Fox, eds.), p. 25. Benjamin, New York, 1974.
11. Nowakowski, M., Kano, S., Romano, T. J., Thorbecke, G. J., and Bloom, B. R., *J. Exp. Med.* in press.

Purification and Cultivation of Monocytes and Macrophages
Paul J. Edelson and Zanvil A. Cohn

1. Introduction

The *macrophage* is a large, phagocytic tissue cell that descends from the circulating blood *monocyte* (1). Both these cells are referred to as *mononuclear phagocytes,* as distinct from the *neutrophil* or polymorphonuclear phagocyte.

Macrophages occur in every species from the starfish to man. In mammals they are dispersed throughout the body, but are particularly accumulated in the spleen, liver, bone marrow, and lungs. They have two key characteristics relevant to *in vitro* work. First, they show an outstanding ability to adhere to glass or plastic surfaces, even in the face of treatment with trypsin or chelating agents. Second, they generally do not divide in culture.

In this chapter, we describe techniques for cultivating mouse peritoneal macrophages and human blood monocytes. Reliable and convenient methods of preparation and maintenance of viable cultures are currently limited to only a few other macrophage sources, beyond these two.

The mouse normally has a population of 2×10^6 to 3×10^6 macrophages resident in its peritoneal cavity which can be directly isolated and placed in culture. It is also possible to inject various inflammatory agents into the cavity before harvesting the cells, but the cells obtained will be quantitatively and qualitatively different from the resident population (see Section 5: Appendix on the Use of Activated Macrophages). Although the normal peritoneal cell population is a mixture of about 60% lymphocytes, 35% macrophages, occasional mast cells, and small numbers of other cells, the exceptional adherence of the macrophages makes it possible to prepare highly purified cell monolayers simply by vigorously washing away the contaminating cells. In the stimulated exudates, contamination with adherent neutrophils and fibroblasts may be more of a problem. The monolayers can be trypsinized to remove contaminating fibroblasts, while neutrophils do not survive in culture overnight. However, they can be phagocytized by the surviving macrophages, complicating interpretation of some experiments by their "internal" contamination of the monolayers.

Circulating monocyte cultures present different problems. First, the low numbers of monocytes present in peripheral blood requires that the white cells be concentrated prior to plating. Second, the enormous numbers of circulating platelets (about 2×10^3 platelets per monocyte) means that even after considerable purification, the monolayer may have 10-fold more platelets than monocytes.

Macrophage cultures have been used for a variety of cell biological and immunological studies. Their use in cell biology is summarized in the recent review by Gordon and Cohn (2), while immunological aspects are dealt with by Steinman and Cohn (3), as well as in other chapters in this volume.

2. Materials

2.1. Collection of Mouse Peritoneal Macrophages

2.1.1. Animals. Mice 25–30 g, of either sex may be used. We routinely use the closed, but not inbred, NCS strain of specific pathogen-free Swiss albino mice, but inbred strains can be used. Cell yields may be somewhat lower with some inbred strains.

2.1.2. Dissection Material

Chloroform

Glass jar or flask, with cover, for sacrificing the animals

Small dissecting board and pins

Dissecting scissors with curved blades, 3-inch

Dissecting forceps without teeth, 1 pair

Dissecting forceps with teeth, 1 pair

Glass Pasteur pipettes, unplugged, sterile

Rubber bulbs

Syringe, 10 ml, sterile

Hypodermic needles, sterile, 23-gauge, 1-inch

Ethanol, 70%

Cotton gauze pads, sterile

Dulbecco's phosphate-buffered saline, without calcium or magnesium (may be purchased as a 10X stock solution from Grand Island Biological Co., Catalogue No. 420)

Plastic test tube, sterile suitable for low-speed centrifugation

2.2. Preparation of Mouse Macrophage Monolayers

Disposable plastic tissue culture petri dishes, sterile (Nunclon-Delta, 30 mm, without air vents, Catalogue No. 1420, distributed by Vanguard International, Box 312, Red Bank, New Jersey)

Medium 199 with Hanks' salts (Grand Island Biological Co., Catalogue No. 115H)

Sodium bicarbonate, 7.5% (Grand Island Biological Co., Catalogue No. 130810)

Fetal calf serum (heat-inactivated at 56°C for 30 min, Millipore filtered).

Tissue culture incubator providing 5% CO_2 atmosphere.

2.3. Collection of Human Blood Monocytes

Heparin, free of preservative, diluted to 1000 units/ml with sterile saline (Connaught Medical Research Laboratories, Toronto, Canada: Sodium Heparin, powdered, 10,000 USP units per vial)

Syringe, 20-ml, sterile

Hypodermic needle, sterile, 19 gauge, 1 inch

Ethanol, 70%

Cotton gauze pads, sterile

Tourniquet

Ficoll−Hypaque mixture: (1) Dissolve 9 g of Ficoll (Pharmacia, approximately 400,000 daltons) in 100 ml of twice distilled water, with stirring. Autoclave. (2) Mix 30 ml of sodium diatrizoate (Winthrop Laboratories, New York: Hypaque-sodium, 50%, w/v) with 14 ml of twice distilled water. If crystals form, solution may be placed in warm water. (3) Mix 24 parts of Ficoll:10 parts of Hypaque.

Eagle's EDTA: (1) Prepare stock solution of EDTA, 150 mM in twice distilled water. (2) Dilute 1:250 with Eagle's balanced salt solution, calcium- and magnesium-free (Grand Island Biological Co., Catalogue No. 415).

2.4. Preparation of Human Monocyte Monolayers

Disposable plastic tissue culture petri dishes, sterile (see Section 2.2).

RPMI 1640 (Grand Island Biological Co., Catalogue No. 187G)

Autologous human serum: heat inactivated at 56°C for 30 min, Millipore filtered

3. Methods

3.1. Preparation of Mouse Macrophage Monolayers. Each animal, in turn, is sacrificed in a closed glass jar containing chloroform-moistened gauze pads. Animals should not all be sacrificed at once. The mouse is then pinned to a dissecting board, with its extremities fully extended. The abdomen is swabbed with 70% ethanol and wiped dry. The lower abdominal skin is tented with the toothed forceps, and a small cut is made. The dissecting scissors, with blades closed, are placed in the incision and spread to separate the abdominal skin from the peritoneum by blunt dissection. If one then firmly holds the lower extremities to the board, the skin may be reflected upward, toward the head, and pulled, to expose the peritoneum. One then injects 2−4 ml of the divalent cation-free saline into the peritoneal cavity. The cavity is then gently massaged with the side of the sterile Pasteur pipette for about 10 sec, care being taken to avoid the liver. The peritoneal wall is then tented with the untoothed forceps, and the tip of the Pasteur pipette is pushed through the membrane into the cavity. The air in the pipette can be blown into the cavity to form a small bubble over the fluid; the pipette can then be used to aspirate the injected saline. About one-half to two-thirds of the injected fluid volume can usually be recovered.

The collected fluid is then centrifuged for 10 min at 400 g at room temperature in an International centrifuge (Model PR-6000), or a similar machine, and the cells are collected in a pellet.

The recovered cells are resuspended in Medium 199 supplemented with 20% fetal calf serum. The medium should include 30 ml of sodium bicarbonate (7.5%) per liter. The cell concentration should be adjusted to 2 × 10^6 cells/ml and 1.5 ml of the suspension be dispensed into each 30-mm tissue culture dish. The dishes are then incubated in a humidified CO_2 incubator for 1–2 hr to allow the macrophages to settle and adhere to the dish floor. The medium is then aspirated, and the plates are rinsed three times with medium 199 without serum, with brisk shaking, to dislodge contaminating adherent cells. Care should be taken to aspirate any medium splashed onto the dish cover. The dishes are then refilled with 1.5 ml of serum-supplemented medium and returned to the incubator.

The monolayers may be used immediately or maintained in culture for several days. Medium can be changed after 48 hr, or sooner if considerable numbers of nonadherent cells have escaped the initial washes. Immediately after plating, the macrophages are generally round, but after 24 hr in culture they should be well-spread, generally somewhat triangular, cells when examined in the inverted microscope.

3.2. Preparation of Human Monocyte Monolayers. Blood is obtained by venepuncture, using about 0.5 ml of heparin (1000 μ/ml) for 20 ml of whole blood, To concentrate the mononuclear cells, layer 10 ml of whole blood over 16 ml of Ficoll–Hypaque mixture, and spin the gradient, at room temperature, at 400 g for 40 min in an International centrifuge (Model PR-6000), or similar machine. The mononuclear cells can be recovered from the band at the plasma–Ficoll–Hypaque interface. These cells are then diluted in 30 ml of Eagle's EDTA and washed twice at 200 g for 10 min (PR-6000) to reduce platelet contamination. The cells are then resuspended in RPMI 1640 + 10% inactivated autologous human serum, at a concentration of 2 × 10^6 cells/ml, and 1.5 ml are dispensed to each 30-mm petri dish.

The monolayers are then treated identically to the mouse cell cultures, except that the cells should not be washed later than 1 hr after plating and are maintained in RPMI 1640 with autologous serum. Human monocytes generally take several days to spread out and begin to look more like typical macrophage cultures.

4. Critical Comments

4.1.1. Other sources of macrophages: Dissociated mouse spleen cells are a disappointing source of macrophages. Many macrophages are not readily dissociated from the organ stroma by the usual physical techniques, while a great many contaminating nonmacrophage adherent cells of this very heterogeneous, hematopoietic tissue remain in culture.

4.1.2. Carbonyl iron: We have found carbonyl iron to be an unreliable agent for the separation of phagocytic cells from mixed lymphoid populations. Certain preparations of carbonyl iron are poorly phagocytized, and tend to adhere to the surface of a variety of cells, including many which are not macrophages. In addition, one must independently assess the extent to which a particular cell mixture has been depleted of macrophages by carbonyl iron treatment, as not all macrophages will reliably ingest or bind this material.

4.1.3. Choice of medium: Several media, including Dulbecco's modified Eagle's medium, can be used in place of Medium 199. Dulbecco's MEM has the advantage that it is somewhat better buffered and so controls the pH of monolayer cultures better than 199.

4.1.4. Serum supplementation: For mouse cells, we use fetal calf serum that has been screened by us to ensure its effectiveness in maintaining the cultures. However, both horse and newborn calf serum are also perfectly usable for mouse cell cultures. One should be cautious with newborn calf serum, as some batches have a naturally occurring bovine antimouse cell antibody which can have significant effects on the physiology of the mononuclear cells (3a).

Human cultures generally require human serum, and autologous serum seems generally the best choice. Mouse cells can be successfully maintained for several days in serum-free medium supplemented with 0.2% lactalbumin hydrolyzate (Grand Island Biological Co., Catalogue No. 164).

4.1.5. Observation of cultures: Cultures are regularly examined by phase microscopy, using an inverted microscope. Healthy cultures have large, well-spread cells firmly adherent to the dish floor. Unhealthy cultures contain many rounded, refractile cells that detach from the dish.

4.1.6. Buffering agents: A bicarbonate–carbon dioxide system seems best for maintaining the pH of these cells. Certain organic buffers, such as TRIS, can have unacceptable effects on macrophages in culture (4).

4.1.7. Assessment of contamination with nonphagocytic cells: One can add 10 μl of India Ink (Higgins Black, No. 4415, Faber-Castell Corp., Newark, New Jersey) to a culture dish and incubate at 37°C for 60 min, to quickly assess phagocytic potential of the monolayer cells. In our experience, about 5% of otherwise normal macrophages may not phagocytize any particular marker particle, so that this test cannot be absolutely relied on to rule out the presence of any macrophages in a given population.

4.1.8. Monolayer preparations for microscopy: For phase contrast microscopy, it is convenient to prepare cultures on sterile glass cover slips (Corning cover glass No. 2, 22 mm diameter). The initial cell suspension can be placed as a bubble over the cover slips, which are held in a sterile petri dish. After attachment, the petri dish can be flooded with medium and reincubated. Cover slips can be fixed in 1.25% glutaraldehyde (Fisher Chemical Co., reagent grade, 50% solution) in phosphate-buffered saline, for 10 min at room temperature. The slips are then rinsed in distilled water, inverted over a drop of water on a glass slide, blotted dry, and sealed with melted paraffin (Bioloid paraffin embedding compound, VWR Scientific Co., San Francisco, California, Catalogue No. 48664-123), or quick-drying nail polish.

The classic method developed for preparing cover-slip cultures is the use of Leighton tubes containing "flying" cover slips on which the cells are plated and which can be removed for microscopy. Leighton tubes can be gassed with a CO_2–air mixture and sealed with screw caps, eliminating the need for a CO_2 incubator. These tubes are also useful for working with infectious agents which cannot be kept in unsealed culture plates.

4.1.9. Alternative method for purifying human monocytes: Huber and Fudenberg (5) and Holm and Hammerström (6) have described techniques for concentrating and purifying human monocytes on bovine serum albumin, based on the method of Bennett and Cohn for the preparation of horse monocytes. The technique, which is no more complex than the one described above, exploits the relatively low density of monocytes to separate them by flotation on a 27% or 28% solution of BSA from lymphocytes and neutrophils. The approach seems sensible and has the attraction that it avoids exposing the cells to such indigestible, and possibly toxic, materials as Ficoll and iopanoic acid.

5. Appendix on the Use of "Activated" Macrophages

Although macrophage activation has a very specific meaning in the context of the studies of macrophage bactericidal activity by Mackaness and his colleagues (7) the term is also used in a broader sense to describe the changes in a macrophage population that participates in an inflammatory process. Since an inflammatory focus is often characterized by the presence of a great *number* of macrophages, one of the earliest techniques for increasing the yield of peritoneal cells from an animal was to induce a sterile inflammation, usually with an intraperitoneal injection, before harvest, and such techniques are still used.

There are two important points to be aware of when using this technique. First, macrophages are not the only cells that will respond to an inflammatory stimulus. Lymphocytes, neutrophils, and other cells may also accumulate locally. While lymphocytes can generally be removed from macrophage cultures by vigorous washing (providing that the cells have been allowed to adhere to the culture surface in the presence of some serum), neutrophil contamination can be quite serious. Neutrophils stick extremely well to glass or plastic, making it almost impossible to wash them away. In addition, they disintegrate rapidly in culture and may be ingested by neighboring macrophages, so that the monolayers may be "internally" contaminated with neutrophil contents. However, since the peak neutrophil response is passed by 48 hr, while the macrophage response is several days slower, one can avoid the problem of neutrophil contamination of inflammatory exudates simply by waiting until day 4 after stimulation to harvest the cells.

The second point is a more serious problem. It seems that when one collects inflammatory cells they are qualitatively different from the cells normally resident in the peritoneal cavity. In addition, cells collected after the injection of different agents may differ among themselves. Recent work has shown that, in addition to the "classical" differences of increased spreading, greater plasma membrane activity (ruffling), and an increased content of lysosomal granules and their hydrolases, there are several additional characteristics that distinguish the "inflammatory" macrophage from the resident cells: (a) A wide spectrum of *neutral proteases* secreted by these cells is recoverable in the culture medium of inflammatory monolayers, while very little activity is usually detectable in unstimulated cultures (8). (b) While all peritoneal macrophages will specifically bind particles that have been coated with an active fragment of the third component of complement, only inflammatory macrophages will *ingest* such particles in the absence of an additional opsonizing antibody (9). (c) Inflammatory macrophages have an increased *pinocytic rate* (10), and (d) a decreased activity of the plasma membrane enzyme 5'-nucleotidase (11). No doubt there are other physiological and biochemical differences between the inflammatory and resident populations still waiting to be detected.

While inflammatory cells can be cultivated as easily, or more easily, than resident cells, and are available in yields of 20×10^6 cells per mouse, or more, they cannot be taken for native unstimulated cells but must be studied as a variety with very different characteristics. Also, since the stimulus used may be a critical variable in the behavior of these cells, the cells should be identified by the inflammatory agent used, along with the dose, route of injection, and timing of the collection.

REFERENCES

1. van Furth, R., *Sem. Hematol.* **7**, 125 (1970).
2. Gordon, S., and Cohn, Z. A., *Int. Rev. Cytol.* **36**, 171 (1973).
3. Steinman, R. M., and Cohn, Z. A. *in* "The Inflammatory Process" (B. W. Zweifach, L. Grant, and R. T. McCluskey, eds., 2nd ed., Vol. 1, p. 450. Academic Press, New York, 1973.
3a. Cohn, Z., and Parks, E., *J. Exp. Med.* **125**, 1091 (1967).

4. Steinman, R. M., and Cohn, Z. A., *J. Cell Biol.* **55**, 186 (1972).
5. Huber, H., and Fudenberg, H. H., *Int. Arch. Allergy Appl. Immunol.* **34**, 18 (1968).
6. Holm, G., and Hammerström, S., *Clin. Exp. Immunol.* **13**, 29 (1973).
7. Blanden, R. V., Lefford, M. J., and Mackaness, G. B., *J. Exp. Med.* **129**, 1079 (1969).
8. Gordon, S., *in* "Mononuclear Phagocytes in Immunity, Infection and Pathology" (R. van Furth, ed.), p. 463. Blackwell, Oxford, 1975.
9. Bianco, C., Griffin, F. M., and Silverstein, S. C., *J. Exp. Med.* **141**, 1278 (1975).
10. Edelson, P., Zweibel, R., and Cohn, Z. A., *J. Exp. Med.* **142**, 1150 (1975).
11. Karnovsky, M. L., Lazdins, J., Drath, D., and Harper, A., *Ann. N. Y. Acad. Sci.* **256**, 266 (1975).

Methods for Detection of Macrophage Secretory Enzymes*

S. Gordon, Z. Werb, and Z. A. Cohn

1. Introduction

Recent studies have shown that macrophages are able to synthesize and secrete a variety of products, including several enzyme activities, during cultivation *in vitro* (1). Lysozyme production is substantial, and this enzyme is secreted continuously by all macrophage populations studied so far (2), whereas several inducible neutral proteinase activities such as plasminogen activators (PA) (3, 4), elastase (5), and collagenase (6) are secreted only after activation of macrophages or after phagocytosis. We have defined secretion of these enzymes in terms of net production *in vitro,* low intracellular levels, less than 20% of the total activity produced per day, and progressive extracellular accumulation during continued cultivation. Some properties of the neutral proteinase activities released by macrophages are summarized in Table 1, and compared with properties of acid proteinase activities, which are mainly distributed intracellularly. Although the biological functions of macrophage secretory enzymes are still unclear, the capacity of these proteinases for specific and restricted cleavage of several major extracellular proteins, at neutral pH, suggests an important role as mediators in the inflammatory response. These products also provide useful enzymic markers to study the mechanism of macrophage activation.

In this chapter we describe assays to measure proteolytic activity against plasminogen—fibrin, elastin, and azocasein, and refer briefly to assays for lysozyme and lysosomal enzymes.

2. Assay Methods

2.1. Lysosomal Enzymes

Acid hydrolases play a major role in intracellular digestion after endocytosis, but may be released extracellularly under certain circumstances (7). Detailed

---

*Abbreviations used: AT-FBS, acid-treated fetal bovine serum; B_z-arg 2N-Nap, α-N-benzoyl-DL-arginine 2-naphthyl amide; CM, conditioned medium; Dip-F, diisopropyl phosphofluoridate; DTT, dithiothreitol; EDTA, ethylenediaminetetraacetic acid; FBS, fetal bovine serum; HBSS, Hanks' balanced salt solution; LPS, lipopolysaccharide; NPGB, 4-nitrophenyl 4′-guanidinobenzoate; PA, plasminogen activator; PMN, polymorphonuclear leukocyte; SBTI, soybean trypsin inhibitor; SDS, sodium dodecyl sulfate.

TABLE 1
Macrophage Proteinase Activities[a]

	Extracellular				Lysosomal	
	Plasminogen activator	Elastase	Collagenase	Neutral proteinases[b]	Cathepsin B1	Cathepsin D
Substrate	Plasminogen	Elastin	Collagen	Azocasein, gelatin proteoglycan	B$_2$-arg 2N-Nap azocasein gelatin proteoglycan	Hemoglobin proteoglycan
pH optimum	Neutral	Neutral	Neutral	Neutral	Acid	Acid
class	Serine	Serine	Metallo-	[Metallo-]	Thiol[c]	Carboxyl
Inhibitors						
DIP-F	+	+	−	−	−	−
EDTA	−	+++	−	−	−	−
NpGB	+	−	−	−	−	−
DTT	+	+	+	+	−	+
Pepstatin	−	−	−	−	−	+
Leupeptin	−	−	−	−	−	−
α$_2$-Macroglobulin	±	+	+	+	+	+
SBTI	−	−	−	−	−	−

[a] Proteolytic activities detected in conditioned media (CM) or cell lysates obtained from thioglycolate-elicited mouse peritoneal macrophages. The number of distinct proteinases is uncertain since substrate and inhibitor profiles have been determined with crude enzyme preparation.
[b] Probably includes several enzymes.
[c] Neutral thiol proteinases have also been reported.

methods for the assay of several of these enzymes, including α-naphthyl acid phosphatase (8), have been described elsewhere (9, 10). We recommend that hydrolases of at least two types be studied including a glycosidase, such as β-glucuronidase, and a proteinase, e.g., cathepsin D, since the intracellular levels and distribution of such enzymes may differ. Fluorimetric (11) or radiolabeled substrates may be useful for measuring low extracellular levels of lysosomal enzymes.

2.2. Lysozyme

Lysozyme is a bulk secretion product that serves as an excellent marker for the mononuclear phagocyte and its total synthetic activity (2). The production rate per cell is remarkably constant, irrespective of cell maturity or activation. To study this product macrophages may be cultivated by standard procedures using medium supplemented with fetal bovine serum, which lacks lysozyme, or with 0.1% (w/v) lactalbumin hydrolysate (Nutritional Biochemicals Corp., tissue culture grade). Human blood monocytes are best cultivated in autologous serum, which itself contains lysozyme. Lysozyme levels in conditioned medium (CM) and cell lysates, prepared in 0.1% Triton X-100, are conveniently assayed from the initial rate of lysis of a suspension of *Micrococcus lysodeikticus* (spray-dried, Miles Laboratories, Inc., Kankakee, Illinois) using a recording spectrophotometer (2). The lysoplate method developed by Osserman and Lawlor (12) is also useful. Dilution in 5% FBS prevents losses of low levels of lysozyme activity. Note that human and rat lysozymes are 3.3- and 2-fold more active, respectively, than hen egg lysozyme. Polyanionic substances readily inhibit lysozyme activity.

2.3. Neutral Proteinases

Neutral proteinase activities are barely detectable in cultures of unstimulated mouse peritoneal macrophages, but relatively high levels of enzyme activities can be induced by intraperitoneal injection of thioglycolate broth (4–6) or by a combined treatment with endotoxin *in vivo* and a phagocytic load of latex particles *in vitro* (4). Even so, macrophage proteinase activities are secreted in trace amounts and sensitive assays are therefore needed for their detection. We describe procedures suitable for two types of assay, a radioactive fibrin-plate method to measure fibrinolysis by intact cells and assays to measure levels of plasminogen activator and other neutral proteinase activities in serum-free conditioned medium and cell lysates. Plaque assays have also been described for detection of fibrinolysis by colonies or single cells (13, 14).

2.3.1. Macrophages

Source. We have used specific pathogen-free NCS mice (Rockefeller colony), of either sex, weighing 25–30 g. Peritoneal cells are harvested by standard methods from control, unstimulated animals or from mice 4 days after intraperitoneal injection of 1 ml of Brewer thioglycolate medium (Difco Labs., Detroit, Michigan, "complete") prepared and stored according to the manufacturer's instructions. Our experience with endotoxin has been mainly with purified preparations of *salmonella abortus equi* lipopolysaccharide (LPS) provided by Professor O. Westphal. The LPS is suspended in sterile saline (1 mg/ml) and sonicated briefly; it has been stored frozen (−20°C) for up to 2 months. The LPS is insoluble and should be resuspended carefully before injection. Peritoneal cells are harvested after 4–5 days. The potency of a particular batch of LPS should be standardized by dose-response experiments. We have obtained optimal macrophage spreading and fibrinolysis after injection of 30 μg of LPS.

Cell Culture. Standard procedures of macrophage cultivation are modified as follows. Peritoneal cell suspensions are plated on regular or ^{125}I-labeled fibrin-coated tissue culture dishes at the following density per square centimeter: unstimulated, 8×10^5; thioglycolate stimulated, 2×10^5; endotoxin stimulated, 5×10^5. The culture medium consists of Dulbecco's modified Eagle's medium (H-21, GIBCO, Grand Island, New York) penicillin and streptomycin supplemented as follows: for culture on uncoated dishes, with 15% acid-treated fetal bovine serum (AT-FBS), for culture on ^{125}I-labeled fibrin-coated dishes, with 10% FBS and 60 μg of soybean trypsin inhibitor (SBTI, fraction VI, Miles, Kankakee, Illinois) per milliliter, to suppress fibrinolysis. Acid treatment of FBS is designed to destroy α_2-macroglobulin, an inhibitor of proteinase activity, and is performed at pH 3.5 with 2 N HCl in isotonic saline for 2 hr at room temperature; the serum is then adjusted to pH 7.4 with 2 M NaOH in isotonic saline and filter-sterilized. The cells are washed and fed fresh medium of the same composition after 4 and 24 hr of incubation.

Phagocytosis. This is employed to enhance fibrinolysis by endotoxin-stimulated macrophages. Polystyrene latex particles (1.01 μm, Dow Diagnostics, Indianapolis, Indiana) are washed thoroughly by centrifugation, resuspended in Dulbecco's medium, and irradiated with ultraviolet light. Macrophages are generally cultivated for 24 hr before phagocytosis. Monolayers are washed twice and incubated in medium containing 5% FBS. Particulate preparations are resuspended in serum-free medium by passage through a syringe and 26-gauge needle and carefully distributed in the culture medium. SBTI (60 μg/ml) is included in the medium during phagocytosis in experiments on radioactive plates. Phagocytosis is observed by phase-contrast microscopy and is stopped when ~ 95% of cells have ingested 20–50 particles per cell. The cells are then washed and placed in fresh medium, as required.

Collection of Conditioned Medium (CM). CM is routinely prepared after 48 hr of cultivation. Wash the monolayers carefully, at least 3 times, with Hanks' balanced salt solution (HBSS) to remove inhibitors and incubate in serum-free Dulbecco's medium supplemented with 0.05–0.2% lactalbumin hydrolysate for 1–4 days. Neuman-Tytell medium (GIBCO, Grand Island, N.Y.) is a more expensive, but particularly rich, serum-free medium that may be preferred for certain purposes. Macrophages can be exposed to repeated cycles of serum-free medium for up to 3 weeks without loss of viability or fall in lysozyme secretion, but such cells may display reduced levels of other activities, such as plasma membrane 5′-nucleotidase. Collect the CM, centrifuge at 500 g for 15 min, and store the supernatant at −20°C until assay.

Preparation of CM for Assay. Although the neutral proteinase activities described are stable to several cycles of freezing and thawing, the enzymes are sticky and easily lost on precipitates and surfaces when dilute solutions are handled in serum-free medium. Enzyme activity is measured directly or after concentration, with different optimal conditions for each activity. PA and elastase activity can often be measured directly, whereas assay of collagenolytic activity usually requires concentration. For this purpose the CM is dialyzed in 10 mM Tris HCl, pH 7.5, containing 2 mM CaCl$_2$ to retain enzyme activity. The sample is then lyophilized and reconstituted in 5–10% of the original volume, with distilled water. This procedure causes little loss of collagenase, but up to 50% loss of elastase. The PA can be concentrated by addition of 0.1 volume of 1 M sodium sulfate, transfer to a dialysis bag, and packing in Sephadex. Azo-caseinase activity is measured after dialysis with or without lyophilization.

Cell lysates. Wash the monolayers twice with HBSS, scrape from the dish with a policeman in 0.5–1 ml of 0.1–0.2% Triton X-100, and store at −20°C. Cells may also be harvested by scraping in isotonic saline and centrifugation, before treatment with Triton X-100. The nuclei can then be removed by low speed centrifugation before freezing. Triton X-100 stimulates PA activity approx. 30%.

2.3.2. Fibrin plate method for assay of fibrinolysis and Plasminogen Activator*

Principle. Plasminogen activator(s) secreted by cells convert the serum zymogen plasminogen to plasmin, a potent fibrinolytic enzyme. Dishes are coated with a thin film of ^{125}I-labeled fibrinogen, which is dried and converted to fibrin by thrombin. Intact macrophages or cell-free fractions are assayed for solubilization of ^{125}I-labeled fibrin in the presence and in the absence of plasminogen.

Purification of fibrinogen. Bovine fibrinogen (Calbiochem) is purified by a modification of Laki's procedure (16) and by ethanol precipitation in the presence of lysine, to reduce contamination with plasminogen (17).

i. Dissolve 4 g of fibrinogen in 400 ml of 0.1 M phosphate buffer, pH 6.4; add 200 ml of distilled water, and leave 6–18 hr on ice. Filter and discard precipitate.

*Adapted from Ref. (15).

ii. Make filtrate 33%, final concentration, with saturated ammonium sulfate, pH 7.0, and stir for 2 hr at room temperature. Centrifuge precipitate. Take up precipitate in about 50 ml 0.6 N NaCl, pH 7.0 and dialyze 3 times in same, at room temperature.

iii. Measure fibrinogen concentration by Lowry method. To 10 mg/ml fibrinogen, in 0.6 N NaCl, pH 7.0, add 5 volumes of 5 mM Na$_2$PO$_4$, 0.12 M lysine, pH 7.0. Bring to 0°C. Add ethanol to 7% final concentration. Stir 30 min in the cold. Centrifuge. Take up precipitate in 10–20 ml of 0.6 N NaCl, pH 7.4, and dialyze in the same buffer. Pass through filter paper and sterilize by Millipore filtration. Measure protein concentration and freeze at −20°C.

Comments: (i) Use plastic containers to minimize clotting. (ii) Repeat ethanol precipitation if significant plasmin contamination remains.

Iodination of Fibrinogen. Iodination is performed by the chloramine T method, using mild conditions to prevent denaturation of fibrinogen, or by the Helmkamp method (18).

Chloramine T Method [adapted from Byrt and Ada (19)]. Add 50 μl of ^{125}I, carrier free, 5 mCi/ml, 50 μl chloramine T (2 mg/ml in 0.3 M PBS, pH 7.4) and up to 250 μl of fibrinogen (3 mg/ml in PBS pH 7.4) and mix at room temperature for 2 min. Add 150 μl of saturated tyrosine and 200 μl of 5% BSA, pH 7.4, and pass the mixture over Sephadex G-25 to remove the bulk of unincorporated ^{125}I. Pool and Millipore-filter the labeled fibrinogen, using BSA to minimize losses. Determine TCA-precipitable radioactivity; typical incorporation efficiency is 70%, 5 × 10^5 cpm/μg protein. Can be stored frozen at −20°C, although the proportion of TCA-precipitable protein may fall rapidly after several weeks of storage.

Preparation of ^{125}I-Labeled Fibrin Plates. Linbro tissue culture plates (24 wells, 16 mm) (New Haven, Connecticut) are most convenient although 35-mm tissue culture dishes can also be used (3). To the desired amount of ^{125}I-labeled fibrinogen, add unlabeled fibrinogen and dilute with distilled sterile water so that 0.3 ml of the final solution contains 5 × 10^4 to 1 × 10^5 TCA-precipitable cpm and 20 μg of unlabeled fibrinogen. Keep the solution warm to prevent precipitation of fibrinogen, and dispense 0.3 ml aliquots with automatic dispenser to Linbro plates. A glass rod is needed to distribute fibrinogen over surface of 35-mm dishes. Dry at 45°C in incubator under sterile conditions for a minimum of 2 days. The radioactive plates can then be stored for several weeks at room temperature or in the cold.

"Activation" of Plates. Incubate each well with 1 ml of Dulbecco's medium + 10% FBS for 2 hr at 37°C to convert fibrinogen to fibrin. Wash twice with HBSS. Plates can also be activated overnight and may be kept 1 day after activation. Wash again before use.

Plasminogen. Purify from human plasma or dog serum by affinity chromatography on lysine–Sepharose or lysine–agarose (Miles Laboratories) according to the method of Deutsch and Mertz (20). The adsorbed protein is washed thoroughly with saline in 0.01 M phosphate buffer, pH 7.4, and the plasminogen is then eluted with 0.2 M ε-aminocaproic acid (EACA) or 0.1 M acetic acid. The EACA is removed by gel filtration on Sephadex G-25 or by dialysis. The plasminogen is assayed with urokinase (Leo Pharmaceutical Products, Denmark) or macrophage CM which contains PA in order to determine the optimal concentration required for assay. Filter, subdivide, and store frozen at −20°C.

Cell-Free Assays. CM and cell lysates are assayed, in duplicate, in a final reaction volume of 0.4 ml (Linbro wells) or 1.0 ml (35-mm dishes), in 0.1 M Tris-HCl buffer, pH 8.0, containing 125 μg of BSA, 5−10 μg of plasminogen, and 10−100 μl of the test fraction. The plates are incubated at 37°C for 1−6 hr, and the solubilized radioactivity is measured in a Packard Gamma Counter, at 2 or 3 time points. Appropriate controls for all reagents and media are included, and the plasminogen-dependent fibrinolysis is determined. Total releasable counts are obtained by incubation in trypsin. The radioactivity released should be proportional to enzyme concentration and time of incubation as long as the solubilization does not exceed approximately 20%.

Assays with Intact Cells. SBTI is added to prevent fibrinolysis prior to assay and media are monitored for breakthrough before each change. To initiate the fibrinolytic assay the monolayer is washed 3 times with HBSS to remove inhibitors and placed in Dulbecco's medium with acid-treated fetal bovine or dog serum, 5−10%, 0.4−2.5 ml per well or dish. Aliquots are removed at intervals and counted to measure solubilization of the fibrin. Controls without cells are included. Cells are observed by phase-contrast microscopy during the assay, which may be extended to 24 hr to detect low levels of activity.

Critical Comments

i. The ^{125}I-labeled fibrin plate assay is a rapid, sensitive, and versatile assay, which can be used to detect plasmin, PA activity in culture fluids, column effluents, SDS gels (3), etc. Its main drawback is lack of standardization. Fibrinolysis can be expressed in arbitrary units (3) or simply as percentage of radioactivity released per unit time. Urokinase reference standards (Leo Pharmaceutical Products, Denmark) are available.

ii. Backgrounds should be less than 1−2% of total radioactivity released per 4 hr, provided fibrinogen and plasminogen are purified and stored with care to prevent contamination with plasmin.

iii. Ensure that plasminogen levels in all assays are optimal, not limiting. Determine the optimal concentration of acid treated fetal bovine or dog serum to be used. Purified plasminogen can also be used to assay PA activity of intact cells.

iv. Use several concentrations of active cells to ensure that fibrinolytic activity is proportional to cell number.

v. Be sure that there are no polymorphonuclear leukocytes (PMN) contaminating the macrophage cultures, since PMN display high levels of fibrinolytic activity. Since PMN die within 6–12 hr of cultivation, it is best to preincubate all cultures for 1 day before assay.

2.3.3. *Collagenase*

Thioglycolate-elicited macrophages secrete rather small amounts of collagenase. Large amounts of conditioned medium and specially prepared substrates are necessary for its assay; methods for this are described elsewhere (6, 21).

2.3.4. *Elastase*

Macrophage elastase has little if any activity when assayed with synthetic substrates, and thus elastin must be used to screen for this enzyme.

Assays Utilizing Radial Diffusion in Agarose Gels Containing Elastin and SDS (5) *Principle.* Elastases bind firmly to elastin, and radial lysis of elastin incorporated in gels provides an easy semiquantitative procedure useful for screening large numbers of samples.

Materials

  Macrophage conditioned medium, concentrated or unconcentrated
  Elastin from bovine ligamentum nuchae, finely pulverized in the dry state with a rotary mill (Fisher Scientific), Micro Mill (Lab Apparatus, Cleveland, Ohio), or a Sorvall tissue homogenizer and passed through a sieve to give a mesh size of 200.
  Tris-HCl buffer, 0.1 M, pH 7.6, containing 1 mM CaCl$_2$
  Agarose
  Sodium azide
  Sodium dodecyl sulfate (SDS), electrophoresis grade
  Glass cover slips, 2 × 3 inches
  Sonicating homogenizer (e.g., Branson, Polytron, Ultraturrax)
  Moist chamber (e.g., food storage box with filter paper moistened with water containing 1% butanol)
  Incubator, 37°C
  Viewing box with dark-ground illumination

Method. Agarose (1 g) is dissolved in 100 ml of Tris-HCl buffer and boiled for 2 min; the mixture is cooled to 65°C. Elastin (100 mg) is moistened with approximately 0.5 ml of 70% ethanol added to the agarose, and the elastin is suspended by a 10-second treatment with the sonicator. SDS (25 mg) is added and the mixture swirled gently to dissolve the detergent. Finally, 0.5 ml of 10% (w/v) sodium azide solution is added to the mixture to retard microbial growth. The elastin suspension is cooled to 50°C and aliquots (6.7 ml) are placed on the glass plates using a plastic pipette or a prewarmed glass pipette. After the agarose has jelled, the plates are stored in a moist chamber at 4°C for at least 1 day prior to use. The plates can be stored for up to 1 month.

For assay of elastase activity, wells (5 mm diameter) are cut into the gel at spacings of about 1.3 cm center to center and samples (up to 30 μl) are placed in each well. Assays are incubated at 37°C in a moist chamber for up to 7 days. Zones of lysis are examined with dark-ground illumination and measured in two perpendicular diameters. Standards of porcine pancreatic elastase are included. Permanent records are kept by fixing and storing plates in 7% acetic acid. Alternatively, the plates may be dried under a sheet of filter paper and stained with Coomassie brilliant blue (400 μg/ml in a solvent consisting of 40% methanol, 40% acetic acid, 20% water) for 10 min, and briefly (1 min) destained in solvent. After rinsing in water and drying, the plates may be kept indefinitely. Note that weak reactions are more easily visible in wet unstained plates than in dried plates.

Assays for Elastinolysis Utilizing Radioactive Elastin as Substrate *Principle.* Insoluble elastin in which aldehydes and cross-links have been labeled by reduction with tritiated NaBH$_4$ provides a suitable substrate for a sensitive, linear assay. The use of sodium dodecyl sulfate, a hydrophobic ligand which makes the substrate more accessible to enzyme, increases the sensitivity of this assay by 5- to 100-fold, depending on the enzyme. The method described is slightly modified from that described by Takahashi *et al.* (22).

Materials

Elastin from bovine ligamentum nuchae, finely powdered to mesh size of 100–200

Sodium borohydride, ^{3}H-labeled (> 100 mCi/mmole)

Sodium borohydride (unlabeled)

NaOH, 1 M

Magnetic stir plate

Glacial acetic acid

Centrifuge with swinging-cup rotor

Tris-HCl buffer, 600 mM, pH 7.6, containing 0.05% sodium azide

Polypropylene centrifuge tubes, 400 μl

Microcentrifuge

Liquid scintillation fluid that will hold 200 μl of aqueous sample

Trypsin, crystalline, 1 mg/ml

Porcine pancreatic elastase, 100 μg/ml

Shaking water bath at 37°C

Method. Elastin (1 g) is suspended in 50 ml of distilled water in a 500-ml conical flask, and the pH is adjusted to 9.2 with NaOH. Tritiated NaBH$_4$ is mixed with 230 mg of unlabeled NaBH$_4$ to approximately 5 μCi/μmole and added to the elastin. This operation *must* be performed in a well-ventilated fume cupboard since *tritium gas* is a by-product of the reaction. The reaction mixture is stirred on a magnetic stirrer for 2 hr, and the reaction is stopped by careful addition of glacial acetic acid, to pH 3. Caution must be exercised since acidification brings about liberation of the residual hydrogen from the $NaBH_4$, and foaming may result. Check pH with pH paper. After stirring for an additional 30 min, the modified elastin is removed by centrifugation and washed with distilled water until the supernatant no longer shows radioactivity. The modified elastin may be stored as a suspension in water or lyophilized.

For assay of elastinolytic acitivity, the elastin is suspended at 2 mg/ml in water, and SDS is added to a final concentration of 0.5 mg/ml. This concentration should be checked by adding various concentrations of SDS and measuring the activity of pancreatic elastase preparations. Excess SDS will inactivate the enzymes. Aliquots of 100 μl (200 μg) of the elastin suspension are placed in microcentrifuge tubes and 600 mM Tris-HCl buffer, pH 7.6 (50 μl), is added. Samples of macrophage culture medium, inhibitors, etc., are added to give a total volume of 300 μl. The tubes are then securely capped, mixed well, and incubated at 37°C in a shaking water bath for 24 hr. Reactions are terminated by spinning in a microcentrifuge at 10,000 g for 5 min; 200 μl aliquots of the supernatant are taken for liquid scintillation counting. In each assay, tubes with trypsin (100 μg) are included to check for nonspecific lysis and with pancreatic elastase, 5 μg/tube, to measure total lysis, as well as the appropriate buffer blanks. Thioglycolate-elicited macrophage cultures secrete elastase activity capable of hydrolyzing up to 0.5 mg of elastin in 24 hr per 10^6 cells. Activities are expressed as micrograms of elastin hydrolysed per hour.

2.3.5. *Proteinase Assays with Azocasein as Substrate*

Principle. Derivatized casein is a sensitive substrate for a variety of proteolytic enzymes including trypsin and plasmin. At pH 5 it is readily hydrolyzed by nonspecific proteinases including enzymes secreted by macrophages. At pH 7.6 little neutral proteinase activity is detectable in thioglycolate macrophage CM before dialysis.

Materials

Casein (Hammersten grade, Mann Research Laboratories)
$NaHCO_3$
$NaNO_2$
Na_3PO_4
Acetic acid
Antifoam emulsion B (Sigma)

Method. Azocasein is prepared essentially as described by Charney and Tomarelli (23), modified by A. J. Barrett (personal communication). Casein (50 g) is dissolved in 1000 ml of 1% $NaHCO_3$, a little at a time. Insoluble material is removed by centrifugation at 5000 g for 10 min.

Sulfanilic acid (5 g) is dissolved in 200 ml of H_2O containing 12.0 ml of 5 M NaOH. $NaNO_2$ is added to this solution and stirred until dissolved. Then 18.0 ml of 5 M HCl is added, and the stirring is continued for 2 min. 18.0 ml of 5 M NaOH is added, and the solution is immediately poured into the casein solution, mixing with a paddle stirrer. This solution turns red as the azocasein is formed. Acetic acid (30%) is added to the mixture with continued stirring until the preparation becomes almost solid and bright orange in color (pH 4). (Persistent foam may be dispersed by gentle stirring with a glass rod dipped in the antifoam emulsion.) The precipitated azocasein is collected by centrifugation (5000 g, 5 min), and the supernatant is discarded. The pellet is resuspended in 300 ml of 1% Na_3PO_4 and 10% Na_3PO_4 added until the azocasein goes into solution (a bright red solution will be obtained). The azocasein is precipitated again with acetic acid and centrifuged; the pellets are redissolved as before. The azocasein solution is dialyzed against distilled water. Finally, the solution is lyophilized for storage.

The azocasein is dissolved, 6 g/100 ml, and the $OD_{366}^{1\%}$ is determined on diluted samples.

For assays of neutral proteinase activity, 0.125 ml of buffer (0.4 M Tris, pH 7.6, containing 20 mM $CaCl_2$) is mixed with 0.25 ml of enzyme solution (concentrated macrophage conditioned medium) in 13 $\times$ 100 mm test tubes. Azocasein (0.125 ml of a 6% solution) is added, and the samples are incubated in a water bath at 40°C for 1–20 hr. The reactions are stopped by the addition of 2.5 ml of 3% (w/v) trichloroacetic acid, and the soluble color is determined at 366 nm after filtration through Whatman No. 1 filter papers. In each assay appropriate blanks and controls are included. Activities are expressed as enzyme producing an increment in OD_{366} of 0.1 per hour.

3. General Comments

Cell culture provides a "closed" system that makes it possible to account accurately for the extra- and intracellular distribution of any product during continued cultivation. A constituent of macrophage CM may be secreted or shed by viable cells, released by damaged cells or derived from serum or other cell sources following modification or activation by macrophages. Adherence of products to cells or the culture vessel and uptake by endocytosis should be kept in mind.

The study of neutral proteinase secretion from macrophages is complicated by other factors. Although high levels of several enzyme activities are accumulated extracellularly over prolonged periods of cultivation, no direct biosynthetic incorporation of a labeled precursor into characterized product has yet been achieved. All the methods described here measure only activity, not enzyme protein. Individual enzyme activities have not been purified and characterized, and the number of distinct proteinases in crude macrophage CM remains unknown. The role of enzyme precursors, activation, and degradation and of plasma and cellular inhibitors remains obscure.

Macrophages from different sources within the same animal, in different states of metabolic activation or from different species, may contain or secrete different enzymes or in different proportions. The methods described here should make it possible to define some of these differences by further study.

ACKNOWLEDGMENTS

We thank Drs. Jay Unkeless, A. Barrett, D. Rifkin, and K. Platzer for helpful advice. Work in our laboratories has been supported by grants from The Rockefeller Foundation Medical Research Council, Nuffield Foundation, and the National Institutes of Health (AI07012 and 01831). Siamon Gordon is a Scholar, Leukemia Society of America, Inc.

REFERENCES

1. Gordon, S., *Science* in press (1976).
2. Gordon, S., Todd, J., and Cohn, Z., *J. Exp. Med.* **139**, 1228 (1974).
3. Unkeless, J. C., Gordon, S., and Reich, E., *J. Exp. Med.* **139**, 834 (1974).
4. Gordon, S., Unkeless, J. C., and Cohn, Z., *J. Exp. Med.* **140**, 995 (1974).
5. Werb, Z., and Gordon, S., *J. Exp. Med.* **142**, 361 (1975).
6. Werb, Z., and Gordon, S., *J. Exp. Med.* **142**, 346 (1975).
7. Davies, P., Page, R. C., and Allison, A. C., *J. Exp. Med.* **139**, 1262 (1974).
8. Axline, S. G., and Cohn, Z., *J. Exp. Med.* **131**, 1239 (1970).
9. Barrett, A. J., *in* "Lysosomes, a Laboratory Handbook" (J. T. Dingle, ed.), p. 46. North-Holland Publ., Amsterdam, 1972.
10. Wiener, E., and Curelaru, Z., *J. Reticuloendothel. Soc.* **17**, 319 (1975).
11. Bowers, W. E., *J. Exp. Med.* **136**, 1394 (1972).
12. Osserman, E. F., and Lawlor, D. F., *J. Exp. Med.* **124**, 921 (1966).
13. Beers, W. H., Strickland, S., and Reich, E., *Cell* **6**, 387 (1975).
14. Jones, P., Benedict, W., Strickland, S., and Reich, E., *Cell* **5**, 323 (1975).
15. Unkeless, J. C., Tobia, A., Ossowski, L., Quigley, J. P., Rifkin, J. B., and Reich, E., *J. Exp. Med.* **137**, 85 (1973).
16. Laki, K., *Arch. Biochem. Biophys.* **32**, 317 (1951).
17. Mosesson, M. W., *Biochem. Biophys. Acta* **57**, 204 (1970).
18. Helmkamp, R. W., Goodland, R. L., Bale, W. F., Spar, I. L., and Mutschler, L. E., *Cancer Res.* **20**, 1945 (1960).
19. Byrt, P., and Ada, G. L., *Immunology* **17**, 503 (1969).
20. Deutsch, D. G., and Mertz, E. T., *Science* **170**, 1095 (1970).
21. Gisslow, M. T., and McBride, B. C., *Anal. Biochem.* **68**, 70 (1975).
22. Takahashi, T., Seifter, S., and Yang, F. C., *Biochim. Biophys. Acta* **327**, 138 (1973).
23. Charney, J., and Tomarelli, R. M., *J. Biol. Chem.* **171**, 501 (1947).

28

Assay of Some Ectoenzyme Hydrolases on Leukocytes

J. W. dePierre and Manfred L. Karnovsky

1. Introduction

In addition to the intensive attention currently being given to such topics as the proteins that comprise part of the structure of cell membranes, the action of lectins at cell surfaces, and the role of immunological receptors on macrophage surfaces, there has been renewed interest in ectoenzymes. Ectoenzymes are defined as those enzymes that are on, or in, the plasma membrane of the cell, with the active sites facing the external medium. They are detected by their attack upon substrates in the external medium when those substrates are in contact with intact cells. The plasma membrane is the only subcellular structure that can be explored without disrupting the cell, so the use of ectoenzyme measurements under various conditions could yield worthwhile information on that organelle. In the descriptions below, three simple cases are outlined: the determination of ecto-ATPase, ecto-5′-nucleotidase, and ecto-p-nitrophenylphosphatase. The ability of intact cells to manifest enzyme activity toward an external substrate is not of itself a demonstration that the enzyme responsible is an ectoenzyme. Some principles, strictures, and *caveats* involved in interpreting the data are given after the description of the assays.

2. Materials

2.1. Chemicals. These should be of reagent grade. The suppliers of special reagents and radioactive substances are indicated in the descriptions of the ectoenzyme measurement procedures below, where each such substance is first mentioned.

2.2. Cells. The techniques with cells in suspension (mentioned below) may be applied to any samples of free-swimming cells. We have utilized neutrophilic granulocytes and elicited macrophages from guinea pigs, rats, and mice [e.g., Oren *et al.* (1)], normal mouse peritoneal macrophages obtained by lavage, and several other cell types, such as human neutrophils obtained by conventional sedimentation methods. Where the cell involved will adhere to glass or plastic, the use of cellular monolayers in the enzyme assay, rather than suspensions, has advantages of purification and scale in some cases. We have found plastic dishes, 35 mm in diameter, to be satisfactory (Falcon Plastics Co., Los Angeles), and the procedure is outlined by Michell *et al.* (2) for the formation and washing of such monolayers. Cell numbers may be determined by conventional means in suspensions, using a hemacytometer. With monolayers, in particular, quantification of cells by means of protein determinations offers some advantages (3). The cell numbers and protein levels cited below are for guinea pig granulocytes and are given only as examples (4).

3. Measurement of Ecto-ATPase

3.1. Cells in Suspension. The assay is based on the observation by Crane and Lipmann (5) that charcoal adsorbs adenosine phosphates but not inorganic phosphate. The standard assay mixture contains 1.2 to 1.8×10^7 intact cells [or an appropriate amount of a homogenate, sonicate, or subcellular fraction of these cells, if one is attempting to prove that the reaction is due to an ectoenzyme, (see below)]. p-Nitrophenylphosphate (5 mM) (Sigma Phosphatase Substrate 104), is added, to avoid inclusion of activity of nonspecific phosphatases in the ATPase measurement, and 1 mM [γ-^{32} P] ATP [synthesized by the method of Glynn and Chappell (6)] in 1 ml of Krebs-Ringer phosphate solution, pH 7.4. The 15 mM inorganic phosphate in KRP does not inhibit the ATPase, since similar results were obtained when this buffering species was replaced with glycylglycine. The assay mixture is incubated at 37°C for 20 or 30 min (shaking is not necessary, but preferable) and then transferred to an ice bucket. After 75 sec, 1 ml of a 10% (w/v) suspension of acid-washed Norit in 10% (w/v) trichloroacetic acid is added to the sample. After another 75 sec in ice, the charcoal is removed by filtration through Whatman No. 1 filter paper. ^{32}P$_i$ in an aliquot of the filtrate is then determined by counting in a liquid scintillation counter. A control without cells is routinely performed, and the assays are done at least in duplicate.

Under these conditions the hydrolysis of ATP by intact cells is linear for at least 30 min and is proportional to cell concentration in the range 0.5 to 3×10^7 cells/ml, at least. The ATPase of homogenates and sonicates is also found to be directly proportional to time and concentration of protein. About 10% of the ATP present is normally hydrolyzed during the incubation period; i.e., the conditions are for saturating substrate.

This assay can easily be scaled down 10-fold by incubating 1.0 to 1.5×10^6 intact cells (or equivalent sonicate, for example), 5 mM p-nitrophenylphosphate, and 1 mM [γ-^{32} P] ATP having five times the usual specific activity, in 0.2 ml of Krebs-Ringer phosphate solution at 37°C for 30 min. The rest of the procedure is unchanged, except that 2 ml of 10% acid-washed Norit in 10% trichloroacetic acid are added to the sample instead of 1 ml.

An important aspect of this assay is that it is specific for the release of the γ-phosphate from ATP. ATPase assays based on the colorimetric determination of released inorganic phosphate must contend with possible contamination from the further breakdown of ADP to AMP and of AMP to adenosine.

3.2. Cells on Monolayers. This procedure is very similar to the assay in suspension, except that the cells are first made into a monolayer. Briefly, 0.4 to 1.8×10^7 intact cells in 1.0 ml of Krebs Ringer phosphate solution, pH 7.4, are added to a plastic tissue culture dish. The preparation (lid on dish) is incubated 30–45 min at 37°C with occasional swirling. The supernatant is then decanted, and the whole dish is washed at least three times by immersion in separate beakers of Krebs-Ringer phosphate solution. This removes nonadherent cells. The monolayers are then covered with 1 ml of medium containing the various substrates and reagents.

The monolayer is then incubated for 20 or 30 min at 37°C in the presence of labeled substrate and p-nitrophenylphosphate (see above). At the end of this period, the supernatant is removed and the monolayer is washed with 1 ml of Krebs-Ringer phosphate solution. After this wash, less than 3% of the added radioactivity remains on the monolayer. Since only about 10% of the added ATP is hydrolyzed, even such a small residual amount of ^{32}P might be significant if the cells took up the product but not the substrate (however, as mentioned below, localization may be determined). The original supernatant and the wash are mixed, 1 ml of this mixture is treated with Norit–trichloroacetic acid as detailed above for the determination of released radioactivity, and the other milliliter is digested at room temperature overnight in 0.5 N NaOH for protein determination. Protein present on the monolayer plate is also measured after dissolution overnight in 1 ml of 0.5 M NaOH. *Total* protein values are used in the calculations. Duplicate or triplicate assays are routinely performed.

This ATPase assay is linear for at least 30 min and over the range of 50 300 μg of protein (0.6 to 3.5 $\times 10^7$ cells) per monolayer plate. ATPase values obtained by this monolayer method are about 95% of the values obtained by assay of the same cells in suspension, suggesting that adhesion to a surface renders few, if any, of the ATPase active sites inaccessible to substrate molecules.

4. Measurement of Ecto-5′-nucleotidase (AMPase)

Since AMP is also adsorbed by charcoal (5), the hydrolysis of AMP is measured in suspension and on monolayers in a manner essentially identical to the assay of ATPase activity. The standard assay mixture contains 1 mM p-nitrophenylphosphate to avoid inclusion of nonspecific phosphatase activity and 1 mM [^{32}P] AMP (Amersham/Searle) in KRP. The 15 mM inorganic phosphate in KRP does not inhibit the AMPase, since similar results are obtained when this buffering species is replaced with Tris buffer. Both in suspension and on monolayers, this assay is found to be linear for at least 30 min and at least over the range of 1 to 8 $\times$ 10^6 cells per assay vessel. Assays are performed in duplicate or triplicate, and the whole procedure can easily be scaled down 10-fold.

5. Measurement of Ecto-*p*-nitrophenylphosphatase

Two methods may be employed to determine the hydrolysis of *p*-nitrophenyl-phosphate. In both procedures 1.0 to 1.5 $\times$ 10^7 intact cells (or an appropriate amount of a homogenate, sonicate, or subcellular fraction) per milliliter of suspension or per monolayer plate is incubated with 1 m*M* substrate in Krebs-Ringer phosphate, pH 7.4, for 20 or 30 min at 37°C. The 15 m*M* inorganic phosphate present in the medium apparently does inhibit *p*-nitrophenylphos-phatase activity to some degree, since the activity is 10–15% higher when this buffering species is replaced with Tris or glycyglycine. In the colorimetric assay the reaction is stopped by adding 3–5 ml of 0.1 *N* NaOH to the suspension or 1 ml of 1.0 *N* NaOH to the monolayer. The optical density at 410 nm is then measured. Background absorbance at this wavelength due to cells alone and to nonenzymic hydrolysis of the substrate are subtracted from the sample readings. In the assay procedure using radioactive substrate (Amersham/Searle) the reac-tion is stopped in the same manner as for the ATPase (*p*-nitrophenylphosphate is also adsorbed onto charcoal), and an aliquot of the filtrate is subsequently counted. The radioactive assay is used chiefly when the presence of a colored reagent would interfere with the colorimetric determination. Direct comparison demonstrated that the assays give identical results. Both procedures were found to be linear for at least 30 min and at least over the range of 0.2 to 3.0 $\times$ 10^7 cells per assay vessel. Duplicates are routinely performed, and the assays can easily be scaled down 10-fold. The *p*-nitrophenylphosphatase measured on monolayers was about 95% of that measured in suspension.

6. Expression of Results

We find it convenient to add about 10^6 cpm in each regular assay tube. It is useful to determine the specific activity of the substrate at the time of each assay. Data may be expressed in comparative or absolute terms; i.e., different cell types or conditions may be compared as percentages or as nanomoles cleaved per milligram of cell protein or per 10^6 cells, for a given time, usually 15 min. The absorbance (*E*) value used for *p*-nitrophenol was 1.84 $\times$ 10^4 (7).

7. Some Strictures That Should Be Considered

7.1. The substrates used for the ectoenzyme assays should not be able to permeate the plasma membrane or should be of very limited permeability.

7.2. The cells should be well washed to avoid complications due to any adsorbed enzyme.

7.3. The cells should be as intact as possible; i.e., optimal conditions should be used for their maintenance, and incubation times should be relatively short. Monitoring by exclusion of trypan blue and determination of the leakage of *known intracellular* enzymes into the external medium helps to assess the integrity of the cells and to ensure that the reaction under study is indeed due to an ectoenzyme.

7.4. The measurements of ectoenzyme activity should be made under conditions of linearity with time. Such linearity would indicate that the cells are not deteriorating, with "leakage" of substrate to the interior or an enzyme to the exterior.

7.5. At saturating levels of external substrate (maximal enzyme action by the intact cells), the effect of disruption of the plasmalemma and of other cellular membranes should be examined. The degree to which such disruptions *increase* the enzymic reactions provides an indication of the proportion of the cellular activity that is truly "ecto." The plasmalemma may simply be a barrier to the substrate with respect to internal enzymes, and saturable transport processes may exist across that barrier. These possibilities must be considered before an enzyme is regarded as "ecto" (4).

7.6. The decision as to whether a substrate added to the medium in which cells are bathed is cleaved by ectoenzymes or simply enters the cell in some fashion, to be hydrolyzed intracellularly, may be made more definitively, as follows: (i) The localization of the products formed in a short time (i.e., intracellular or extracellular) can be determined. If the products are predominantly extracellular, an ectoenzyme is indeed indicated. (ii) The effect of nonpenetrating (highly charged) inhibitors, preferably those that form a covalent bond with membrane proteins, may be determined. If the nonpenetrating reagent inhibits the enzymic reaction, involvement of an ectoenzyme is strongly indicated.

7.7. It should be recognized that there are differences in ectoenzyme activities between cell types within a species (8). For a given cell type values may depend upon species or the previous history of the cells (9). For example, guinea pig granulocytes have abundant ecto-AMPase, whereas human granulocytes lack that ectoenzyme. In mice, normal peritoneal macrophages have ecto-AMPase, while peritoneal cells elicited with caseinate are devoid of the enzyme (9).

The strictures given above are not explored further here. They have been dealt with previously (4). The actual approach to measuring the reaction of putative ectoenzymes of intact cells with external substrates is exemplified by the cases given. The investigator is left to interpret the *caveats* offered above and to employ one or more methods of proof that a given enzymic action is really ectoenzymic.

REFERENCES

1. Oren, R., Farnham, A. E., Saito, K., Milofsky, E., and Karnovsky, M. L., *J. Cell Biol.* **171,** 484 (1963).
2. Michell, R. H., Pancake, S. J., Noseworthy, J., and Karnovsky, M. L., *J. Cell Biol.* **40,** 216 (1969).
3. Lowry, O. H., Rosebrough, N. J., and Randall, R. J., *J. Biol. Chem.* **193,** 269 (1951).
4. dePierre, J. W., and Karnovsky, M. L., *J. Biol. Chem.* **249,** 7111 (1974).
5. Crane, R. K., and Lipmann, F., *J. Biol. Chem.* **201,** 235 (1953).
6. Glynn, I. M., and Chappell, J. B., *Biochem. J.* **90,** 147 (1964).
7. Kedzy, F., and Bender, M., *Biochemistry* **1,** 1097 (1962).
8. dePierre, J. W., and Karnovsky, M. L., *J. Biol. Chem.* **249,** 7121 (1974).
9. Karnovsky, M. L., Lazdins, J., Drath, D., and Harper, A., *Ann. N. Y. Acad. Sci.* **256,** 266 (1975).

A Nonspecific Esterase Strain for the Identification of Monocytes and Macrophages

I. R. Koski, D. G. Poplack, and R. M. Blaese

1. Introduction

The identification of monocytes and macrophages in mixed lymphoid cell populations frequently presents problems for investigators, particularly those who are not experienced morphologists or in situations where clear visualization of the cell is obscured. A variety of methods have been employed to aid the identification of this cell type, including phagocytosis of easily visualized particles (yeast, polystyrene-latex beads, etc.) and various histochemical reactions that take advantage of the macrophages' rich complement of lysosomal enzymes. Nonspecific esterases catalyze the reaction

$$R\text{-}COOR' + HOH \rightarrow RCOOH + R'OH$$

and many investigators have demonstrated the presence of such enzymes in macrophages (1–6). This chapter describes our modification of a staining technique for nonspecific esterase originally described by Yam, Li, and Crosby (7).

The method is useful for the identification of macrophages and monocytes in fixed smears and touch preparations of mixed lymphoid cell preparations and is particularly valuable for distinguishing macrophages and monocytes from lymphocytes in mixed populations containing lymphoid cells coated with erythrocytes in various cell surface receptor assays (e.g., Fc, EAC).

2. Materials

2.1. Equipment: Coplin staining jars; Glass pipettes, 5 ml; Slide holders (slide grip, Peel-A-Way Plastics, VWR Scientific No. 4844-002); Screw-cap glass bottle, 100 ml; Fluted filter paper (No. 58, Schleicher and Schuell, fast speed, 0.008 thickness)

2.2. Fixative solution: Na_2HPO_4, 20 mg; KH_2PO_4, 100 mg; distilled water, 30 ml; acetone, 45 ml; formaldehyde (30%), 25 ml. Mix reagents thoroughly and adjust pH to 6.6. Keep refrigerated. Fixative solution can be reused 2 or 3 times before discarding.

2.3. Pararosaniline solution: pararosaniline hydrochloride (Sigma No. P-

3750), 1.0 g; 2 N HCl (warm), 25 ml. Store this stock solution in refrigerator.

2.4. 4% Sodium nitrite solution: sodium nitrite, 100 mg; distilled water, 2.5 ml. Prepare fresh for each use.

2.5. $M/15$ Sorenson's phosphate buffer (pH 6.3): Na_2HPO_4, 2.128 g; KH_2PO_4, 6.984 g; distilled water, 1000 ml.

2.6. α-Naphthyl butyrate solution: α-naphthyl butyrate (Sigma N-8000), 1.0 g; dimethyl formamide (Mallinckrodt spectrophotometric grade or Sigma D-4254), 50 ml. Mix reagents in a glass bottle using a glass pipette. Keep solution in freezer (it will not freeze). Protect from light.

2.7. Methyl green counterstain (0.5%): methyl green (Fisher No. 76110), 500 mg; distilled water, 100 ml. Store in refrigerator and filter before use.

3. Staining Procedure

3.1. Prepare smears in serum for best morphology.

3.2. Fix slides in cold fixative in Coplin jar for 30 sec.

3.3. Rinse by transferring slides carefully through four jars of distilled water.

3.4. Air-dry slides for 30 min.

3.5. Using fluted filter paper, filter approximately 1 ml of pararosaniline solution.

3.6. Mix filtered solution with an equal volume of freshly prepared 4% sodium nitrite for hexazotization. Allow to stand for 1 min before use.

3.7. Mix in sequence: $M/15$ phosphate buffer, pH 6.3, 44.5 ml; hexazotized pararosaniline, 0.25 ml; α-naphthyl butyrate solution (glass pipette), 3.0 ml.

3.8. Filter into Coplin jar (use only once).

3.9. Stain slides in Coplin jar by placing jar in 37°C water bath for 45 min.

3.10. Rinse slides carefully, as before, in distilled water.

3.11. Drain slides and counterstain with 0.5% methyl green for 15 sec.

3.12. Rinse in distilled water.

3.13. Air-dry for 30 min and cover slip with Permount.

Suggestions

1. Follow procedure without interruption.

2. For best results, fix and stain slides within 24 hr of preparation.

3. Store unfixed and unstained slides at room temperature since condensation of water vapor on cold slides may alter morphology and staining characteristics.

4. Interpretation and Comments

Nonspecific esterase-containing cells are easily distinguishable by the presence of multiple intensely red-stained granules in the cytoplasm compared with the green counterstain of the esterase-negative cells (Fig. 1). Nonspecific esterase activity is very strong in monocytes, macrophages, histiocytes, and megakaryocytes and very weak or absent in neutrophils, basophils, eosinophils, myeloblasts, promyolocytes, and erythroblasts (7). It is also usually absent from lymphocytes and plasma cells, although occasionally these cells will contain a single intensely stained granule. The technique has been successfully applied in studies of human, monkey, mouse, rat, and guinea pig cells. It can also be used in combination with other stains (e.g., Giemsa) when more detailed visualization of the esterase-negative cells is desired.

Correlation of monocyte count using this nonspecific esterase stain with other morphological or functional assays of monocyte number is generally very good. A combined procedure of latex bead phagocytosis followed by nonspecific esterase staining usually reveals a slightly higher percentage of cells containing esterase than those actively engaged in latex bead phagocytosis. A direct correlation has been demonstrated between the number of esterase-staining cells present and the degree of killing observed in a monocyte-mediated assay of antibody-dependent cellular cytotoxicity (8). Approximately 85–90% of peripheral blood esterase containing monocytes also have demonstrable receptors for IgG-Fc, and 98–100% of esterase-positive monocytes from inflammatory exudates have such Fc receptors. The esterase staining of monocytes is particularly valuable in these receptor assays since frequently the entire cell surface is

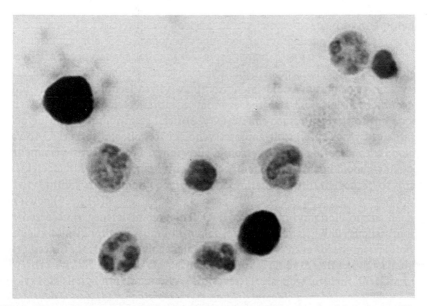

Fig. 1. Smear of dextran-sedimented human peripheral blood stained for nonspecific esterase activity. The field contains two intensely stained monocytes, 2 esterase-negative lymphocytes, and 5 esterase-negative neutrophils.

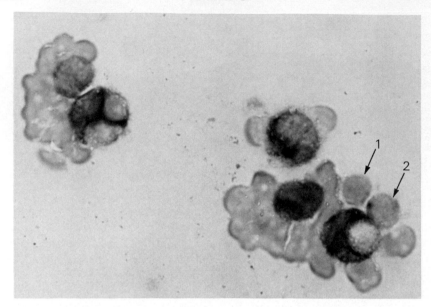

Fig. 2. Fc receptor assay employing IgG antibody-coated human erythrocytes and human peripheral blood mononuclear leukocytes. Five monocytes are coated with adherent erythrocytes. The arrows indicate lymphocytes that are not distinctive in the photomicrograph because of the black and white photography. Lymphocyte 2 contains a single esterase-positive granule.

covered by one to four layers of erythrocytes and only the histochemical reaction demonstrating esterase in the center of the rosette allows identification of the rosetted cell as a monocyte (Fig. 2).

REFERENCES

1. Koelle, G. B., *J. Pharmacol. Exp. Ther.* **103,** 153 (1951).
2. Grogg, E., and Pearse, A. G. E., *Br. J. Exp. Pathol.* **33,** 567 (1952).
3. Gall, E. A., *Ann. N. Y. Acad. Sci.* **73,** 120 (1958).
4. Gropp, A., and Hupe, K., *Virchows Arch. Pathol. Anat. Physiol.* **331,** 641 (1958).
5. Hosoda, S., and Takase, S., *Nature (London)* **190,** 927 (1961).
6. Leder, L. P., *Blut* **16,** 86 (1967).
7. Yam, L. T., Li, C. Y., and Crosby, W. H., *Am. J. Clin. Pathol.* **55,** 283 (1971).
8. Poplack, D. G., Bonard, J. D., and Blaese, R. M., *Fed. Proc., Fed. Am. Soc. Exp. Biol.* **34,** 823 (1975).

30

Measurement of Phagocytosis by Macrophages*

Joyce M. Cox and Thomas P. Stossel

1. Introduction

One of the major characteristics of macrophages is their capacity to engulf particulate matter, thereby constituting an indispensable host defense mechanism against invasion by microorganisms and other alien materials (1).

Phagocytosis has been measured in a number of different ways. Frequently the extent of phagocytosis is determined microscopically and is expressed either as the number of particles per cell or as the average number of cells containing particles. Besides being tedious, this method is inaccurate because of the tendency of many particles to aggregate and/or adsorb to the outside of the cell without being ingested. Methods that involve inactivation of a population of bacteria by phagocytes can also be considered only semiquantitative because of the complexity of the systems utilized. Rates of metabolic responses to phagocytosis, such as O_2 consumption and hexose monophosphate shunt activity has been used as an index of phagocytic rates (2) in view of the observations that these parameters parallel the amount of ingestion that has occurred (2–4, 10). Although the use of such metabolic indicators of ingestion is convenient because it permits the study of a wide range of test particles since separation of particles from cells is not required, the metabolic activities of resting cells contribute background activity and certain chemical and biological agents can stimulate cellular metabolism without the occurrence of particle uptake (5). The best assays for ingestion involve direct measurement in phagocytes of particles that permit detection by chemical techniques. Such systems have been devised with polystyrene or polyvinyltoluene particles (3, 6), radioactively labeled bacteria (4, 7, 8), starch particles (4) or immune complexes (9). The method presented here involves the use of diisodecyl phthalate particles containing oil red O. Macrophages and other phagocytes ingest oil droplets containing oil red O stabilized with a variety of substances. Spectrophotometric determination of oil

*This work was supported by U.S. Public Health Service Grant HL-19429, Contract HL 15157, and an Established Investigatorship of the American Heart Association (to Dr. Stossel).

red O in the cells after uningested particles have been removed by differential centrifugation provides a quantitative measure of phagocytosis (10–12). Control experiments with this system have demonstrated proportionality of ingestion rate with particle concentration at low particle:cell ratios and independence of ingestion rate with respect to particle concentration at high particle:cell ratios. Complete inhibition of ingestion is obtained by incubating cells and particles together at 0°C or with a high concentration of metabolic inhibitors. The method is quantitative and allows for measurement of initial *rate* as opposed to capacity of ingestion, the utility of which has been established (4, 6, 11). Depending upon the particle surface and cell types selected, the rate of phagocytosis varies. *Escherichia coli* lipopolysaccharide-coated oil red O droplets are not ingested by macrophages unless the particles are first allowed to react (opsonized) with fresh serum.

The opsonic activity of serum for lipopolysaccharide-coated oil red O particles involves the fixation of C3 by means of the alternative complement system (11–13): Therefore, measurement of the initial rate of uptake of these particles constitutes a precise assay for the opsonic activity of serum mediated by this pathway.

2. Materials

2.1. Preparation of Phagocytes

Sodium chloride, 0.9% (normal saline)

Modified Krebs-Ringer phosphate medium (KRP), pH 7.4 NaCl, 0.15 M, 100 parts KCl, 0.154 M, 4 parts. Phosphate buffer, pH 7.4, 12 parts prepared from Ca 3 parts of 0.10 M Na_2HPO_4 and 1 part of NaH_2PO_4, adjusted to pH 7.4; $MgSO_4$, 0.15 M, 1 part; $CaCl_2$, 0.11 M, 1 part; add slowly with stirring to avoid precipitation.

The final solution is adjusted to pH 7.4 with 1.0 M NaOH.

2.2. Preparation of Diisodecyl Phthalate Containing Oil Red O Particles

Diisodecyl phthalate (Coleman, Matheson-Bell, Cleveland, Ohio)

Oil red O (Allied Chemical Corp., Morristown, New Jersey)

Escherichia coli lipopolysaccharide, 10 mg/ml in normal saline (Serotype 026:B6, Boivin preparation, Difco, Detroit, Michigan) Catalogue no. 3920-25

fresh serum

2.3. Ingestion Assay

Macrophages 5–10% (v/v) in KRP (see Section 3.2)

Opsonized particles (see Sections 3.3–3.5)

Wash solution: 1 mM N-ethyl maleimide (Nutritional Biochemicals Corp.) in 0.15 M NaCl

p-Dioxane

3. Methods

3.1. Principle of Assay. Macrophages (or other phagocytes) are fed oil red O-containing oil droplets, coated with *E. coli* lipopolysaccharide. It is necessary to opsonize these particles by treating them with fresh serum in order for ingestion to be optimized. The rate of ingestion of the opsonized particles by the cells is initially constant for 10 min for rabbit pulmonary macrophages. After cells and particles have been incubated for the selected time interval, the uningested oil particles, because of their low density, are efficiently separated from the cells containing ingested particles by centrifugation: the cells sediment and the unengulfed particles float. Oil red O is extracted from the washed cell pellets with dioxane and spectrophotometrically measured.

3.2. Preparation of Phagocytes. The phagocytosis assay can be used for any phagocyte including blood phagocytes (PMN, bands, and monocytes), peritoneal phagocytes (PMN + macrophages), alveolar macrophages, and even amoebae. Cells may be stimulated by an appropriate method if desired or simply collected as present in body cavities or on the surface of organs and tissues. In either instance, the cells are collected by lavage with 0.15 M NaCl and centrifuged at about 100 g for 10 min. A sample is removed for differential count at this point as cell morphology is still well preserved. If the pellets appear to contain erythrocytes, they are lysed as follows: the pellet is resuspended in 2.0 ml of 0.9% sodium chloride after which are added in quick succession, 20.0 ml of H_2O and 2.0 ml of 9.0% sodium chloride. The tubes are then centrifuged again at 100 g for 10 min. The cell buttons are suspended in ice-cold 0.15 M NaCl, pooled, and washed once with 0.15 M NaCl (centrifuged 500 g for 10 min). If a delay in performing the assay is anticipated, most phagocytic cells can be left for some time in cold 0.15 M NaCl which is better than buffered media with divalent cations, as the latter allow for clumping of cells. The final cell buttons are suspended in any buffered isotonic medium with divalent cations (Krebs–Ringer phosphate, Hanks' balanced salt solution, etc.) at a concentration of 5–10% (v/v) or 20,000–60,000 mm³. A sample is taken for cell count or protein at this time.

3.3. Preparation of Diisodecyl Phthalate and Oil Red O. Approximately 2 g of oil red O is added to 50 ml of diisodecyl phthalate in a large porcelain mortar and ground with a pestle. The saturated suspension is centrifuged in glass tubes (top speed in a Sorvall or International clinical centrifuge) to remove undissolved dye (which can be reutilized). The dye-containing oil is stable and can be stored indefinitely at room temperature. Since the amount of dye in the oil varies, a factor is computed that converts optical density to milligrams of oil to permit normalization and comparison of results. Ten microliters of oil red O–diisodecyl phthalate is added to 10 ml of dioxane, and the optical density at 525 nm is determined. The following formula gives the conversion factor (mg/OD).

$$\frac{0.95}{\text{OD}} = \frac{\text{(the density of the oil)}}{\text{(the actual reading)}}$$

3.4. Preparation of Particles. To prepare the droplets, 40 mg of *E. coli* lipopolysaccharide are dissolved into 3 ml of balanced salt solution in a 10–15-ml glass or thick-walled plastic test tube. The LPS is dispersed by brief sonication (any model sonifier will do). One milliliter of the oil–oil red O is layered over the aqueous LPS solution, and the mixture is sonified. The sonifier probe should be just below the oil–aqueous interface; the length of sonication is about 90 sec, just until the tube becomes hot to handle. The output can be low–the sonication details are unimportant except that it is better to err on the side of sonicating too long. The final preparation should look like a strawberry milkshake. The particle suspension can be used immediately (after cooling) or frozen. Brief sonication after thawing is advisable.

3.5. Opsonization. The particles are opsonized, usually just before the ingestion step, by adding an equal volume of fresh human serum and incubating at 37°C for 15–30 min. The rate of C3 deposition varies with the species of origin of the serum–it is complete within 15 min in guinea pig serum, 20–30 min in human or rabbit serum. If the particles are allowed to sit indefinitely in serum at 37°C, proteolytic activity slowly removes the opsonically active C3. Therefore, the opsonized particles must be kept cold, frozen or washed (see below) until use. Opsonized particles can be frozen and thawed and are still palatable to the phagocytes.

3.6. Ingestion (Individual Tube Method). To assay ingestion, 0.2 volume of opsonized particle suspension (prewarmed to 37°C) is added to 0.8 volume of cell suspension (also prewarmed). The reaction can be started by adding either particles to cells or cells to particles. The reaction can be run in siliconized glass 15-ml conical centrifuge tubes in a system of total volume 1 ml (in which case 0.2 ml of particles is added to 0.8 ml of cell suspension). After 5 min, during which the tubes are occasionally tapped to keep the actors in suspension, 6 ml of ice-cold isotonic saline containing 1 mM N-ethyl maleimide (126 mg/liter), which poisons the cells and stops ingestion. The tubes are centrifuged at 250 g (1000 rpm for 10 min in a centrifuge with 19-cm radius). The rim of uningested particles at the top is dislodged by shaking the tube vertically; the supernatant is discarded, but the pellets are not completely drained. The small amount of residual supernatant is used to suspend the cell pellet by tapping the bottom of the tube. More NEM-saline is added, and the washing is repeated. After the second wash the supernatant is discarded, the tubes are inverted to drain the pellets, and finally the sides of the tubes are wiped with tissue. The cell pellets are disrupted and oil red O is solubilized by addition of 1 or more milliliters of dioxane with tapping or vortexing of the tubes. The extracts are centrifuged at 500 g for 15 min to remove debris, and the optical density of the extracts is read in a colorimeter or spectrophotometer at a wavelength of 525 nm against a dioxane blank.

3.7. Ingestion—Batch Aliquot Method for Time Course. If a time course of uptake is desired, it is convenient to incubate a larger volume of reaction mixture and remove samples at different times. Cell suspension, 4.0 ml (6–10% in KRP) is prewarmed to 37°C in a 25–50 ml siliconized flask or plastic vial; 1.0 ml of particles is added to start the reaction. The flasks are placed on a shaker in a 37°C water bath, and 0.5 ml is transferred in duplicate at 0, 3, 6, and 9 min to 12-ml conical centrifuge tubes in ice containing 5–6 ml of 1 mM N-ethyl maleimide in isotonic saline. The rest of the assay is done as described above.

3.8. Calculation of Results

$$\text{Initial ingestion rate} = \frac{(OD_{525})\ (\text{conversion factors})}{[(\text{cells} \times 10^7)/\text{ml}]\ (\text{time of incubation})}$$

Where initial ingestion rate is in milligrams of oil per 10^7 cells per minute and the time of incubation is in minutes. (For the conversion factor see Section 3.3.)

4. Interpretation of Data and Critical Comments

This assay allows for the accurate determination of the initial rate of ingestion and thus allows for precise quantification of phagocytosis. The oil emulsion is easily prepared and relatively inexpensive. Diisodecyl phthalate is convenient for the assay because its density is low enough to facilitate separation of uningested particles from the cells, but is not low enough to make the cells float. The phagocytes are not unduly stressed by the procedure, since cells that have been through the wash procedure can be reincubated at 37°C with shaking for as long as 90 min and still retain 100% of the oil red O present at the end of the washing.

It is important when measuring phagocytosis to be able to distinguish between particles adsorbed to the surface of phagocytes or trapped between phagocyte clumps and particles actually internalized. This ambiguity is usually controlled through the determination of zero time controls or by incubation with metabolic inhibitors that block ingestion but not nonspecific adsorption and trapping. High concentrations of inhibitors completely inhibit oil red O uptake.

Other advantages of the method presented here include the facts that complete extraction of oil red O from the washed cell pellets can be visually monitored and that, since the hydrocarbons are only minimally metabolized (14), metabolic experiments may be performed concurrently. The spectrophotometric reading in the visible range obviates the need for spectral quality solvents and minimizes the unrecognized absorption of light by materials present in cellular extracts. Ingestion can also be monitored visually by observing Wright's stained smears. The methanol in the stain elutes the oil, and ingested particles appear as lucent vacuoles whereas extracellular particles are removed (15). This approach can be used to determine which cells in a mixed population are phagocytic.

The assay is most specific for determining differences in cell populations from a single source examined at the same point in time. There is marked variation in test results performed on different days or with different animals because of the many factors that contribute to the final value. Absolute differences in maximal rates of uptake may reflect differences in homogeneity of cell population and protein content per cell. Differences may also arise secondary to variability in the opsonizing power of the serum used.

REFERENCES

1. Metchnikoff, E., "Immunity in Infectious Diseases" (English trans. by F. G. Binnie), Cambridge Univ. Press, London, 1905.
2. Sbarra, A. J., and Karnovsky, M. L., *J. Biol. Chem.* **234,** 1355 (1959).
3. Roberts, J., and Quastel, H., *Biochem. J.* **89,** 150 (1963).
4. Michell, R. H., Pancake, S. J., Noseworthy, J., and Karnovsky, M. L., *J. Cell Biol.* **40,** 216 (1969).
5. Cohn, Z. A., and Morse, S. I., *J. Exp. Med.* **111,** 688 (1960).
6. Weisman, R. A., and Korn, E. D., *Biochemistry* **6,** 485 (1967).
7. Root, R. K., Rosenthal, A. S., and Balestra, D. J., *J. Clin. Invest.* **51,** 649 (1972).
8. Ulrich, F., *Am. J. Physiol.* **220,** 958 (1971).
9. Ward, P. A., and Zvaifler, N. J., *J. Immunol.* **111,** 1771 (1973).
10. Stossel, T. P., Mason, R. J., Hartwig, J., and Vaughan, M., *J. Clin. Invest.* **51,** 615 (1972).
11. Stossel, T. P., *J. Cell Biol.* **58,** 346 (1973).
12. Stossel, T. P., Alper, C. A., and Rosen, F. S., *J. Exp. Med.* **137,** 690 (1973).
13. Stossel, T. P., Field, R. J., Gitlin, J. D., Alper, C. A., and Rosen, F. S., *J. Exp. Med.* **141,** 1329 (1975).
14. Bollinger, J. N., *J. Pharmacol. Sci.* **59,** 1084 (1970).
15. Altman, A., and Stossel, T. P., *Br. J. Haematol.* **27,** 241 (1974).

31

The Gold Uptake Assay

Christopher Meade, Peter Lachmann, and Diane Lowe

1. Introduction

Supernatants prepared by incubating lymphocytes from sensitized animals with antigen produce a number of changes in macrophage populations (1, 2). These changes have been loosely termed "macrophage activation." Pinocytosis is of particular interest as a parameter of "macrophage activation" because changes in the rate of pinocytosis occur relatively early after exposure to active lymphocyte supernatants (24 hr) (3). Furthermore, a relationship has been demonstrated between rate of pinocytosis and rate of lysosome formation (4), lysosomes being formed by fusion of pinocytic vesicles with vesicles from the Golgi body (5).

As a pinocytosis marker, Au-198 colloid has several advantages. It is relatively nontoxic and stable to aggregation in biological media (6). Once taken up by the macrophage, colloidal gold is quantitatively retained for at least 24 hr (7), and there is relatively little uptake by lymphocytes or polymorphonuclear leukocytes, which are frequently also present in macrophage populations (8, 9). Compared with other isotopes, ^{198}Au is not expensive, and being a gamma emitter may be counted without elaborate sample preparation.

As an *in vitro* assay for cell-mediated immunity, the main practical advantage of the gold uptake assay is that relatively smaller quantities of lymphocyte products are required to stimulate macrophage pinocytosis than are required to inhibit migration inhibition (3).

In our laboratories, the gold uptake assay has been used to detect sensitivity to purified protein derivative (PPD), ovalbumin, and basic protein in guinea pigs using either peritoneal exudate cells or blood cells as indicator populations (3, 9) and has also been used to assay an antigen-specific factor produced *in vivo* during a delayed hypersensitivity response in the sheep, again using a guinea pig peritoneal exudate cell-indicator population (10).

2. Materials

i. Au-198 colloid, particle size 5–20 nm (Radiochemical Centre, Amersham, Bucks, England, item GCSIP). The colloidal gold is supplied in a stabilizer containing per milliliter 20 mg of gelatin and 200 mg of glucose. If the isotope is supplied in an inconveniently small volume it may be necessary to dilute the batch further with this stabilizer for storage.

ii. Medium TC199 (Wellcome Reagents Ltd, Beckenham, Kent, England, item TC22 or GIBCO Biocult, Washington Road, Paisley, Scotland, item E-12). Media are made up in deionized water and are Millipore-filtered before use.

iii. Sodium bicarbonate solution, 4.4% (Wellcome Reagents Ltd., item TC27)

iv. Streptomycin sulfate (Dista Products, Liverpool, England)

v. Crystapen benzylpenicillin sodium (Glaxo Laboratories, Greenford, England)

Preparation of exudate cells also requires the following.

vi. Bayol 85 (Esso Ltd). This is sterilized at 160°C for 2 hr in bottles with silicone rubber-lined caps before use.

Preparation of peripheral blood does not require items ii, iii, and vi, but also requires the following.

vii. Heparin, preservative free (Evans Medical)

viii. RPMI 1640 (GIBCO Biocult, item H-18)

ix. Ficoll, MW ~400,000 (Pharmacia, Uppsala, Sweden), kept as a 9% stock solution sterilized by Millipore filtration

x. Triosil 75 (Nyegaard and Co., AS Oslo, Norway) kept away from light as a solution (Triosil 34) made by mixing 20 ml of Triosil 75 with 24.2 ml of deionized water

xi. Fetal calf serum (GIBCO Biocult, item 614)

3. Apparatus

i. Sterile plastic tubes, 10 X 75 (Falcon item 2038). Falcon do not supply closures for these tubes, which must be obtained from Luckham Ltd, Labro Works, Burgess Hill, England (item LP3/S). Alternatively 11 X 70 mm sterile plastic tubes from Nunc, Algade 8, 000 Roskilde, Denmark, item N-1090-1, have proved to be satisfactory. These are sold with a closure.

ii. Nonsterile tubes, 10 X 70 mmm, and closures (Luckham, item LP3)

iii. Roller culture apparatus. The "large model" supplied by Leec Ltd, Colwick, Nottingham, England has proved to be satisfactory. The drum of this machine rotates at 1 revolution per 8 min, maintaining the culture tubes at 5° to the horizontal.

iv. Hamilton automatic syringe (Hamilton, Reno, Nevada).

v. Test tube rack suitable for 10 mm diameter tubes (Denley Instruments, Bolney, Sussex, item R115).

vi. Syringes, 10 ml

vii. Automatic syringe or dispenser suitable for dispensing 1-ml volumes (e.g., Jencons Repette).

Preparation of blood or exudate cells also requires the following.

viii. Anesthetic (e.g., ether or Penthrane) soaked cotton wool wad in beaker

ix. 19G1 and 19G2 needles

x. Sterile plastic universal containers (Sterilin Ltd, Richmond, Surrey, England, item 128.C)

xi. Sterile glass universal containers

xii. Syringes, 20 and 50 ml. For exudate cell preparation, a retort stand and clamp to hold the 50-ml syringes are also required.

Preparation of lymph node cell supernatants also requires the following.

xiii. Sterile dissection equipment, e.g., large and small scissors and forceps

xiv. Fur clippers

xv. Wash bottle of 70% alcohol

xvi. Sterile petri dishes (Sterilin)

xvii. Two syringes with sterile bent 26-gauge needles attached (for teasing nodes)

xviii. Sterile tubes, 50 ml (e.g., Falcon, item 2070)

xix. Nylon mesh (Nybolt 80 μm nylon microfilament mesh, J. Stainer and Co, Manchester Wireworks, Sherbourn Street, Manchester, item 17). This is autoclaved before use.

xx. Sterile tissue culture tubes, 15 ml (Falcon, item 3026)

A centrifuge (preferably cooled) capable of spinning with g forces down to 100 g is required for preparing exudate cells. Some centrifuges may have to be placed in series with a suitable potentiometer (e.g., Variac) to achieve sufficiently low speeds.

4. Method

Exudate cells and blood contain both lymphocytes capable of producing pinocytosis-stimulating substances and macrophages (or in blood; monocytes) capable of responding to such substances. The gold uptake assay can therefore be performed both as a "direct assay," in which the blood or exudate cells are taken from a primed animal, and gold uptake stimulator (GUS) is produced in the same culture in which it is detected, or as an "indirect assay," in which GUS is produced *in vivo* (10) or by incubation of primed lymphocytes with antigen in a separate culture, and is then added to exudate cells from an unprimed animal. A macrophage monolayer may be preferred to the complete exudate as the indicator cell population.

4.1. **Indirect Assay.** This is illustrated in Fig. 1. All cultures are performed in TC199 supplemented with 15% normal guinea pig serum (NGPS), 100 units of

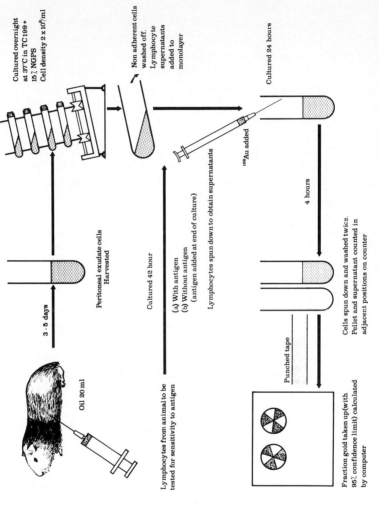

Fig. 1. Scheme illustrating indirect assay using gold uptake stimulator. NGPS, normal guinea pig serum.

Oil 20 ml

3 - 5 days

Peritoneal exudate cells
Harvested

Cultured overnight
at 37°C in TC199 +
15% NGPS
Cell density 2 x 10⁶/ml

Non adherent cells
washed off.
Lymphocyte
supernatants
added to
monolayer

Lymphocytes from animal to be
tested for sensitivity to antigen

Cultured 42 hour

(a) With antigen
(b) Without antigen
(antigen added at end of culture)

Lymphocytes spun down to obtain supernatants

¹⁹⁸Au added

Cultured 24 hours

4 hours

Punched tape

Cells spun down and washed twice.
Pellet and supernatant counted in
adjacent positions on counter

Fraction gold taken up (with
95% confidence limit) calculated
by computer

benzylpenicillin, 100 μg of streptomycin per milliliter, and 0.22% sodium bicarbonate. NGPS is used either fresh or after storage at $-70°$C. Lymph nodes are teased under medium supplemented with 15% serum, but cold serum-free Medium 199 (supplemented with bicarbonate and antibiotics) has proved to be satisfactory for brief washing procedures.

4.1.1. Preparation of Lymph Node Cell Supernatants. The guinea pig is anesthetized and exsanguinated by cardiac puncture. The fur is shaved from the region under the arms and legs and from the neck and chest region. The shaved areas are damped with alcohol (largely to prevent any loose fur from entering dissection sites), and the popliteal, axillary, brachial, cervical, and inguinal lymph nodes are excised under sterile conditions and placed in a petri dish of medium. The lymph nodes are separated from any attached fat, transferred to a fresh petri dish, and teased apart under ice-cold Medium 199 supplemented with 15% NGPS. The teased cells and debris are separated by passage through a medium-dampened sterile nylon mesh placed over a 50-ml Falcon tube. Cells are washed twice in ice-cold medium 199, spinning 5 min at 250 g for each wash, then a small sample is mixed with 2 parts of 0.1% trypan blue in saline and the yield of viable cells is counted. (Typically, viability is between 50 and 80%.) Viable cells, 2×10^7/ml, are cultured in 4-ml aliquots of medium 199 with 15% NGPS in 15-ml tissue culture tubes gassed with 5% CO_2:95% air. The tubes are rotated at 1 revolution/8 min for 42 hr at $37°$C. At the end of the culture period, the suspension is spun 5 min at 500 g, and supernatants from cells incubated without antigen are reconstituted with antigen.

4.1.2. Preparation of Exudate Cells. A normal guinea pig is held upside down, so that its viscera fall forward, and 20 ml of sterile "Bayol" oil are injected into the space thus left in the peritoneum. After 3–5 days the animal is exsanguinated by cardiac puncture. The blood is placed in a glass universal container (glass giving better clot retraction) and used as a source of NGPS later in the assay. The dead animal is then left a further 10 min (not longer) to permit coagulation of small vessels in the peritoneum so that a relatively blood-free exudate cell population may be obtained. Cervical dislocation may be necessary to ensure death even after a very large volume of blood has been removed. After 10 min, the guinea pig is pinned out and a long ventral incision into the skin, but not the body wall, is made. The skin is reflected, and the body wall over the peritoneum is lifted with forceps. Ice-cold Medium 199 is squirted into the peritoneum with a 50-ml syringe and 19Gl needle, taking care to keep the needle point well away from the viscera. The peritoneum is shaken vigorously, and the skin is pinned out so the body wall is stretched, leaving a gap between body wall and viscera at the side of the peritoneum. Cells, oil, and medium collecting in this gap are withdrawn using a 19Gl needle by applying gentle suction with a 50-ml syringe. The syringe is inverted in the retort stand, so that oil floats above the medium and cells. The cells may then be removed and stored in plastic universal containers kept in ice. This procedure is repeated until the peritoneum has been washed with about 100 ml of medium. The cells are then washed 3 times with ice-cold Medium 199, centrifugation for 7 min at 100 g being used for each washing step. Finally they are counted and adjusted to 2 × 10^6/ml in Medium 199 with 15% NGPS. Cell yield from one guinea pig is usually about 2 × 10^8 cells. Viability is almost 100%.

    4.1.3. Preparation of Monolayers and Measurement of Pinocytosis. One-milliliter aliquots of 2 × 10^6/ml exudate cells are cultured overnight in medium 199 with 15% NGPS in 10 × 75 mm sterile tissue culture tubes gassed with 95% air–5% CO_2. The tubes are rotated at 1 revolution/8 min at 37°C. Most of the macrophages, but only a few polymorphs and hardly any lymphocytes, attach to the tube wall under these conditions. The tubes are very briefly agitated with a Whirlimixer and nonadherent cells are poured off. One milliliter of lymphocyte test supernatant is then added, and the tube is recapped and cultured with rotation for a further 24 hr at 37°C. The correct degree of agitation to disturb the lymphocytes without damaging macrophages requires some experience, and experimenters may wish to set up the assay first using whole exudate cell populations rather than purified macrophage monolayers as indicators. In this case, after overnight culture exudate cells are spun down 7 min at 100 g, the supernatants are poured off, and the test lymphocyte supernatants are added. Alternatively, 0.5-ml aliquots of exudate cells, 4 × 10^6/ml, in NGPS to give a final concentration of 15%, are mixed with 0.5 ml of test supernatant factor. The tubes are gassed and capped as before, and cultured at 37°C for 40 hr with rotation.

    When 24 hr have elapsed 0.2 μg of ^{198}Au, about 0.1 μCi/μg, is added to the cultures. Radioactive gold is usually supplied from Amersham at 5 mg/ml in stabilizer. A solution containing 10,000 counts/sec/ml and 20 μg/ml gold is prepared immediately before use by mixing "hot" gold from a new batch with "cold" gold from a decayed batch. A 23-gauge needle held vertically gives a 10-μl drop sufficiently accurately for the purposes of this assay, and makes it unnecessary to contaminate micropipettes with very hot isotope. Ten microliters of this radioactive colloidal gold is added to each culture tube using a Hamilton automatic syringe, and the tubes are replaced on the rotator at 37°C.

    Four hours after addition of isotope, the cells are harvested by spinning the culture tubes for 5 min at 500 g, decanting the supernatant into a nonsterile plastic tube (LP3) and washing the adherent monolayer twice with 1-ml aliquots of Medium 199. The monolayer is spun down 5 min at 500 g for each wash, and the tubes are drained carefully by being inverted over absorbent paper in a test tube rack. The first supernatant and the washed adherent cells are counted in a suitable gamma counter in the order monolayer, supernatant; so that it is unnecessary to allow for radioactive decay when calculating the fraction of isotope taken up. This fraction is given by

$$\frac{(X - \text{background})}{(X - \text{background}) + (Y - \text{background})}$$

where X represents the counts given by the tube containing cells, Y, the counts given by the tube containing supernatant, and background, the background counts. In our laboratories output from the SC-20 scalers of our Wallac 800000 counter, in the form of 8-hole punched tape, is fed into a computer which calculates the mean fraction of gold taken up for groups of replicates, and the 95 confidence limits of such uptake. Count data may be treated in either square root or logarithmic transformation for statistical analysis, in order to homogenize variance. A computer program, suitable for use with the Wallac machine output only, is available from Professor P. J. Lachmann, Royal Postgraduate Medical School, London (written in Algol for the Elliott 4000 computer in cooperation with Professor I. D. P. Wooton) or from Dr. C. J. Meade, Transplantation Biology Section, Clinical Research Centre, Harrow, Middlesex (written in Fortran in cooperation with Dr. C. J. Sanderson).

4.2. Direct Assay. Exudate cells are prepared as in the indirect assay, but are taken from primed rather than normal animals and cultured with or without antigen. The cells are set up at 2×10^6/ml on a rotator at $37°C$, as in the indirect assay, but are then not disturbed until after 42 hr of culture, when gold is added as before. Cells are harvested after a further 4 hr as before.

Direct Assay Using Guinea Pig Blood Cells. Blood is withdrawn from the heart through a 19G2 needle into a well heparinized syringe. It is then diluted with an equal volume of Medium 199 and gently layered over 10 ml of a sterile Ficoll/Triosil mixture. This mixture is made by mixing 10 parts of Triosil 34 with 24 parts of 9% Ficoll solution.

Medium, cells, and Ficoll/Triosil are spun at high speed (3000 g) for 30 min when red cells pass through the Ficoll/Triosil layer. The cells remaining at the interface are carefully removed with as little Ficoll/Triosil as possible, washed twice in Medium 199 (spinning 7 min at 200 g in each wash), counted, adjusted to 5×10^6/ml in RPMI 1640 plus 15% NGPS or fetal calf serum (no NGPS is produced as a by-product of this procedure), and cultured at $37°C$ with rotation in 10×75 mm plastic tissue culture tubes gassed with 95% air: 5% CO_2. As before, 10 μl of gold is added after 24 hr, and the cells are harvested in the standard manner 48 hr after the beginning of the culture.

As it stands, this method is not applicable to human blood.

5. Interpretation of Data

Animals showing delayed hypersensitivity show stimulation of gold uptake in either direct or indirect assays with relatively small quantities of specific antigen, whereas antigen effects on cells from unprimed animals or animals primed against a different antigen are normally negligible (3). An exception is purified protein derivative of tuberculin (PPD), which in high concentrations (much higher than those required to stimulate gold uptake in unprimed animals) will stimulate gold uptake by normal exudate cells. Possibly this reflects a weak mitogenic activity.

In lymph from sheep primed with bacillus Calmette-Guérin (BCG) the major GUS activity was associated with material of molecular weight approximately 70,000 (by Sephadex chromatography) in fractions that did not contain significant amounts of IgG. Like migration inhibition, gold uptake stimulation was enhanced by specific antigen (10).

The activity present in supernatants prepared by incubating primed lymph node lymphocytes with PPD was also largely associated with properties different from those of conventional antibody, but not different from those of the so-called "migration inhibitory factor" (3).

However, just as lymphocyte [methyl-^{3}H]thymidine uptake may be stimulated by antigen–antibody complexes as well as a nonantibody "mitogenic factor" (11) and macrophage migration may be inhibited by such complexes as well as by nonantibody "migration inhibition factor" (MIF) (12, 13), so gold uptake may be stimulated by antigen–antibody complexes, as shown by a stimulation of normal exudate cell gold uptake with antigen in the presence of specific antiserum, but not normal serum (9). The "direct" assay is thus useful for assaying cellular hypersensitivity where antibody production is known to be negligible, or for *in vitro* assay of "reactivity" (including cellular hypersensitivity) to an antigen. However, for distinguishing between cellular hypersensitivity and humoral effects in the indirect gold uptake assay, great care should be taken to remove immunoglobulins (by either gel filtration or selective ammonium sulfate precipitation) from the supernatant before the assay is performed.

Very high concentrations of either lymphocyte supernatants (in the indirect assay) or antigen (in the direct assay) produce less stimulation of gold uptake than do slightly lower concentrations. A similar phenomenon is seen in lymphocyte transformation, where again there is an optimum antigen concentration. It is therefore necessary to work within a suitable range of antigen or lymphocyte supernatant concentrations. In practice this range is very large and the existence of a "prozone" effect is not a serious limitation. For those antigens we have tested [ovalbumin and basic protein in guinea pigs immunized with these antigens in complete Freund's adjuvant (CFA); PPD in guinea pigs immunized with BCG or CFA], antigen concentrations between 0.1 μg/ml and 10 μg/ml have been most useful in the direct test, and lymphocyte supernatants are generally tested at dilutions between 1:2 and 1:64. Supernatants with high titers of GUS generally also have high titers of MIF, but the concentration of lymphocyte supernatant required to produce a significant effect is about 50-fold less in the GUS assay compared with the MIF assay. The dose-response curve of lymphocyte supernatants is usually linear between dilutions of about 1:2 and 1:64, giving a useful dilution range of about 32-fold for quantitative experiments.

Pinocytosis (like many other parameters of macrophage function) is affected by the protein concentration in the medium. The level of serum present in gold uptake assay cultures is sufficiently high so that only very large increases in added protein concentration produce any significant increase in rate of gold uptake, but it may be necessary to control for protein concentration when assaying small amounts of GUS in the presence of large quantities of protein.

If it is suspected that test supernatants or antigens will affect indicator cell viability or numbers, ^{51}Cr incorporation can be simultaneously followed as a control. ^{51}Cr is not taken up by pinocytosis (14). Sodium chromate labeled with ^{51}Cr (Radiochemical Centre, Amersham, item CJSIP) is mixed into the "diluted gold stock" so that the final concentration of chromium is 0.025 μg/ml, specific activity 100 μCi/μg (i.e., providing about 100 counts/second per 10 μl). The assay is then continued as before. Counts in cells and supernatant attributable to gold and chromium are separable by pulse height analysis. Overlap between channels must be corrected using the formulas

$$G = \frac{g - (b \times c)}{1 - (a \times b)} \quad \text{and} \quad C = \frac{c - (a \times g)}{1 - (a \times b)}$$

where G and C are "true" counts, and g and c are observed counts in the "gold" and "chromium" channels, respectively, a is the fractional overlap of "gold" counts into the "chromium" channel, and b is the fractional overlap of "chromium" counts into the gold channel. The fraction of chromium taken up is calculated in a way analogous to gold uptake.

In practice, none of our test supernatants have ever had an effect on ^{51}Cr-labeled chromate uptake, but the technique might be valuable when potentially toxic antigens are being assayed.

Culture of exudates or monolayers of exudate macrophages with gold for 4 hr gives 3–15% gold uptake. When the guinea pigs are BCG primed, this should be at least doubled in the presence of 10 μg of PPD per milliliter. Over 24 hr, 5 × 10^6/ml white cells from peripheral blood take up 2–20% gold, which again should be at least doubled by 10 μg of PPD per milliliter when the cells come from primed animals. However, in one or two experiments a very high apparent gold uptake and a very poor stimulation of such uptake has been obtained. This has been traced to use of old preparations of "diluted gold stock," which have been left several days before use, and may be due to aggregation of gold colloid particles. Another hazard, clumping of guinea pig peripheral blood cells when placed on the Ficoll/Triosil, has been traced to inadequate heparinization of the syringe used for taking blood.

When attention is paid to the above points, the assay has proved to be simple and very reproducible in our hands.

REFERENCES

1. Nath, I., Poulter, L. W., and Turk, J. L., *Clin. Exp. Immunol.* **13**, 455 (1973).
2. Nathan, C. F., Karnovsky, M. L., and David, J. R., *J. Exp. Med.* **133**, 1356 (1971).
3. Meade, C. J., Lachmann, P. J., and Brenner, S., *Immunology* **27**, 227 (1974).
4. Cohn, Z. A., and Benson, B., *J. Exp. Med.* **121**, 835 (1965).
5. Cohn, Z. A., Fedorko, M. E., and Hirsch, J. G., *J. Exp. Med.* **123**, 757 (1966).
6. Gosselin, R. E., *J. Gen. Physiol.* **39**, 625 (1956).
7. Cohn, Z. A., and Benson, B., *J. Exp. Med.* **122**, 455 (1965).
8. Roser, B., *Aust. J. Exp. Biol. Med. Sci.* **43**, 553 (1965).
9. Meade, C. J., Soluble factors in lymphocyte-macrophage interaction. Ph.D. Thesis, University of Cambridge, 1974.
10. Lowe, D. M., and Lachmann, P. J., *Scand. J. Immunol.* **3**, 423 (1974).
11. Bloch-Shtacher, N., Hirschhorn, K., and Uhr, J. W., *Clin. Exp. Immunol.* **3**, 889 (1968).
12. Spitler, L., Huber, H., and Fudenberg, H. H., *J. Immunol.* **102**, 404 (1969).
13. Bloom, B. R., and Bennett, B., *Science* **153**, 80 (1966).
14. Ronai, P. M., Studies on the rejection of radioisotope labelled grafts. Ph.D. Thesis, University of Sydney, 1967.

Horseradish Peroxidase as a Marker for Studies of Pinocytosis

Ralph M. Steinman *

1. Introduction

Pinocytosis, the uptake of fluid droplets by cells, is a widespread phenomenon. Immunologists suspect that activated macrophages (1) and blast-transformed lymphocytes (2) exhibit increased pinocytic activity. More recently, it has been shown that lymphocyte surface determinants may be selectively interiorized by pinocytosis following interaction with specific ligands (3, 4). The importance of "drinking" in the physiology of cells is still unclear; but these immunological examples suggest at least that alterations in pinocytic activity reflect changes in the cell's functional state. Accordingly, it is fitting for this book to consider methods for identifying and quantitating pinocytosis in cultured cells.

Historically, direct observations of cells by phase-contrast microscopy provided the means for identifying and studying pinocytic activity. Lewis (5) discovered the phenomenon in mammals when he noted that cells in culture, especially macrophages, generated phase-lucent vesicles at their ruffling margins. Cohn and his colleagues (reviewed in 6, 7) have studied these vesicles in more detail. They identified several agents that modify pinocytosis, by counting the number of vesicles as an index of pinocytic activity; and they elaborated in detail the relation of incoming fluid droplets to other elements of the vacuolar system. Phase contrast observations are helpful when examining heterogeneous populations, and when screening various agents for their effects on pinocytosis. However, vesicle counts are a tedious and possibly misleading means for quantitative work on the rate of fluid entry. It is clear that many pinocytic vesicles fall below the limit of resolution of the light microscope, that vesicles vary greatly in diameter and thus enormously in volume, and that incoming vesicles shrink rapidly following fusion with lysosomes (e.g., 8). Thus the number of vesicles may bear little resemblance to the rate at which fluid is moving into the cell in bulk, and may reflect alterations in the fate vs production of pinocytic droplets.

*The author is a Scholar of the Leukemia Society of America; and Irma T. Hirschl Career Scientist.

For these reasons, a variety of marker materials have been employed for quantitative work, e.g., colloidal gold (9, 10), iodinated proteins (11–14) and polyvinylpyrrolidone (14, 15), tritiated sucrose (16), and inulin (17). In each case, the marker apparently is incapable of direct transport and/or permeation across the plasma membrane, so that entry into the cell occurs by bulk or vesicular means. To characterize a marker in any given cell system, it is important to distinguish whether the material is entering solely in the fluid phase of pinocytic droplets (fluid phase pinocytosis) vs attached to the incoming vesicle membrane (adsorptive pinocytosis). Markers that adsorb to the cell surface are probably dangerous for quantitative work, since their rate of entry may be influenced by a number of factors other than the rate of vesicle or fluid entry. For example, the percentage of the administered load that is interiorized will depend on the number and affinity of surface binding sites as well as the concentration of marker; the test material, because it interacts with the cell surface, may itself stimulate and/or retard vesicle fluid entry so that it is not a marker, but a determinant of pinocytic activity; finally the quantitative assay must distinguish between surface bound vs interiorized marker, and this is often difficult.

The marker we favor for studies of pinocytosis is the glycoprotein enzyme, horseradish peroxidase (HRP). We have used it on cultures of mouse peritoneal macrophages (18) as well as continuous fibroblast lines (19). Paul Edelson (personal communication) has also applied it to Chinese hamster ovary and human lymphoid lines. The main advantage of the HRP model is that it appears to be interiorized in the fluid phase only, without prior binding to the cell surface. Initially this conclusion was made by quantitating the amount of cell-bound HRP after administration of varying concentrations of enzyme for one time interval, or one concentration of enzyme for varying intervals. Cell binding was directly proportional to the concentration and time of exposure (Fig. 1). Had HRP undergone a significant adsorptive step, the binding of marker to cells should have shown evidence of saturation with increasing HRP concentrations, and binding should have proceeded more rapidly during the initial period of exposure (Fig. 1). The latter features are seen during protein uptake by amoeba, where adsorptive pinocytosis is well known (20). This approach did not exclude the possibility that some HRP entered the cell by an adsorptive mechanism, e.g., the number and/or affinity of surface binding sites may have been small, or the rate of entry of that portion of the cell surface binding HRP may have been large. These possibilities seem unlikely in view of a recent analysis we made using stereologic techniques (8). We measured the volume of cytochemically reactive, i.e., HRP-containing, pinocytic vesicles. The rate at which the pinocytic vesicle space expanded with time was found to be very similar to that predicted from quantitative measurements of solute uptake, assuming entry only in the fluid phase.

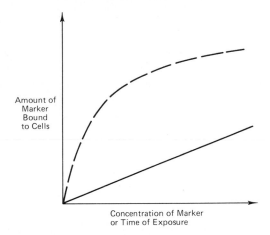

Fig. 1. During fluid phase pinocytosis (———), the amount of marker bound to the cells increases linearly with the concentration of marker in the culture medium, and the time of exposure. Cell-bound markers would all be located in the vacuolar system. In adsorptive pinocytosis (– – –), cell binding is likely to show evidence of saturation with increasing concentrations of marker; also the kinetics of binding includes an early rapid adsorptive step. The measured amount of cell-bound marker consists of material on the cell surface as well as in the vacuolar apparatus. The amount of marker bound to cells is much greater during adsorptive pinocytosis.

Our studies have established several other advantages of the HRP system.

1.1. Cell-bound HRP can be quantitated by a sensitive, reliable, and simple enzymic assay that detects concentrations of nanograms per milliliter. Sensitivity is critical here since the actual amounts of solute interiorized during fluid phase pinocytosis is minute relative to the load; e.g., each hour, a million cultivated resident mouse peritoneal macrophages take in just 0.01% of the administered load per milliliter. Similar uptakes are obtained whether one employs the enzymic assay or radioiodonated HRP. The former, however, obviates the expense and difficulties involved in radiolabel techniques. It may seem dangerous *a priori* to rely on enzymatic activity in a quantitative assay, but so far HRP has proved to extremely stable; e.g., it can be maintained fully active in detergents and extreme dilutions.

1.2. Although HRP does bind to plastic tissue culture vessels, most can be removed by appropriate washes, such that the residual dish-bound enzyme is less than 10% of the amount interiorized by the cells. Therefore uptake measurements can be performed on cell monolayers directly in the culture vessel. Compared to suspension cultures, monlayers are easier to process and to visualize.

1.3. A 2–3 hr exposure to HRP does not appear to perturb the cultivated macrophage or fibroblast. Pinocytic activity, measured by the simultaneous addition of other markers is not altered (8, 19); cell morphology, ATP levels, and growth potential are normal (19), and the actual dimensions of the pinocytic vesicle and secondary lysosome compartments remain at equilibrium (8).

1.4. Cell-bound HRP is readily visualized by a reliable and sensitive, light and electron microscopic, cytochemical technique (21). Cytochemistry helps one to establish that cell-bound enzyme is within the vacuolar system, to screen heterogeneous populations, and to estimate roughly the degree of pinocytic activity.

1.5. Adequate supplies of HRP can be obtained from commercial sources at reasonable prices. The Sigma type II preparation we use costs \$54 per gram which allows one to do thousands of assays on the populations we studied. At least 10 different lots have been used with similar results.

1.6. After uptake, HRP is inactivated in the lysosomal apparatus with first-order kinetics and at relatively slow rates ($t_{1/2}$ of 7–9 hr in cultured mouse cells) (18, 19). Examination of the fate of pinocytosed enzyme thus provides an indication of the ability of the lysosomal system to destroy ingested materials.

2. Materials

2.1. Horseradish peroxidase (HRP) (Sigma Chemical Co., Type II, Catalogue No. P-8250). This consists of several peroxidase isoenzymes, the relative amounts of which vary from lot to lot. Small amounts of nonenzymically active protein are also detected by immunoelectrophroesis. Nevertheless, the type II preparation provides data that are identical to those obtained with an immunoelectrophoretically pure one, e.g., Sigma type VI–tested with an antiserum to Sigma type II. Several other companies market HRP but we have not employed their preparations as yet.

The enzyme is readily soluble, and is maintained frozen as a Millipore-filtered stock solution at 10–20 mg/ml normal saline, or phosphate-buffered saline. Millipore filtration removes small amounts of particulates and maintains sterility. There is no loss of enzymic activity for many months, even with repeated freezing and thawing.

2.2. Hydrogen peroxide (H_2O_2): The stock solution for cytochemistry is 30% (v/v) Superoxal (J. T. Baker Chemical Co.). For the enzymic assay, the superoxal is diluted in water to give a 0.3% stock. This retains activity for months at 4°C.

2.3. o-Dianisidine (Sigma, Catalogue No. D-3127), dissolved fresh each day in absolute methanol at 10 mg/ml. This compound is carcinogenic.

2.4. 3,3′-Diaminobenzidine tetrahydrochloride (DAB) (Sigma, Catalogue No. D-8126). It too is carcinogenic.

2.5. Sodium phosphate buffer, 0.10 M, pH 5.0

2.6. Tris buffer, 0.05 M, pH 7.6

2.7. Triton X-100 (Sigma). A 5% (w/v) stock solution is made in water and diluted in water to 0.05% prior to use.

2.8. Fixative for cytochemistry: We use 1.25–2.5% glutaraldehyde in phosphate-buffered saline or 0.1 M sodium cacodylate, pH 7.4.

3. Methods

3.1. The Enzymic Assay. For calibrating the enzymic assay, standard solutions are made fresh at levels of 1–20 ng/ml. The diluent is phosphate-buffered saline, supplemented with 1 mg of bovine serum albumin per milliliter or 1% (v/v) fetal calf serum. Otherwise the diluted enzyme loses activity within hours.

The substrate solution for the assay is prepared fresh daily in an opaque bottle by mixing 3 reagents in the following proportions: (a) 6.0 ml of sodium phosphate buffer, (b) 0.06 ml of 0.3% hydrogen peroxide, (c) 0.05 ml of 10 mg/ml o-dianisidine.

We measure the rate at which colored, oxidized o-dianisidine (absorbing at 460 nm) accumulates with time using the recording apparatus of a Gilford Model 240 spectrophotometer. The initial rate of the reaction is directly proportional to enzyme concentration (Fig. 2), and this linear relationship passes through the origin.

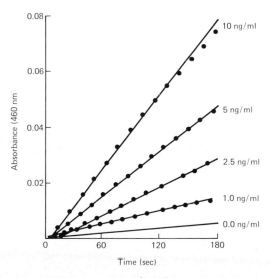

Fig. 2. Detection of horseradish peroxidase (HRP) by enzymic assay. The oxidation of o-dianisidine by HRP and H_2O_2 is followed with a recording spectrophotometer at 460 nM. The reaction rate is directly proportional to the concentration of enzyme present. [Reproduced with permission of *Journal of Cell Biology* from Steinman *et al.* (19)].

The instrument is adjusted for maximum sensitivity according to the directions embossed on the recorder; 0.100 absorbance is the full-scale range, and 1.0 the ratio control; 0.1 ml of varying standard HRP solutions are dispensed into 1.25-ml quartz cuvettes, 1 cm path length; 0.9 ml of substrate solution is then added with a 5.0-ml disposable pipette, controlled with a Propipette bulb. The cuvettes are mixed by inversion, and the rate of color development is followed at 460 nm. The kinetics are linear for 1–3 min for concentrations less than 20 ng/ml. Higher concentrations provide adequate data if the very first points are used. Alternatively, one can assay 0.01 ml, or a dilution of the unknown.

The cells to be used should be assayed to check that they lack endogenous peroxidatic activity. Also, standard solutions should be prepared using cell lysates as diluent to be certain that the lysate does not influence enzymic activity.

3.2. Administration of HRP to Cells. We have worked mainly with cells grown in monolayer culture. Suspension cultures can also be assayed, though washing off the non-cell-bound HRP at the end of the uptake period is more tedious. Enzyme is diluted in tissue culture media at a concentration suitable for obtaining readily detectable uptakes—considering the time of exposure, and number and activity of the cells. For example, we use concentrations of 0.1–1.0 mg/ml and 0.5–1 hr exposures in cultures of 2 to 10×10^5 mouse macrophages or L cells.

After the exposure to HRP, the cells are washed 5 times, usually in phosphate-buffered saline. As mentioned above, a small residual of dish-bound HRP remains, but this does not contribute significantly to most uptake experiments. To be certain, though, it is well to run dish controls. Here enzyme is administered to dishes that have been exposed to culture media without cells, or better still, dishes from which the cells have been removed, e.g., by scraping, lysis, trypsinization, or local anesthetics.

The washed cells are then lysed in an appropriate volume of 0.05% Triton X-100 in water, and the enzymic assay is run. If the lysates cannot be assayed in 1–2 hr, it is best to add some serum or to dilute in PBS–1% serum, whereupon the enzyme is stable for the rest of the day.

3.3. Expression of Data. The enzymic assay provides a rate of change in OD_{460} , which is converted to a concentration of enzyme in nanograms per milliliter, using appropriate standards. This concentration is then multiplied by the total volume of cell lysate, times any dilution factor, to yield the total uptake per dish. The dish control is subtracted to give cell uptake. Cell mass can be expressed in terms of cell number, cell DNA, or cell protein, and generally uptake rates are expressed on a per hour basis.

3.4. Cytochemistry. The Graham–Karnovsky procedure (21) is simple, sensitive, reliable, and can be used for both light and electron microscopic studies. The substrate is prepared fresh and consists of 0.5 mg of DAB per milliliter in 0.05 M Tris, pH 7.6, to which is added enough Superoxal (30% H_2O_2) to give a final concentration of 0.01%. Washed monolayers are fixed for 5 min at room temperature in 1.25–2.5% glutaraldehyde in PBS or 0.1 M sodium cacodylate buffer, pH 7.5. The monolayers are rinsed in buffer and stained for 10 min at room temperature with the substrate mixture (18, 19). Controls involve the omission of H_2O_2 and/or the DAB. The cells are washed again in buffer and processed further for electron microscopy, or they are rinsed in distilled water and mounted at one's convenience for phase contrast microscope level; although many HRP-filled secondary lysosomes are too small to be resolved, there are always some which can be visualized as brown granules, especially in the perinuclear region. For photographic records, it is good to photograph the same field by both phase contrast and bright field microscopy. Generally lysosomes are not visible by the latter technique unless cytochemically reactive.

3.5. Inactivation of HRP. To assess the ability of cells to inactivate HRP, cells are returned to HRP-free culture medium for varying times. Then one follows the level of cell-bound enzyme, enzyme in the culture medium, and cell viability. In mouse cells, HRP is inactivated with first-order kinetics, the $t_{1/2}$ being 7–9 hr. Obviously, the total amount of HRP in the culture diminishes. Radioiodinated HRP may be employed to demonstrate full recovery of label and to corroborate that digestion of HRP is typical of lysosomal degradation, i.e., that it is accompanied by the release of label into the culture medium as amino acids or small peptides (12, 18).

4. Critique and Comment

4.1. The Enzymic Assay. The assay conditions are not stringent. The concentrations of H_2O_2 and o-dianisidine are in adequate excess for the levels of HRP that will be assayed, and they could be increased severalfold more without affecting the result. The enzyme has a broad pH optimum of 4.5–5.5. The key is to have linear kinetics and to show that oxidation of o-dianisidine is H_2O_2 dependent.

4.2. The Cells. The cells we have studied lack endogenous peroxidatic activity and do not alter the activity of added HRP, but these features must always be ascertained beforehand. The cell population must be homogeneous to interpret quantitative data. Within a given population, cytochemical criteria can be employed to show that most cells are participating in the pinocytic activity being quantitated. If the cells are not homogeneous, it is important to establish that the "other" cells neither bind HRP nor influence the activity of the cells being measured. Finally, HRP exposure should not have toxic effects; useful criteria are dye exclusion, growth inhibition, alternation of major functional and morphological properties.

4.3. Uptake of HRP. Careful studies of uptake vs exposure time and concentration of HRP must be obtained to ensure that uptake is via the fluid phase, and that there is no significant adsorption of enzyme to the culture vessel. These studies must be repeated whenever a new variable is introduced. Another feature of fluid phase pinocytosis is that it is highly temperature dependent with little or no uptake at 4°C (19). One must also show that HRP inactivation is relatively slow and therefore does not significantly affect the uptake data. The uptake data must make sense for fluid influx; e.g., somewhere around 0.01% or less of the administered load per milliliter per million cells per hour; or if possible, estimate the volume of medium cleared by the cells vs the total cell volume. Finally, quantitating pinocytic activity is still a new approach, so that data with another marker are appropriate.

4.4. Cytochemistry. Exclude the presence of endogenous peroxidatic activity first. Catalases may also produce electron miscroscopic reaction product when diaminobenzidine is the substrate. Catalase DAB activity is dependent upon alkaline pH and glutaraldehyde fixation (22). Electron microscopic cytochemistry is especially helpful in visualizing pinocytic vesicles and small lysosomes, in excluding surface binding of enzyme, in proving that exposure to HRP does not alter cell morphology, and in comparing the pinocytic activity from cell to cell.

REFERENCES

1. Blanden, R. V., *J. Reticuloendothel. Soc.* **5,** 179 (1968).
2. Hirschhorn, R., Brittinger, G., Hirschhorn, K., and Weissman, G., *J. Cell Biol.* **37,** 412 (1968).
3. Taylor, R. B., Duffys, W. P. H., Raff, M. C., and de Petris, S., *Nature (London), New Biol.* **233,** 225 (1971).
4. Unanue, E. R., Perkins, W. D., and Karnovsky, M. J., *J. Exp. Med.* **136,** 885 (1972).
5. Lewis, W. H., *Bull. Johns Hopkins Hosp.* **49,** 17 (1931).
6. Gordon, S., and Cohn, Z. A., *Int. Rev. Cytol.* **36,** 171 (1973).
7. Steinman, R. M., and Cohn, Z. A., *in* "The Inflammatory Process" (B. W. Zweifach, L. Grant, and R. T. McCluskey, eds.), 2nd ed., Vol. 1, p. 449. Academic Press, New York, (1974).
8. Steinman, R. M., Brodie, S. E., and Cohn, Z. A., *J. Cell Biol.* **68,** 665 (1976).
9. Gosselin, R. E., *J. Gen. Physiol.* **39,** 625 (1956).
10. Wills, E. J., Davies, P., Allison, A. C., and Haswell, A. D., *Nature (London), New Biol.* **240,** 58 (1972).
11. Ryser, H., Aub, J. C., and Caulfield, J. B., *J. Cell Biol.* **15,** 437 (1962).
12. Ehrenreich, B. A., and Cohn, Z. A., *J. Exp. Med.* **126,** 941 (1967).
13. Ryser, H. J.-P. *Science* **159,** 390 (1968).
14. Williams, K. E., Kidston, E. M., Beck, F., and Lloyd, J. B., *J. Cell Biool.* **64,** 123 (1975).
15. Williams, K. E., Kidston, E. M., Beck, F., and Lloyd, J. B., *J. Cell. Biol.* **64,** 113 (1975).
16. Wagner, R., Rosenberg, M., and Estensen, R., *J. Cell Biol.* **50,** 804 (1971).
17. Bowers, B., and Olszewski, T. E., *J. Cell Biol.* **53,** 681 (1972).
18. Steinman, R. M., and Cohn, Z. A., *J. Cell Biol.* **55,** 186 (1972).
19. Steinman, R. M., Silver, J. M., and Cohn, Z. A., *J. Cell Biol.* **63,** 949 (1974).
20. Schumaker, V. N., *Exp. Cell Res.* **15,** 314 (1959).
21. Graham, R. C., Jr., and Karnovsky, M. J., *J. Histochem. Cytochem.* **14,** 291 (1966).
22. Herzog, V., and Fahini, H. D., *J. Cell Biol.* **60,** 303 (1974).

33

Purification of Human Granulocytes and Production of the Corresponding Monospecific Antisera

Adel A. F. Mahmoud

1. Introduction

"Anti-leukocyte sera" produced by immunizing animals with white cells from other species have been available since the days of Metchnikoff (1). This has added little to our knowledge, however, as peripheral blood leukocytes are a heterogeneous cell population. The neutrophil, which is the most abundant leukocyte in the peripheral circulation, was the first cell to which specific antibodies were obtained; this facilitated studies of its kinetics (2), regulation (3) and function (4). Next came the isolation of relatively pure suspensions of lymphocytes from lymph nodes, thoracic duct, and peripheral blood and the subsequent production of anti-lymphocyte sera, which have played a major role in elucidation of the function of these cells (5, 6). Furthermore, two major lymphocyte subpopulations have been identified by specific antibodies raised against surface determinants (7). Attempts to produce antisera against macrophages have met with only partial success because of incomplete specificity (8, 9).

Recently, highly specific antisera have been produced against cells of the polymorphonuclear granulocyte series (basophils, eosinophils, and neutrophils) and their precursor cell, the myeloblast, and this is the matter of particular concern in this discussion. Although the granulocytes are heterogeneous morphologically, cytochemically, and functionally, the lack of purification procedures for the different cell types has hampered progress in their immunological characterization, and to some extent in the elucidation of their function. The recent development of techniques for the separation and purification (10, 11) of the different cells of this series has facilitated the production of antisera specific for basophils, eosinophils and neutrophils as well as myeloblasts. This presentation will describe in detail the methodology for obtaining purified cells of each of the three subtypes of mature human granulocytes and of their precursor cell and for producing monospecific antisera against them. The methodology of purification of these cells was first developed using cells obtained from the laboratory mouse (12), and was later adapted to the isolation and purification of human cells (10, 13). The following variables were used to ensure the purification of specific cells and the production of potent antisera.

    1.1. The basic theoretical principle of the purification procedure is derived from the general sedimentation law. The heterogeneous nature of the granulocytes enabled its use in the purification of specific cell types.

    1.2. Neutrophils were obtained from normal human donors, but the other cells were acquired from those with clinical conditions that induce a marked increase in that cell type.

    1.3. Antisera to mature granulocytes (neutrophils and eosinophils) had no detectable effect on immature bone marrow precursor cells of experimental animals (2, 14). This led to the production of antisera against human myeloblasts obtained from patients with different leukemic conditions; such antisera had no effect on the mature granulocytes (10).

The discussion to follow will concentrate on the processing of human cells, although references will be given for the use of animal materials.

2. Materials and Equipment

For the bleeding of human donors, purification of granulocytes, and preparation of monospecific antisera, the following materials are required.

2.1. Bleeding of Donors

    2.1.1. Plastic disposable syringes, 30 ml, with 20-gauge needles (Becton Dickinson and Company, Rutherford, New Jersey)

    2.1.2. Heparin solution. Two strenths are needed: Lipo-hepin 20,000 U/ml (Riker Laboratory, North Ridge, California) for bleeding donors, and sodium heparin injection, USP 1000 U/ml (The Upjohn Company, Kalamazoo, Michigan) for handling the cells after bleeding.

    2.1.3. Bleeding kit containing tourniquet, antiseptic swabs, and Band-aids.

2.2. Separation of Red Cells

    2.2.1. Polypropylene centrifuge tubes, 50 ml (Falcon, Catalogue No. 2070, Falcon Plastics, Oxnard, California)

    2.2.2. Dextran, 200,000–275,000 MW (Sigma Chemical Co., St. Louis, Missouri)

    2.2.3. Sodium ethylenediamine tetraacetate (EDTA) (J. T. Baker Chemical Co., Phillipsburg, New Jersey)

    2.2.4. Ammonium chloride (Allied Chemical, General Chemical Division, Morristown, New Jersey)

    2.2.5. Pyrogen-free 0.9% sodium chloride solution (Baxter Laboratories, Division of Travenol Laboratories, Inc., Morton Grove, Illinois)

    2.2.6. Sterile distilled water

    2.2.7. Phosphate-buffered saline, pH 7.4.

    2.2.8. Serological pipettes, 5 and 10 ml (Falcon, Catalogue No. 7543 and 7551).

2.3. Purification of Eosinophils and Neutrophils

2.3.1. Hypaque sodium 50% (w/v) brand of sodium diatrizoate USP (Winthrop Laboratories, Division of Sterling Drug, Inc., New York, New York)

2.3.2. Distilled water

2.3.3. Polypropylene centrifuge tubes, 50 ml (Falcon, Catalogue No. 2070).

2.3.4. White cell counting pipettes and chambers

2.3.5. Turk's solution [2% acetic acid (20 ml/liter) colored pale violet with gentian violet] or Coulter counter for total nucleated cell counts.

2.3.6. Discombe's fluid: 1 part 2% aqueous eosin solution (Eosin Y, Fisher Co., Fairlawn, New Jersey), 1 part acetone, and 8 parts distilled water.

2.3.7. Tetrachrome blood stain (Harleco, Philadelphia, Pennsylvania) and buffer solution, pH 6.4–6.5 (Fisher Scientific Co.)

2.3.8. Normal human serum

2.4. Preparation of Antisera

2.4.1. Two adult male or female New Zealand albino rabbits, weighing 5–6 kg, for each cell type used

2.4.2. Freund's complete adjuvant with H37Ra mycobacteria (Bacto, Difco Laboratory, Detroit, Michigan)

2.4.3. Glass syringes, 10 ml, and 3-way connectors for mixing the cells with the adjuvant

2.4.4. Vacutainer tubes 20 ml size (Fisher Scientific Co.) with attached needles for bleeding

2.4.5. Polypropylene tubes, 50 ml (Falcon, Catalogue No. 2070)

2.4.6. Polystyrene tubes for storage of antisera, 5 and 10-ml (Falcon, Catalogue No. 2054 and 2057)

2.4.7. Packed group O red blood cells. These cells should be washed 6 times in large volumes of phosphate-buffered saline before they are used for absorption.

3. Methods

3.1. Leukocyte Preparation

3.1.1. Blood Sample. Venous blood, 30 ml, is drawn into a plastic syringe containing 10,000 units of heparin (0.5 ml of Lipo-hepin). The blood is mixed by inversion and then transferred to a 50-ml polypropylene tube (Falcon, No. 2070) containing the following: 6 ml of 5% dextran in 0.9% sodium chloride, 0.8 ml of 4.0% aqueous sodium EDTA, and 300 units of heparin. The sample is mixed by inversion and allowed to settle for 30 min at 22°C (ambient air temperature). This procedure allows the red cells to sediment to the bottom of the tube with leukocyte-rich plasma supernatant on top. The supernatant plasma is transferred with serological pipettes to another 50-ml centrifuge tube.

3.1.2. Hemolysis of Red Cells. Add to the leukocyte-rich plasma, 3 times its volume 0.87% ammonium chloride solution, mix by inversion and then centrifuge at 100 g for 10 min at 4°C. The supernatant is removed and the leukocyte button, free of red cells, is resuspended in heparinized phosphate-buffered saline. Tubes containing cell suspensions should be kept on ice during counting and preparation of the density gradients.

3.1.3. Counting of Cells. Total cell counts can be done by the Coulter counter or in white cell pipettes by diluting the leukocyte suspension with Turk's fluid. Absolute eosinophil counts are done by using Discomb's fluid as a diluent in white cell pipettes. For differential counts small amounts of the leukocyte suspension are mixed with equal volumes of human serum and smears are stained with the tetrachrome stain.

3.2. Purification of Cells

3.2.1. Ten milliliters of the leukocyte suspension is layered carefully over an equal volume of a solution of sodium diatrizoate (Hypaque 50) diluted as described below for the specific cell type required, in 50-ml Falcon No. 2070 tubes. Care should be exercised that the two solutions remain separate, with a clear line of demarcation at the interface.

3.2.2. For human neutrophils the Hypaque 50 solution is diluted 1 part Hypaque to 2.1 parts distilled water.

3.2.3. For human eosinophils the Hypaque 50 solution is diluted 1 part Hypaque to 1.7 parts distilled water.

3.2.4. The tubes are centrifuged at 400 g for 40 min at 4°C. At the end of this period the cells are found in two different areas: one at the interface of the phosphate-buffered saline and the Hypaque solution, and the other in a pellet at the bottom of the tube.

3.2.5. The phosphate-buffered saline, the cells at the interface, and the Hypaque solution are aspirated carefully, leaving the cell pellet at the bottom. This pellet is then resuspended in heparinized phosphate-buffered saline, washed twice in 20–30 ml of the buffer by centrifugation at 100 g for 10 min, and resuspended in fresh buffer.

3.2.6. Total and differential cell counts are then performed as described above [3.1.3].

3.2.7. Basophil and myeloblast donors: Basophils were obtained from a patient with chronic myelogenous leukemia who had a total peripheral leukocyte count of 75,000/mm³ with a differential count of 32% basophils, 62% blasts, 2% myelocytes and 4% lymphocytes. Attempts at purification of the basophils caused their degranulation, and so the leukocyte suspension was injected into rabbits as obtained. In recent experiments, however, we have been able to show that human basophils differ in their migration through Hypaque solutions from the other granulocytes (A. A. F. Mahmoud, unpublished observations). Leukocyte suspensions containing 32% basophils and 30% eosinophils were layered over Hypaque solution (1 part Hypaque to 1.7 parts distilled water) and centrifuged as described before. This procedure resulted in preferential separation of the two granulocyte cell populations; eosinophils constituted 90% of the cells at the pellet, and 62% of the cells at the interface were basophils. Patients with myelogenous leukemia during relapse with over 90% of their peripheral white cell count as myeloblasts were the donors of these cells. No purification step was necessary, as the leukocyte suspension contained 95% myeloblasts after the sedimentation of red cells.

3.3. Preparation of Antisera

3.3.1. Immunization Schedule. At least two rabbits should be used for the production of a pool of antiserum against each cell type. Between 8 and 10×10^7 cells per rabbit are suspended in 1 ml of phosphate-buffered saline and mixed well with an equal volume of Freund's complete adjuvant. The mixture is divided into 4 equal aliquots and injected subcutaneously into both axillae and groins. Using the same procedure each rabbit is immunized twice more at 1-week intervals along its back and in the axillae and groins.

3.3.2. Bleeding of Rabbits and Separation of the Antisera. One week after the third immunizing dose, the rabbits are bled 3 times every other day. The blood is left to clot at 37°C for 1 hr, then overnight at 4°C. Sera are then separated, pooled, and stored at 20°C until further use.

3.4. Testing the Potency and Specificity of Antisera.

Several techniques have been used to test the potency and specificity of antisera. References are included for the agglutination (2), cytotoxicity (15), basophil degranulation (16), and immunofluorescence tests (17). The crude antisera were first tested for potency, then subjected to a series of absorptions before assessing their specificity. All antisera were absorbed twice with an equal volume of packed group O red blood cells for 1 hr at room temperature and overnight at 4°C. Other minor antibody components against contaminating cells were similarly absorbed with the corresponding cells. Usually about 2×10^8 cells were incubated with 1 ml of serum and the absorption protocol for the red cells was followed. Specificity of the antisera was then evaluated by specific and cross-absorption studies using different purified cell preparations.

3.5. Antisera against Animal Granulocytes.

The studies from which the above-described methods were derived concentrated on the use of human material for raising different anti-granulocyte sera. As several animal models have proved to be easy to handle and useful investigative tools, references are given below for the methodology of obtaining different cell lines from animals and for the techniques of purifying the cells.

3.5.1. The Mouse. Neutrophils can be obtained from normal animals as described by Simpson and Ross (2) and purified on a Hypaque 50 gradient, 1 part Hypaque and 2.2 parts distilled water (A. A. F. Mahmoud, unpublished observations). Eosinophils obtained from schistosome- or *Trichinella*-infected animals (12, 18) can be purified on a Hypaque 50 gradient, 1 part Hypaque and 2 parts distilled water (12).

3.5.2. The Rat. Relatively pure preparations of neutrophils can be obtained from the peritoneal cavity using proteose peptone stimulation (2). Eosinophils have been obtained from normal animals and purified on human serum albumin gradients (18). We are now attempting the purification of rat granulocytes via Hypaque 50 density gradients.

3.5.3. The Guinea Pig. Reference (29) includes a detailed description of the methods for obtaining neutrophils and eosinophils and purifying them.

4. Comments

4.1. The most critical step in our technique is the purification of cells on the Hypaque gradient. It should be emphasized that the density of the Hypaque solution and distilled water can vary from one laboratory to another. In the initial attempts, therefore, several different gradients should be used, the amount of distilled water added to the Hypaque 50 solution being varied within 0.2–0.6 ml above or below the level recommended in this article. We have found that this preliminary run is essential in order to establish the particular conditions necessary for purification of the cells in each laboratory. Once these conditions are defined, reproducibility of the technique becomes merely a matter of accurate measurement of Hypaque and distilled water.

4.2. The preferential purification of a specific cell type on density gradients under standardized conditions depends mainly on two factors: the proportion of the required cell type in the original suspension and the density of the gradient. Cell suspensions with less than 15–20% of the particular cell type needed are difficult to process by the methods outlined above. When there are adequate numbers of cells, the density of the gradient under the conditions described is the factor that will determine the yield and purity of cell preparations obtained. While higher cell yields are obtained with slightly less dense gradients, it is at the expense of the purity of the cells. In contrast, slightly denser gradients will result in fewer but more highly purified cells in the pellet. Finally, it is essential to assess the condition and viability of the purified cells by dye exclusion, morphological, and functional criteria.

4.3. The monospecific antisera produced by the above methodology have helped to define the immunological identity of the granulocyte within the white blood cell series. Evidence for the immunological specificity of the basophils, eosinophils, neutrophils, and myeloblasts was obtained from *in vitro* work using human material (10) and from both *in vitro* and *in vivo* animal experiments (2, 10, 14). These cell-specific antibodies also react with cells obtained from normal donors and from patients with a variety of different clinical conditions. Thus these antisera recognize antigenic determinants common to each cell line.

4.4. Evidence from *in vitro* studies with human cells and *in vivo* animal experiments has shown that the antisera are stage specific insofar as the maturity of the cells is concerned. Antisera raised against the mature basophil, eosinophil, and neutrophil contain no cytotoxic or agglutinating activity against the myeloblasts. Conversely, anti-myeloblast serum had no effect on mature cells (10). Treatment of animals with anti-eosinophil or anti-neutrophil sera led to virtual elimination of the corresponding mature cells but had no effect on their bone marrow precursors (2, 14).

4.5. While anti-neutrophil sera have been available for some time to study the effects of neutrophil depletion in experimental animals, it is only recently that similar studies were feasible with antieosinophil sera (14, 21, 22). The anti-eosinophil serum has been used to study the kinetics of the eosinophil response associated with the granulomatous reaction around schistosome eggs (14). Depletion of the mature eosinophils enabled investigations into the regulation of eosinopoiesis and the possible role of humoral regulatory factors (23). Furthermore, the anti-eosinophil serum helped in defining the effector cell in the *in vitro* cytotoxicity assay against the immature forms of the schistosomes (24) and in demonstrating that by depletion of eosinophils, animals which were previously immune to schistosome infection lost their resistance (21).

ACKNOWLEDGMENT

The author extends sincere thanks to Dr. Kenneth S. Warren for his continual encouragement and painstaking advice during the preparation of this chapter.

REFERENCES

1. Metchnikoff, E., *Ann. Inst. Pasteur (Paris)* **13**, 737 (1899).
2. Simpson, D. M., and Ross, R., *Am. J. Pathol.* **65**, 79 (1971).
3. Shadduck, R. K., and Nagabhushanam, N. G., *Blood* **38**, 559 (1971).
4. Cochran, C. G., *Adv. Immunol.* **9**, 97 (1968).
5. Lance, E. M., Medawar, P. B., and Taub, R. N., *Adv. Immunol.* **17**, 2 (1973).
6. Böyum, A., *Scand. J. Clin. Lab. Invest.* **21**, Suppl. 97, 77 (1968).
7. Raff, M. C., *Nature (London)* **242**, 19 (1973).
8. Unanue, E. R., *Nature (London)* **218**, 36 (1968).
9. Boros, D. L., and Warren, K. S., *J. Immunol.* **107**, 534 (1971).
10. Mahmoud, A. A. F., Kellermeyer, R. W., and Warren, K. S., *Lancet* **2**, 1163 (1974).
11. Day, R. P., *Immunology* **18**, 955 (1970).
12. Mahmoud, A. A. F., Warren, K. S., and Boros, D. L., *J. Exp. Med.* **137**, 1526 (1973).
13. Mahmoud, A. A. F., Kellermeyer, R. W., and Warren, K. S., *N. Engl. J. Med.* **390**, 417 (1974).
14. Mahmoud, A. A. F., Warren, K. S., and Graham, R. C., Jr., *J. Exp. Med.* **142**, 560 (1975).
15. Engelfriet, C. P., and Britten, A., *Vox Sang.* **11**, 334 (1966).
16. Ishizaka, T., Tomeoka, H., and Ishizaka, K., *J. Immunol.* **106**, 705 (1971).

17. Lamelin, J. P., Lisowska-Bernstein, B., Matter, A., Ryser, J. E., and Vassali, P., *J. Exp. Med.* **136,** 984 (1972).
18. Warren, K. S., Karp, R., Pelley, R. P., and Mahmoud, A. A. F., *J. Infect. Dis.* in press.
19. Archer, G. T., and Hirsch, J. G., *J. Exp. Med.* **118,** 277 (1963).
20. Gleich, G. J., and Loegering, D. A., *J. Lab. Clin. Med.* **82,** 523 (1973).
21. Mahmoud, A. A. F., Warren, K. S., and Peters, P. A., *J. Exp. Med.* **142,** 805 (1975).
22. Gleich, G. J., Loegering, D. A., and Olson, G. M., *J. Immunol.* **115,** 950 (1975).
23. Mahmoud, A. A. F., Stone, M. K., Kellermeyer, R. W., and Warren, K. S., *Clin. Res.* **23,** 524A (1975).
24. Butterworth, A. E., Sturrock, R. F., Houba, V., Mahmoud, A. A. F., Sher, A., and Rees, P. H., *Nature (London)* **256,** 727 (1975).

Fluorescence Microscopy of Lymphocytes and Mononuclear Phagocytes and the Use of Silica to Eliminate the Latter

Anthony C. Allison

1. Introduction

Ehrlich (1) pioneered the use of dyes to study living animal cells. He introduced vital dyes, such as neutral red, and observed their selective concentration in certain cell types and within particular cytoplasmic organelles. Among the cells that he studied were peripheral blood leukocytes, and he distinguished certain cells readily taking up dyes, which we now know to be monocytes, from other cells taking up very little dye, including lymphocytes. His observations, which showed how specifically compounds are distributed in the body, provided the basis for his later pharmacological researches, in which he sought dyes taken up selectively by pathogenic organisms, killing them or inhibiting their multiplication (2). When lysosomes were discovered, it was recognized that the intracellular granules vitally stained by neutral red are lysosomes (3).

During the period of classical cytology, about the turn of the century, vital staining for mitochondria was often used. With the development of phase-contrast and electron microscopy and cellular biochemistry, the attention of the new generation of cell biologists after the last World War was turned to these techniques, and great advances were made. However, all these methods have limitations. Phase-contrast microscopy has limited resolving power, and the distinction between lysosomes and other intracellular organelles in leukocytes cannot always be made with confidence. Electron microscopy can be carried out only on fixed and dehydrated preparations, and cellular chemistry on disrupted cells. In both cases some measure of distortion is inevitable, and there are many situations in which it is still of interest to observe living cells, either freshly prepared or cultured *in vitro*. Since lysosomes play important roles in leukocytes, it is useful to have a selective vital stain for these organelles. Neutral red staining and conventional microscopy are applicable, but now that fluorescence microscopes are available in most immunological laboratories, the superior definition given by fluorescence microscopy of lysosomes in vitally stained cells can be exploited. In this way the pattern of lysosomes in different cell types and changes associated with processes such as lymphocyte transformation and macrophage activation can be observed. This approach is useful to monitor techniques such as the depletion of mononuclear phagocytes from a cell population. In view of renewed interest in lysosomotropic drugs, fluorescence microscopy is again being used to follow the intracellular fate of drugs and toxins. Another application of fluorescence microscopy is to estimate the proportion of living cells in a population by their capacity to split fluorescein esters (4). This is useful with lymphocytes, for example, in histocompatibility typing (5) and in macrophages (6).

Since mononuclear phagocytes play an important part in the defenses of the body against microorganisms and interact with lymphocytes in immunity, it is helpful to have methods for selective depletion of macrophages *in vivo* and *in vitro*. It has long been known that silica is highly cytotoxic for macrophages in culture (7). Other agents, such as carrageenin, have limitations because relatively high concentrations are required to kill macrophages, whereas lower concentrations stimulate the cells to synthesize and release hydrolases (8). The cells may, in addition, be stimulated to secrete other factors, many of which are now known. Carrageenin also has other effects, such as activation of complement by the alternative pathway and activation of Hageman factor (9), making it difficult to interpret the results of administration, especially *in vivo*. Carrageenin is taken up by pinocytosis, so that it can enter most cell types. To achieve selective depletion of macrophages, we therefore prefer to use silica particles, which are taken up only by phagocytic cells, do not activate complement or induce enzyme secretion from mononuclear phagocytes, and are highly cytotoxic for these cells. Silica can be used *in vitro* and, with certain reservations, *in vivo*, where the activity is greater and more prolonged than that of conventional blocking agents, such as carbon or Thorotrast. Examples of the use of silica for investigating some immunological problems are discussed in Section 4.

2. Materials

2.1. Acridine Orange. Most commercial samples are mixtures, as can be shown by chromatography. The purest commercial sample we have obtained is Euchrysine 3R from G. T. Gurr, London, but some others, although impure, have been satisfactory for fluorescence microscopy.

2.2. Fluorescein Esters. These can be purchased from Eastman Organic Chemicals, Rochester, New York. Various esters are supplied, of which the most convenient is fluorescein dibutyrate.

2.3. Silica. As a pure mineral, silica (silicon dioxide) occurs in three main crystal forms or isomers: quartz, tridymite, and cristobalite; other rare crystalline variants are coesite and stishovite, both found in meteorite craters. The fibrogenic and cytotoxic activities of silica samples depend on the size and composition of the particles and the state of their surfaces (whether natural or changed by hydration, heating, or some other reaction). With particles of comparable size, fibrogenic and cytotoxic activities decrease somewhat in the following order: tridymite, cristobalite, quartz, coesite. Stishovite, which lacks the tetrahedral structure of other crystal forms, resembles in its structure and properties the rutile form of titanium dioxide; it is neither fibrogenic nor cytotoxic.

Since tridymite and cristobalite are not readily obtainable, most experiments are carried out with quartz particles small enough to be respirable and to be taken up by phagocytosis, i.e., in the range 1 to 5 μm in diameter. Different samples of quartz vary in their biological effects. Research into the biological effects of asbestos has been facilitated by the availability of international standard samples of the various fiber types. Efforts are now being made to obtain a large sample of high-quality quartz of suitable size that could be used as an international standard sample. In recent years a German sample, Dörentrup No. 12, <5 μm, has been used in several laboratories. Although the quality of this material is not as high as would be desired, it is cytotoxic for macrophages and has the expected *in vivo* effects.

A commercially supplied quartz is No. 216 Min-U-Sil, which can be purchased from Whittaker, Clarke and Daniels, Inc., White Plains, New York. Samples of this material have been found by Dr. Pooley, University of Cardiff, to have surface contamination with iron oxide, which affects biological activity. This can be eliminated by boiling in 1 N hydrochloric acid until no further green color is observed, washing in distilled water until there is no further reaction for chloride, and drying the silica thoroughly for storage.

3. Methods

3.1. Acridine Orange Fluorescence Microscopy. Five milligrams of dye is dissolved in 5 ml of Hanks' solution to make up a stock solution of 1/1000 (w/v). This is kept in a dark bottle in a refrigerator, and a fresh stock solution is added to 500 parts of culture medium.

Cells can be stained in suspension or, preferably, on cover slips. Cultures of macrophages adherent to cover slips can be obtained in Leighton tubes or by inserting cover slips into Petri dishes when cultures of peritoneal or other macrophages are being established.

Cells must be alive and metabolizing normally when stained. They are therefore incubated for 30 min at 37°C in their normal suspension or culture medium containing a final concentration of 1 in 5×10^5 (w/v) acridine orange. The staining should be carried out in the dark (e.g., in a CO_2 incubator), and washing should be performed in subdued light. When stained, suspensions of cells are centrifuged, washed once in medium at room temperature, and resuspended in culture medium lacking the dye. Washing reduces the green background fluorescence and cell damage by photosensitization. A small drop of suspension is placed on a clean, high quality slide, and a cover slip is lowered on it gently. The preparation is sealed with wax or nail varnish. Cover slips with adherent cell suspensions are readily rinsed with medium lacking dye, mounted in the living state, and sealed to prevent evaporation. The preparations are then examined by fluorescence microscopy.

3.2. Fluorescein Dibutyrate. Five milligrams of the dibutyrate are dissolved in 1 ml of acetone and diluted in culture medium (e.g., medium 199 containing 10% newborn calf serum for macrophages) to a final concentration of 15 μg of fluorescein dibutyrate per milliliter. The cells are incubated in the medium at 37°C for 15 min, washed once in medium lacking the dye, and mounted in fresh medium, as described in the previous section, for observation. As before, the incubation with fluorescein dibutyrate should be in the dark, and the washing should be in subdued light, never direct sunlight. Fluorescence microscopy is carried out with any convenient system for fluorescein, e.g. Zeiss Universal microscope with HBO 200 mercury lamp with BG 38 and BG 12 primary filters and a Zeiss secondary filter No. 47.

3.3. Silica. Silica is dry-sterilized in a hot-air oven and suspended in Hanks' solution for *in vivo* administration (this, being equilibrated with air, does not become alkaline in the absence of CO_2) or in culture medium for use with cell suspensions or cultures. Clumps of silica should be dispersed by ultrasonic vibration a few minutes before use; they can cause embolism when injected intravenously, and they can result in uneven distribution of silica *in vitro*. It is preferable to have some serum in the medium to coat the silica particles and prevent early cytotoxicity. Usually 10% calf or fetal calf serum is satisfactory. The surface properties of aqueous suspensions of silica particles change, even when stored at −20°C, so that it is advisable to use suspensions not more than 3 days old to obtain reproducible cytotoxicity.

The amount of silica that can be administered intravenously varies with the species of experimental animal and silica sample. With two quartz samples we have found that mature mice tolerate intravenous injections of 3 mg well; rats tolerate at least 10 mg. Intraperitoneal doses of 25 mg in mice or 200 mg in rats have marked effects on local macrophages, as well as effects on other sites.

The concentration of silica required to kill macrophages varies with the sample. With Dörentrup No. 12 quartz, addition to the culture medium of 50 μg (10^6 macrophages) per milliliter kills the majority of the cells within 12 hr of incubation at 37°C. However, incubation in 20 μg/ml results in little cell killing but an increase in the concentration of nonlysosomal enzymes, such as leucine-2-naphthylamidase and lactate dehydrogenase. The stimulating effects of small doses of silica on macrophages must be borne in mind when interpreting experiments *in vivo* as well as *in vitro*.

Incubation of human peripheral blood mononuclear cells with silica (100 μg/ml Dörentrup No. 12) for 48 hr kills more than 95% of phagocytic cells. Counts of B and T lymphocytes by membrane immunofluorescence and E rosetting, responses to PHA and capacity to kill Chang cells sensitized with antibody (K cell activity) are unaffected by the silica treatment (E. J. O'Rourke and S. B. Halstead, personal communication).

4. Interpretation of Data

4.1. Acridine Orange Fluorescence. After staining of living cells, acridine orange is concentrated in lysosomes, which therefore fluoresce orange-red because of molecular stacking of the dye molecules bound to a specific glyco-lipid constitutent of lysosomes. Lower concentrations of dye molecules accumulate in the nucleus, which fluoresces green. This is convenient because at the same time the distribution and features of the lysosomes and nucleus are demonstrable, and these differ in different cell types and with stimulation of the cells.

The most intense lysosomal fluorescence is observed in cells of the mononuclear phagocytic series. Peripheral blood monocytes show prominent orange-fluorescing lysosomes around the nucleus, as well as fairly large nuclei fluorescing pale green. Peritoneal and alveolar macrophages show larger numbers of lysosomes, especially when the former have been cultured under conditions stimulating lysosome formation (for example, exposure of mouse macrophages to bovine serum). The lysosomes are predominantly perinuclear, and few are seen in the peripheral cytoplasm, including pseudopodia where ruffled membrane activity and macropinocytosis are taking place. After phagocytosis large secondary lysosomes show moderately intense orange fluorescence, and when mononuclear phagocytes are stimulated by an agent that induces selective release of lysosomal enzymes into the medium, such as the type-specific polysaccharide and peptidoglycan of streptococcal cell walls, lysosomes are seen near the periphery of the cells and extending into pseudopodia (6).

Polymorphonuclear leukocytes show much less intense, red cytoplasmic fluorescence and green fluorescence of their lobed nuclei. Small lymphocytes show intense green fluorescence of their condensed nuclei and a small number of bright, orange-fluorescing lysosomes, usually found on one side of the nucleus. When lymphocytes are stimulated by mitogens, the nucleus enlarges and fluoresces less intensely, and the number of lysosomes is considerably increased. These show intense fluorescence, usually concentrated around the Golgi region to one side of the nucleus. Plasma cells show moderate numbers of lysosomes, often arranged like beads around the Golgi region.

Lysosomal fluorescence has several practical uses. Because mononuclear phagocytes show intense lysosomal fluorescence that can readily be identified under the low power of the light microscope, the technique is convenient for monitoring the effectiveness of procedures for depleting these cells. Second, observations on the lysosomes of mononuclear cells complement biochemical studies of different types of activation (8). Third, acridine orange fluorescence is a rapid and convenient way to follow the course of lymphocyte transformation. Although this should again be carried out in parallel with biochemical studies, it is now becoming clear that incorporation of labeled thymidine should not be the only criterion of transformation. For example, a "lymphocyte chalone" appears to be cold thymidine, which dilutes the label incorporated into DNA, and some reported effects of macrophages on tumor cell multiplication again seem to be the result of dilution of label. It is therefore desirable that other criteria be used, and microscopic examination of cells can reveal unexpected complications of experiments, including cell death or contamination. Dead cells show diffuse green fluorescence after acridine orange staining and can readily be identified.

One of the limitations that must be borne in mind is when cells cultured on cover slips are infected with viruses or subjected to some other types of insult, they become detached into the medium. They are not then represented in the final cover slip preparation. It is, however, possible to recover such cells by centrifugation of the medium.

4.2. Fluorescein Ester Staining.   Living cells are able to hydrolyze the ester to liberate fluorescein, which shows strong green cytoplasmic fluorescence, in mononuclear phagocytes and lymphocytes as well as other cell types. Dead cells are unable to split the ester and are unstained. This procedure is useful for assessing the viability of cultured macrophages after exposure to toxic agents or stimuli (6) and for histocompatibility typing with small numbers of lymphocytes (6). This technique along with others, such as liberation into the medium of the cytoplasmic enzyme lactate dehydrogenase, appear to be more reliable indicators of cell death than release of ^{51}Cr, because at least two-thirds of the ^{51}Cr is not bound to cytoplasmic macromolecules and might be released without cell death.

4.3. Applications of Silica *in Vitro*.   That silica is cytotoxic for mouse macrophages in culture was demonstrated by Marks (11). It has since been recognized that there are two distinct types of cytotoxic effects (12). Rapid cytotoxicity occurs when relatively large amounts of silica are added to macrophages in a serum-free medium. Within 1 hr of exposure many cells are damaged. This appears to be due to interaction of silica with the plasma membranes of the macrophages and is the counterpart in nucleated cells of silica hemolysis. Rapid cytotoxicity can be inhibited by coating the silica particles with proteins, pulmonary surfactant (phosphatidylcholine) or other materials. Inhaled or intravenously injected silica particles are soon coated with surfactant or serum proteins. Particles are ingested by macrophages with a protein coat demonstrable by immunofluorescence. Soon the protein coat is digested and the surface of the silica particles is free to react with the membrane surrounding the secondary lysosomes in which the particles are enclosed. With the doses of silica recommended, the majority of macrophages are killed within 6 hr. Silica particles greater than 1 μm in diameter are not taken up by lymphocytes, even after transformation, so that the killing of macrophages is selective.

Unlike chrysotile asbestos, silica does not induce the selective release of lysosomal enzymes from viable cells. In macrophages dying of exposure to silica, there is simultaneous release of lysosomal and cytoplasmic marker enzymes. Small doses of silica do not kill the cells but stimulate the synthesis of nonlysosomal marker enzymes, such as lactate dehydrogenase and leucine-2-naphthylamidase. In such cells mechanisms controlling intracellular bacterial multiplication are impaired. Thus, *Mycobacterium tuberculosis* organisms grow better in such cells than in untreated cells (13). This explains the well known aggravation of tuberculosis in humans and experimental animals by silica inhalation. Alveolar macrophages from animals that have inhaled silica inactivate bacteria less well than normal macrophages (14). *In vitro* treatment of macrophages with silica inhibits their phagocytic capacity (15). Silica treatment of spleen cells from immune donors decreased their capacity to prevent growth of tumor cells with which they were injected into syngeneic mice (16). Keller (17) reported that proteose–peotone-induced peritoneal exudate cells from rats inhibited the proliferation of tumor cells in culture. Elimination of functional macrophages by silica resulted in unrestricted tumor-cell multiplication. Keller concluded that nonspecifically activated macrophages have cytostatic effects on tumor cells, in addition to relatively weak cytotoxic effects.

4.4. *In Vivo* Administration of Silica. Intravenous injection of 3 mg of silica into mice decreases the clearance of colloidal carbon from the blood (15, 18). The inhibition of carbon clearance was observed as soon as 2 hr after silica injection and persisted for the 3 days studied, longer than the blockade induced by nontoxic materials. This suggests that macrophages in contact with circulating blood are killed, or incapacitated for several days, by silica. Related to this effect is the observation that yellow fever virus was more slowly cleared from the circulation in mice after intravenous injection of silica than in control mice (19). After intravenous injection of silica, mice showed decreased resistance to infection with virulent blood forms (trypomastigotes) of *Trypanosoma cruzi*. In treated animals both the level of parasitemia and mortality rate were significantly increased over those of control mice inoculated only with the parasites (18).

After intravenous injection of silica, mononuclear cells containing silica particles are seen in peritoneal washouts. Some of these cells are killed, and there is a variable depletion of the mononuclear phagocyte population that can be recovered without stimulation. Presumably cells bearing silica pass from the blood stream to the peritoneal cavity, and vice versa. The effects of intraperitoneal injection of silica on local macrophages are much more dramatic, with vacuolation and killing of large numbers of cells. The importance of mononuclear cells in controlling virus infection can be illustrated by experiments with silica. Adult mice survive intravenous or intraperitoneal injections of herpes simplex virus type 1, but after intraperitoneal injection of silica the virus produces a lethal hepatitis (20); Kupffer cells provide a barrier to the spread of the infection in adult, but not in newborn, mice. With several viruses, much larger inocula are required to establish infection by the intraperitoneal than the intravenous route. After intraperitoneal inoculation of silica, much less Friend virus is required to establish an infection than in uninoculated mice (21), and we have found this to be true also of Semliki forest virus and encephalomyocarditis virus. Thus a high proportion of the virus inoculated into the peritoneal cavity, or presumably introduced into other tissue spaces, is inactivated by macrophages.

Silica has also been used to study the role of macrophages in the induction and expression of immunity. Pernis and Paronetto (22) reported that silica administered to rabbits 2–13 weeks before ovalbumin increased antibody formation. In contrast, silica injected intravenously into mice 1–3 days before sheep erythrocytes (SRBC) depressed the number of anti-SRBC plaques in the spleen (15). Silica given 2 hr before, or any time after, the antigen did not significantly affect the antibody response. Inoculation of silica 2 days before allogeneic cells depressed the induction of cell-mediated immunity as shown by the capacity of spleen cells to lyse ^{51}Cr-labeled allogeneic cells *in vitro*. After intravenous injection of silica the basal level of labeled thymidine incorporation into spleen cells was increased, and concanavalin A stimulation of the incorporation was first increased and then depressed. Miller and Zarkower (14) reported that in mice after inhalation of silica spleen cells showed a diminished mitogenic response to lipopolysaccharide (the reduced index of stimulation being at least partly due to the high basal level of incorporation).

Pearsall and Weiser (16) reported that single doses of silica given to mice intravenously 3 days to 4 hr before skin grafting resulted in highly significant prolongation of allograft survival; silica administration 1–4 days after grafting had no significant effect, but single or multiple injections of silica during the efferent phase of the reaction, 5 or more days after grafting, again prolonged graft survival. As mentioned in Section 4.3, Pearsall and Weiser found that silica treatment of immune cells before mixture with tumor cells and inoculation into syngeneic recipients reduced the ability of the immune cells to inhibit tumor growth. They concluded that macrophages contribute both to the afferent and efferent phases of allograft and tumor rejection, presumably to the first by transporting or processing antigen and to the latter by effector activity against allograft target cells. The observations of Pearsall and Weiser on skin grafts have been confirmed by Rios and Simmons (23), who found also that the effects of silica could be counteracted by administration of poly-2-vinylpyidine 1-oxide, which prevents silica toxicity of macrophages.

Further evidence for the participation of host-cell macrophages in adoptive immunity against syngeneic SV40-induced tumor cells in mice was obtained by Zarling and Tevethia (24). Tumor cells and immune spleen cells transferred to recipients after intravenous injection of silica induced tumors much more frequently than in untreated recipients. Injection of BCG into subcutaneous sites of tumor growth in rats can lead to regression of small tumors in these and other sites, indicating systemic immunization. Intraperitoneal injections of silica (with or without intravenous injection) can prevent the induction of this type of immunity (25, 26).

These examples suffice to show that silica is a useful tool in analyzing the role of macrophages in the afferent and efferent limbs of the immune response. Silica effects on macrophages *in vivo* are relatively short lived, lasting a few days in the case of intravenous injection, so that the timing and route of silica injection can markedly influence its effects. The effects of different silica samples may also vary, and care must be taken that they are not contaminated with bacterial endotoxins or other extraneous materials that can influence immune reactivity. The availability of an international standard sample of silica, uncontaminated, of good quality and in the size range 1 to 5 μm, would help to ensure uniformity of results in different laboratories. Use of silica is the most selective and efficient way of depleting macrophages at present available, and many possible applications to immunology can be envisaged.

REFERENCES

1. Ehrlich, P., *Biol. Zentralbl.* **6**, 214 (1887).
2. Marquardt, M., "Paul Ehrlich." Heinemann, London, 1949.
3. Allison, A. C., and Young, M. R., *in* "Lysosomes in Biology and Pathology" (J. T. Dingle and H. B. Fell, eds.), Vol. 2, p. 600. North-Holland Publ., Amsterdam, (1969).
4. Rotman, B., and Papermaster, B. W., *Proc. Natl. Acad. Sci. USA* **55**, 134 (1966).
5. Bodmer, W., Tripp, M., and Bodmer, J., "Histocompatibility Testing," p. 341. Munksgaard, Copenhagen, 1967.
6. Davies, P., Page, R. C., and Allison, A. C., *J. Exp. Med.* **139**, 1262 (1974).
7. Allison, A. C., Harington, J. S., and Birbeck, M. *J. Exp. Med.* **124**, 141 (1966).
8. Davies, P., and Allison, A. C., *in* "Lysosomes in Biology and Pathology" (J. T. Dingle and R. T. Dean, eds.), Vol. 5, p. 61. North-Holland Publ., Amsterdam, 1976.
9. Schwartz, H. J., and Kellermeyer, J. J., *Proc. Soc. Exp. Biol. Med.* **132**, 1021 (1969).
10. Allison, A. C., and Davies, P., *in* "Mononuclear Phagocytes in Immunity, Infection and Pathology" (R. van Furth, ed.), p. 487. Blackwell, Oxford, 1975.
11. Marks, J., *Br. J. Ind. Med.* **14**, 81 (1957).
12. Allison, A. C., *Ann. N. Y. Acad. Sci.* **221**, 299 (1974).
13. Allison, A. C., and Hart, P. d'A., *Br. J. Exp. Pathol.* **49**, 465 (1968).
14. Miller, S. D., and Zarkower, A., *J. Immunol.* **113**, 1533 (1974).
15. Levy, M. H., and Wheelock, E. F., *J. Immunol.* **115**, 41 (1975).
16. Pearsall, N. N., and Weiser, R. S. *J. Reticuloendothol. Soc.* **5**, 107 (1968).
17. Keller, R., *J. Exp. Med.* **138**, 625 (1973).
18. Kierszenbaum, F., Knecht, E., Budzko, D., and Pizzimenti, M. C., *J. Immunol.* **112**, 1839 (1974).

19. Zisman, B., Wheelock, E. F., and Allison, A. C., *J. Immunol.* **107,** 236 (1971).
20. Zisman, B., Hirsch, M. S., and Allison, A. C., *J. Immunol.* **104,** 1155 (1970).
21. Larson, C. L., Ushujima, R. N., Baker, R. E., M. B., and Gillespie, C. A., *J. Natl. Cancer Inst.* **48,** 1403 (1972).
22. Pernis, B., and Paronetto, F., *Proc. Soc. Exp. Biol. Med.* **110,** 390 (1962).
23. Rios, A., and Simmons, R. L., *Transplantation* **13,** 343 (1972).
24. Zarling, J. M., and Tevethia, S. S., *J. Natl. Cancer Inst.* **50,** 149 (1973).
25. Chassoux, D., and Salomon, J. C., *Int. J. Cancer* **16,** 515 (1975).
26. Baldwin, R. W., Hopper, D. G., and Pimm, M. W., *Ann. N. Y. Acad. Sci.* in press (1976).

Measurement of Fc Receptors on Human Monocytes

Fred S. Rosen

1. Introduction

Antibody that is cytophilic for monocytes and macrophages has been detected in the serum of guinea pigs, rabbits, mice, and man (1–3). These macrophage receptors for Fc may be essential for noncomplement-dependent phagocytosis, antibody-dependent cell-mediated cytotoxicity, macrophage "arming," and antigen processing and presentation. Cytophilic antibodies in the guinea pig and mouse are of the IgG_2 class whereas in man IgG_1 and IgG_3 subclasses display this property (4). The following description is based on work with human monocytes, antibodies, and erythrocytes to form rosettes that detect the Fc receptor. Detailed descriptions of a mouse system are available (5).

2. Materials

2.1. Collection of Monocytes and Monolayers
Syringes and needles
Heparin
Dextran, 3% in saline
Hanks' balanced salt solution containing 5×10^{-4} M $MgCl_2$ and 1.3×10^{-3} M $CaCl_2$
Refrigerated centrifuge at 4°C
Disposable tissue culture wells, 16 mm (Linbro Scientific Corp., New Haven, Connecticut)

2.2. Preparation of Erythrocytes for Rosetting
Human erythrocytes, type O, Rh+
$Na_2{}^{51}CrO_4$
Incomplete Rh antibody
Water bath, 37°C
Hanks' balanced salt solution
Centrifuge
Gamma counter

3. Methods

Blood, 40 ml, is drawn into a syringe containing 20 ml of 3% dextran in saline and 1000 units of heparin. The erythrocytes are allowed to settle for 1 hr at room temperature. The plasma is expressed from the syringe into conical, siliconized centrifuge tubes, and the white cells are sedimented at 300 g for 10 min at 10°C. The white cell pellet is then washed twice in Hanks' balanced salt solution. Leukocytes, 15,000–20,000 per cubic millimeter, are suspended in Hanks' balanced salt solution, and 0.4 ml are poured onto 16-mm Linbro tissue culture trays. After 30 min at room temperature, nonadherent cells and Hanks' solution are suctioned off and the monolayer is washed 4 times with fresh Hanks' solution.

Type O Rh+ blood, 40 ml, is drawn into a syringe with 1000 units of heparin, and immediately centrifuged; the red cells are washed 3 times in saline, and once in Hanks' solution. They are then suspended in an equal volume of Hanks' solution to give a hematocrit of 50%. A half volume of $Na_2{}^{51}CrO_4$ (1 mCi/ml) is mixed with the red cell suspension for 15 min at room temperature. The red cells are washed 3 times in Hanks' solution, and a final 16% suspension of ^{51}Cr labeled erythrocytes is prepared. Anti-Rh antiserum is diluted 1:16 in Hanks' solution. One volume of antiserum is incubated with 3 volumes of 16% ^{51}Cr labeled erythrocytes for 1 hr at 37°C. The red cells are then washed 3 times with Hanks' solution and then suspended at a concentration of 4% (v/v). Of the 4% red cell suspension, 0.4 ml is added to each monolayer and incubated for 2 hr at room temperature. Unbound red cells are then removed by aspiration. The monolayers are washed 4 times with Hanks' solution and then assayed for ^{51}Cr.

REFERENCES

1. Berken, A., and Benacerraf, B., *J. Exp. Med.* **123,** 119 (1966).
2. Lay, W. H., and Nussenzweig, V., *J. Exp. Med.* **128,** 991 (1968).
3. Lo Buglio, A. F., Cotran, R. S., and Jandl, J. H., *Science* **158,** 1582 (1967).
4. Abramson, N., Gelfand, E. W., Jandl, J. H., and Rosen, F. S., *J. Exp. Med.* **132,** 1207 (1970).
5. Unkeless, J. C., and Eisen, H. N., *J. Exp. Med.* **142,** 1520 (1975).

36

Methods for the Study of
Macrophage Fc and C3 Receptors

Celso Bianco*

1. Introduction

This chapter describes methods for the detection of plasma membrane receptors for the Fc portion of the IgG molecule and for fragments of the third component of complement (C3) by means of rosette formation with sheep erythrocytes. Although the emphasis is on monocytes and macrophages, the reagents can be used for the identification of these receptors on any cell type. The distribution of plasma membrane receptors for C3 among several cell types has been recently reviewed (1).

Table 1 summarizes the distribution of Fc and complement receptors. The receptor for Fc of IgG is present on all "professional" phagocytes and is essential for immune phagocytosis (12), but the function of these receptors on nonphagocytic cells is unclear.

C3 receptors are also present on a variety of cells (1), and their role in phagocytosis has been recently clarified. In the absence of IgG, C3 is insufficient to promote particle ingestion by any cell except by the activated macrophage (5, 13). However, C3 may act synergistically with small amounts of IgG, which are themselves insufficient to promote phagocytosis (3).

C3, a complement component, is cleaved sequentially by two enzymes during the process of complement activation: (a) C3 convertase cleaves C3 in two fragments, C3b, a large fragment that attaches to cell membranes, and C3a, which remains in the fluid phase; (b) C3b can be acted upon by the C3b inactivator enzyme, and only a small fragment, C3d remains associated with the cell membrane; C3c, the large fragment, is liberated in the fluid phase (reviewed in 14).

Two types of C3 receptors have been described (7). The CRI (or *b*) receptor binds to the C3b fixed to the erythrocyte membrane after cleavage by the C3 convertase. The CRII (or *d*) receptor binds to the fragment that remains attached

*Scholar of the Leukemia Society of America.

TABLE 1
Receptors for the Fc Fragment of IgG and for Fragments of C3 on Several Cell Types

Cell type	Species	Receptor type			
		Fc	CRI $(b)^a$	CRII $(d)^a$	References[b]
Monocytes	Human	+	+	+	(2, 3)
Macrophages (peritoneal cavity)	Mouse	+	+	−	(4)
Activated macrophage	Mouse	+	+	−	(5)
Macrophage (lung)	Human	+	+	−[c]	(6)
Granulocytes	Human	+	+	−	(7)
B lymphocytes	Mammals	+	+	+	(7–9)
T lymphocytes	Mouse	−[d]	−	−	(8)
Erythrocytes	Human and primates	−	+	−	(10)
Erythrocytes	Nonprimate mammals	−	−	−	(10)
Platelets	Human and primates	−	−	−	(10)
Platelets	Nonprimate mammals	−	+	−	(10)

[a]Receptors of the CRI (b) type can bind C4b and C3b, but not C3d; CRII (d) type receptors bind C3d and C3b, but not C4b.
[b]More extensive references can be found in references cited.
[c]The CRII (d) receptor activity may be detected or not, according to the method used to prepare the erythrocyte complexes (6).
[d]Mouse activated T cells have been shown to bind IgG (11).

to the erythrocyte membrane after digestion by the C3b inactivator. The following scheme summarizes the reactions:

E IgM C14 (binds to b receptor) + C2 → E IgM C142

E IgM C142 + C3 → C3a + E IgM C1423b   (binds to b and d receptor)

E IgM C1423b + C3b inactivator → C3c + E IgM C1423d   (binds to d receptor)

Table 2 shows the presumed forms of C3 on erythrocyte complexes routinely prepared in this laboratory.

Mouse peritoneal macrophages bind only complexes containing C3 in the form of C3b (15). Lymphocytes bind both C3b and C3d (7, 9).

The fate of erythrocyte complexes offered to mouse peritoneal macrophages provides an indication of the state of activation of these cells (5) (Table 3). Attachment or ingestion, and the degree of ingestion of the erythrocyte complexes, depend both on the nature of the complex and on the state of the macrophages: (a) Activated mouse peritoneal macrophages, obtained after intra-

TABLE 2
Receptor-Binding Properties of Complexes of Erythrocytes with Antibody and Complement

Erythrocyte complex[a]	Source of complement[b]	Binds to plasma membrane receptor type		
		Fc	CRI (b)[c]	CRII (d)
E(IgG)		+	−	−
E(IgM)		−	−	−
E(IgM)C(3b)	C5-deficient mouse serum, 10 min 37°C	−	+	+
E(IgM)C(3d)	C5-deficient mouse serum, 60 min 37°C	−	−	+
E(IgM)C14	Partially purified[d]	−	+	−
E(IgM)C1423b	Partially purified[d]	−	+	+
E(IgM)C1423d	Partially purified, followed by source of C3b inactivator[e]	−	−	+

[a]Sheep erythrocytes coated with IgM or IgG fraction of rabbit antibodies, as described in Section 2.
[b]Complement preparations are described in Section 2. When the time of incubation is not specified, it is 30 min at 37°C.
[c]See footnote a in Table 1.
[d]Human or guinea pig.
[e]Heat-inactivated serum or purified preparation (see Section 2).

TABLE 3
Fate of Erythrocyte Complexes Added to Unstimulated or Activated[a] Mouse Peritoneal Macrophages

Erythrocyte complex	Fate of complexes on macrophages	
	Unstimulated	Activated
E(IgG)	Ingestion (1000–2000)[b]	Ingestion (2000–3000)
E(IgM)C	Attachment (500–2000)	Ingestion (200–1000)
E or E(IgM)	No interaction	No interaction

[a]Macrophages obtained 4 days after ingestion of endotoxin or Brewer's thioglycolate medium i.p.
[b]Index, number of erythrocytes attached to or ingested by 100 macrophages.

peritoneal injection of Brewer's thioglycolate medium or endotoxin, ingest a larger number of IgG-coated erythrocytes than do resident peritoneal macrophages (6). Activated mouse peritoneal macrophages ingest E(IgM)C, while unstimulated macrophages will only bind these particles.

Ingestion of E(IgM)C is, within the limits of the assay, an all or none phenomenon. Consequently, it is the most convenient marker of macrophage activation for studies carried out at the individual cell level.

Recent studies have shown that other properties, such as pinocytic rates (16) and secretion of plasminogen activator and other proteases (17–20), also are different in the resident peritoneal cells compared to macrophages obtained after inflammatory stimuli. These are described in other sections of this book.

2. Materials

2.1. Reagents

2.1.1. Veronal-buffered saline with glucose, Ca^{2+} and Mg^{2+} (VBG): NaCl, 16.6 g; glucose, 25.0 g; Na-5,5-diethylbarbiturate, 1.02 g; H_2O, 800 ml. Adjust pH to 7.35 with 1 N HCl. Add 1 ml of a stock solution containing 1 M $MgCl_2$ and 0.15 M $CaCl_2$ in H_2O. Add 1 g of gelatin dissolved in about 10 ml of hot water and adjust final volume to 1000 ml. Keep cold to avoid contamination.

2.1.2. Hanks' balanced salt solution (Hanks') (Grand Island Biological Co., New York)

2.1.3. Dulbecco's modified Eagle's minimum essential medium (Dulbecco's MEM) (Grand Island Biological Co., New York)

2.1.4. Hypaque–Ficoll mixture: Lymphocyte Separation Medium (Bionetics, Bethesda, Maryland)

2.1.5. Glutaraldehyde 2%, used for specimen fixation. Dilute 50% stock (Fisher Scientific Co., Fair Lawn, New Jersey) in phosphate-buffered saline

2.1.6. EDTA (disodium ethylenediamine tetraacetate). Prepare 0.1 M solution in H_2O. Adjust pH to 7.35 with NaOH. This solution is isotonic.

2.1.7. Suramin (FBA Pharmaceuticals, New York, New York). Inhibits the action of the serum enzyme C3b inactivator.

2.1.8. ^{51}Cr, as sodium chromate, sterile in isotonic saline (Amersham-Searle Co., Arlington Heights, Illinois, 10 mCi/ml). The half-life of ^{51}Cr is 27.8 days.

2.2. Antisera and Serum Products 2.2.1. Antibodies to Sheep Erythrocytes. IgG and IgM fractions of rabbit antisera to sheep erythrocytes (E) can be prepared by chromatography on DEAE-cellulose followed by gel filtration on Sephadex G-200. They can also be obtained commercially from Cordis Corporation, Miami, Florida.

The antisera should be tested by hemagglutination against 0.25% E, and the lowest nonagglutinating dilution determined. Since the methods described below require a 5% E suspension, the dilution used should contain 20 times more antibody than the dilution obtained in the hemagglutination test.

Special attention should be given to the possible presence of IgG in the IgM fraction, which can be determined by passive hemagglutination of the E (IgM) with a high-titer heavy-chain specific antiserum to rabbit IgG. The commercial preparations vary and should be tested before a large batch is acquired.

2.2.2. Mouse Complement. The best source is inbred mice genetically deficient in C5 (21). Among those, the AKR/J are very convenient. Other C5-deficient mice are the A/J and the DBA/2J. Pooled serum from other inbred and outbred strains can also be used because mouse complement is generally poorly lytic at the concentration necessary for good C3 fixation. The mice are anesthetized with ether, and bled either by cutting the axillary vein or by heart puncture. Blood is collected into glass test tubes. The tubes should be stoppered to avoid drying and consequent hemolysis. After 15 min at room temperature the tubes are left in ice for 1 hr and then centrifuged at 1000 g for 15 min. The serum is collected and either used immediately or stored up to 90 days at −70°C. Freezing and thawing should be avoided.

2.2.3. Partially Purified Human and Guinea Pig Complement Components. These can be obtained from Cordis Laboratories, Miami, Florida. Each vial should be reconstituted with 5 ml of cold distilled water; the volumes mentioned in the following sections refer to these solutions. C1, C4, C2, and C3 are the components needed.

2.2.4. Source of C3b Inactivator for the Preparation of E(IgM)C3d. Human blood is allowed to clot at 37°C for 1 hr, then spun at 1000 g for 15 min. The serum is collected and heat inactivated for 30 min at 56°C; EDTA is added to a final concentration of 10 mM. The serum is then absorbed in the cold with 1/5 volume of packed E.

2.3. Cells *2.3.1. Indicator Erythrocytes (E).* Sheep erythrocytes (E) in Alsever's, less than 2 weeks old, are used as indicator erythrocytes. They are washed 3 times with large volumes of Hanks' and resuspended to a 5% packed cell volume in Hanks'. This suspension contains approximately 10^9 cells/ml. It should be prepared fresh on the day of the experiment.

For use in experiments with human leukocytes, the E 5% should be treated for 1 hr at 37°C with 1 mg of trypsin per milliliter, then washed in Hanks' containing 1 mg of soybean trypsin inhibitor per milliliter. This procedure prevents binding of E to human T cells (22).

2.3.2. Monocytes and Macrophages. The preparation of monocyte and macrophage monolayers on cover glasses is described in detail by Edelson and Cohn in Method 26.

For the detection of macrophage activation with the E(IgM)C, we have used recently explanted mouse peritoneal macrophages as well as cells cultivated for

24, 48, or 72 hr. Cells in culture show higher activity. The most consistent results are obtained after 24 hr in culture.

2.3.3. Lymphocytes. These can be obtained from any lymphoid organ by teasing, or from peripheral blood by differential flotation in Hypaque–Ficoll. Five milliliters of peripheral blood collected in heparin is diluted with 5 ml of Hanks', and carefully layered on top of 10 ml of Hypaque–Ficoll. The tube is centrifuged for 40 min at 400 *g* (measured at the interface) at 12°C. Lymphocytes and monocytes localize in the interface while erythrocytes and granulocytes are pelleted.

2.3.4. Other Cells. Methods for obtaining other cells are described elsewhere in this book.

3. Methods

3.1. Preparation of the Indicator Erthrocytes *3.1.1. (E(IgG).* Combine 1 ml E 5% + 1 ml of the appropriate dilution of IgG anti-E in Hanks'. Incubate 30 min at 37°C. Wash 3 times by centrifugation and resuspend in 10 ml of Dulbecco's for E(IgG) 0.5%.

3.1.2. E(IgM). Add 2 ml of E 5% + 2 ml dilution of IgM anti-E in Hanks'. Incubate 30 min at 37°C. Wash once. Resuspend in 2 ml of VBG; 1 ml is washed twice and resuspended to 10 ml with Dulbecco's MEM; and 1 ml is used for the preparation of E(IgM)C.

3.1.3. E(IgM)C (Prepared with Mouse Complement). Add 1 ml of E(IgM) 5% in VBG to 1 ml of AKR serum 1/5 in VBG containing 2 mg/ml Suramin. Incubate 10 min at 37°C. Add cold VBG. Wash 3 times in the cold. Resuspend the pellet in 10 ml of Dulbecco's for E(IgM)C 0.5%.

Note: E(IgM)C prepared as above contains mostly C3b and reacts with receptors type CRI and CRII. The addition of Suramin is not essential, but in its absence some C3b will be converted to C3d during the 10 min incubation period. E(IgM)C3d is prepared in the following way: The Suramin is omitted; the period of incubation extended to 30 min. This E(IgM)C should be further incubated for 30 min with mouse serum diluted 1:1 in saline, in the presence of 10 m*M* EDTA. E(IgM)C3d reacts only with receptor type CRII.

3.1.4. E(IgM)C14 (Prepared with Partially Purified Complement Components, from Human or Guinea Pig Serum). Add 1 ml of E(IgM) 5% in VBG to 1 ml Cl. Incubate 45 min in ice bath, then 5 min at 37°C. Spin in the cold, discard supernatant. Add 0.5 ml of cold VBG, 1 ml of cold C4. Incubate 30 min at 0°C. Wash 3 times in the cold. Resuspend in 10 ml of Dulbecco's MEM.

3.1.5. E(IgM)C1423b. To 1 ml of E(IgM)C14 (5%) add 1 ml of C2 + 1 ml of C3. Incubate for 45 min at 30°C. Wash twice in the cold. Resuspend in 10 ml of Dulbecco's MEM (final concentration of 0.5%).

3.1.6. E(IgM)C1423d. Add 1 ml of E(IgM)C1423 5% to 1 ml of heat-inactivated (56°C, 30 min) human or guinea pig serum 1:2 in saline containing 0.01 M EDTA. (The sera should be preabsorbed with 1/5 volume of packed E for 10 min in the cold.) Incubate for 45 min at 37°C. Wash twice. Resuspend in 10 ml of Dulbecco's MEM.

3.1.7. Chromium Labeling. In a plastic disposable tube mix: 50 μl of packed (300 g, 10 min) erythrocyte complex; 50 μl of Hanks'; 100 μCi of ^{51}Cr. Incubate 40 min at 37°C with occasional shaking. At the end of the incubation period add 1 ml of Dulbecco's MEM. Layer the suspension carefully on top of 5 ml Hypaque–Ficoll. Spin at 500 g for 15 min. Discard supernatant. Wash once in Dulbecco's MEM. Incubate 30 min at 0°C. Wash 3 times. Resuspend to 10 ml (0.5% final concentration) in Dulbecco's MEM.

3.2. Assays *3.2.1. Monolayers (Monocytes and Macrophages).* Monolayers of monocytes and macrophages are prepared on glass cover slips. The cover slips can be kept in petri dishes and should be washed vigorously by immersion in a container of fresh medium, in order to remove nonadherent cells. Erythrocyte complexes are added either to the dish or as a "bubble" directly on top of the cover slip sitting on a dry dish. A final concentration of erythrocytes between 0.2 and 0.5% should be used. Ideally, the assay should be carried out in serum-free medium. After 1 hr of incubation at 37°C, the cover slips are washed by immersion in Dulbecco's MEM and fixed with glutaraldehyde 2% for 10 min at room temperature. Before glutaraldehyde fixation, duplicate cover slips are washed for 15 sec in Hanks' diluted 1:5 in water to lyse erythrocytes external to the phagocytes. For visual examination, cover slips are mounted unstained for phase microscopy, or are stained with Giemsa. When ^{51}Cr-labeled erythrocytes are used, cover slips are counted directly in a gamma counter.

3.2.2. Cell Suspensions (Lymphocytes). Add 0.5 ml of cell suspension (2 × 10^6/ml) and 0.5 ml of the erythrocyte complex (0.5%) to 5-ml plastic test tube. Spin at 40 g for 5 min. Incubate in 37°C water bath without disturbing the pellet, and examine the sample in a counting chamber.

4. Interpretation of Data and Critical Comments

4.1. Discrimination between Binding and Ingestion of the Indicator Erythrocytes. Binding of the erythrocytes [especially E(IgM)C] to monocytes and macrophages is often so intense that it is impossible to determine by visual observation in the microscope if ingestion has occurred. The hypotonic lysis of erythrocytes bound to the surface of the leukocyte, as suggested in Section 3.2.1, is essential for accurate results. Other methods, such as NH_4Cl, have the inconvenience that the partially damaged erythrocyte may be ingested during lysis, leading to invalid results.

4.2. Attachment and Phagocytic Indices. Frequently, the most illuminating results are obtained when the percentage of leukocytes binding or ingesting erythrocytes and the number of erythrocytes bound or ingested per leukocyte are both determined. We define the index as the number of erythrocytes bound or ingested by 100 macrophages.

4.3. Controls. The Quality of Reagents. The quality of some of the reagents utilized in the above described tests is critical. Some comments about each of them follow; controls for the nonspecific attachment and ingestion of the erythrocytes should be included in each experiment.

4.3.1. Sheep Erythrocytes. Old E (more than 2 weeks in Alsever's) often bind to mouse macrophage monolayers. Erythrocyte complexes maintained in synthetic media for more than 24 hr behave similarly, even when prepared with fresh E. This is not observed with lymphocytes for which complexes prepared up to a week in advance are appropriate. For use with human lymphocytes, the E should be trypsinized.

4.3.2. Antibodies against E. Minimal contamination of IgG in the E(IgM)C preparation promotes ingestion by the mouse peritoneal macrophages. This contamination is usually insufficient to induce ingestion of the E(IgM) without complement. Ingestion of E(IgM)C by unstimulated mouse macrophages should always be considered as an indication of IgG contamination.

4.3.3. Complement. Instability of the complement activity is the most common source of problems, and batches of frozen complement should always be pretested for activity.

4.4. Visual Examination Versus Chromium Assay. The ^{51}Cr assay is very convenient when large numbers of samples have to be examined. However, the following points should be considered: (a) Erythrocytes may bind nonspecifically to cover slips. Serum pretreatment of cover slips prevents the binding. (b) The method is not sensitive when very low numbers of erythrocytes are involved. (c) The isotope requires many precautions. We strongly suggest that the initial standardization of the system be made visually.

REFERENCES

1. Bianco, C., *in* "Biological Amplification Systems in Immunity" (N. K. Day, and R. A. Good, eds.). Plenum, New York, 1976.
2. Huber, H., Polley, M. J., Linscott, W. D., Fudenberg, H. H., and Müller-Eberhard, H. J., *Science* **162**, 1281 (1968).
3. Ehlenberger, A. G., and Nussenzweig, V., *Fed. Proc,. Fed. Am. Soc. Exp. Biol.* **34**, 854 (1975).
4. Lay, W. H., and Nussenzweig, V., *J. Exp. Med.* **128**, 991 (1968).
5. Bianco, C., Griffin, F. M., and Silverstein, S. L., *J. Exp. Med.* **141**, 1278 (1975).
6. Reynolds, H. Y., Atkinson, J. P., Newball, H. H., and Frank, M. M., *J. Immunol.* **114**, 1813 (1975).
7. Ross, G. D., and Polley, M. J., *J. Exp. Med.* **141**, 1163 (1975).
8. Bianco, C., and Nussenzweig, V., *J. Exp. Med.* **132**, 702 (1970).
9. Eden, A., Miller, G. W., and Nussenzweig, V., *J. Clin. Invest.* **52**, 3239 (1973).
10. Nelson, D. S., *Adv. Immunol.* **3**, 131 (1963).

11. Anderson, C. L., and Grey, H. M., *J. Exp. Med.* **139,** 1175 (1974).
12. Rabinovitch, M., *in* "Mononuclear Phagocytes" (R. van Furth, ed.), p. 299. Philadelphia, 1970.
13. Mantovani, B., Rabinovitch, M., and Nussenzweig, V., *J. Exp. Med.* **135,** 780 (1972).
14. Ruddy, S., and Austen, K. F., *J. Immunol.* **107,** 742 (1971).
15. Griffin, F. M., Bianco, C., and Silverstein, S. C., *J. Exp. Med.* **141,** 1269 (1975).
16. Edelson, P. J., Zwiebel, R., and Cohn, Z. A., *J. Exp. Med.* **142,** 1150 (1975).
17. Unkeless, J., Gordon, S., and Reich, E., *J. Exp. Med.* **139,** 834 (1974).
18. Gordon, S., Unkeless, J. C., and Cohn, Z. A., *J. Exp. Med.* **140,** 995 (1974).
19. Werb, Z., and Gordon, S., *J. Exp. Med.* **142,** 346 (1975).
20. Werb, Z., and Gordon, S., *J. Exp. Med.* **142,** 361 (1975).
21. Cinader, B., Dubisky, S., and Wardlaw, A. C., *J. Exp. Med.* **120,** 897 (1964).
22. Weiner, M. S., Bianco, C., and Nussenzweig, V., *Blood* **42,** 939 (1973).

Activation of Macrophages in Suspension Culture

W. Hallowell Churchill, Willy F. Piessens, and John R. David

1. Introduction

Previous studies have shown that macrophages incubated *in vitro* in monolayer cultures with lymphocyte mediators become activated as shown by having enhanced phagocytosis and adhesiveness, enhanced ruffled membrane activity and motility (1), enhanced bacteriostatic and bactericidal capacity (2, 3), and enhanced cytotoxicity for tumor, but not for normal, target cells (4). However, activation of macrophages as monolayer cultures has several disadvantages. First, a 3-day activation period is required to demonstrate enhancement of some of these functions (e.g., cytotoxicity). Second, the number of macrophages remaining in the monolayers after the activation period varies from experiment to experiment. Third, because of the biological effect of lymphocyte mediators on macrophage adhesiveness, more macrophages are present in the plates incubated with active than in those incubated with control supernatants. Therefore, if results are to be expressed per cell number, numerous cultures have to be carried out in parallel so that the experimental results can be studied in one set of plates, and the number of macrophages determined by measurement of adhering protein or DNA in a parallel set of cultures.

The method described below of activating macrophages in suspension culture appears to have several advantages. First, the activation period required to demonstrate enhancement of certain functions, such as cytotoxicity, is shorter. Second, a larger number of cells can be more conveniently handled by this technique. Third, because macrophages do not have to be recovered from monolayers, multiple functions can be tested simultaneously on the same pool of cells.

Macrophages activated in suspension culture appear to be indistinguishable from macrophages activated by monolayer techniques. They have increased adhesiveness (unpublished observations), glucosamine incorporation is enhanced (5), their migration is inhibited, and their cytotoxicity for tumor targets is enhanced (6). This method of activation is currently being used to study changes in macrophage membranes associated with activation and the mechanisms by which this event takes place.

2. Materials and Equipment

2.1. Materials for Inducing Peritoneal Exudate Cells. These were described by David and David (7).

2.2. Materials for Collection of Peritoneal Exudate Cells (PEC). These were described by David and David (7).

2.3. Materials for Preparing Supernatants Rich in Lymphocyte Mediators. The materials and those for preparing partially purified fractions from these supernatants were described by Remold et al. (8).

2.4. Materials for Activating Macrophages in Suspension Culture

    a. Spinner flasks, 50 ml size (Catalogue No. 1969-00050 or 25 ml size (Catalogue No. 1960-00025), both from Bellco Glass Inc., Vineland, New Jersey)

    b. Magnetic stirrer plates: Bell-Stir Multi-Stir 4-position magnetic stirrer (Catalogue No. 7760-06005, from Bellco Glass Inc, Vineland, New Jersey)

    c. Minimal essential medium, Eagle (MEM) (Catalogue No. 109; from Grand Island Biological Co., GIBCO, Grand Island, New York)

    d. Fetal calf serum, stored frozen

    e. Antibiotic–antimycotic mixture (100X), containing penicillin (10,000 U/ml), fungisone (25 μg/ml), and streptomycin (10,000 μg/ml) (Catalogue No. 524, GIBCO)

    f. L-Glutamine solution (200 mm) (Catalogue No. 503, GIBCO)

    g. Sodium bicarbonate solution (7.5%, Lot No. 508, GIBCO)

2.5. Materials for Preparing Supplementatry Macrophage Food Solution

    a. MEM containing 1% antibiotic–antimycotic solution

    b. MEM amino acids (50X) (GIBCO, Catalogue No. 113)

    c. Dextrose, 2.5 M

    d. Fetal calf serum

    e. NaOH, 1 N

    f. L-Glutamine

Mix 163 ml of (a), 2.80 ml of (b), 0.63 ml of (c), and 9 ml of (d). Adjust the pH of the mixture to 7.3 with (e), Millipore filter, and incubate for 24 hr to check sterility. Add 1.43 ml of (f) prior to use.

2.6. Other Materials

    a. Detergent for tissue culture glassware, 7X (Linbro Chemicals, Hamden, Conn.)

    b. Millipore filters (0.45 μm pore size) (Catalogue No. HAWPO2500, Millipore Corp., Bedford, Massachusetts)

3. Methods

3.1. Preparation and Sterilization of Materials. All glassware is cleaned in a detergent made for tissue culture glassware (such as 7X, Linbro Chemicals), after which it is thoroughly rinsed with distilled water. Glassware and pipettes are sterilized by dry heat (175°C for 4 hr) or by steam autoclave. Mineral oil and 1% casein can be autoclaved. The antigen preparation, lymphocyte supernatants and other solutions which cannot be autoclaved, can be sterilized by filtration through Millipore filters. The filters are washed with 20 ml of normal saline prior to use to remove traces of detergent.

3.2. Harvest of Peritoneal Exudate Cells. The following procedure is a modification of a method previously described by David and David (7). Peritoneal exudates are induced by intraperitoneal injection of either 30 ml of light mineral oil or 20–25 ml of 1% casein and collected after 72 hr (oil) or 96 hr (casein). Starving the animals the night before the exudates are harvested will decrease the risk of perforating a viscus during the collection procedure. Guinea pigs anesthetized by CO_2 or ether are sacrificed by exsanguination from cardiac puncture. The abdomen is shaved, then the peritoneal surface is exposed by a midline skin incision. Hanks' balanced salt solution (HBSS), 150–200 ml, is injected intraperitoneally, and the fluid containing the exudate cells is then drained via a trocar and a polyethylene tube into a 250-ml centrifuge bottle.

Spin the bottles at 5°C at 450 g for 12 min (1300 rpm in a PR2 No. 259 head). Aspirate the supernatant by vacuum, then resuspend the peritoneal exudate cells and transfer the exudates from each bottle to a 12-ml centrifuge tube and wash once with HBSS by spinning for 5 min at 5°C at 250 g (900 rpm, No. 253 head in a PR2). Inspect the cell pellets, discard any that appear contaminated, and pool the remaining cells. The cell pool is washed once more, resuspended in tissue culture medium (MEM containing 20% fetal calf serum, 1% L-glutamine, and 1% antibiotic mixture), and then counted.

3.3. Preparation of Mediator-Rich Supernatants. The method by which mediator-rich or control supernatants can be obtained from cultures of lymphocytes stimulated with either antigen or concanavalin A (Con A) has been described by Remold et al. (8, 9). At 2–3 weeks after sensitization, draining lymph nodes are removed from guinea pigs and teased into a single cell suspension. One-half of the lymphocytes thus obtained are incubated with antigen or Con A as previously described. The cell-free supernatant from the antigen or Con A-stimulated culture will be referred to as mediator-rich supernatant. The supernatant from the other half of the lymphocytes, cultured without antigen, will be referred to as the control supernatant. Antigen or Con A is added to the control supernatant immediately after the cells have been removed by centrifugation.

The supernatants are dialyzed against 5 volumes of MEM for 12 hr and then kept at 4°C until used. Fractions free of antigen or Con A are prepared by Sephadex G-100 chromatography as described by Remold et al. (9).

3.4. Preparation of Suspension Cultures of Peritoneal Exudate Cells (PEC). Bellco spinner flasks are filled with either mediator-rich or control supernatants made to contain 20% fetal calf serum, 1% L-glutamine, and 1% antibiotics. PEC are then added to a final concentration of 4.0 million/ml. The side arms of the flasks are either cotton plugged or loosely capped. The suspension flasks are placed on a magnetic stirrer in a CO_2 incubator. The stirrer is adjusted to turn at the minimum possible speed (about 60 rpm). Cells can be removed via the sidearms to study macrophage functions after variable periods of activation. To minimize the possible effects of variable utilization of nutrients, the cultures are supplemented with macrophage food, after each 24-hr incubation period (the volume added being 1/10 of the volume remaining in the spinner flask at that time). If necessary, the pH of the suspension fluid is adjusted to 7.4 with isotonic $NaHCO_3$ after 24- and 48-hr incubation.

4. Interpretation of Data and Critical Comments

4.1. Evidence of Macrophage Activation. Evidence of macrophage activation in suspension culture has been obtained by the following assays: enhancement of cellular adhesiveness to culture vessels, enhancement of glucosamine incorporation, inhibition of migration and enhancement of macrophage-mediated tumor cytotoxicity (1, 5, 6).

4.2. Yield of Cells. The number of cells that can be recovered from the spinner cultures decreases with increasing periods of incubation. Under optimal conditions recovery at 24 hr is about 75%, at 48 hr 53%, and at 72 hr 30% of the initial cell concentration. At any given time the recoveries of activated and control PEC are similar. Cell recovery may drop if the volume in the spinner flask is too small or if, because of shifts in rotor speed resulting from fluctuating electrical current, the stirring bar either stops or stirs too fast. Each size spinner flask has optimal conditions that have to be determined empirically. For example, with the 50-ml flask, optimal volume is about 30 ml, but experiments can be done in a 20-ml volume. With the 30-ml spinner flask, optimal volume is 20 ml, but experiments can be done with as little as 12 ml.

4.3. Cell Viability. Viability is routinely greater than 90% after 24- and 48-hr culture.

4.4. Optimum Dose of Mediators. Depending on the method of preparing the lymphocyte-rich supernatant, it may be necessary to adjust the concentration of the mediator in the activating supernatants. Fractions from supernatants prepared from Con A-stimulated lymphocytes are more potent than fractions from antigen-stimulated lymphocytes.

4.5. Attempts to Conserve Materials by Decreasing the Volume of the Suspension Cultures. The methods as described require rather large quantities of lymphocyte mediators and macrophages. We are evaluating the possibility of conserving materials by the use of standard glass culture tubes (size 1.6 mm inside diameter) and a Model MS-7 Tri-R microsubmersible magnetic stirrer

(Tri-R Instrument, Rockville Center, Maryland). Our preliminary studies suggest that such a culture system may work with 5–10 ml of culture media containing lymphocyte mediators. The optimal conditions in this system remain to be determined.

REFERENCES

1. Nathan, C. F., Karnovsky, M. L., and David, J. R., *J. Exp. Med.* **133**, 1356 (1971).
2. Fowles, R. E., Fajardo, I. M., Leibowitch, J. L., and David, J. R., *J. Exp. Med.* **138**, 952 (1973).
3. Leibowitch, J. L., and David, J. R., *Ann. Immunol. Inst. Pasteur* **124c**, 441 (1973).
4. Piessens, W. F., Churchill, W. H., Jr., and David, J. R., *J. Immunol.* **114**, 293 (1975).
5. Sober, S. J., Haynie, M., Inman, F. P., and David, J. R., *Fed. Proc., Fed. Am. Soc. Exp. Biol., Abstr.* **35**, 489 (1976).
6. Churchill, W. H., Jr., Piessens, W. F., Sulis, C. A., and David, J. R., *J. Immunol.* **115**, 781 (1975).
7. David, J. R., and David, R. A., *in* "*In Vitro* Methods in Cell-Mediated Immunity," (B. Bloom and P. Glade, eds.), p. 249. Academic Press, New York, 1970.
8. Remold, H. G., Katz, A., Haber, E., and David, J. R., *Cell. Immunol.* **1**, 133 (1970).
9. Remold, H. G., David, R. A., and David, J. R., *J. Immunol.* **109**, 578 (1972).

The ^{51}Cr Release Assay as Used for
the Quantitative Measurement of Cell-Mediated Cytolysis *in Vitro*

K. Theodor Brunner, Howard D. Engers, and Jean-Charles Cerottini

1. Introduction

The ^{51}Cr release assay is based on the observation that the radioactive chromate (^{51}Cr$_2$O$_4{}^{2-}$) ion, following diffusion through the cell membrane is retained in the cytoplasm for a relatively extended period of time. Thus ^{51}Cr release from a labeled target cell into the supernatant fluid does not occur unless the cell membrane is sufficiently damaged to allow the efflux of intracellular molecules. While little is known concerning the biochemical properties of the isotopically labeled material that is released, it has been shown that such material is not subsequently reincorporated into undamaged cells. Since direct target cell lysis is the only parameter measured, the cells involved in mediating this process may be referred to as cytolytic effector cells.

The ^{51}Cr release assay system represents a simple, rapid, and quantitative means of testing for cell-mediated cytolysis (CMC), and has been useful in the detection of cytolytic activities of the different effector cell types involved in CMC model systems [see Ref. (1) for review]. These include target cell lysis by (a) cytolytic T lymphocytes (CTL); (b) lymphoid-like K cells, monocytes, or polymorphonuclear cells (all requiring the presence of IgG antibody); (c) activated macrophages, and (d) undefined lymphoid cells responsible for "natural" CMC.

Although the test cannot be used to detect effector cell activity at the single cell level, its use under appropriate conditions does allow an empirical estimation of the relative effector cell frequency in different populations. This quantitative aspect has been particularly useful for studies concerning (a) the generation and differentiation of CTL, (b) the relative number of human peripheral blood K cells detected in both normal individuals and patients, and (c) the molecular mechanism of CMC.

The application of the assay is limited by the availability of appropriate target cells, i.e., target cells that exhibit a relatively low spontaneous isotope release. In general, long-term assays are not feasible, although 24-hr incubation periods have been used successfully in selected systems. Another limitation is the relatively large number of target cells required. With the specific activity of ^{51}Cr currently available, up to 10^4 labeled target cells per tube are often required to obtain a measurable reaction.

The following sections describe one specific application of this technique, namely the detection and quantitation of CTL activities in murine model systems of allograft and tumor immunity.

2. Materials and Equipment

2.1. Materials

1. Dulbecco's modified Eagle's medium (DMEM) (virtually any minimal essential medium is adequate).
2. Fetal bovine serum (FBS), heat inactivated at 56°C for 45 min (Flow Laboratories, Irvine, Scotland)
3. TD buffer: Tris-phosphate buffer; 8 g of NaCl, 0.38 g of KCl, 3 g of Tris, 0.1 g of anhydrous Na_2HPO_4 in 1 liter of distilled H_2O, adjusted to pH 7.4 with HCl
4. Na_2 $^{51}CrO_4$, sterile, pyrogen free, 1 mCi/ml, with a minimum specific activity of 200 mCi of Cr per milligram (EIR, Würenlingen, Switzerland)
5. Plastic or glass, flat or round-bottomed disposable assay tubes (10X 55 mm) U- or V-bottomed plastic microplates may also be used.
6. HEPES buffer solution, 1 M in DMEM, pH 7.2 (N-hydroxyethylpiperzine-N-2-ethanesulfonic acid; Calbiochem, San Diego, California)
7. Phosphate-buffered saline (PBS), pH 7.2
8. Automatic pipettes
9. Hemocytometer or other means of determining cell numbers (such as Coulter counter)

2.2. Equipment

1. CO_2 incubator or a gas-tight box that can be gassed, sealed, and placed in a conventional 37°C incubator
2. Centrifuge
3. Gamma counter (for enhanced sensitivity, a liquid scintilation counter can be used)

3. Methods

3.1. Target Cells. Many different cell types have been successfully used as target cells in the ^{51}Cr release test. However, considerable variations in sensitivity to lysis are encountered, ranging from highly sensitive lymphoid tumor cells (maintained in ascitic form or as cultured cell lines), lymphoblast cell lines, mitogen-induced lymphoblasts, and macrophages, to less sensitive cells like lymphocytes and a variety of malignant or normal, freshly isolated, short- or long-term cultured cells, such as fibroblasts and nonlymphoid tumor cells. Generally, nonadherent cells are more sensitive to lysis than glass (or plastic) adherent cells. Target cells frequently used in the mouse are lymphoma or mastocytoma cells kept in logarithmic growth phase in suspension cultures or serially passaged in ascitic form in the syngeneic strain. Cell cultures serving as a source for target cells are usually maintained in DMEM or medium RPMI-1640 supplemented with 10% FCS.

3.2. Source of CTL. Cells from the spleen, lymph nodes, peritoneal cavity, peripheral blood, or thoracic duct of mice injected with allogeneic cells may be used as a source of CTL. To induce strong CTL responses, recipient mice may be injected intraperitoneally with 30×10^6 viable ascites tumor cells, and the spleen or peritoneal cells harvested 10–12 days later. Increased CTL activities are observed when phagocytic and/or adherent cells are removed from the immune peritoneal cell populations. CTL may also be obtained by transfer of lymphoid cells into lethally irradiated allogeneic recipients. Usually, 50×10^6 spleen, lymph node, or thymus cells are injected intravenously, and the transferred cells present in the recipient's spleen are harvest 4 days later. Augmented CTL activities may be generated *in vitro* in allogeneic mixed lymphocyte cultures (MLC) or in syngeneic mixed lymphocyte-tumor cell cultures (MLTC) (see Method 69).

3.3. ^{51}Cr Labeling of Target Cells

3.3.1. Nonadherent Target Cells. Target cells maintained as suspension cultures or in ascitic form, or mitogen-induced lymphoblasts, are washed once with culture medium, and the supernatant is aspirated to leave 0.1–0.2 ml of medium. Add to this pellet 0.2 ml of TD buffer–5% FBS. Then, add 0.1 ml Na$_2$^{51}CrO$_4$ solution (1 mCi/ml; specific activity 200 or more mCi/mg) per 2×10^6 target cells and incubate at 37°C for 30–45 min with occasional gentle shaking. The labeled cells are then washed 3 times with assay medium containing 5–10% FCS–10 mM HEPES, with an absolute minimum of pipetting, and finally adjusted to 50,000 viable cells per milliliter.

3.3.2. Adherent Target Cells. Cell cultures grown as monolayers in Falcon 3013 (or equivalent) tissue culture flasks (2 to 5×10^6 cells/flask) are washed once with fresh medium. Two milliliters of culture medium containing 0.2 ml of Na$_2$^{51}CrO$_4$ (1 mCi/ml, specific activity 200 mCi/mg or more) are then added per flask, and the cultures are incubated at 37°C for 1–2 hr. The cells are then trypsinized, washed twice, distributed into flat-bottomed tissue culture tubes (10 $\times$ 60 mm) or Falcon 3040 (or equivalent) microtest plates (5×10^3 cells per tube or well), and incubated for 4–24 hr before use.

Cells cultured as monolayers may also be first trypsinized and then labeled in suspension as described in section 3.3.1. Similarly, ^{51}Cr-labeled macrophages, peritoneal (exudate) cells or Ficoll-purified peripheral blood leukocytes may be labeled in suspension and dispensed into flat-bottomed tubes or microplates; the nonadherent cells are removed by washing after 2 to 24 hr of incubation.

3.4. Assay Procedure

3.4.1. Nonadherent Target Cells. Aliquots of the ^{51}Cr-labeled target cell suspension containing 10^4 cells are pipetted in 0.2-ml volumes into round-bottomed plastic tubes (12×55 mm) or in 0.1-ml volumes into microtiter MR24 (or equivalent) U-bottomed microplates. Equal volumes of various dilutions of suspensions of effector cells generated *in vivo* or *in vitro* are then added to the target cells to yield ratios of lymphocytes to target cells of 100, 30, 10, 3, and 1. For short-term (e.g., 3 hr) assays, the tubes or plates may be centrifuged at 200 g for 60 sec before incubation at 37°C in a CO_2 incubator, (tubes may be gassed with 5% CO_2 in air, stoppered, and incubated in a water bath or ordinary incubator). After the chosen incubation period (generally 3 hr), 0.6-ml volumes of PBS are added to the tubes, and 0.5-ml volumes of the supernatant fluid are collected for counting after centrifugation of the tubes at 600 g for 5 min. Samples of supernatant fluid (100 μl) from microplate wells are removed directly by automatic pipette. Released ^{51}Cr is determined in a well-type gamma counter (it should be noted that ^{51}Cr can also be estimated using liquid scintillation counting techniques, which yield up to a 5-fold enhancement in counting efficiency over standard gamma counting values) [see Ref. (2) for details]. For a standard 3-hr test, spontaneous release values (target cells incubated without effector cells) range from 5 to 15%, with maximal lysis in the order of 75–90% of the total isotope incorporated. Maximal release using the tube method is defined either by freeze-thawing 3 times (0.2 ml of target cells + 1.8 ml of H_2O) or the plateau value observed at an excess of effector cells, whichever is higher. Maximal release from target cells placed in microplate wells is determined by adding a given volume of detergent (for instance, 0.5% NP 40) and removing a sample for counting after 1 hr of incubation.

3.4.2. Adherent Target Cells. The prelabeled target cells incubated in flat-bottomed tubes or microplate wells are carefully washed twice by aspirating the fluid with an automatic pipette or by tilting and shaking the tubes or plates followed by addition of fresh culture medium. After removal of the medium, 0.1–0.2-ml volumes of various dilutions of suspensions of effector cells generated *in vivo* or *in vitro* are then added to the target cells, usually at lymphocyte to target cell ratios of 100, 30, 10, 3 and 1. For short-term assays (3 hr), the tubes or plates may be centrifuged at 200 g for 60 sec before incubation at 37°C in a CO_2 incubator (tubes may be gassed with 5% CO_2, stoppered, and incubated in a water bath or ordinary incubator). After the chosen incubation period, 0.1–0.2 ml volumes of the supernatant fluid are removed by automatic pipette for counting in a well-type gamma counter. Maximal release from control target cells incubated without effector cells is determined as described in Section

3.4.1. For certain systems, it may be necessary to count both the supernatants and the cell pellets to obtain an accurate measurement of total ^{51}Cr activity present per individual assay tube or well.

3.4.3. "Direct Assay" with Adherent Target Cells. Instead of first preparing target monolayers by preincubating labeled adherent cells in flat-bottomed tubes or microplate wells and then adding effector cells, as described in Section 3.4.2., adherent target cells may also be trypsinized, labeled, and then mixed directly with effector cells in round-bottomed tubes or microplate wells. Such a direct assay is of course more efficient and less variable, since the number of target cells per tube or well is constant. In some systems, sensitivity to lysis of such freshly trypsinized target cells is in fact found to be similar to the one of preincubated monolayers, and spontaneous release of label is not increased.

3.5. Quantitation of Results. The percentage of specific lysis is calculated for each lymphocyte to target cell ratio tested using the formula

$$\frac{\text{experimental }^{51}\text{Cr release} - \text{spontaneous release}}{\text{maximal release} - \text{spontaneous release}} \times 100$$

where spontaneous release is determined with or without normal lymphocytes present, and experimental release is that seen in the presence of immune lymphocytes. Maximal release is the plateau value observed in the presence of an excess of immune lymphocytes or the value observed after either freeze-thawing or detergent treatment of control target cells.

The specific ^{51}Cr release values thus obtained are then plotted versus the $\log_{10}$ of the lymphocyte-to-target cell ratio using semilog graph paper [see Ref. (1) for details]. A curve linear between 20 and 80% lysis is usually observed, with a lytic unit (LU) arbitrarily defined as that number of lymphocytes required to yield 50% lysis of the given number of target cells in the chosen incubation time. Using this value, one can then calculate the number of LU present in 10^6 cells or per culture and/or organ tested. As proposed by several authors, quantitative results can also be obtained by using modifications of the standard ^{51}Cr release assay (3, 4).

4. Comments

There are several critical comments that should be made concerning the ^{51}Cr release assay when used as a measure of cell-mediated cytolysis. (a) The use of 5% FBS–TD buffer to ^{51}Cr label the target cells appear to permit a more rapid, increased ^{51}Cr uptake as compared to a conventional tissue culture medium. (b) It should be stressed that labeled cells are generally more fragile than normal cells, and they should be manipulated as gently as possible (e.g., it may be advantageous to use centrifugation through a 50–100% FBS step gradient to wash the cells instead of repeated centrifugations). (c) The geometry of the assay tube (or microplate well) is important. While round-bottomed tubes or wells appear to be optimal, overcrowding conditions with increased effector cell numbers are reached earlier than in the flat-bottomed tubes originally described. Adequate cell-to-cell contact may also be assured by rocking of flat-bottomed culture tubes or vessels. V-bottomed microplates may yield higher cytotoxic values than U-bottomed microplates under conditions where cell-to-cell interaction is limited by low target cell numbers. (d) Target cells are generally considered satisfactory for the ^{51}Cr release assay if they incorporate between 0.1 and 1 cpm per cell (hence permitting the routine use of between 1,000 and 10,000 target cells per individual assay). In addition, they should exhibit a spontaneous release value of less than 20% over the desired test interval, generally 3–6 hr (certain target cells that can be utilized for such short-term assays are frequently unsuitable for overnight assays). (e) Generally, control spontaneous release tubes should contain only target cells and assay medium (DMEM–5% FBS–10 mM HEPES), and usually they yield results identical to those tubes where normal lymphoid cells have been included. However, in some systems at relatively high lymphocyte-to-target cell ratios, nonimmune cell populations can yield reduced or enhanced spontaneous release values, presumably owing to a protective effect or "natural" CMC activity, respectively. The method given above for the calculation of specific cytolysis would appear to be the most adequate for short-term assay conditions, where the spontaneous release rate should be less than 20%. However, as discussed by Berke and Amos (5), in those systems where spontaneous release values are exceedingly high (greater than 30%, for example), it may be more appropriate (in order to avoid overcompensating for the high background values) to use the formula

$$\frac{\text{experimental release} - \text{spontaneous release}}{\text{total incorporation}} \times 100$$

or simply

$$\frac{\text{experimental } or \text{ spontaneous release}}{\text{total incorporation}} \times 100$$

For undefined systems, it is recommended that the actual experimental values be presented.

REFERENCES

1. Cerottini, J.-C., and Brunner, K. T., *Adv. Immunol.* **18,** 67 (1974).
2. Herscowitz, H. B., and McKillip, T. B., *J. Immunol. Methods* **4,** 253 (1974).
3. Dunkley, M., Miller, R. G., and Shortman, K. J., *Immunol. Methods* **6,** 39 (1974).
4. MacDonald, H. R., *Eur. J. Immunol.* **5,** 251 (1975).
5. Berke, G., and Amos, D. B., *Transplant. Rev.* **17,** 71 (1973).

Measurement of the Efflux of ^{86}Rb and ^{14}C-Nicotinamide from Target Cells during Cell-Mediated Cytolysis: An Early Index of Membrane Permeability Changes

Christopher S. Henney

1. Introduction

Early attempts at quantitating the lymphocyte-mediated destruction of target cells was hampered by the subjectivity of assessing cell death by morphological criteria and by the possible replication of target cells in the assay system. Both these shortcomings were overcome by the innovative procedure of incorporating radioisotopically labeled markers into the target cell. The variety of markers employed to data has been impressive, but ^{51}Cr-labeled sodium chromate, first used in this context by Brunner *et al.* (1) has received by far the widest employment. Cells incubated with ^{51}Cr-labeled sodium chromate in physiological solution readily incorporate the radioisotope, and, in the absence of membrane injury, most cell types yield it sparingly. The efflux of ^{51}Cr from lymphocyte-damaged cells correlates well with cytolysis as assessed by inclusion of vital dye (1, 2).

isotope was released in a macromolecular form, associated with peptides and/or protein (3). Furthermore, using labels of various molecular sizes, it was found that the rate of marker release from lymphocyte-damaged cells was an inverse function of the size of the marker. These observations imply that lymphocytes induce discrete "holes," which initially allow ions, but not macromolecules, to leak out. These findings suggested that the great proportion of time expended in ^{51}Cr release assays is used, not in the insertion of a lesion in the target cell, but in the subsequent leakage of macromolecular ^{51}Cr. It was thus reasoned that markers which did not become associated with constituents of high molecular weight might provide a more rapid index of membrane permeability changes in a damaged target cell. Additionally, it is conceivable that markers of low molecular weight might detect lesions inserted by the effector lymphocyte which never "progress" to a size that allows passage of macromolecules. Among such lesions might be those repaired by the metabolic activities of the target cell.

It is against this background that studies on the efflux of low-molecular-weight markers from target cells during cell-mediated cytolysis have been pursued. The practicality of two such labels, ^{86}Rb, an analog of K, and ^{14}C-nicotinamide, has been established (3, 4); their use in a T cell-mediated lytic system will be described here.

The assay to be described is one of general applicability. Its principal impact lies in its ability to detect membrane permeability changes in a target cell population (and thus the cytotoxic action of lymphoid cells) over a very short time framework (10–40 min).

2. Materials and Methods

2.1. Medium. The medium in which effector and target cells were prepared, and in which the lytic assays were carried out, was minimal essential Eagle's medium with Earle's salts (Microbiological Associates, Bethesda, Maryland) containing 2 mM glutamine, 100 U of penicillin and 100 μg of streptomycin per milliliter, and 10% heat-inactivated (56°C, 40 min) fetal calf serum (Microbiological Associates). This medium is referred to in the text as MES.

Comments: The only essential features of the medium in short-term ($<$ 2 hr) assays are divalent cations and a pH of approximately 7.4. Ca^{2+} are absolutely required for cytolysis, and a synergistic effect is noted when Mg^{2+} are added (5). Approximately 1 mM concentrations of each cation are optimal. Serum is not required, although its presence does reduce the rate of spontaneous efflux of isotopic markers. The medium used here is one that supports cytolysis in the longer-term assays that are necessary when ^{51}Cr or ^{3}H-thymidine are used as target cell labels.

2.2. Effector Cells. Spleens were removed aseptically from adult C57BL/6 mice (Jackson Laboratories, Bar Harbor, Maine) 10–12 days after intraperitoneal immunization with 10^7 P815-X2 mastocytoma cells in serum-free medium. Single-cell suspensions were made by pressing small pieces of the spleen through a stainless stell mesh (size 60, wire diameter 0.0075 inch; L. E. Jones, Inc., Baltimore, Maryland). The cell suspension was centrifuged (300 g, 5 min, International Centrifuge Model PRJ), and the cell pellet was resuspended in MES and centrifuged at 200 g for 15 sec. The splenic capsule and cell debris pelleted under these conditions were discarded and the supernatant was recentrifuged (300 g, 5 min). The resulting cell pellet was washed 3 additional times. The number of viable lymphocytes in the cell suspension (usually of the order of 10^8/spleen) was calculated by vital dye exclusion criteria (erythrocin B).

Spleen cells from unimmunized C57BL/6 mice were prepared in exactly the same manner as controls.

Comments: Although for reasons of convenience spleen cells are often taken as an effector cell source, other lymphoid cell populations can be used. Peritoneal exudate populations, for example, often have a higher cytolytic activity per cell, particularly when immunization is by the intraperitoneal route.

2.3. Target Cells. P815-X2 mastocytoma cells of the DBA/2 strain were carried in ascitic form in adult male mice by weekly intraperitoneal passage of 10^7 cells. Ascitic fluid, 5–7 days after passage of 10^7 cells, was harvested into a syringe containing 100 units of heparin (Abbott Laboratories, North Chicago, Illinois). The cells were washed once (300 g, 5 min) in serum-free Eagle's medium and were than resuspended at a viable cell concentration of 3×10^7 cells/ml in MES.

2.3.1. Incorporation of [86]Rb. [86]Rb was purchased from New England Nuclear (Boston, Massachusetts) as [86]RbCl containing 10 mg of Rb per milliliter in 0.5 M HCl (specific activity approximately 2 mCi/mg). This preparation was neutralized by the addition of an approximately equal volume of 0.5 M NaOH, and was then diluted with Tris-buffered saline, pH 7.4, to give total solids of 0.4 mg Rb/ml.

To 10^7 P815 cells in 0.3 ml of MES was added 100 μCi of ^{86}Rb, and the cell suspension was incubated at 37°C for 45 min. The cells were then washed (300 g, 5 min) 4 times using a 30-fold excess of MES on each occasion, and suspended to a concentration of 10^6 viable cells/ml in MES. Cells prepared in this manner gave 2000–4000 cpm/10^5 cells.

Comments: (a) The incorporated ^{86}Rb in MES (as cpm per cell) was found to be a linear function of isotope added (over the range 10–200 μCi), and time of incubation (10–120 min). As ^{86}Rb is an analog of K, total cellular uptake is a function of the sum of extracellular K and Rb. (b) ^{86}Rb is not readily available commercially in a carrier-free form. (c) In measurements of cell-mediated cytotoxicity, ^{86}Rb has some obvious advantages over its K isotope analogs, the most obvious of which is its relatively long half-life ($T_{1/2}$ = 18.7 days) compared with [42]K ($T_{1/2}$ = 12.4 hr).

2.3.2. Incorporation of [^{14}C]-Nicotinamide. The labeling of P815 cells with [^{14}C]-nicotinamide was accomplished by culturing 10^7 P815 cells in 10 ml of MES in an atmosphere of 5% CO_2–95% air at 37°C. Cultures were established for 16–24 hr in a 10-cm diameter polystyrene petri dish (Falcon Plastics, Oxnard, California) (4) or in a 16 $\times$ 125 mm plastic tube (Falcon Plastics), in the presence of 50 μCi [carbonyl-^{14}C]nicotinamide (Amersham Searle Corp., Arlington Heights, Illinois) from a stock solution containing 60 Ci/ml in Tris-buffered saline pH 7.4. The cells were then washed (300 g, 5 min) 3 times in MES and adjusted to a viable cell concentration of 10^6 cells/ml in MES. Cells prepared in this manner yielded 5000–7000 cpm per 10^5 cells after three cylces of freeze-thawing.

Comments. Predictably, the degree of isotope incorporation per cell was found to be a function of cell concentration, time of culture (over a period 2–30 hr), and of exogeneous nicotinamide concentrations. The conditions chosen are those empirically arrived at by Martz *et al.* (4) to be suitable for P815 target cells.

2.4. Cytotoxic Assay. Cytotoxic assays were routinely carried out in 12 X 75 mm plastic tubes (Falcon Plastics) in a reaction volume of 1 ml of MES. Serial dilutions of lymphoid cells from either immune or normal donors were added to 10^5 isotopically labeled target cells to give lymphocyte:target cell multiplicities ranging from 100:1 to 1:1. The cell suspensions were mixed by gentle agitation and the tubes than centrifuged (300 g, 1 min) before incubating at 37°C in an atmosphere of 5% CO_2–95% air for periods of time up to 90 min. At the termination of culture, the tubes were centrifuged (300 g, 5 min) and 0.5-ml aliquot of cell-free supernatant was removed, using an automatic pipette (Selectapette, Schwarz-Mann Co., Orangeburg, N.Y.); the isotopic content was assessed by γ-(^{86}Rb) or β-(^{14}C-nicotinamide) scintillation counting.

Comments: (a) The volume of the assay is unimportant. Indeed, ^{86}Rb and ^{14}C-nicotinamide release assays can be conveniently carried out in microcytotoxicity plates (Dynatech Laboratories, Inc., Division of Cooke Engineering, Alexandria, Virginia) using a total reaction volume of 200 μl of MES (6). In this case 10^4 target cells are commonly used together with the same multiplicity of lymphocytes as employed in the tube assay. The reaction volume sampled at the termination of the culture is usually 100 μl. The feature limiting the minimal number of target cells that can be employed is the amount of isotope incorporated. For both α- and β-emitting isotopes, there should be approximately 1000 cpm/unit target cells.

(b) Brief centrifugation before culture is not essential, although it does augment the rate of lysis, presumably by decreasing the time required for cell–cell interaction.

(c) The procedure used in this laboratory to count ^{14}C-nicotinamide fluids is as follows: 0.5 ml of cell-free supernatant is added to 10 ml of a dioxane-based scintillator, such as Bray's solution (7) or Aquaflour (New England Nuclear, Boston Massachusetts).

(d) When ^{86}Rb or ^{14}C-nicotinamide flux are measured as an assessment of target cell membrane permeability changes, significant differences in isotope release between cultures containing immune lymphocytes and those containing norma lymphocytes can be seen within 10 min at 37°C (3, 4). An empirically useful time for carrying out Rb and nicotinamide flux assays with P815 target cells is 40 min; the spontaneous leakage of both labels (^{86}Rb approximately 40% per hour; ^{14}C-nicotinamide 10–15% per hour) usually precludes culture periods longer than 90 min for ^{86}Rb and 180 min for nicotinamide.

(e) The incremental flux of both ^{86}Rb and ^{14}C-nicotinamide caused by immune C57BL/6 spleen cells was totally abolished after treatment of the effector population with an antiserum against thy 1.2 alloantigens (AKR anti-C_3H thymus) in the presence of rabbit complement. Thus, in this system both ^{86}Rb and ^{14}C-nicotinamide release are measurements of a T effector cell function.

(f) If rates of ^{86}Rb (or ^{14}C-nicotinamide) flux are to be made at various times, it is essential to sample the amount of non-cell-associated label at time zero. Failure to measure time zero values will often give spuriously nonlinear flux at the early time points. No measurement at time zero is required if cultures are all to be terminated at one time and when comparisons with cultures containing normal spleen cells are made.

2.5. Evaluation of Cytotoxicity. The evaluation of target cell lysis is best discussed in relation to data generated in a typical experiment. One such experiment measuring ^{86}Rb release is shown in Table 1; the same arguments would apply to ^{14}C-nicotinamide release.

Between 10^5 and 3×10^6 immune spleen cells were incubated for 40 min with 10^5 ^{86}Rb labeled target cells. As can be seen (Table 1), the suspension of 10^5 target cells in this experiment contained 4172 cpm. After 40 min at 37°C, the percent extracellular isotope ranged from 10.9% (3×10^6 normal lymphocytes present) to 29.0% in the presence of 3×10^6 immune spleen cells.

That portion of cell death caused by immune lymphoid cells, and usually referred to as percent specific cytolysis, is calculated by different laboratories in various ways. Table 1 gives examples of the two methods most commonly employed in ^{51}Cr release assays. The simplest evaluation is made by subtracting percent isotope release in the absence of lymphocytes (or in the presence of normal lymphoid cells) from that observed in the presence of immune cells.

An alternative method, introduced by Brunner *et al.* (1) is to use the formula:

$$\frac{\% \text{ lysis with immune cells} - \% \text{ lysis with normal cells}}{\% \text{ lysis after freeze-thaw} - \% \text{ lysis with normal cells}} \times 100$$

for calculations of specific cytolysis. This equation allows that not all the cell-associated counts are available following cell lysis and chooses to equate the total isotope with that compartment released by freeze-thawing. Additionally the percent of isotope released with normal cells is subtracted both from the numerator and denominator of the equation.

Comments: (a) This laboratory prefers to record specific cytolysis simply as the difference in percent isotope release between cultures containing normal and immune spleen cells. Using this criterion for specific cytolysis and a 40-min assay period before assessment of ^{86}Rb flux, we have been able to establish a linear relationship between: (i) percent specific cytolysis and time (10, 20, 40 min) and (ii) Log target cells specifically killed and log immune lymphocytes added. A slope of 1.0 is obtained if the total number of lymphocytes in the culture is kept constant by the addition of normal spleen cells. These parameters are identical to those established in the same system using a 4-hr ^{51}Cr assay (8).

(b) Although the correction of Brunner *et al.* does not markedly affect the value of percent specific cytolysis in situations where spontaneous leak is low (as

TABLE 1

Evaluation of ^{86}Rb Release from P815 Target Cells in the Presence of Normal and Immune C57BL/6 Spleen Cells[a]

Lymphoid cell source	Lymphocyte: target cell	^{86}Rb in supernatant after 40 min (cpm)[b]	% Isotope flux, 0–40 min	% Specific cytolysis	
				$\left(\dfrac{\text{immune}}{\text{total}} - \dfrac{\text{normal}}{\text{total}}\right) \times 100$[c]	$\dfrac{(\text{immune}) - (\text{normal})}{(\text{freeze-thaw}) - (\text{normal})} \times 100$[d]
Immune[e]	30:1	1210	29.0	18.1	26.2
	10:1	990	23.8	12.9	18.6
	3:1	704	16.9	6.0	8.6
	1:1	586	14.1	3.2	4.5
Normal[e]	30:1	455	10.9		

[a] Input 10^5 target cells: 4172 cpm; cells frozen and thawed: 3338 cpm. Values given are mean counts per minute of triplicate cultures; replication was invariably <5%.

[b] As 1 ml of reaction volume was used, and only 0.5 ml of supernatant was sampled, these values are 2 times actual cpm measured.

[c] Specific cytolysis was calculated simply as the difference in percent flux between immune and normal cultures, using the total cell-associated counts added at time zero at 100%.

[d] Specific cytolysis was calculated by the method of Brunner et al. (1) as described in the text. Three cycles of freeze-thawing cells released 80% ^{86}Rb.

[e] Spleen cells from immune C57BL/6 mice were obtained 10 days after 3×10^7 P815 cells intraperitoneally. Control cultures contained spleen cells from unimmunized controls. ^{86}Rb flux in the rpesence of normal spleen cells did not vary significantly with lymphocyte number over the range of 0 to 3×10^6 lymphocytes.

is the case with P815 cells for 4-hr ^{51}Cr release), the use of their formula to evaluate lysis in ^{86}Rb assays (where spontaneous release is 40% per hour) is a controversial issue (8, 9). Clearly, the lower denominator used yields a substantially higher value for "percent specific cytolysis" than is obtained by other methods. Additionally, although there is good correlation between ^{51}Cr release and cell death (as measured either by vital dye exclusion criteria or by loss of cloning efficiency), no such relationship has been established between cell death and the flux of ^{86}Rb of ^{14}C-nicotinamide. These considerations dictate that the principal usage of this cytotoxic assay system be for evaluations of minimal membrane permeability changes in very brief reaction periods, rather than for enumerating cell lysis.

(c) There is no indication that significant reutilization of [86]Rb (or ^{14}C-nicotinamide) occurs within 90-min assay times. Thus, no corrections need be applied for uptake of previously released marker by the cells in culture.

3. Summation

The measurement of [86]Rb (or ^{14}C-nicotinamide) flux across the membrane of target cells cultured with homologous immune lymphocytes affords a sensitive, reproducible, and, above all, rapid assessment of lymphocyte cytotoxicity. There remains, moreover, the theoretical possibility that ^{86}Rb flux assays will detect target cell lesions which anneal or are too small to allow ^{51}Cr release (10, 11).

ACKNOWLEDGMENTS

Several colleagues are to be thanked for helping to develop the methodology reported here. They include J. Eric Bubbers, Marshall Plaut, and particularly Carl A. Geyer, who carried out the experiment reported in Table 1.

This work was supported by Grant AI 10280 from the National Institute of Allergy and Infectious Disease and Contract NO1-CB-43965 from the National Cancer Institute. The author is the recipient of a Research Career Development Award from the National Institute of Allergy and Infectious Disease. This is communication No. 212 from the O'Neill Memorial Research Laboratories.

REFERENCES

1. Brunner, K. T., Mauel, J., Cerottini, J.-C., and Chapuis, B., *Immunology* **14**, 181 (1968).
2. B. Bloom and P. Glade (Eds.), "*In Vitro* Methods in Cell-Mediated Immunity." Academic Press, New York, 1971.
3. Henney, C. S., *J. Immunol.* **110**, 73 (1973).
4. Martz, E., Burakoff, S., and Benacerraf, B., *Proc. Natl. Acad. Sci. U.S.A.* **71**, 177 (1974).
5. Plaut, M., Bubbers, J. E., and Henney, C. S., *J. Immunol.* **116**, 150 (1976).
6. Thorn, R., Palmer, J. C., and Manson, L. A., *J. Immunol. Methods* **4**, 301 (1974).

7. Bray, G. A., *Anal. Biochem.* **1**, 279 (1960).
8. Henney, C. S., *Transplant. Rev.* **17**, 37 (1973).
9. Stulting, R. D., and Berke, G., *Cell Immunol.* **9**, 474 (1973).
10. Henney, C. S., *Nature (London)* **249**, 456 (1974).
11. Ferluga, J., and Allison, A. C., *Nature (London)* **250**, 673 (1974).

Guidelines for the Microcytotoxicity Assay

Carol O'Toole and Edward A. Clark

Men do not stumble over mountains, but over molehills. Confucius
The falling drops at last will wear the stones. Lucretius

1. Introduction

Cellular immunity denotes an anamnestic response by lymphoid cells to specific antigens. *In vitro* such responses can be measured by specific lysis of target cells bearing the antigen(s) used for sensitization (1–4). This specific reactivity should be distinguished from nonspecific target-cell lysis such as that mediated by nonsensitized granulocytic cells, which release hydrolytic enzymes during *in vitro* incubation (5, 6).

The microcytotoxicity assay introduced by Takasugi and Klein in 1970 (7) has been widely used to detect cellular immunity in animals to alloantigens (7–9) and to virally (10–12) and chemically (13–16) induced syngeneic tumors, and in man to detect immunity to a variety of histological types of neoplasms (17–21). However, the results obtained by different investigators lack concordance in both qualitative and quantitative interpretation. As a result, whether or not this assay can be used to detect tumor-specific antigens still requires definitive proof in the majority of tumor systems so far studied. The precise methodology being employed lacks standardization (22). In addition, the patient material under study has frequently lacked adequate definition as to tumor stage, duration of the disease, and treatment the patient has received prior to being tested for cellular immunity. In these circumstances the clinical relevancy of the results obtained cannot be evaluated. The purpose of this report is to examine the steps of the microassay that might account for technical variation and to establish some guidelines for standardizing the assay system.

The methodology presented has been used to study cell mediated immunity in patients with transitional cell carcinoma of the bladder (TCC) (18). Lymphoid cell preparations from certain patients with TCC show a significant selective cytotoxicity for allogeneic target cells derived from TCC. Both short-term cultures and established cell lines from TCC can be used as target cells. The assay has been standardized by using reference cell lines as targets and by titrating the effector:target cell ratio used in every experiment. The assay is reproducible and has been used successfully to monitor patients through the clinical course of the disease. The method is also economic in the quantity of lymphoid cells required, this being particularly important when studying patients with radiotherapy-induced lymphopenia. Using the test conditions described here, the microcyto-toxicity assay has been found to have clinical relevance. The incidence of cellular immunity to TCC has been shown to relate to tumor burden, a response being detected most often in patients with localized tumor and a short disease history. The assay has prognostic value in that remaining tumor can be detected early after surgery (18).

2. Materials

2.1. Target Cells

2.1.2. Human. Primary cultures were established from explant fragments of a variety of normal and neoplastic tissues. To detect cellular immunity to TCC, several established cell lines were used as reference target cells: T24 (23), RT4 (24), and J82 derived from TCC; HCV-29 (J. Fogh, unpublished) originated from nonmalignant transitional epithelium; MEL-1 derived from metastatic cutaneous melanoma; 2T (25) from osteogenic sarcoma and Chang (26) origi-nated from normal liver. The target cells used as specificity controls for TCC are summarized in Table 1.

2.1.2. Rat. Two 3-methylcholanthrene-induced rat fibrosarcomas, LMM1 originating in Lewis strain tissue culture passage (TC 11) and FMF1 of Fisher strain origin (TC 27), were used to demonstrate *in vitro* cytotoxicity to alloanti-gens. The tumors were maintained *in vivo* by serial subcutaneous passage in syngeneic hosts. The cells tested were from *in vivo* passages 7–11.

2.2. Effector Cells

2.2.1. Human. Blood samples were obtained from patients with clinically verified TCC. The clinical evaluation of these patients included tumor stage (27), grade (28), known duration of disease, and previous therapy. Control blood samples were obtained from patients with other neoplasms or with infections or from health normal donors (Table 1).

2.2.2. Rat. Normal Lewis and Fisher rats were used as normal syngeneic donors. Lewis rats were made hyperimmune to Fisher non-Ag-B alloantigens by multiple monthly subcutaneous injections of Fisher normal or tumor cells. Fisher rats were immunized to Lewis non-Ag-B alloantigens by two monthly subcutaneous injections of 10^6 LMMI cells.

2.3. Solutions

2.3.1. Tris-Ammonium Chloride (29). 9 volumes of 0.83% NH_4Cl plus 1 volume of Tris buffer (20.59 g Tris base/liter, pH adjusted to 7.65 with HCl), final pH 7.2. Used at $4°C$.

TABLE 1
Controls Used in Microcytotoxicity Assay for Cellular Immunity to
Transitional Cell Carcinoma

Effector cell level	Target cell level
Normal healthy	Cell lines
	HCV-29, nonmalignant bladder epithelium
Chronic cystitis	Chang, normal liver
Interstitial cystitis	MEL-1, metastatic cutaneous melanoma
Urethritis	2T, osteogenic sarcoma
Carcinoma	
Breast	Primary cultures
Cervix	Bladder epithelium
Ovary	Bladder fibroblasts
Prostate	Lung fibroblasts
Melanoma, cutaneous and ocular	Carcinoma kidney
	Adenocarcinoma of rectum metastatic
	to bladder
Metastatic tumor to bladder	
from carcinoma	
Colon	
Prostate	
Adenocarcinoma of rectum	

2.3.2. Gelatin (L936). Dissolved at 37°C in Tris-buffered Hanks' solution to give 3% gelatin solution (w/v). Used at 37°C. Made by Peter Leiner and Sons, Tree Forest, Glamorgon, Wales.

2.3.3. Tissue Culture Medium. For human cells: Medium 199 with Hanks' salts containing 10 % fetal calf serum (FCS), heat inactivated at 56°C for 1 hr, antibiotics (100 IU penicillin and 100 μg streptomycin/ml), and 0.3 mg glutamine per milliliter, pH 7.2. For rat cells: Dulbecco's modified Eagle's medium containing 15% heat-inactivated FCS, 25 mM HEPES buffer, antibiotics, glutamine; pH 7.2. Media used at 37°C.

2.3.4. Tris-Buffered Hanks' Solution. one volume of Tris buffer (20.2 g of Trizma HCl, 2.65 g of Trizma base in 1 liter of distilled water) plus one volume of Hanks' balanced salt solution (BSS) used at 37°C.

2.3.5. Trypsin Solutions. For human cells: trypsin-Versene, 0.2 g EDTA dissolved in 1 liter Ca^{2+}- and Mg^{2+}-free PBS, pH 7.2, stored at 4°C. Just before use 2.5 ml of 1% trypsin (frozen stock) is added to 50 ml of buffer. For rat cells: 2.5% trypsin (GIBCO) diluted 1:10 in Ca^{2+}- and Mg^{2+}-free Hanks' BSS pH 7.2 containing 25 mM HEPES buffer, frozen in aliquots and thawed just before use.

2.3.6. May–Grünwald Stain. Solution of May-Grünwald stain (0.3 g of powdered stain in 100 ml of methanol, pure acetone-free) diluted 1:1 with methanol just before use. Preparations are stained for 10 min, washed with water for 5 min, counterstained with 5% Giemsa solution in distilled water for 5 min, rinsed with distilled water, and air dried.

2.3.7. Turks' Stain. 40 mg of gentian violet plus 12.5 ml of acetic acid in 200 ml of distilled water.

3. Protocol for Microcytotoxicity Assay (Fig. 1)

3.1. Preparation of Target Cells. The availability of established cell lines has facilitated standardization of the assay. The cells have an excellent viability and a plating efficiency ≥90%. They show a predictable doubling time in culture and can be characterized morphologically. When primary tissue culture cells are used

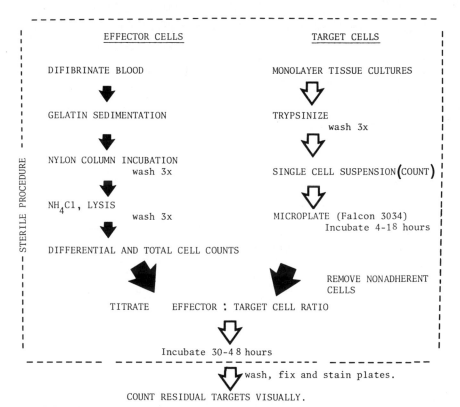

Fig. 1. Protocol for microcytotoxicity assay. Cytotoxicity is estimated as % reduction $(1-P/C) \times 100$. Where P is the mean number of surviving targets after exposure to patients' effector cells and C is the mean number of surviving targets after exposure to control effector cells.

as targets in this assay, their plating efficiency and doubling time should be evaluated before testing. The cultures should be passaged at least once to eliminate contaminating leukocytic cells. The cells are harvested from mono-layer cultures by trypsinization and washed 3 times in tissue culture medium containing 10% FCS. This is necessary to remove residual trypsin, which will decrease viability and cause poor plating efficiency. The cells are then counted in 0.05% Trypan blue solution, to assess total number and viability. Cells are dispersed into Falcon 3034 microplates (Falcon plastics, Oxnard, California) to give 50–150 cells per well. The cells can be accurately dispensed using a Hamilton Luer tip 500-μl syringe (Hamilton, Whittier, California) with an automatic dispenser attachment and attached to a 22-gauge needle. Alternatively, a tuberculin syringe with attached Yale 25-gauge needle may be used.

To dispense targets evenly, clumped cells must be removed to leave a single-cell suspension. Care should be taken to keep suspensions well mixed to avoid settling of cells prior to plating. Dispensing the cells in a volume >10 μl tends to give more even plating than smaller volumes. We have found a volume of 20 μl/well to give optimal cell attachment and survival of targets. The plates are incubated 4–18 hr at 37°C to allow cell adherence. In order to prevent posi-tional effects, i.e., slower cell growth in the outer wells of the plate, high humidity and a good buffering system are vital. HEPES buffer is recommended for obtaining a constant pH. If a bicarbonate buffer is used, care must be taken to maintain a constant 5% CO_2 level in the incubator (e.g., charging the CO_2 after each opening and closing of the incubator). It is recommended that the plates be incubated in a humidity level higher than in the normal incubator. This is most simply achieved by placing the plates in the vapor phase above a saturated sponge in a plastic box with loosely fitting cover.

After incubation the plates are inverted for 20 min under incubation condi-tions, and the medium is then gently removed. Cell attachment should be checked using a phase-contrast inverted microscope. It is important to estimate the number of attached cells at this stage so that the concentration of effector cells added can be accurately adjusted to maintain uniform effector:target cell ratios for each effector:target combination in the assay. Ideally, the number of target cells attached to each well should not exceed 100–150, otherwise visual counting tends to become laborious and counting errors can result. If fewer than 30 cells are plated, well variation may influence the significance of results.

3.2. Preparation of Effector Cells. The method for purifying human lymphoid cells has been described in detail previously (30). From each donor, 30–50 ml of defibrinated blood are obtained. This is conveniently done in a 125-ml Erlenmeyer flask containing three 2-inch steel paper clips. The de-fibrinated blood is mixed gently with a 3% gelatin solution at a ratio 3:1 (v/v) in a measuring cylinder and incubated at 37°C for 60 min. During this time the bulk of the erythrocytes sediment. The leukocyte-plasma supernatant is then removed and added to a loosely packed nylon wool column (3 g of nylon evenly packed in a 50-ml chemical separating funnel). The plasma supernatant should be distributed evenly so that no dry areas remain in the nylon wool; media containing 10% FCS should be added if necessary. The column is placed at 37°C in a humidified air +5% CO_2 for 30 min. Nonadherent cells are then eluted from the nylon wool column by washing with 50 ml of Tris-buffered Hanks' (TH) solution containing 2.5% FCS. The cells are sedimented at 700 g for 10 min; the pellet is resuspended in 40 ml of TH+2.5% FCS and centrifuged at 400 g for another 10 min. This last (washing) step is repeated twice. The cells are then resuspended in 2 ml of TH+2.5% FCS and mixed with 0.83% Tris ammonium chloride solution at a 1:8 ratio (v/v). The NH_4Cl solution should be precooled at 4°C. The mixture is kept at 4°C for a maximum period of 10 min. (Red cell lysis should be checked visually during this period.) The cell suspension is diluted 1:1 with TH + 10% FCS and centrifuged at 400 g for 10 min. The cells are then washed 3 more times in TH+2.5% FCS. The total number of mononuclear cells is estimated by counting in Turk's stain. Differential counts should be made on cytocentrifuge preparations of each donor's "purified" effector cells. These are stained with May—Grünwald—Giemsa. At least 500 cells are counted per preparation.

This method of preparing effector cells involves primarily physical separation of lymphoid cells from other cell types, with a minimum use of chemical additives. Care should be taken during the NH_4Cl lysis step, as prolonged treatment or incubation temperatures above 10°C cause membrane damage to lymphoid cells (31). We have routinely incubated effector cell preparations overnight after separation to permit recovery from handling procedures before testing in the microcytotoxicity assay. The cells are incubated at 37°C in tissue culture medium with 10% FCS at a concentration of 1×10^6 cells/ml in air + 5% CO_2.

The procedure described here for obtaining human lymphoid cells has been found superior to the use of Ficoll density separation methods (32). Lymphoid cells prepared on Ficoll were found to produce a generalized cytotoxicity on all target cell types tested. However, this was observed only with incubation periods exceeding 30 hr (33). As Ficoll is known to act as a mitogen for mouse lymphoid cells (34), its use in cytotoxicity assays involving incubation periods of 2—3 days should be critically examined.

Rat effector cells are prepared from spleens by gently teasing them apart in tissue culture medium. The cells are washed and resuspended in Tris-ammonium chloride at 4°C for 10 min. The cells are then washed thrice and viability checked by Trypan blue dye exclusion. If viability is low the cells are resuspended in low ionic strength buffer (31) to permit clumping of dead cells, followed by filtration through cotton. Adherent cells are removed by incubating the cell preparations on a column of loosely packed cotton in a 6-ml syringe barrel. (The column should be saturated in sterile distilled water and washed with tissue culture medium containing 20% FCS prior to use.) The cells are added to the column at a concentration of 10^8/ml in a 2-ml volume and incubated at 37° for 30 min in humidified air +5% CO_2. The nonadherent cells are then eluted. Nylon column purification is done according to Julius *et al.* (35). Purity of the effector cell preparations is checked on cytocentrifuge preparations as described for human lymphoid cells.

   3.3. Plating of Effector Cells. The medium is removed from the target cells, and the number of adherent cells is estimated. It is important to keep the target cells moist and maintain the pH prior to adding the effector cells. This is conveniently done by adding 10 μl of medium to each well. Each effector cell preparation should be tested at a minimum of two ratios to each target cell type in the assay. We routinely use a maximum ratio of 500:1 and doubling dilutions thereof. The number of lymphoid cells added per well must be based on the actual number of adherent targets at this stage. At least six wells should be used for each test parameter, including targets incubated with medium alone. Control effector cell preparations should be tested wherever possible on the same test plate as the tumor patients' effector cells. Optimal culture conditions are obtained with a 20-μl incubation volume per well.

   The experimental incubation time is 30–48 hr. After longer intervals the background cytotoxicity and well-to-well variation tend to rise. This may be due to *in vitro* sensitization (36) or to unfavorable culture conditions due to cell death and exhaustion of the media. At the termination of the experiments, the microplates are inverted for 20 min under incubation conditions, and then the medium is gently removed. Residual effector cells and debris are removed by flooding the plates with phosphate-buffered saline pH 7.2 and mixing gently. Removal of debris should be checked microscopically and washing repeated if necessary. The plates are then stained with May–Grünwald–Giemsa, and the residual targets are counted visually. Visual counting is facilitated by projecting the well image onto a microprojection screen attached to an inverted microscope (Reichert). A significant advantage of visual counting is that viable cells can be distinguished from nonviable cells. Accuracy in counting can be improved by dividing the well image into quadrants on the screen.

4. Interpretation of Data

   4.1. Experimental Design. To test for cellular immunity, as many effector and target cell controls as is technically possible should be used in each experiment. The controls listed in Table 1 have been used when testing effector cells from patients with TCC for specific reactivity. As normal controls have often been observed to differ in reactivity (37), it is advisable to test more than one normal donor in each experiment. The normal controls should be aged matched with the tumor patients. Ideally, clinical controls should be included in each experiment; these should be matched for stage of disease and therapy received with the tumor patient being tested for specific cellular immunity.

At the target cell level, the normal tissue component for the particular histological type of tumor should be included wherever possible. This will help to define whether reactivity observed relates to tissue type or malignancy per se. To define specificity for a particular histological tumor type, at least one target cell from an unrelated neoplastic tissue should be included. Table 2 illustrates an experiment using three types of target cells. T24 and J82 derived from transitional cell carcinoma, HCV-29 from nonmalignant transitional epithelium, and MEL-1 from cutaneous melanoma. The test included two patients with TCC and one age-matched normal control. The data on the medium control wells are presented, but are not used in the estimation of cytotoxicity. It can be seen that the numbers of residual cells for all targets are somewhat lower after incubation with the control donor's cells as compared to the medium controls. There is no evidence, however, that this effect is selective for any of the four target cells used. It is also not clear whether the effect is an actual killing of targets or is due to reduced cell division in the wells containing the normal donor's cells. The reduction caused by normal donor's cells shows a slight titration effect, greater at the higher effector cell concentration on three of the four targets.

In this experiment two types of cytotoxic activity by TCC patients' effector cells are revealed. Patient A shows a highly significant effect only on TCC targets with no effect on nonmalignant bladder epithelium or an unrelated neoplasm. It should be noted that individual A had a localized TCC at the time of test. Patient B's cells produced a generalized effect on all four targets; this patient had metastatic TCC at the time of test. These two types of cytotoxicity are clearly significant as compared to either the normal donor LA38 or to the media control. The question arises what should be used as a control base line for estimation of cytotoxicity. We feel the media control values should be presented; they are an important monitor of the viability and growth condition of the target cells, and they reflect the degree of nonselective cytotoxicity present in the assay. Increased growth of target cells in the presence of some effector cell preparations is often reported; this can result from better buffering in the presence of lymphoid cells and indicates suboptimal culture conditions in the media only wells.

The results presented in Table 3 illustrate an experimental model in the rat. Unlike in the human, normal donor controls syngeneic to the tumor are readily available. However, effector cell preparations from the same inbred strain may differ in cytotoxic activity against both allogeneic and syngeneic targets. For example, A's untreated spleen cells kill syngeneic target LMM1 significantly better than spleen cells from a normal Lewis donor. A was not age-matched to the normal control and had been in the animal quarters for over a year longer.

TABLE 2

Cytotoxicity Reactions Produced by Effector Cells of Patients with
Transitional Cell Carcinoma of the Bladder (TCC)

Target[a]	Effector cell conc./well ($\times 10^4$)	Surviving targets/well[b] (mean ± SD)			% Reduction[c]
		Patient	Control	MC[b]	
T24		A	LA38		
	5.0	56±14	120±28	148±9	53[d]
	2.5	75±15	128±22		41[d]
		B			
	5.0	34±17		138±16	72[d]
	2.5	75±22			41[d]
J82,		A	LA38		
TC 35	5.0	2±2	20±6	33±6	91[d]
	2.5	7±3	21±5		67[d]
		B			
	5.0	5±3		28±6	77[d]
	2.5	5±3			76[d]
HCV-29,		A	LA38		
TC 80	5.0	72±11	62±10	80±8	0
	2.5	82±11	71±16		0
		B			
	5.0	26±6		84±10	58[e]
	2.5	28±8			61[e]
MEL-1,		A	LA38		
TC 30	5.0	90±27	84±12	125±17	0
	2.5	119±25	102±24		0
		B			
	5.0	58±14		101±20	31[d]
	2.5	79±26			23[e]

[a]For origin, see materials Section 2.1.
[b]MC, medium control, targets incubated alone. A, TCC T1M2, untreated (localized superficial tumor); B, TCC metastatic to bone; LA38, normal healthy control. Incubation time, 46 hr.
[c]Percent reduction compared to control lymphocyte donor.
[d]$p < 0.001$.
[e]$p < 0.01$.

An analogous example in man has been reported in which laboratory workers showed in general more reactivity against cultured tumors than nonlaboratory normal controls (37).

Animal B and its syngeneic effector cell control donor were age matched and showed no significant difference in reactivity toward a syngeneic tumor target FMF1. If a single target, such as FMF1, had been used in this experiment to test

TABLE 3
Allogeneic Cytotoxicity to Rat Fibrosarcomas

Spleen cell effectors	Target	Effector cell conc./well ($\times 10^5$)	Surviving targets/well (mean ± SD)		MC[c]	% Reduction[d]
			Experimental[a]	Syngeneic control[b]		
Untreated, 26-hr incubation	LMM1[e]		A			
		1.0	8±6	79±13		90[g]
		0.5	48±18	137±13		65[g]
					222±45	
			B			
		1.0	30±11			62[g]
		0.5	93±22			30[h]
	FMF1[f]		A			
		1.0	2±1	19±7		95[g]
		0.5	18±8	47±19		62[h]
					257±31	
			B			
		1.0	26±14			0
		0.5	27±25			45
Cotton column and nylon column purification 42-hr incubation	LMM1		A			
		1.0	165±51	268±16		38[h]
		0.5	263±53	306±46		14
					467±26	
			B			
		1.0	181±29			32[g]
		0.5	290±34			5
	FMF1		A			
		1.0	12±16	114±42		89[g]
		0.5	27±12	129±30		79[g]
			367±49			
			B			
		1.0	113±50			1
		0.5	146±40			0

[a]A, Lewis anti-Fisher, hyperimmune; B, Fisher anti-Lewis, immune.
[b]Control syngeneic to target cell tested.
[c]Medium control, targets incubated alone.
[d]% Reduction compared to syngeneic control.
[e]Lewis fibrosarcoma, see Section 2.1.2.
[f]Fisher fibrosarcoma, see Section 2.1.2.
[g]$p < 0.001$.
[h]$p < 0.01$.

untreated spleen cells, the results could have been interpreted as a specific killing by animal A of FMF1, whereas in fact the use of a second target showed the effect to be entirely nonspecific. This effect is also shown by patient B in Table 2 and demonstrates the critical importance of using adequate target cell controls.

The effect produced by animal A's cells in Table 3 indicates the necessity for using age-matched controls in this type of assay. Incubation of the effector cell suspensions on cotton and nylon columns reduced but did not eliminate this nonspecific effect.

When results are compared to the medium control, it is clear that in this example the greatest portion of the cell reduction is nonselective. If medium controls were not presented, the data would misrepresent the portion of the cytotoxic reaction due to specific cellular immunity. The percentage of the nonselective killing compared to the medium control was reduced but not eliminated by purification of cells on cotton and nylon columns. The specific killing of animal A against FMF1, however, remained strong. The fact that animal B did not show strong specific killing of LMM1 could be due to insufficient immunization or due to allelic differences in the histocompatibility antigens known to be present in the Lewis and Fisher strains (38). Comparison of results to the medium control also indicate that the FMF1 tumor is more sensitive than the LMM1 tumor. This may also explain why specific cytotoxicity was detected with animal A, but not animal B, effector cell preparations and again emphasizes the need for *several* syngeneic or allogeneic tumor controls when studying allogeneic or tumor-associated reactions.

4.2. Composition of Effector Cell Preparations. A summary based on differential counts of the effector cell preparations obtained from normal donors and patients with TCC is shown in Table 4. The method of cell purification yielded $\geqslant 95\%$ cells of lymphoid morphology for normal donors and patients with

TABLE 4

Cellular Content of Effector Cell Preparations (Mean ± SD) from Patients with Transitional Cell Carcinoma of the Bladder (TCC)

		TCC[a]		
	Normal healthy	Localized	Metastases	Tumor-free post radio-therapy
Lymphocytes	95 ±3	96.5± 2	74 ± 12[b]	93.5 ± 5.7
Neutrophils	1.2 ± 1.5	1 ± 1	5.6 ± 5.7[c]	0.9 ± 1.3
Eosinophils	2.2 ± 1.8	0.4 ± 0.5[c]	15 ± 16[c]	2.7 ± 4.9
Basophils	1.6 ± 1.9	0.9 ± 0.6	2.3 ± 2.5	2.4 ± 1.6
Monocytes	0.3 ± 0.36	0.26 ± 0.28	0.2 ± 0.4	0.2 ± 0.24
Immature cells	0.08 ± 0.22	0.46 ± 0.6[c]	0.7 ± 0.7[c]	0.45 ± 0.6[c]
Promyelocytes	0.28 ± 0.07	0.5 ± 1.3[c]	2.7 ± 5.6[c]	0.3 ± 0.6

[a]Results were based on a minimum of 20 donors per group.
[b]$p < 0.001$.
[c]$p < 0.01$.

localized TCC. However, increased numbers of immature cells were recovered in preparations from all patients with TCC. In particular, in patients with widespread disease, preparations contained significantly elevated proportions of eosinophils, neutrophils, and promyelocytes (39). While cellular immunity to TCC could be detected with effector cells from patients with localized TCC, those with widespread disease, such as patient B in Table 2, frequently showed a generalized cytotoxicity for all target cell types tested (39). The method described can therefore best detect cellular immunity to TCC when relatively pure effector cell preparations are available.

Similarly, in allogeneic and syngeneic animal systems, cellular immunity can be better detected after removal of adherent cells on cotton or nylon columns (Table 3). Further efforts should now be made to clearly define the cell populations involved (33, 40, 41) in cell-mediated immunity.

To conclude, standardization of this assay requires optimal tissue culture incubation conditions, adequately characterized target cells, a method of effector cell preparation that does not influence target cell survival, clinically defined patient material, concurrent testing of appropriate effector and target cell controls, and titration of the effector:target cell ratio for each donor/target combination.

REFERENCES

1. Cerottini, J.-C., and Brunner, K. T., *Adv. Immunol.* **18,** 67 (1974).
2. Canty, T. G., and Wunderlich, J. R., *J. Natl. Cancer Inst.* **45,** 761 (1970).
3. Golstein, P., Wigzell, H., Blomgren, H., and Svedmyr, E., *J. Exp. Med.* **135,** 890 (1972).
4. Brondz, B. D., Egorov, I. K., and Drizlikh, G. I., *J. Exp. Med.* **141,** 11 (1975).
5. Lundgren, G., Zukoski, C. F., and Möller, G., *Clin. Exp. Immunol.* **3,** 817 (1968).
6. Edelson, P. J., and Cohn, Z. A., *J. Exp. Med.* **138,** 318 (1973).
7. Takasugi, M., and Klein, E., *Transplantation* **9,** 219 (1970).
8. Mullen, Y., Takasugi, M., and Hildemann, W. H., *Transplantation* **15,** 238 (1973).
9. Biesecker, J. L., Fitch, F. W., Rowley, D. A., Scollard, D., and Stuart, F. P., *Transplantation* **16,** 421 (1973).
10. Lamon, E. W., Skurzak, H. M., and Klein, E., *Int. J. Cancer* **10,** 581 (1972).
11. Hayami, M., Hellström, I., Hellström, K. E., and Yamanouchi, K., *Int. J. Cancer* **10,** 507 (1972).
12. LeClerc, J. C., Gomard, E., Plata, F., and Levy, J. P., *Int. J. Cancer* **11,** 426 (1973).
13. Colnaghi, M. I., Menard, S., and Della Porta, G., *J. Nat. Cancer Inst.* **47,** 1325 (1971).
14. Lamon, E. W., and Wigzell, H., *Transplantation* **18,** 368 (1974).
15. Kearney, R., Basten, A., and Nelson, D. S., *Int. J. Cancer* **15,** 438 (1975).
16. Baldwin, R. W., Embleton, M. J., and Robins, R. A., *Int. J. Cancer* **11,** 1 (1973).
17. Currie, G. A,, and Gage, J. O., *Br. J. Cancer* **28,** 136 (1973).
18. O'Toole, C., Unsgaard, B., Almgard, L. E., and Johansson, B., *Br. J. Cancer,* Suppl. I, **28,** 266 (1973).
19. De Vries, J. E., Rumke, P. H., and Bernheim, J. L., *Int. J. Cancer* **9,** 567 (1972).
20. Hellström, I., Hellström, K. E., Sjögren, H. O., and Warner, G. A., *Int. J. Cancer* **7,** 1 (1971).

21. Diehl, V., Jereb, B., Stjernswärd, J., O'Toole, C., and Ahstrom, L., *Int. J. Cancer* 7, 277 (1971).
22. Bean, M. A., Bloom, B. R., Heberman, R. B., Old, L. J., Oettgen, H. F., Klein, G., and Terry, W. D., *Cancer Res.* 35, 2902 (1975).
23. Bubenik, J., Baresova, M., Viklicky, V., Jakoubkova, J., Sainerova, H., and Donner, J., *Int. J. Cancer* 11, 765 (1973).
24. Rigby, C. C., and Franks, L. M., *Br. J. Cancer* 24, 746 (1970).
25. Ponten, J., and Saksela, E., *Int. J. Cancer* 2, 434 (1967).
26. Chang, R. S., *Proc. Soc. Exp. Biol. Med.* 87, 440 (1954).
27. UICC Union Internationale Contre Le Cancer, "Cancer of the Urinary Bladder." Karger, Basel, 1963.
28. Bergkvist, A., Ljungkvist, A., and Moberger, G., *Acta. Chir. Scand.* 130, 371 (1965).
29. Boyle, W., *Transplantation* 6, 761 (1968).
30. O'Toole, C., Helmstein, K., Perlmann, P., and Moberger, G., *Int. J. Cancer* 16, 413 (1975).
31. Shortman, K., von Boehmer, H., Lipp, J., ånd Hopper, K., *Transplant. Rev.* 25, 163 (1975).
32. O'Toole, C., *Natl. Cancer Inst. Monogr.* 37, 19 (1973).
33. O'Toole, C., Stejskal, V., Perlmann, P., and Karlsson, M., *J. Exp. Med.* 139, 457 (1974).
34. Möller, G., Coutinho, A., Gronowicz, E., Hammarström, L., and Smith, E., *in* "The Role of Mitogens in Immunobiology 1975." In press.
35. Julius, M. H., Simpson, E., and Herzenberg, L. A., *Eur. J. Immunol.* 3, 645 (1973).
36. Schellekens, P. T., and Eijsvoogel, V. P., *Clin. Exp. Immunol.* 38, 17 (1968).
37. Takasugi, M., Mickey, M. R., and Terasaki, P. I., *Cancer Res.* 33, 2898 (1973).
38. Mullen, Y., and Hildemann, W. H., *Transplant. Proc.* 3, 669 (1971).
39. Unsgaard, B., and O'Toole, C., *Br. J. Cancer* 31, 301 (1975).
40. Special Technical Report, *Scand. J. Immunol.* 3, 521 (1974).
41. *Transplantation Review* (G. Moller, ed.), 25 (1975).

Estimation of Human Cell-Mediated Cytotoxicity by Lymphocyte Titration and Automated Image Analysis

Thomas R. Hakala, Paul H. Lange, and Elwin E. Fraley

1. Introduction

The *in vitro* cytotoxic activity of lymphocytes is estimated by determining target cell survival after exposure to lymphocytes. In conventional cell-mediated cytotoxicity (CMC) assays, the number of target cells surviving exposure to lymphocytes at a selected concentration is compared to the number of target cells surviving exposure either to control lymphocytes at the same concentration or to medium alone. Reduction in target cell survival caused by the test lymphocytes, expressed as a percentage of target cell reduction (% TCR), is commonly used as an index of the lymphocyte's cytotoxic activity. However, % TCR is not proportional to lymphocyte cytotoxic activity. For example, doubling the cytotoxic activity of lymphocytes which caused a 60% reduction in target cell survival could not possibly cause 120% reduction in target cell survival. Because % TCR is not proportional to lymphocyte cytotoxic activity, quantitative comparisons between the activity of lymphocytes having a very strong or very weak cytotoxic activity is not practical.

Titration of lymphocyte concentration in order to achieve some selected reduction in target cell survival does allow an estimate of lymphocyte cytotoxic activity proportional to that activity. Because the cytotoxic activity of lymphocytes from different donors differ widely, lymphocytes must be tested at many different concentrations in order to determine the concentration that will cause a selected reduction in target cell survival. Because lymphocyte titration requires the testing for cytotoxicity at multiple lymphocyte concentrations, enumeration of surviving target cells is greatly increased.

In the cell-mediated cytotoxicity assays described by Takasugi and Klein (1) and the Hellström's (2), target cells surviving exposure to lymphocytes are counted optically and manually. Manual optical counting is slow and therefore expensive. It is subject to operator errors, and practical constraints limit the number of target cells that can be counted per well.

In order to remove the necessity for manual optical counting, target cells have been labeled with various radioactive compounds. Artifacts introduced by the labeled compound or the radioactivity itself may hamper the interpretation of the results. The time required for the preparation of samples and counting limits the number of tests which can be performed in a given time. In order to reduce the artifacts introduced by heavy labeling of the target cells while obtaining sufficient radioactive disintegration to allow statistically significant analysis of the results, the number of target cells is often increased, and as a consequence the demands for lymphocyte effector cells are simultaneously increased.

While titration of lymphocytes to estimate lymphocyte cytotoxic activity has theoretical advantages over the conventional CMC assays, lymphocyte titration has not usually been employed because of the increased demands for target cell enumeration. The recent availability of commercial electrooptical devices for the counting of adherent target cells has made practical the following application of lymphocyte titration for estimation of cytotoxic activity *in vitro*.

2. Materials and Methods

2.1. Equipment

2.1.1. Vertical laminar flow biohazard hood (Baker Company, Inc., Biddeford, Maine)

2.1.2. CO_2 incubator (Webco, Inc., Silver Springs, Maryland)

2.1.3. Centrifuge, Model PR6 (Damon/IEC Division, Needham Heights, Massachusetts)

2.1.4. Inverted phase-contrast microscope

2.1.5. Magnetic stirrer

2.1.6. Leveling platform (custom fabricated)

2.1.7. Syringe, 500 μl, Luer tip (Hamilton Company, Reno, Nevada, No. 1750)

2.1.8. Needle, 21-gauge, 3-inch, point style No. 3 (Hamilton Company, No. KF-721)

2.1.9. Repeating dispenser (Hamilton Company, No. PB 600-1)

2.1.10. Gyrotory shaker (New Brunswick Scientific Company, New Brunswick, New Jersey, No. G-2 and AG2-125)

2.1.11. Wintrobe cannula

2.1.12. Controlled Histoplate washer (custom fabricated; modified from a design of D. Aoki and M. Takasugi, Department of Surgery, University of California, Los Angeles)

2.1.13. Image analyzing computer, Quantimet 720 with teletype drive and paper tape punch (Cambridge-Imanco, Monsey, New York)

2.1.14. Calculator, Hewlett-Packard 9830 with paper tape reader, plotter, external tape cassette, and thermal printer (Hewlett-Packard, Loveland, Colorado)

2.2. Supplies

2.2.1. Scalp vein needle, 18-gauge (Abbott Laboratories)

2.2.2. Nylon fiber [Fenwal Laboratories, Morton Grove, Illinois, No. FT242(4C2906)]

2.2.3. Erlenmeyer flask, 125 ml, screw top (Bellco Glass Inc., Vineland, N.J.)

2.2.4. Zip-Lok plastic bags

2.2.5. 72-Well Costar Histoplate (Cooke Engineering, Alexandria, Virginia, No. 4-236-72)

2.2.6. Plastic tissue culture flasks, 30 ml and 250 ml (Falcon Plastics, Los Angeles, California)

2.2.7. Plastic screw-top centrifuge tubes, 15 ml and 50 ml sterile (Falcon Plastics)

2.3. Reagents

2.3.1. Basic media: Waymouth, R PMI-1640, L-15 media reconstituted from the powdered form (GIBCO, Grand Island, New York) supplemented with penicillin—100 units/ml, streptomycin, 100 μg/ml, Bacto-tryptose phosphate broth (Difco, No. 0060-01), 10%, sodium pyruvate, 100 X (Microbiological Associates, Bethesda, Maryland, No. 13-115), 1 ml/100 ml, nonessential amino acids, 100 X (GIBCO, No. 114), 1 ml/100 ml, L-glutamine, 2 mM (General Biochemicals, Chagrin Falls, Ohio, NRC10510.) The choice of medium is determined by the growth characteristics of the target cells.

2.3.2. Tissue culture medium: Basic medium plus 10% fetal calf serum (FCS) (Reheis, Kankakee, Illinois)

2.3.3. MNC medium: Basic medium plus 25 mM HEPES buffer (N-2-hydroxyethylpiperazine-N-2-ethane; General Biochemicals, No. 130440)

2.3.4. Trypsin: versene solution: Versene solution: 1 liter contains 8 g of NaCl, 0.4 g of KCl, 0.2 g of Versene. A 0.125% solution of trypsin 1:250 (General Biochemicals, No. 70720) is made in the Versene solution, allowed to stand overnight at 4°C and sterilized by filtration through a 0.22 μm Millipore filter.

2.3.5. Gelatin solution (3%) in Tris-buffered Hanks' solution: Tris buffer: Trizma HCl (Sigma Biochemicals), 20.20 g; Trizma base (Sigma), 2.65 g; Distilled water, 1000 ml. One volume of sterilized Tris buffer is combined with 1 volume of Hanks' solution (GIBCO) and supplemented with penicillin (100 units/ml) and streptomycin (100 μg/ml) to produce Tris-buffered Hanks' solution (TBH). Dissolve 1.5 g of Deionized Bone Gelatin, Type L-936 (P. Leiner and Sons, America, Inc., St. Claire Shores, Michigan), as obtained from the manufacturer, in 50 ml of Tris-buffered Hanks' solution. Dissolution of gelatin is hastened by heating in a water bath; after gelatin is completely dissolved, it is kept from gelling by heating at 37°C in a water bath. The gelatin solution is prepared fresh for each lymphocyte separation (3).

2.3.6. Ficoll-Hypaque Solution. A 9% (w/v) solution of Ficoll (Pharmacia) in water is prepared and sterilized by filtration through a 0.22 μm Millipore filter. Sterile 50% Hypaque solution (Winthrop Laboratories) is diluted to 33.9% with sterile water. Ten parts of the Ficoll solution are combined with 24 parts of the Hypaque solution. The final density of this solution should equal 1.077 ± 0.001. This Ficoll–Hypaque solution should be stored at approximately 4°C in a light-proof container.

2.3.7. Crystal violet: A 0.1% solution of crystal violet (Curtin Scientific No. GX55) is made in distilled water.

3. Procedures

3.1. Target Cell Plating. Tissue culture medium is decanted from target cells grown in Falcon 30- or 250-ml tissue culture flasks. The adherent monolayer of cells is washed briefly with approximately 3 ml of sterile, phosphate-buffered saline (pH 7.4). Approximately 5–10 ml of 0.125% trypsin–Versene solution (37°C) is added to the flask. Dispersion of the target cell monolayer into single cells is monitored using the inverted, phase-contrast microscope and usually proceeds within 1–3 min. Approximately 10 ml of tissue culture medium is added to the flask, and the cells are transferred to a centrifuge tube and washed twice in tissue culture medium. After sedimentation following the final wash, the cells are suspended in MNC medium supplemented with 10% FCS.

The concentration of the target cells is adjusted to 100–250 cells per 10 μl of medium. (The exact concentration of target cells must be determined empirically by the percentage of target cells that adhere to the bottom of the Histoplate after a 24-hr incubation.) The target cell suspension is transferred to square glass bottles containing a small, magnetic spin bar and placed on top of a magnetic stirrer. A square bottle is used in preference to a round bottle so that during agitation a turbulent motion is induced in the suspension to ensure uniform distribution of the target cells in the suspension. Care must be taken so that surface of the magnetic stirrer does not become so hot as to damage the target cells. Using the 500-μl syringe, 21-gauge needle (No. KF-721), and repeating dispenser, 10-μl aliquots of the target cell suspension are dispensed into each of the 72 wells of the Costar Histoplate (see Fig. 1). The wells of the Histoplate are arranged in an array consisting of 6 horizontal rows and 12 vertical columns. Target cells are added to the wells horizontally across the plate. Additional medium is dispensed into the corners and along the edges of the Histoplate in order to supplement the moisture inside the closed plate. The covered Histoplate together with a moistened sponge is placed into a self-sealing Zip-Lok bag and incubated on a leveling

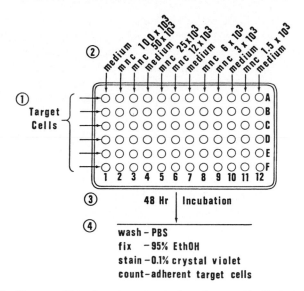

Fig. 1. Diagram of lymphocyte concentration placement in the test plate.

platform overnight in a humidified atmosphere of 5% carbon dioxide in air at 37°C.

3.2. Lymphocyte (MNC) Preparation. Venous blood, 50 ml, is collected without anticoagulant using a syringe and scalp vein needle. This blood is immediately transferred into a sterile 125-ml screw-top Erlenmeyer flask containing paper clips that have been bent open slightly. Blood is defibrinated by rotating the flask on a New Brunswick gyrotory shaker at 250 rpm for 10 min at room temperature. The Erlenmeyer flask is clamped to the platform of the shaker at a 45° angle so that during rotation turbulent flow occurs in order to assure satisfactory defibrination. The defibrinated blood is mixed with the 3% gelatin solution in a ratio of 1:3 (gelatin solution:blood). Mixing is accomplished by inversion in a graduated cylinder, after which the foam is aspirated from the top with suction through a sterile Pasteur pipette. Red cells are allowed to sediment from the suspension during an incubation of approximately 30 min at 37°C. (4) The leukocyte-containing supernatant fluid is then removed with a sterile pipette and the cells are sedimented by centrifugation at 1200 rpm, at room temperature for 10 min. The cells are gently resuspended in approximately 20 ml of the original serum:gelatin solution and transferred to a sterilized glass column containing approximately 1 g of scrubbed nylon fiber (5). Care should be taken that the leukocyte suspension is in contact with the nylon fiber throughout the column. The column is incubated for 30 min at 37°C. Nonadhering cells are gently washed from the column in a downward flow using approximately 30 ml of MNC medium. The collected cells are pelleted by centrifugation and resuspended in approximately 10 ml of the original solution. This suspension is then transferred to a 15-ml Falcon centrifuge tube and underlain with 4 ml of the Ficoll–Hypaque solution using a Wintrobe cannula. This gradient is then centrifuged at 1200 rpm at room temperature for 20 min such that a force of 400 g is applied at the Ficoll–Hypaque interface according to the method of Böyum. (6)

The majority of red blood cells are sedimented during the initial sedimentation in the presence of gelatin. Incubation on the nylon fiber removes most monocytes and polymorphonuclear neutrophiles. The final centrifugation over a Ficoll–Hypaque barrier removes residual red blood cells.

3.3. Lymphocyte Titration Assay. The lymphocyte suspension is adjusted to a concentration of 10×10^6 cells per milliliter in MNC medium (without FCS). Six serial 2-fold dilutions are prepared in MNC medium. (Final concentrations are from 10^5 to 1.6×10^3 lymphocytes per 10 μl) At each concentration 10 μl of lymphocytes are added to the six wells of each column as indicated in Fig. 1. MNC medium without lymphocytes is added to columns 1, 4, 7, 10, and 12 to allow estimation of target cell survival in the presence of medium alone (without lymphocytes). The Histoplate containing the target cells and lymphocytes is then replaced in the Zip-Lok plastic bag together with the moistened sponge and replaced in the incubator on the leveling platform. Incubation is carried out for 40–48 hr, after which the plate is inverted to allow effector cells and nonadherent target cells to fall away from the bottom of the well.

The removal of effector cells and nonadherent target cells is completed using a device that delivers 72 individual low-pressure jets of phosphate-buffered saline to each of the wells of the Histoplate for a preselected time interval (usually 3–6 sec) (Fig. 2). Uniform plate washing is important in achieving reproducible results. Immediately after washing, the plates are immersed in 95% ethanol and allowed to fix for 2 min or more. The ethanol is washed off by immersion in tap water, and the cells are stained using a 0.1% solution of crystal violet. Staining is carried out for more than 30 sec, after which the excess crystal violet is removed by immersion in tap water. The dye used in staining must be frequently filtered to remove precipitated debris that will interfere with electrooptical counting. The plates are blown dry using a jet of filtered compressed air.

Stained adherent target cells are counted using the Quantimet 720 Image Analyzing Computer. The Histoplate is placed in the microscope, and the image of target cells in an entire well is projected onto a Vidicon tube. This image is displayed on a TV-type display so that gross technical errors of contamination may be detected by the operator.

Objects are counted on the basis of the level of grayness and size of the detected image. The level of grayness is selected so that the nucleus, but not the cytoplasm, is detected. In this way continuous target cells may be counted

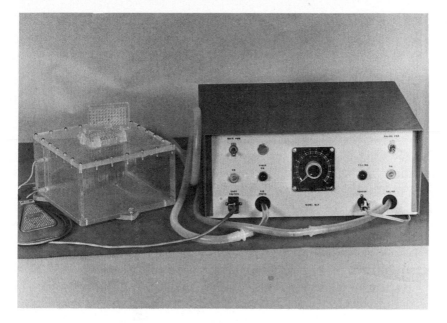

Fig. 2. Controlled Histoplate washer.

separately. Occasional adherent lymphocytes are differentiated from the target cells on the basis of size. The number of target cells counted is transferred to a teletype and simultaneously is punched on a paper tape. Information identifying the target cell and lymphocyte donor for each plate is entered manually on the teletype (and simultaneously on the paper tape).

Data encoded on paper tape is entered into the calculator via a paper tape reader. The mean number of target cells surviving in each of the columns is calculated.

The mean number of target cells surviving in each of the columns containing lymphocytes is compared to the mean number of target cells surviving in the wells incubated without lymphocytes (medium base line). Target cell growth in the Histoplate and microtest plate differs depending upon the position of the well in which the target cells are grown (7). Target cell growth is greater toward the center of the plate. In order to compensate for this variation in target cell growth, the medium base line of target cell growth in wells containing medium alone is extrapolated from the observed target cell growth in the medium containing columns bounding the selected lymphocyte-containing columns. For example, the percentage of target cell survival for column 2 (Fig. 1, 100×10^3 lymphocytes/well) is based on the expected target cell growth in medium extrapolated between columns 1 and 4 and is calculated as follows:

$$\frac{\% \text{ Target cell survival in column 2}}{(100 \times 10^3 \text{ lymphocytes/well})} = \frac{TCS_2}{TCS_1 + [(TCS_4 - TCS_1)/3]}$$

where TCS_2 is the mean number of target cells surviving in column 2, TCS_1 is the mean number of target cells surviving in the medium control wells of column 1, and TCS_4 is the mean number of target cells surviving in the medium control well to wells of column 4.

The expression $\frac{1}{3} (TCS_4 - TCS_1)$ equals the slope of the line between mean target cell survival in column 1 and in column 4. $TCS_1 + \frac{1}{3} (TCS_4 - TCS_1)$ equals the anticipated target cell survival for target cells grown in column 2 had there been no lymphocytes in the wells. The percentage of target cell survival in the presence of lymphocytes in column 3 (50×10^3 lymphocytes per well) is calculated as

$$\frac{TCS_3}{TCS_1 + \frac{2}{3} (TCS_4 - TCS_1)}$$

Target cell survival following exposure to the lymphocytes at 25×10^3 and 12.5×10^3 (columns 5 and 6) would be calculated on the basis of the extrapolated medium base line calculated between mean target cell survival found in columns 4 and 7.

The percentage of target cell survival is plotted versus lymphocyte concentration (Fig. 3) and from this the number of lymphocytes required to cause a 50% reduction in target cell survival is estimated by extrapolation. For convenience in plotting the cytotoxic activity of lymphocytes with widely different activities, the number of lymphocytes required to cause a 50% reduction in target cell survival is concerned to a logarithm to the base 2 and called a lymphocyte lethal dose 50 (LLD_{50}). The LLD_{50} is calculated as follows:

$$LLD_{50} = -\log_2 L/200,000$$

where L is the number of lymphocytes required to reduce target cell survival by 50%.

The number of lymphocytes required to reduce the target cell survival by 50% is divided by 200,000, so that the resulting LLD_{50} is expressed as a small positive number. Calculation of percentage of target cell survival and LLD_{50} is performed automatically by the calculator.

4. Critical Comments

In order to obtain reproducible results, great care must be taken to ensure uniformity in lymphocyte preparation, target-cell propagation, and manipulation during the assay. Fetal calf serum is purchased in lots of sufficient size so that tests can be performed for at least a year before changing fetal calf serum lots.

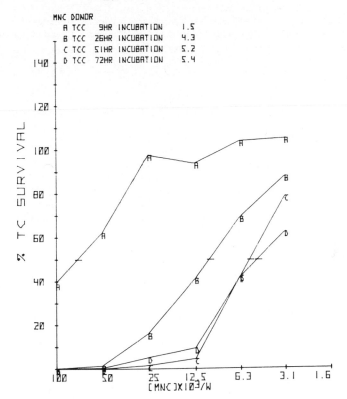

Fig. 3. Calculator-generated plot of percentage of target cell survival versus lymphocyte concentration (lymphocyte titration curves). Lymphocytes from the same donor, a patient with transitional cell carcinoma of the bladder (TCC), were incubated for the times indicated upon target cells derived from TCC.

Mechanical defibrination is carried out to ensure that all blood samples are subjected to a uniform amount of agitation.

The automated plate washer significantly reduces variation between duplicate tests. When this automated plate washer is employed, the LLD_{50}'s obtained from duplicate assays seldom vary by more than 0.3 LLD_{50} unit. When hand-washing of the plates is carried out, this difference may increase to as much as 0.6 to 0.8 LLD_{50} unit.

The application of this lymphocyte titration assay to serial estimation of CMC in patients with bladder and kidney carcinoma has been described elsewhere (8, 9).

ACKNOWLEDGMENTS

This study was supported in part by research funds of the Veterans Administration, American Cancer Society Institutional Grant, Minnesota Medical Foundation, United States Public Health Service Training Grant AMO5514-08, National Cancer Institute Grant CA13095-03, and National Bladder Cancer Project Grant CA1551-02.

REFERENCES

1. Takasugi, M., and Klein, M., *Transplantation* **9,** 219 (1970).
2. Hellström, I., Hellström, K. E., Sjögren, H. O., and Warner, G. A., *Int. J. Cancer* **7,** 1 (1972).
3. O'Toole, C., Perlmann, P., Unsgaard, B., Almard, L. E., Johansson, B., Moberger, G., and Edsmyr, F., *Int. J. Cancer* **10,** 92 (1972).
4. Coulson, A. S., and Chalmers, D. G., *Lancet* **1,** 468 (1964).
5. Greenwalt, T. J., Gajewski, M., and McKenna, J. L., *Transfusion* **2,** 221 (1962).
6. Böyum, A., *Scand. J. Clin. Lab. Invest.* **21,** 97, Suppl. (1968).
7. Takasugi, M., Mickey, M. R., and Teresaki, P. I., *Natl. Cancer Inst. Monogr.* **37,** 77 (1973).
8. Hakala, T. R., Lange, P. H., Elliott, A. Y., and Fraley, E. E., *J. Urol.* in press.
9. Hakala, T. R., Lange, P. H., and Fraley, E. E., *Cancer Res.* in press.

Determination of Cell-Mediated Cytotoxicity by
the [125] I-Labeled Iododeoxyuridine Microcytotoxicity Assay

Robert K. Oldham and Ronald B. Herberman

1. Introduction

Many *in vitro* assays to measure cell-mediated cytotoxicity have been described (1–15). The central need is for an assay that is technically reproducible, reasonably simple to perform and applicable in a wide variety of laboratories. We will describe here the [125] I-labeled iododeoxyuridine ([125] IUdR) method for evaluating cellular cytotoxicity. This method has been utilized by ourselves and others as a microcytotoxicity assay method measuring cell-mediated cytotoxicity over 24–48 hr incubation periods both in animal tumor systems and in man (16–20). These labeled target cells can also be used to assess antibody-mediated cytotoxicity (21). The assay as it is described here involves the prelabeling of the appropriate target cells, but this assay has also been utilized in a postlabeling assay as a measure of target cells remaining in the well after incubation with appropriate effector cells (21).

[125] IUdR is incorporated into target cell nuclear DNA in place of the sterically similar thymidine. An inhibitor of thymidylate synthetase, fluorodeoxyuridine (FUdR), is added so that cells preferentially take up the [125] IUdR in place of thymidine. This assay offers several potential advantages over many of the existing assay methods. The objectivity and ease of an isotopic method is preferable to the subjective visual counting method. This assay can be used for both monolayer and suspension cell systems as long as the cells proliferate and thereby incorporate [125] IUdR (21, 22). After incorporation of this isotope into the target cell, there is no spontaneous release from living cells and very little reutilization. Therefore, release of this isotope into the supernatant is a direct reflection of cell death and lysis. The only exception to this statement is when whole cells lost adherence and are released into the supernatant, thereby decreasing the amount of radioactivity in the adherent cells and contributing to the counts per minute in the supernatant. By merely centrifuging the supernatants, one can determine whether whole cells are present; if not, the [125] IUdR counted in the supernatant is a direct measure of lytic events in the labeled target cell (19).

We initially evaluated the use of trypsin as described by Klein and Perlmann (23) and Hirata (24) to preferentially lyse target cells that have undergone immune membrane damage, thinking that trypsin might increase the sensitivity of this assay. In a rat tumor system and in human microcytotoxicity, we did not find any additional advantage of trypsinization of the target cells as opposed to directly measuring isotope release (17, 18). In a mouse tumor system trypsin has been helpful (25).

2. Materials and Methods

This method can be equally adapted for cellular cytotoxicity assays in petri dishes, Linbro Plates (Linbro FB-16-24-TC, Bellco Glass Co., Inc., Vineland, New Jersey), or in the smaller Microtest II plates. The assay as described here has been performed in the Microtest II plates (Falcon Plastics, Los Angeles, California), which minimizes the number of target cells and effector cells needed to perform such assays.

2.1. Materials and Equipment

2.1.1. Plastic tissue culture flasks, T-60 (250 ml) and T-30 (30 sterile ml), (Falcon Plastics, Los Angeles, California)

2.1.2. Graduated conical plastic centrifuge tubes, sterile, 50 ml (Falcon Plastics)

2.1.3. Plastic pipettes, sterile

2.1.4. Counting tubes for gamma counting or vials for scintillation counting

2.1.5. Microtest II plates (No. 3040, Falcon Plastics)

2.1.6. Biopette (1-ml Biopette, Schwarz/Mann, Orangeburg, New York)

2.1.7. RIA Microharvest Tips (Cooke Engineering, Rockville, Maryland) Other equipment includes the following

2.1.9. 8-Pronged aspirator and 8-pronged dispenser devices for the Microtest II plates (NIH Shop, Bethesda, Maryland). These are fabricated to fit an aspirator vacuum line or a dispensing syringe. The latter delivers equal volumes to each well.

2.1.10. Hamilton dispensing syringe (Hamilton Co., Reno, Nevada)

2.1.11. Standard microscope with hemacytometer

2.1.12. Coulter counter (Model Z, Coulter Electronics, Hialeah, Florida)

2.1.13. Incubator with 5% CO_2 humidified atmosphere, 37°C

2.1.14. Mash II automatic harvester (Microbiological Associates, Bethesda, Maryland)

2.1.15. Gamma counter (Beckman Biogamma, Irvine, California)

2.1.16. Beta scintillation counter (Isocap 300, Searle Analytic Inc., Des Plaines, Illinois

2.2. Solutions and Chemicals

2.2.1. Incubation Media. A variety of incubation media can be utilized for this test. The tissue culture media in which the cells are normally carried are satisfactory for the assay. Our assays are all done in RPMI 1640 (NIH Media Unit, Bethesda, Maryland) with 20% fetal bovine serum (Grand Island Biological Co., Grand Island, New York). Hanks' balanced salt solution (BSS) is utilized to wash the cells (NIH Media Unit).

2.2.2. Trypsin. (a) 0.25% crystalline trypsin (Worthington Biochemical Co., Freehold, New Jersey) was used to trypsinize cells at the end of the assay. (b) 0.25% crude trypsin (NIH Media Unit) was used as needed to detach cells for labeling.

2.2.3. HEPES Buffer. Hepes Buffer (Microbiological Associates, Bethesda, Maryland) can be utilized at concentrations of 25 mM in addition to the CO_2 buffering system of the medium for additional buffering capacity during the incubation period.

2.2.4. Antibiotics. All of our cell lines are carried on antibiotic-free media for their propagation. For the assay the media utilized are supplemented with penicillin (100 μg/ml) and streptomycin (100 μg/ml) (NIH Media Unit).

2.2.5. ^{125}I-Labeled Iododeoxyuridine (^{125} IUdR) (New England Nuclear, Boston, Mass., or Amersham Searle, Arlington Heights, Illinois). Stock solutions of 50 μCi/ml are prepared on arrival by dilution with RPMI 1640. The stock solution is stored at 4°C.

2.2.6. Fluorodeoxyuridine (FUdR). 10^{-5} Molar stock solutions were prepared. This chemical has been obtained from Hoffmann-La Roche, Nutley, New Jersey, as well as from the NIH Chemotherapy Branch. FUdR stock solution is kept at 4°C, but the FUdR concentrated solution (10^{-2} M) is held frozen at −70°C.

2.2.7. Aquasol Beta Scintillation Fluid (New England Nuclear, Boston, Massachusetts). Because water is present in the samples to be counted, a scintillation fluid that will tolerate water is necessary.

2.3. Effector Cell Preparation. Lymphocytes can be prepared by a variety of methods for use in this assay. We have used the standard Ficoll–Hypaque gradient technique of Böyum (26) as well as the Plasmagel sedimentation–nylon column technique to prepare lymphocyte preparations. Platelet aggregation can be enhanced by adenosine diphosphate (ADP), which facilitates platelet removal on Ficoll–Hypaque gradients. The addition of carbonyl iron to eliminate phagocytic cells from the lymphocyte band has also been used (27). These methods and the methods for preparing mononuclear cells from the lymphoid organs of rodents are listed below.

2.3.1. Ficoll–Hypaque. Peripheral blood (60 ml) was drawn in syringes containing 2000 units of preservative-free heparin (Fellows Manufacturing Co., Inc., Anaheim, California). The heparinized blood was diluted 2-fold with phosphate-buffered (pH 7.4) isotonic saline (PBS) or Hanks' BSS and carefully placed on Ficoll–Hypaque gradients as originally described by Böyum. These gradients were prepared in 50-ml clonical graduated Falcon tubes and centrifuged at 400 g at the interface. Such cell preparations contain 95–100% small to medium mononuclear cells from heparinized human blood. Esterase-positive monocytic cells comprised approximately 5–20% of these preparations depending on how carefully the lymphocyte layer was aspirated (28). Preparations from rat peripheral blood contain 95% or more small lymphocytes. As with all methods using Ficoll–Hypaque gradients, removal of a significant number of cells below the lymphocyte layer will increase the number of esterase-positive cells in the preparation. Significant platelet contamination is present in these preparations.

2.3.2. Ficoll–Hypaque/ADP Iron. Lymphocytes were also purified by the method of Faguet (27). Heparinized blood (60 ml) was incubated in the presence of adenosine diphosphate (ADP) (Nutritional Biochemical Corp., Cleveland, Ohio) and carbonyl iron (GAF Corp., New York, New York) for 30 min at 37°C. The ADP is made up in a stock solution of 97 mg/100 ml of Hanks' BSS, and 0.2 ml of stock solution is added for each 20 ml of diluted blood. Carbonyl iron is used at a concentration of 16 mg per milliliter of diluted blood. The blood was then placed on Ficoll–Hypaque gradients in the usual manner. Centrifugation at 400 g for 40 min was carried out. Preparations derived from this manner contained fewer platelets and very few esterase-positive cells as compared to the Ficoll–Hypaque gradient technique described above.

2.3.3. Plasmagel–Nylon Column. Plasmagel (R. Bellon Laboratory, Neuilly, France) (10 ml) was mixed with 60 ml of heparinized blood, and the erythrocytes were allowed to sediment for 1 hr at 37°C. The leukocyte-rich plasma was aspirated, washed, and placed on a warm (37°C) nylon column (1–2 g of sterile nylon in a 12-ml plastic syringe barrel that had been equilibrated with warm medium) for 30 min. The nonadherent cells were eluted with warm Hanks' BSS. Although the cell yield is quite a lot lower with this preparation method (30–40% versus 50–70% for Ficoll–Hypaque gradients), it results in an almost pure population of mononuclear cells with few esterase-positive cells, but again with significant platelet contamination.

2.3.4. Preparation of Cells from Rat Spleen and Lymph Nodes. Cell suspensions were prepared by gently macerating spleens or lymph nodes in sterile plastic petri dishes in Hanks' BSS until the cells were disaggregated from the stroma. Cells were then aspirated with a 10-ml pipette, passed through a sterile layer of gauze, washed twice, centrifuged and diluted in RPMI 1640 with FBS and counted.

2.4. Preparation of Target Cells

2.4.1. Adherent Monolayers. Cells were normally grown in T-60 flasks. Single-cell suspensions were prepared by one of two methods: (a) When the cells were loosely adherent, the addition of Hanks' BSS (without Ca^{2+} and Mg^{2+}) with shaking, gave detachment of the cells, and these could be removed and counted. (b) For strongly adherent cells, 0.25% trypsin (NIH Media Unit) (1–2 ml) is added with incubation at 37°C for 1–10 min (depending on the rate of cell detachment). The cell suspension is then diluted with medium containing 10%

fetal bovine serum to neutralize the trypsin, and the cells are counted. The cell suspension from a confluent T-60 flask is diluted in 3 ml of complete media, and 0.5 ml is added to each T-30 flask, giving a subconfluent monolayer in the smaller flask. Complete medium, 2.5 ml, is added to the T-30 flask and it is placed in the incubator for 2–4 hr to allow the cells to attach to the plastic. ^{125}IUdR, 2.5 μCi (occasionally larger amounts are needed to label certain cell lines), is added to the flask after the cells become adherent. FUdR is included in the labeling medium to give a final concentration of $10^{-6}M$ in the medium with the cells to be labeled. Labeling time from 4 hr to overnight at $37°C$ may be utilized depending on the cell line and the number of counts per minute desired in the cells. Generally, 1000 cpm per well is needed for adequate counts to be in cells and supernatant at the end of the assay. Obviously the rate of DNA synthesis, the amount of isotope, and the incubation time as well as isotype toxicity are all considerations relative to the number of counts in the labeled targets (19).

After labeling, the flask is removed from the incubator, the supernatant is poured off, and the monolayers are gently washed twice with Hanks' BSS to remove excess isotope. Cells are then detached from the monolayer as described earlier. If trypsin is utilized, it must be inhibited with media containing fetal bovine serum. The radioactive cell suspension is then diluted to the appropriate concentration.

2.4.2. Suspension Cells. For suspension cells, labeling directly in the T-30 flask or in tubes with similar amounts of IUdR results in adequately labeled target cells (18, 22). For suspension cells, all steps requiring separation of supernatant from cells (such as washing the cells) must be done by centrifugation, in contrast to the monolayer where the supernatants are poured off.

2.5. Assay Procedure. From the appropriately diluted labeled cell suspension, usually 10^3 to 10^4 cells in 0.1 ml of complete media are added to each well of a Microtest II plate. An aliquot of target cells should be counted before plating to determine whether adequate labeling has occurred. If labeling is inadequate, a greater number of target cells can be used (see above).

The labeled target cells are allowed to attach to the Microtest II plate (2–4 hr). Lymphocyte suspensions may be prepared while target cells are becoming adherent. After attachment of the labeled target cells to the wells, the supernatants containing released isotope and unattached target cells are removed by the aspirator device very gently, without disturbing the monolayer, and 0.1 ml of complete medium is added to each well with the dispensing device.

The lymphocytes prepared as described earlier can then be diluted to the appropriate concentration, usually with ratios of lymphocytes:target cells plated in the range of 25:1 up to 250:1. The lymphocytes in 0.1 ml are then dispensed into the plate with a Hamilton dispensing syringe. Replicates of at least four, and preferably six, for each group should be prepared.

The mixtures can be incubated at 37°C in a humidified CO_2 incubator after dispensing, but centrifugation of the mixture in the plates at 300 rpm for 2 min lightly packs the cells, promoting the lymphocyte target cell interaction. From 12–60 hr incubations have been utilized in this assay. Although the first part of the incubation period was previously done on a rocker, the small volume of the Microtest II plate wells allows for very little cell motion, and it appears that rocking is unnecessary for effective release of the isotope. With the centrifugation step described above, rocking is obviously superfluous. Three harvesting techniques are currently available.

2.5.1. Well Punch. Supernatants are removed gently by aspiration with the aspirator device, the monolayer is washed once with Hanks' BSS, and the plate is allowed to dry. The plate is then sprayed with an adhesive plastic spray (Aeroplast Spray Adhesive), and the well bottom is punched out with a hand punch (fabricated to fit the well from steel stock—NIH Shop). Each well bottom may then be placed in plastic counting tubes for counting.

2.5.2. Mash II. For suspension cells, direct harvesting on the automatic Mash II harvesting apparatus allows the retention of the labeled cells on the filter paper, and the released isotope in the supernatant can be discarded or collected in counting tubes. For monolayer cells, 0.1 ml of 0.25% trypsin (Worthington Biochemical Co.) must be added to detach the cells from the plastic after removal of the supernatant. With both types of cells, one can count the radioactivity in both the supernatant and the cell button.

2.5.3. Supernatant Aliquot. Aliquots of the supernatants can be removed with a 0.1-ml Biopette or with the RIA "tips" after centrifugation of the plate and the aliquot of the supernatant counted to determine the counts per minute released.

The three methods give essentially the same results, but the calculations differ for each of the three methods by virtue of the fact that the well-punch harvesting method yields counts per minute of the cells remaining adherent to plastic at the end of the assay, whereas the supernatant aliquot method measures released isotope into the supernatant. The Mash II harvester provides the values of both supernatant and target cells in a single extraction. By taking the counts per minute of plated target cells in other wells in separate plates done at the start of the assay, the total counts incorporated into the target cells is known. Therefore, with each of the three harvesting methods, if two of the three values are known (total cpm, target cell cpm, supernatant cpm), the other can be determined and the percent release calculated. The radioactivity can be measured by either of two counters with comparable results.

Gamma counter (Beckman Biogamma)—counts per minute are determined directly from sample.

Beta counter (Isocap 300, Searle Analytic Inc.)—counts per minute are determined by adding scintillation fluid, allowing to set at room temperature overnight to decrease chemoluminesence, and counting the secondary emissions.

2.6. Calculation of Results. As outlined above, one can determine the counts per minute in the supernatant and the cells and the total counts per minute in the test system (any two of these values allows calculation of the third value by subtraction). The percent cytotoxicity then is calculated as shown below. A cytotoxic index can also be calculated with just the counts per minute (cpm) of the adherent cells at the end of the assay, but the first method is preferred (18):

$$\% \text{Cytotoxicity} = \frac{\text{cpm supernatant}}{\text{cpm total}} \times 100$$

$$\text{Cytotoxic index} = \frac{\text{cpm remaining in the cells of experimental group}}{\text{cpm remaining in the cells of control group}}$$

In the calculation of percent cytotoxicity, the significance of difference between experimental and control values can be determined by students' T test. For the cytotoxicity index the values can be put on scattergrams, and significant differences between different groups relative to a control determined by the Welch modification of students' T test (28). The percent cytotoxicity figure is a direct measure of cell lysis in the system and is less affected by small numbers (low cpm) in the assay as compared to the cytotoxic index (18).

2.7. Experimental Design Considerations. The technical aspects of this cytotoxicity assay are rather simple, and both in animal systems and in the human this assay is quite reproducible (standard errors between replicates of less than 2%). For interpretable results, one of the most important considerations is the experimental design of each experiment. It is critically important to include in each experiment the lymphocytes from a number of unselected normal controls. It is equally important to include a number of different target cell lines, each known to be susceptible to cytotoxicity by some effector cells so that adequate target cell controls are available for interpretation of the test. Last, it is preferable that two separate systems be simultaneously tested. For example, if carcinoma of the breast and melanoma are to be tested, then target cells from each type of tumor should be available, and the specificity of each lymphocyte preparation therefore can be more appropriately evaluated. Another factor affecting the interpretation of this assay is the susceptibility of the target cell lines to lysis or to detachment from the wells. Interpretation of the results in the absence of knowledge of these factors as listed above is extremely difficult.

3. Critical Comments

[125] IUdR is an excellent marker to measure target cell lysis. As with any nuclear label, the release of the isotope into the supernatant or its absence in the monolayer is strong evidence of cell lysis. If one has excluded the presence of

detached cells in the supernatant by centrifugation, appearnace of the isotope in the supernatant is direct evidence of cell lysis. This is in contrast to labels, such as ^{51}Cr and ^{3}H-proline and other amino acids, which can be released without cell lysis. Reutilization of ^{125}IUdR is minimal in contrast to some of the labeled amino acids (18, 19).

The main disadvantage of this particular isotope is that synthesis of DNA, and hence replicating cells, are necessary for its incorporation; therefore, cells with metabolic but not replicative activity, and cells with slow replication rates incorporate little or no ^{125}IUdR into the nucleus and therefore their labeling index (the amount of radioactivity in a given number of target cells) is too low to be useful for cytotoxicity assays. An additional problem with ^{125}IUdR is its inherent toxicity, which must be assessed for each target cell (19, 20).

Because this isotope requires replicating cells, tissue culture target cells are the predominant cell type utilized in this assay. All the difficulties associated with tissue culture target cells, such as the possibility of acquisition or loss of membrane antigens in culture, change in the lysability and expression of antigens with culture, changes in antigenic expression with the phases of the cell cycle, and other factors may influence the results.

The use of trypsin after the incubation to increase the release of radioactivity from cells previously damaged by the effector cells is a method to increase the amount of release of isotope. In our hands, in the systems examined, trypsin did not give positive results not already positive without the trypsin except with certain mouse tumor lines (18, 25).

As with other variations of the microcytotoxicity assay an appropriate base line must be chosen against which to measure activity. Since cells from both unimmunized (may have natural activity) and immunized individuals (may have both immune and natural activity) may be cytotoxic, neutral base lines are needed (29, 30). The media control is especially poor for ^{125}IUdR, since the background release in media control wells is quite variable from experiment to experiment and the release is highly dependent on the number of target cells plated. At low target cell numbers, the media control release values can be quite high (75%), much greater than the release in wells containing effector cells. An autologous control, where unlabeled target cells in equivalent numbers to the effector cells are added to the unlabeled target cell, can be used. Except at extremely high attacker/target (A/T) cell ratios ($>$ 500/1) this neutral background is quite stable (25). In animal model systems we have used adult thymus cells from normal or immune animals since, when added in A/T ratio similar to the lymphocytes, they give little or no activity compared to the autologous control. Not being a tissue culture cell, depletion of nutrients at high A/T ratios is not a problem with thymus cells (29, 30).

In the human assays, we have used the least active normal as the background in most studies. One can calculate cytotoxic indices and use the least active normal as the base line. All the values for normals and for patients can be scatter-grammed against the least active normal, and the degree of activity in each population can be compared against the common base line (28). Alternatively, the median of several normals on each day can be used as the base line, and the experimentals can be related to this value (31).

Most of the problems discussed above are not unique to this assay, but are common to most microcytotoxicity assays (31, 32) and apply in general to most *in vitro* assays of cell-mediated immunity.

REFERENCES

1. Rosenau, W., and Moon, H. D., *J. Natl. Cancer Inst.* **27**, 471 (1961).
2. Takasugi, M., and Klein, E., *Transplantation*, **9**, 219 (1970).
3. Hellström, I., Hellström, K. E., Sjögren, H. O., and Warner, G. A., *Int. J. Cancer* **7**, 1 (1971).
4. Jagarlamoody, S. M., Aust. J. C., Tew, R. H., and McKhann, C. F., *Proc. Natl. Acad. Sci. U.S.A.* **68**, 1346 (1971).
5. Brunner, K. T., Mauel, J., Cerottini, J.-C., and Chapuis, B., *Immunology* **14**, 181 (1968).
6. Canty, T. G., and Wunderlich, J. R., *J. Natl. Cancer Inst.* **45**, 761 (1970).
7. Holm, G., and Perlmann, P., *Immunology* **12**, 525 (1967).
8. Hellström, I., and Hellström, K. E., *Fed. Proc., Fed. Am. Soc. Exp. Biol.* **32**, 156 (1973).
9. Bubenik, J., Perlman, P., and Helmstein, K., *Int. J. Cancer* **5**, 39 (1970).
10. O'Toole, C., Perlmann, P., and Unsgaard, B., *Int. J. Cancer* **10**, 77 (1972).
11. Bloom, E. T., Ossorio, R. C., and Brosman, S. A., *Int. J. Cancer* **14**, 326 (1974).
12. Heppner, G. H., Stolbach, L., and Byrne, M., *Int. J. Cancer* **11**, 245 (1973).
13. Fossati, G., Colnaghi, M. I., and Della Porta, G., *Int. J. Cancer* **8**, 344 (1971).
14. Bean, M. A., Pees, H., and Rosen, G., *Natl. Cancer Inst. Monogr.* **37**, 41 (1973).
15. Bean, M. A., Pees, H., and Fogh, J. E., *Int. J. Cancer* **14**, 186 (1974).
16. Cohen, A. M., Burdick, J. F., and Ketcham, A. S., *J. Immunol.* **107**, 895 (1971).
17. Oldham, R. K., Siwarski, D., McCoy, J. L., Plata, E. J., and Herberman, R. B., *Natl. Cancer Inst. Monogr.* **37**, 49 (1973).
18. Oldham, R. K., and Herberman, R. B., *J. Immunol.* **111**, 1862 (1973).
19. LeMevel, B. P., Oldham, R. K., Wells, S. A., and Herberman, R. B., *J. Natl. Cancer Inst.* **51**, 1551 (1973).
20. Seeger, R. C., Rayner, S. A., and Owen, J. J. T., *Int. J. Cancer* **13**, 697 (1974).
21. LeMevel, B. P., and Wells, S. A., *J. Natl. Cancer Inst.* **50**, 803 (1973).
22. Ting, C. C., Bushar, G. S., Rodrigues, D., and Herberman, R. B., *J. Immunol.* **115**, 1351 (1975).
23. Klein, G., and Perlmann, P., *Nature (London)* **199**, 451 (1963).
24. Hirata, A. A., *J. Immunol.* **91**, 625 (1971).
25. Ting, C. C., and Herberman, R. B., personal communication, 1975.
26. Böyum, A., *Scand. J. Clin. Lab. Invest.* (Suppl. 97) **21**, 1 (1968).
27. Faguet, G. B., *Biomedicine* **21**, 153 (1974).
28. Oldham, R. K., Djeu, J. Y., Cannon, G. B., Siwarski, D., and Herberman, R. B., *J. Natl. Cancer Inst.* **55**, 1305 (1975).

29. Oldham, R. K., Ortaldo, J. R., Holden, H. T., and Herberman, R. B., *J. Natl. Cancer Inst.* (1975). Submitted.
30. Oldham, R. K., Ortaldo, J. R., and Herberman, R. B., *J. Immunol.* (1975). Submitted.
31. Herberman, R. B., Oldham, R. K., and Connor, R. J., this volume, Method 44.
32. Herberman, R. B., and Oldham, R. K., *J. Natl. Cancer Inst.* **55,** 749 (1975).

Tritiated-Proline Microcytotoxicity Assay for the Study of Cellular and Humoral Immune Reactions Directed Against Target Cells Grown in Monolayer Culture*

Michael A. Bean, Yoshihisa Kodera, and Hiroshi Shiku

1. Introduction

In vitro assays for cell-mediated cytotoxicity are in wide use for the investigation of the immune reaction(s) of experimental animals and cancer patients to their tumor cells. The microcytotoxicity test (MCT) originally described by Takasugi and Klein (1) takes advantage of the characteristic of most solid tumors to grow attached to the surface of a culture vessel as "monolayer cultures." Under the conditions of the assay, target cells and lymphoid cells are coincubated for a period of time (24–72 hr) and then the lymphoid cells and dead or dying target cells that have detached from the microtest-well bottom are washed away. Thus, this assay depends on cell detachment as an indicator of target cell death. The number of remaining target cells is enumerated visually after staining. The number of target cells present at the termination of the assay is considered to be the number of target cells surviving and is compared with the number of target cells present in control wells. This assay and the modification of it (2) are now widely used to measure cell-mediated immunity to target cell antigens.

Many investigators, however, have developed radioisotope assays because of difficulties inherent to the original MCT (3–13). Briefly, these difficulties are as follows: (a) Since living, dividing tissue culture cells are used as targets, there is a component of cell growth during the assay. Therefore, the number of cells present at the end of the assay will reflect both cell destruction and effects on cell growth, such as cytostasis (6, 14). (b) Many nonimmunological factors contribute to growth of the target cells in the microwells, different target cells

---

*Abbreviations used: MCT, microcytotoxicity test; MEM, minimal essential medium; FBS, fetal bovine serum; PHA, P/S, phytohemagglutinin; penicillin and streptomycin; NEAA, nonessential amino acids; PBS, phosphate-buffered saline; cpm, counts per minute; PC, peritoneal cells; EBSS, Earle's balanced salt solution; F-H, Ficoll–Hypaque.

grow at different rates, and there is a difference in the growth fraction between short-term and established cell cultures. Also, the division rate of target cells may be influenced by pH, humidity, CO_2 gradients, and "feeder effects" caused by the addition of effector cells. (c) Visual counting of remaining tumor target cells is time consuming, tedious, and sometimes subjective. Because of these difficulties we devised a modification of the MCT utilizing ^{3}H-proline-prelabeled target cells in order to have a truer estimate of target cell death and to eliminate the tedious and time-consuming subjective visual counting of remaining cells.

In this assay (see Fig. 1), the number of target cell counts per minute (cpm) remaining after incubation with effector cells, serum, or combinations thereof is used as an indicator of the number of target cells surviving. And, by using prelabeled target cells, we eliminate the contribution of cell growth to the test result (6–8, 14). We have found ^{3}H-proline to be particularly well suited for this purpose for the following reasons: (a) A minimum of handling of the cultures is required as the cells are labeled prior to trypsinization and seeding. (b) There is no reutilization of the isotope, as a considerable excess of nontoxic unlabeled proline is readily available as a medium supplement in the form of nonessential amino acids. This is not the case for other commonly used labeling techniques. (c) High levels of label are incorporated throughout the nucleus and cytoplasm of the target cell with little toxicity compared to DNA precursor labels where the isotope is (i) concentrated in the nucleus and (ii) has chemical toxicity. (d) Cultures in all phases of growth, of human and nonhuman origin, and from short- and long-term culture adequately and easily incorporate ^{3}H-proline in contrast to ^{125}I-iododeoxyuridine (4), which can be used only with some difficulty with early cultures of human tumors where the growth fraction is small or where medium conditions are not optimal for cell division (11). (e) ^{3}H-Proline is adequately retained through the long assay periods in contrast to ^{51}Cr which, although used successfully with some monolayer culture cells (12, 15), has a high rate of spontaneous release (14). (f) ^{3}H-Proline has a long half-life allowing plates to be processed at the investigator's convenience, in contrast to an isotope such as technetium 99m, which has a half-life of 6 hr (13) and thus would decay 8 half-lives in the course of a 48-hr assay (less than 0.02% of starting label would remain), not to mention the decay of isotope that would occur during the processing and counting of the well bottoms from a relatively complicated experiment.

We have found this ^{3}H-proline MCT to be a useful tool in the study of cellular immune reactions in murine systems to both allograft and syngeneic tumor antigens (8, 9), of human cell-mediated immune responses to tumor cells (7) and antibody-dependent cell-mediated cytotoxicity directed against alloantigens, blood group antigens, and to melanoma-associated antigens (10).

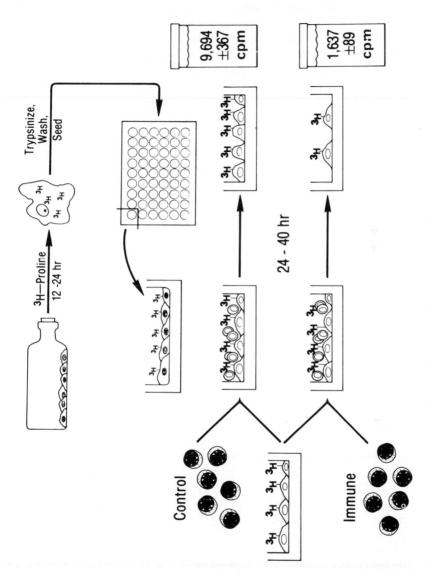

Fig. 1. Tritiated-proline microcytotoxicity assay.

2. Materials

2.1. Tritiated-Proline Stock Solution. ^{3}H-Proline [obtained from either New England Nuclear, Boston, Massachusetts (NET-323 L-proline-2,3-^{3}H-N) or from Schwartz BioResearch, Orangeburg, New York (L-proline-5-^{3}H)] with specific activities of 20–50 Ci/mmole is made into a stock solution of 100 μCi/ml in the labeling medium described below, with sufficient extra 10 × MEM added to balance the salts diluted by the carrier solution (0.01 N HCl). The solution is then filtered through a 0.45-μm filter for sterilization, aliquoted, and stored at −20°C.

2.2. Labeling Medium. Eagle's minimal essential medium (MEM) of any brand name with Earle's balanced salt solution (EBSS) is adjusted to contain 15% prescreened fetal bovine serum (FBS), 100 units of penicillin (P), and 100 μg of streptomycin (S) per milliliter, and 2 mM final concentration of freshly reconstituted lympholyzed glutamine. No nonessential amino acids (NEAA) (which contains proline) is added to this solution. If using some other medium, check to make sure that it does not already contain proline.

2.3. Medium for Assay. The medium for use in the MCT consists of MEM supplemented with P/S, 2 mM glutamine, and 1% NEAA (normal tissue culture concentration). The NEAA contributes unlabeled proline at a final concentration of 11.5 μg/ml. Calculations show that this provides a ratio of greater than 10^6 unlabeled to labeled proline molecules. The medium is adjusted to contain 10% heat-inactivated prescreened FBS. For use in murine experiments, 2-mercaptoethanol is added at 5 × 10^{-5} M (8, 9).

2.4. Medium for Washing Microtest Plates. Calcium- and magnesium-containing phosphate-buffered saline (PBS), pH 7.2, containing either 5% FBS or calf serum is used for washing the microtest plates.

2.5. Fetal Calf Serum. Samples of FBS from several different companies are screened for suitability in the microtest systems. This screening procedure consists of testing human and murine established and short-term tumor cell cultures for plating efficiency and support of cell growth. In addition, the sera are tested to determine their ability to support proliferation of both human leukocytes and murine lymph node cells to PHA and in mixed-leukocyte culture while giving low spontaneous background stimulation. Once a suitable batch has been selected it is stored frozen (−20°C) and used exclusively for assays over a period of 6 months to a year.

3. Methods

3.1. Labeling of Target Cells
3.1.1. A T 30 (25 cm^2) or T 60 (75 cm^2) tissue culture flask containing monolayer target cells in good growth phase are selected for labeling (60–80%

confluence is best, but both extremely light and extremely heavy cultures will label adequately for the test).

3.1.2. The medium from the tissue culture flask is decanted and the monolayer is washed gently with 37°C labeling medium 3 times with 10 ml each for T 60's and with 3 ml each for T 30's. The final wash is left on the monolayer until ready for the next step.

3.1.3. When ready, the flask is labeled with 50 μCi/ml of ³H-proline in labeling medium by decanting the wash fluid and adding either 5 ml for a T 60 flask or 2 ml for a T 30 flask. The flasks are then usually incubated overnight (18 hr) so that incorporation of label into the target cells can proceed. We have found both shorter and longer labeling periods (8–24 hr) to also be satisfactory depending upon the metabolism of the target cells.

3.2. Trypsinization and Seeding of Target Cells

3.2.1. At the end of the labeling period decant the radioisotope-containing solution.

3.2.2. Gently wash the monolayer of tumor cells in the T 60 3 times each with 10 ml of 37°C labeling medium to which 2% NEAA have been added as an excess of unlabeled proline (3 ml each time for a T 30). Decant third wash when ready to trypsinize.

3.2.3. Add 10 ml of fresh trypsin solution (0.25%) or Tryptar (Armour Pharmaceuticals, 0.05% in Puck's saline A) and incubate at 37°C with gentle shaking until the tumor cells detach from the surface. Remove the trypsinized cell suspension, and neutralize the trypsin by adding to labeling medium with 2% NEAA.

3.2.4. Centrifuge the cells into a pellet at 150–200 g at room temperature, decant the supernatant fluid, resuspend the pellet, add medium, and repeat centrifugation. After removing the last supernatant, gently resuspend the pellet and then add 2–3 ml of assay medium. Mix well and transfer to a 15-ml siliconized glass or plastic centrifuge tube and allow to stand for 2–3 min at room temperature in order for any clumps to settle. Starting at the meniscus, gently remove 1.5–2.5 ml of supernatant, avoiding clumps. Count viable cells with 0.1 ml of cell suspension plus 0.1 ml of trypan blue and adjust to a final concentration of 10^5 cells/ml for dispensing into wells of Falcon Microtest II plates (No. 3040) in 10-μl volumes using a Hamilton microliter syringe resulting in 1000 target cells/well. Odd rows are seeded first and then even rows. The microtest plates are prefilled with 0.1 ml of assay medium before adding the labeled target cells in order to give a more even distribution of target cells across the bottom of the microtest plate wells.

3.2.5. The microtest plates prefilled with 0.1 ml of test medium and 10 μl of labeled target cells can be used immediately by the addition of effector cells in 0.1 ml of assay medium or the plates can be incubated overnight before the addition of effector cells.

3.3. Experimental Design. All test combinations to be compared are performed within one microtest plate. Samples are tested in replicates of 4 or 5 wells in a cluster.

3.3.1. Murine Models. For assaying cell-mediated cytotoxicity in the mouse models (8, 9), effector cells are tested at a high dose of 250,000 cells/well with doubling dilutions as needed and as the availability of cells permits. Wells containing no effector cells, nonimmune effector cells, and effector cells immune to an unrelated antigen are also included as controls on any given target cell. Cytotoxicity or the survival fraction is then determined in reference to the number of target cell cpm remaining after incubation with the test effector cells compared to the number of target cell cpm remaining after incubation with nonimmune effector cells. These same effector cell combinations are run simultaneously on an unrelated target cell for proof of specificity and for detection of nonselective effects such as occur with *in vitro*-sensitized effector cells.

3.3.2. Human Models. For assaying cell-mediated cytotoxicity (7) with human blood leukocytes or lymph node cells, tests are run under similar conditions to those described for the murine models. However, controls are not as easily defined. We try to include, at minimum, effector cells from two unselected normal healthy donors and from two patients with unrelated diseases in addition to the "test" patient(s) effector cells within any given experiment. Comparison is then made to the activity of the normal donors on a given target cell. And, at minimum, two unrelated target cells are tested. Fibroblast cultures are considered unsatisfactory for control target cells as they are not very susceptible to spontaneous cytolysis or to PHA-induced destruction by human effector cells.

For detection of lymphocyte dependent antibody (10), assays are performed with the following variations: Preselected active normal donors are used as a source of effector cells and used at 250,000/well in replicates of 4 with 1000 ^{3}H-proline-labeled target cells/well. After seeding the target cells and prior to or soon after the addition of effector cells, heat-inactivated human normal and test serum are added to the respective wells. Dilutions of serum to give a final concentration of 1:20 and less are added in 10-μl aliquots and serum tested at the 1:5 dilution is added neat at 0.05 ml/well. The plates are then incubated 24–40 hr at 37°C in a 5% CO_2 in humidified air atmosphere. An important control for assessment of the activity of the more concentrated serum dilutions is the inclusion of titrations of FCS in addition to that already contained in the assay medium, as high concentrations of serum may give feeder effects depending on the target cell being tested.

3.4. Effector Cell Preparation *3.4.1. Murine Effector Cells.* Mice are killed by cervical dislocation. To obtain unfractionated peritoneal cells (PC), a transverse midventral incision is made and the abdominal muscles and fascia are exposed. Through a 26-gauge needle, 5 ml of EBSS with 2.5% FBS and 25 U of heparin per milliliter is injected into the peritoneal cavity. After gentle agitation, the fluid is aspirated and pooled in siliconized tubes. The unfractionated PC are washed twice in EBSS with serum and resuspended in assay medium. To obtain nonadherent PC, unfractionated PC are incubated in T 60 glass flasks at 3×10^6 to 5×10^6 cells/ml in 10–15 ml assay medium for 2 hr at 37°C. The supernatant is then transferred to another flask and again incubated for 2 hr at 37°C. The cells remaining in the supernatant after the second incubation are referred to as "nonadherent PC." Spleen and lymph node cells are prepared by gentle teasing to spill the cells. The cells are then washed twice in EBSS with serum and resuspended in assay medium. Clumps are removed by spontaneous sedimentation. For assays with murine cells, 2-mercaptoethanol is always included in the media used to process the cells and the assay medium at 5×10^{-5} M, as it increases both viability and activity of the effector cells (8, 9).

3.4.2. Human Effector Cells Preparation. Lymphoid effector cells are purified in two ways. Freshly drawn venous blood is defribinated in sterile Erlenmeyer flasks containing 3-mm glass beads. For Ficoll–Hypaque separation (10), an aliquot of 20 ml of defribinated blood is diluted with an equal volume of PBS, underlayered with 10 ml of Ficoll–Hypaque (FH) solution of specific gravity 1.077, and centrifuged at 400 g at the interface for 40 min at room temperature. The interface is aspirated, diluted with EBSS containing 2.5% FBS, and centrifuged at 500 g for 10 min to collect the cell pellet. These cells are then resuspended at 4 to 8×10^6 cells/ml in assay medium and incubated in glass tissue culture flasks for 1 hr in order to remove the adherent cells. The unattached cells are then washed twice more prior to use.

Effector cells purified by gelatin sedimentation are prepared as described previously (7). One part of 3% edible gelatin (Peter Leiner and Sons, Glamorgan, England) in Hanks' balanced salt solution is added to three parts of defribinated blood, and the mixture is incubated upright in an appropriate sized sterile plastic syringe for 45–60 min at 37°C. The supernatant serum containing leukocytes is then incubated on scrubbed nylon fiber for 30 min at 37°C. After elution with EBSS containing 2.5% FBS, the cells are sedimented by centrifugation and resuspended in a small volume of medium. For Tris-NH$_4$Cl treatment, the effector cells in 2 ml of medium are treated with 16 ml of pH 7.2 Tris-NH$_4$Cl (0.83% NH$_4$Cl) for 5 min at 37°C and then washed three times.

The final effector cell preparations with either method routinely contain more than 95% mononuclear cells as determined by staining with crystal violet in acetic acid and by tetrachrome staining of air-dried smears. Viability is always greater than 98% as measured by trypan blue exclusion.

The Ficoll–Hypaque prepared effector cells are used in the assay for antibody-dependent cell-mediated cytotoxicity. The gelatin preparation is used for the cell-mediated cytotoxicity assays. However, recent work has shown that the Tris-NH$_4$Cl treatment reduces effector cell activity in ADCMC, and therefore this preparative technique will have to be modified for future studies of CMC in humans (10, 20).

3.5. Termination of the MCT. The microtest plates are washed by inverting them and gently shaking to allow the medium to drop out. They are then returned to the upright position and submerged into a pan twice the height of the microtest plates filled with 37°C PBS containing 5% FBS. This step is then repeated twice; after the final shaking, the surface of the microtest plate is blotted dry and the plates are returned to the upright position and allowed to dry before processing (2 hr or longer at room temperature). Washing of the test plates without serum in the wash medium will result in loss of some viable target cells from the well bottom (6), even with unlabeled target cells.

3.6. Processing of Microtest Plate Well Bottoms for Liquid Scintillation Counting. After the microtest plates are thoroughly dry, they are sprayed with Fluoroglide (film bonding grade, Chemplast, Inc., Wayne, New Jersey) to prevent isotope loss. The well bottoms are punched out by means of a hand-operated can punch press (Roper-Whitney, Rockford, Illinois, with a cutting dye 6.528 mm in diameter and a punch 6.350 mm in diameter). Hyamine of hydroxide (Packard Instrument Co.), 0.3 ml, is then added at room temperature to the scintillation vials containing well bottoms for 30 min prior to the addition of scintillation fluid. The scintillation fluid is a toluene base with PPO and dimethyl POPOP. The vials are then capped tightly and kept at 4°C for 24 hr in order to completely solubilize the protein and for the well bottoms to dissolve in the toluene. Addition of the Hyamine of hydroxide is not an absolute requirement, but will nearly double the cpm, resulting in less counting time. We are currently in the process of changing to Mini Vials for reduced costs.

4. Interpretation and Comments

Using this assay we measure the target cell cpm remaining after incubation of prelabeled target cells with lymphoid cells, antibody, etc., as a measure of the number of target cells surviving treatment. Under properly controlled conditions, detachment of target cells is a reliable measure of cell death (cytolysis) and is reflected as a net loss of target cells from the surface. This has been confirmed by trypan blue staining of the detached cells, by release of ^{3}H isotope into the medium, and by time-lapse cinemaphotography in addition to replating experiments. It should be obvious, however, that cell detachment need not always be a reflection of cell death (e.g., as in the case of the commonly used trypsinization procedures for passage of monolayer culture cells).

A consideration that must be kept in mind when discussing isotope assays is the difference between prelabeling and postlabeling. Investigators have used postlabeling of target cells with a variety of isotopes including ^{51}Cr (16) and even ^{3}H-proline (17) in order to quantitate objectively the number of target cells remaining at termination of the assay. Postlabeling with isotope can be viewed as an improvement over visual counting but does not negate the difficulties inherent to the original MCT (1) caused by target cell growth. However, the use of such an assay in conjunction with a prelabel assay should allow the investigator to make assessments of the cytostatic component of effector cell activity (17).

We have found that selection of FBS for these assays is especially important for clear-cut experimental results. We select sera for high plating efficiency and support of growth of cultured cells and for low spontaneous stimulation of blastogenic response of lymphocytes. Use of a single lot of such serum over time will result in less day-to-day variation in assays, and the addition of effector cells to the target cells will have little or no feeder effect. In cases where the target cells were plated in less than optimal medium, we had observed that quite often the addition of control effector cells would increase the plating efficiency of the target cells and result in more target cell CPM remaining in the presence of effector cells than there were in the medium alone owing to conditioning of the medium caused by the lymphoid cells. Controls for each assay include medium alone, lymphoid cells alone, serum alone, and combinations thereof. All these are important internal controls. We calculate percent survival in reference to the number of target cell cpm remaining after incubation with the experimental lymphocytes compared to the target cell cpm remaining in the control donor lymphocyte wells.

No definite statements can be made at this time as to what is the "correct" procedure for purification of human blood leukocytes for demonstration of cell-mediated cytotoxicity, as it is apparent that different preparative techniques produce effector cells containing different proportions of T, B, null, and non lymphocytic cells in addition to giving different absolute yields and different results in the same and different microcytotoxicity tests (18). We had thought previously (6, 7) that gelatin sedimentation of red blood cells with incubation of the leukocyte-rich plasma on nylon followed by lysis of the residual red blood cells by Tris-NH_4Cl was the best method, but must now reconsider this matter, as we have found the Tris-NH_4Cl treatment reduces significantly the effector cell lytic activity in antibody-dependent cell-mediated cytotoxicity (10). Thus, in the human bladder tumor system where antibody-dependent cell-mediated cytotoxicity has been implicated as an effector system (15, 19), the effector-cell preparative technique commonly used for these studies diminishes the sought-after activity (7, 10, 15). It would appear from preliminary work in our laboratory (10) and elsewhere (20) that while NH_4Cl inhibits the lytic function of K cells it does not inhibit their binding to target cells. Therefore, it is possible that activity may still be detected in the Takasugi and Klein MCT (1) through the binding of effector cells to the target cells producing a cytostatic influence through the mechanism of contact inhibition. Experiments are in progress to clarify these issues.

ACKNOWLEDGMENTS

Work supported in part by the United States Public Health Service Grants CA-19165 and CA-08748 and by Virginia Mason Research Center Grant No. 229.

REFERENCES

1. Takasugi, M., and Klein, E., *Transplantation* **9**, 219 (1970).
2. Hellström, I., and Hellström, K. E., *in* "*In Vitro* Methods in Cell-Mediated Immunity" (B. R. Bloom and P. R. Glade, eds.), p. 409. Academic Press, New York, 1971.
3. Jagarlamoody, S. M., Aust, J. C., Tew, R. H., and McKhann, C. F., *Proc. Natl. Acad. Sci. U.S.A.* **68**, 1346 (1971).
4. Cohen, A. M., Millar, R. C., and Ketcham, A. S., *Transplantation* **13**, 57 (1972).
5. Hashimoto, Y., and Sudo, H., *Gann* **62**, 139 (1971).
6. Bean, M. A., Pees, H., Rosen, G., and Oettgen, H. F., *Natl. Cancer Inst. Monog.* **37**, 41 (1973).
7. Bean, M. A., Pees, H., Fogh, J. E., Grabstald, H., and Oettgen, H. F., *Int. J. Cancer* **14**, 186 (1974).
8. Shiku, H., Bean, M. A., Old, L. H., and Oettgen, H. F., *J. Natl. Cancer Inst.* **54**, 415 (1975).
9. Shiku, H., Kisielow, P., Bean, M. A., Takahashi, T., Boyse, E. A., Oettgen, H. F., and Old, L. J., *J. Exp. Med.* **141**, 227 (1975).
10. Kodera, Y., and Bean, M. A., *Int. J. Cancer* **16**, 579 (1975).
11. Oldham, R. K., Djeu, J. Y., Cannon, G. B., Siwarski, D., and Herberman, R. B., *J. Natl. Canc. Inst.* **55**, 1305 (1975).
12. Berke, G., Ax, W., Ginsburg, H., and Feldman, M., *Immunology* **16**, 643 (1969).
13. Barth, R. F., and Gillespie, G. Y., *Cell. Immunol.* **10**, 38 (1974).
14. Perlmann, P., and Holm, C., *Adv. Immunol.* **11**, 117 (1969).
15. O'Toole, C., Stejskal, V., Perlmann, P., and Karlsson, M., *J. Exp. Med.* **139**, 457 (1974).
16. Levy, N. L., Seigler, H. F., and Shingleton, W. W., *Cancer* **34**, 1548 (1974).
17. Bataillon, G., Pross, H., and Klein, G., *Int. J. Cancer* **16**, 255 (1975).
18. Bean, M. A., Bloom, B. R., Herberman, R. B., Old, L. J., Oettgen, H. F., Klein, G., and Terry, W. D., *Cancer Res.* **35**, 2902 (1975).
19. Hakala, T. R., Lange, P. H., Castro, A. E., Elliot, A. Y., and Fraley, E. E., *N. Engl. J. Med.* **291**, 637 (1974).
20. Yust, I., Smith, R. W., Wunderlich, J. R., and Mann, D., *J. Immunol.* **116**, 1170 (1976).

Statistical Analysis and Selection of
Baseline Controls in Cytotoxicity Assays

Ronald B. Herberman, Robert K. Oldham and Robert J. Connor

1. Introduction

Considerable variation exists among laboratories and investigators in the procedures used to describe and analyze the results of cytotoxicity studies. This variation occurs with ^{51}Cr release assays (1–3) and other isotopic assays (4–7), as well as with the visual microcytotoxicity assays (8–10).

While differences occur throughout the entire handling of the cytotoxicity results, the most prominent areas of disparity are: the selection of a base-line control, the formula and procedures describing cytotoxicity, and the statistical methods for testing the results. The various decisions made on these points have a large impact in the reported magnitude of the immune reactivity and on the apparent specificity of the reactions.

For some time (11), we have been concerned about the effects of these issues on the interpretation of results in cytotoxicity assays. In the analyses recommended here, procedures have been used that tend to take into account problems inherent in the assays and tend to reflect the true differences between "experimental" groups. These procedures, we believe, are conservative and, hence, provide numbers that are often considerably smaller than those reported elsewhere. This disparity may be due to an underestimation by these conservative procedures or due to others magnifying the differences, or more likely to a combination of these factors.

2. Methods

There are two aspects to our recommended statistical treatment of the data, the descriptive procedures and the testing procedures. These are given below using a "baseline control" and a "total incorporation value," both of which must be defined. Our recommendations for these are presented later (see Sections 2.4, 3.1., and 3.4).

2.1. Descriptive Statistics

2.1.1. In ^{51}Cr release assays, the results are most often reported using the percent increase in cytotoxicity from some "baseline control" percent cytotoxicity. We follow this practice for the ^{51}Cr release assay and also for other isotopic assays (6) and use

$$\text{"Baseline control" \% cytotoxicity} = \frac{\text{cpm}_{bc} - \text{cpm}_{bk}}{\text{cpm}_t - \text{cpm}_{bk}} \times 100$$

and

$$\text{\% Increase in cytotoxicity} = \frac{\text{cpm}_{exp} - \text{cpm}_{bc}}{\text{cpm}_t - \text{cpm}_{bk}} \times 100$$

where cpm_{bc} is the average of the four replicate counts per minute of isotope released into the supernatant for the baseline control in the experiment; cpm_{bk} is the average for the counter background; cpm_t is the average for the total counts per minute incorporated into the cells at the onset of the experiment; and cpm_{exp} is the average counts per minute released into the supernatant for an "experimental" individual tested in the experiment. The selection of the baseline control is discussed in Sections 2.4 and 3.4, and the selection of total incorporation for the denominator is discussed in Section 3.1. To indicate roughly the variability of the percent increase, an approximate standard error is calculated. The formula for this is

$$\frac{\text{cpm}_{exp} - \text{cpm}_{bc}}{\text{cpm}_t - \text{cpm}_{bk}} \left[\left(\frac{\text{Var}(\text{cpm}_{exp})}{n_{exp}} + \frac{\text{Var}(\text{cpm}_{bc})}{n_{bc}} \right) \middle/ (\text{cpm}_{exp} - \text{cpm}_{bc})^2 \right.$$
$$\left. + \left(\frac{\text{Var}(\text{cpm}_t)}{n_t} + \frac{\text{Var}(\text{cpm}_{bk})}{n_{bk}} \right) \quad (\text{cpm}_t - \text{cpm}_{bk})^2 \right]^{1/2}$$

where $\text{Var}(X)$ is variance of X and n_X represents the number of replicates for the X average (12).

Note that in many cases the formula is simplified by dropping the second term, because the second term usually is small relative to the first (i.e., the total incorporation average is usually much greater than its standard deviation whereas the experimental individual's average is often not very much greater than its standard deviation). However, this simplification can give deceptively small standard errors when the increase in cytotoxicity is substantial.

2.1.2. Often in visual microcytoxocity assays (8–10) and occasionally in isotopic assay (4, 7) the results are expressed by a cytotoxic index. We do this using the formula

$$\text{Cytotoxic index (C.I.)} = \frac{\text{cpm}'_{exp}}{\text{cpm}'_{bc}}$$

where cpm'_{exp} is the average of four replicates of cells or counts per minute *remaining* in cells at the end of the incubation period of an "experimental" individual, cpm'_{bc} is the average remaining in the cells of four replicates of the experiment's baseline control, and $cpm'_X + cpm_X = cpm_t$ defined earlier. A common variant of this measure is the percent reduction which is

$$\text{Percent reduction} = (1 - \text{C.I.}) \times 100$$

As a guide for the variability of this measure, an approximate standard error can be calculated. The formula for the standard error is analogous to the one given for the percent increase in cytotoxicity. It is

$$\frac{cpm'_{exp}}{cpm'_{bc}} \left(\frac{[\text{Var}(cpm'_{exp})]}{n_{exp}} \middle/ (cpm'_{exp})^2 + \frac{[\text{Var}(cpm'_{bc})]}{n_{bc}} \middle/ (cpm'_{bc})^2 \right)^{1/2}$$

Note that the above two descriptive measures, percent increase in cytotoxicity and cytotoxic index, are recommended, along with their standard errors, only to describe or report the experimental results.

2.2. "Testing" Procedures.   In the cytotoxicity assays, the average results for each individual in an experiment are compared with the average results of the baseline control for that experiment. Our philosophy is that a significant test (p <0.05) allows us to characterize differences in reactivity as "true"; we then pool the results over experiments to obtain the proportion of "true differences." The proportions can be tested with the $2 \times k$ contingency table method for comparison of several proportions (12).

The differences in reactivity between an experimental group and the base-line control are tested using the four cpm's observed for each by Welch's modification of student's t test (12). Any differences that have a p value less than 0.05 in this test are called true differences (they can be significantly more or less reactive than the baseline control). Note that the tests are based on the raw cpm's of each group, not the descriptive measures of Section 2.1 (e.g., percent increase in cytotoxicity).

2.3. Data Transformation and Editing.   In our experience with data obtained in cytotoxicity studies, we have observed that the variation of the raw counts (as measured by the standard deviation) has tended to be proportional to the average of the counts. This relationship suggests that a logarithmic transformation of the data be used to stabilize the variance (see 12). Thus, as part of our statistical "testing" of the data, logs are taken of the raw counts before any calculations are done. Note, however, the results are reported using the original values (e.g., the formula for percent increase in cytotoxicity uses the raw counts).

Also we have learned that occasional disparate values occur. Hence we use a data-editing procedure (13) to detect such disparate values ("outliers"). This provides us with an objective method to test for extreme values among the quadruplicate values obtained for each individual tested. Values found extreme at the 0.01 level are deleted. (See Section 3.2 for further discussion on this topic.)

2.4. Baseline Control. The selection of a baseline control in the above calculations is important. For the short-term ^{51}Cr release (14) [and for other isotopic assays with some target cells obtained from experimental animals (6)] the "autologous control" have been a satisfactory choice as a baseline control. For this control, unlabeled target cells are used in place of (at the same concentration) the attacker lymphoid cells.

A similar baseline control, which has been quite satisfactory in our tests with animal target cells, is the use of normal thymus cells as nonreactive lymphocytes in place of attacker lymphoid cells (R. K. Oldham, J. Ortaldo, and R. B. Herberman, unpublished observations).

The baseline controls most widely used for the human studies and one which also has been most satisfactory for some animal target cells (C.-C. Ting and R. B. Herberman, unpublished observations) is a control with lymphocytes from normal individuals. We have elected, in studies where the autologous control cannot be used, to "randomly select" (see Section 3.4) one to five normal adults for testing in each experiment and up to quite recently have used the "least active" of these as the baseline normal control (7). However, there are several problems with this approach. For example, experiments with several normals will tend to give more "true actives" than those with few normals. Therefore, we now recommend that the normal with the median activity among the normals be selected as the baseline control (i.e., if we rank normals by increasing reactivity, the median active normal is the $\frac{1}{2}(n+1)$th one for n odd and the $\frac{1}{2}n$th one for n even). This procedure is not without its problems (e.g., it is more likely to give a high estimate for nonreacting normals), but it is simple to apply and it gives a relatively consistent baseline from experiment to experiment even if the number of normals varies. We believe the benefits of other approaches (e.g., the mean of the normals, or the least active normal with an adjustment for the number of normals) are outweighed by their complexity.

3. Critical Comments

3.1. In ^{51}Cr release assays, there is considerable variation among laboratories in the term used in the denominator of the formula to calculate percent cytotoxicity. The most frequently used values are those designed to represent the maximum ^{51}Cr that can be released from the cells upon total lysis. Many laboratories have felt this to be desirable, since with most target cells, at least 10% of the incorporated isotope remains in the cell sediment regardless of the lysis procudure used. Although we previously used the values obtained by freezing and thawing the target cells three (15) or four times (16, 17), we have recently abandoned this in favor of using the total counts per minute incorporated into the target cells. This is because some target cells are rather resistant to lysis by freezing and thawing, and some are also resistant to lysis by incubation in distilled water or treatment with agents like saponin or Triton (other procedures used in some laboratories to achieve "maximal" lysis). Furthermore, the same cell line may vary considerably among experiments in its susceptibility to damage by these procedures. In some cases, these procedures cause a release of only 50–60% of the ^{51}Cr. The use of such values in the formula yield high and variable baseline control and experimental levels of cytotoxicity. In some instances, using low maximum release values as denominator in the formula gives experimental percent cytotoxicity levels above 100%, clearly indicating the artificiality of the "maximum" lysis determined by a method quite independent of that used in the test.

In the same vein, many investigators subtract the baseline control counts per minute from the denominator in the formula to calculate percent cytotoxicity (e.g., 1). This formula is equivalent to percent reduction

$$\text{Percent reduction} = \frac{\text{cpm}'_{bc} - \text{cpm}'_{exp}}{\text{cpm}'_{bc}}$$

$$= \frac{\text{cpm}_{exp} - \text{cpm}_{bc}}{\text{cpm}_{t} - \text{cpm}_{bc}}$$

since $\text{cpm}'_X + \text{cpm}'_X = \text{cpm}_t$. This has little effect when the baseline control is low, e.g., less than 10%. However, with high baseline controls, as sometimes seen, e.g., with cryopreserved human leukemia cells (16), this procedure substantially reduces the denominator and magnifies the experimental percent cytotoxicity by as much as 2- or 3-fold.

3.2. Our experience with these assays is that occasional experimental errors occur and give rise to disparate or extreme values among replicate observations. When such errors are recognized, the values are discarded because they clearly do not reflect the true reactivity. Unfortunately all such errors are not detected, and thus, when we observe an extreme value among the replicates, it is likely to be the result of some unnoticed technical error. Rather than subjectively deleting such values, we recommend that a statistical test for "outliers" (extreme observations) be used. The procedure we have adopted (13) uses the results of the whole experiment in evaluating extreme observations for each individual's quadruplicate set of values. Because deleting an observation among a set of replicates is difficult (when no technical error is known to have occurred), we consider a value to be an "outlier" and delete it only when the test gives a p value of 0.01 or less; also we carry out the entire analysis both with and without the outliers included. In this way we can see whether there are substantial differences in the results, which would make interpretation of the experiment difficult, and if so, include reference to the discrepancy in our presentation of the results.

3.3. We feel that it is preferable to describe the results using percent increase in cytotoxicity rather than cytotoxic indices or percent reduction relative to control. Although the percent increase in cytotoxicity is generally used in ^{51}Cr release assays, the other terms are much more widely used in visual microcyto-toxicity assays (8–10) and in assays with other isotopes (4, 7). It should be pointed out that both the cytotoxic index and the percent reduction are different from, but related to, percent increase in cytotoxicity. Only the percent cytotoxicity uses as denominator the total cells or cpm in these cells that are added into the test. Since those values are always much higher than those remaining at the end of the incubation period in the baseline controls (the denominator in the cytotoxic index or percent reduction), the percent cyto-toxicity in the experimental group above that in the baseline control is usually much lower than the percent reduction. When the percent cytotoxicity of the baseline control is high, this magnifies the difference, sometimes to a remark-able extent (e.g., see 5). This can be seen from the fact that

$$\frac{\text{percent reduction}}{\text{percent increase in cytotoxicity}} = \frac{\text{cpm}_t}{\text{cpm}_t - \text{cpm}_{bc}}$$

(assuming cpm_t is much larger than cpm_{bc}) and hence the greater cpm_{bc}, the greater the ratio.

Note that our statistical testing procedures are unaffected by these considera-tions because we use the raw data (transformed) in our tests, not these measures.

3.4. We have become increasingly concerned about the baseline control to be used in cytotoxicity assays. Comparisons, particularly in visual microcyto-toxicity assays (e.g., 9, 10), are often made relative to the medium control. Our experience is that this is often an artificial control, bearing little relationship to the values seen in groups with attacker cells of any type present. Frequently, particularly in the isotopic assays, and when the target cells are not in a state of optimal viability, we have seen much higher percent cytotoxicity values in the medium control than in other controls (e.g., 18). This is probably related to the frequent need for target cells, in order to maintain viability, to be in the presence of a higher cell concentration than that present in the medium control. Conversely, in the visual microcytotoxicity assay with some target cells, addition of lymphocytes from any source will give cytotoxicity above the medium control. This may be due to sensitivity of these target cells to depletion of essential components in the medium by the lymphocytes. The development of the autologous control was to correct for these problems and yet retain a neutral base-line. This has worked well in the short-term ^{51}Cr release assay, where frequently the values obtained with lymphocytes from some normal individuals are not significantly different from the autologous control (19, 20). In the assays involving incubation for 24–48 hr, with some target cells, particularly at high A/T ratios, the autologous controls may be unsatisfactory (C.-C. Ting and R. B. Herberman, unpublished observations). In those systems, and rather routinely in the long-term assays in human tumor systems, where it is more difficult to assess the adequacy of the autologous control, we have used lymphocytes from normal adult donors as controls. This type of control remains the most common one used for visual microcytotoxicity assays. However, when this control is used, it is important to do so in a manner that will still allow examination of cytotoxic reactivity of normal individuals. It has recently become quite clear that many normal rodents (19, 20) and humans (7, 17, 21, 22) have cytotoxic reactivity against a variety of tumor or tissue culture target cells. In the human microcytotoxicity assays, we have handled this problem by testing in each experiment several normal donors chosen at random (i.e., without any selection according to previous testing in the assay). The median reactive normal against each cell line is recommended for use as the baseline control. This will permit, within an experiment, differences in reactivity among normals as well as among patients to be studied. This procedure also permits comparison of data among different experiments as to whether, as a population, normal controls are as reactive as cancer patients against a given target cell. The median reactive normal control provides a more stable baseline than most others that are now used. However, we still do not consider this to be an optimal solution. When different laboratories performed assays with the same attacker and target cells (23), it was necessary to arbitrarily to select a common baseline, one normal individual, to adequately compare the results. It would be preferable, both for comparisons of results among experiments within a laboratory and for comparison of results between laboratories, to use a standard reagent as baseline in each experiment. We are now investigating the use of a cryopreserved pool of normal lymphocytes as the baseline for each test.

When the median reactive normal or a randomly selected normal donor, is used as the baseline, it is then quite possible to see both normals and patients with cytotoxic indices significantly above 1, or negative values for percent reduction (23). This type of outcome should be reported in any analysis, but not arbitrarily set to zero percent reduction, as has been frequently done. The use of multiple normal individuals in an experiment is also important in that it decreases the possibility of seeing "specific" reactivity of a cancer patient against a tumor line based on the choice of one normal control with low reactivity against that line.

3.5. It is quite useful to perform tests using more than one A/T ratio for each attacker cell population. This permits the generation of dose–response curves and more accurate quantitative comparison of reactivity among different attackers. Although this works quite well in most short-term ^{51}Cr release assays (e.g., 24) and in the proline assay (7), good dose–response relationships are often not seen in the visual microcytotoxicity assays. This presumably is due to technical problems in the assays and physical effects of the different numbers of cells in the wells. In any event, using more than one A/T ratio may complicate interpretation of results, particularly when the same attacker population is significantly more reactive than the control at one A/T ratio and significantly less reactive than the baseline control at another (e.g., see 23). Despite these complexities, we recommend that multiple doses of effector cells be used.

REFERENCES

1. Brunner, K. T., Mauel, J., Cerottini, J.-C., and Chapius, B., *Immunology* 14, 81 (1967).
2. Canty, T. G., and Wunderlich, J. R., *J. Natl. Cancer Inst.* 45, 761 (1970).
3. Simpson, E., O'Hopp, S., and Wunderlich, J., *Transplantation* 8, 734 (1974).
4. Cohen, A. M. Burdick, J. F., and Ketcham A. S., *J. Immunol.* 107, 895 (1971).
5. Oldham R. K., *in* "Conference and Workshop on Cellular Immune Reactions to Human Tumor-Associated Antigens" (R. B. Herberman, and C. E. Gaylord, eds.), *Natl. Cancer Inst. Monogr.* 37, 125 (1973).
6. Oldham, R. K., and Herberman, R. B., this volume, Method 42.
7. Oldham, R. K., Djeu, J. Y., Cannon, G. B., Siwarski, D., and Herberman, R. B., *J. Natl. Cancer Inst.* 55, 1305 (1975).
8. Hellström, I., and Hellström, K. E., *in* "*In Vitro* Methods in Cell-Mediated Immunity" (B. R. Bloom and P. R. Glade, eds.), p. 409. Academic Press, New York, 1971.
9. Takasugi, M., Mickey, M. R., and Terasaki, P. I., *Natl. Cancer Inst. Mongr.* 35, 77 (1973).
10. Bloom, E. T., Ossorio, R. C., and Brosman, S. A., *Int. J. Cancer.* 14, 326 (1974).
11. Herberman, R. B., and Gaylord, C. E., eds., *Natl. Cancer Inst. Monogr.* 37, (1973).
12. Armitage, P., "Statistical Methods in Medical Research." Wiley, New York, 1971.
13. Quesenberry, C. P., and David, H. A., *Biometrika* 48, 375 (1961).
14. Herberman, R. B., Nunn, M. E., and Holden, H. T., this volume, Method 45.
15. Oren, M. E., Herberman, R. B., and Canty, T. G., *J. Natl. Cancer Inst.* 46, 621 (1971).
16. Rosenberg, E. B., Herberman, R. B., Levine, P. H., Halterman, R. H., McCoy, J. L., and Wunderlich, J. R., *Int. J. Cancer.* 9, 648 (1972).
17. Rosenberg, E. B., McCoy, J. L., Green, S. S., Donnelly, F. C., Siwarski, D. F., Levine, P. H., and Herberman, R. B., *J. Natl. Cancer Inst.* 52, 345 (1974).
18. Ting, C.-C., Bushar, G. S., Rodrigues, D., and Herberman, R. B., *J. Immunol.* 115, 1351 (1975).
19. Herberman, R. B., Nunn, M. E., and Lavrin. D. H., *Int. J. Cancer.* 16, 216 (1975).
20. Nunn, M. E., Djeu, J. Y., Glaser, M., Lavrin, D. H., and Herberman, R. B., *J. Natl. Cancer Inst.* 56, 393 (1976).
21. Oldham, R. K., Siwarski, D., McCoy, J. L., Plata, E. J., and Herberman, R. B., *Natl. Cancer Inst. Monogr.* 37, 49 (1973).
22. Takasugi, M., Mickey, M. R., and Terasaki, P. I. *Cancer Res.* 33, 2898 (1973).
23. Bean, M. A., Bloom, B. R., Herberman, R. B., Old, L. J., Oettgen, H. F., Klein, G., and Terry, W. D., *Cancer Res.* 35, 2902 (1975).
24. Cerottini, J.-C., Engers, H. D., MacDonald, H. R., and Brunner, K. T., *J. Exp. Med.* 140, 703 (1974).

Cytotoxicity Inhibition Assay for Analysis of Specificity of Cell-Mediated [51]Cr Release Cytotoxicity

Ronald B. Herberman, Myrthel E. Nunn, and Howard T. Holden

1. Introduction

It has been generally very difficult to define the specificity of cell-mediated immune reactions. In most studies of specificity, effector cells have been tested against a variety of target cells of antigenic preparations. The same antigen would then be considered to be present on all cells that gave positive reactions in the direct tests and to be absent on those that gave negative reactions. This procedure has suffered from two fundamental problems: (a) Cells with sub-threshold amounts of antigen or otherwise lacking susceptibility to immune cells would be classified as antigen negative. (b) Immune reactions may occur against a particular antigen on one cell and against different antigens on other cells. By direct testing, it would be possible to distinguish only reactions against common antigens from those against multiple antigens by isolation and comparison of the antigens on different cells.

For the cell-mediated ^{51}Cr release cytotoxicity assay, it has been possible to develop the cytotoxicity inhibition assay (1) to examine the specificity of the reactions in more detail and to at least partially overcome the two problems mentioned above. The inhibition assay was based on the general observation in the ^{51}Cr release assay that, over a considerable range, the percentage of cytotoxicity is directly proportional to the A/T (attacker:target cell) ratio (2). Addition of unlabeled target cells bearing the same antigens as those recognized on the ^{51}Cr-labeled target cells produced competitive inhibition and a decrease in detected ^{51}Cr release proportional to the number of added unlabeled cells. In contrast, addition of unlabeled cells lacking the relevant antigens would not be expected to produce significant inhibition of ^{51}Cr release.

This assay was first used to analyze the specificity of the cell-mediated cytotoxicity against a syngeneic rat lymphoma induced by Gross leukemia virus (1). Studies in this tumor system (1, 3) and of the immunity induced by inoculation of murine sarcoma virus into C57BL/6 mice (4, 5) have demonstrated that the antigens detected by cell-mediated cytotoxicity were quite distinct from the known serological specificities. The inhibition assay has also been quite useful in analyzing the specificity of the natural cell-mediated cytotoxicity in mice (6–9) and rats (3) against tumor cells and in man against lymphoid tissue cultured cell lines (10, 11). This method has also been applicable to analysis of the specificity of mouse histocompatibility antigens detected by cell-mediated ^{51}Cr release cytotoxicity (12–14). By a modification of the procedure, Sendo *et al.* (15) have looked for specificities recognized both by immune cells and by antibodies.

2. Materials

2.1. Water bath, 37°C

2.2. Centrifuge, refrigerated

2.3. Rocker platform, 10″ × 10″ (Bellco, Vineland, New Jersey, Catalogue No. 7740-10010), with stainless steel stray (10″ × 10″) to hold the petri dishes (NIH Shop).

2.4. Incubator, CO_2, humidified, 37°C

2.5. Gamma scintillation counter (Biogamma, Beckman Instruments Inc., Fullerton, California)

2.6. Petri dishes, plastic. For test: 35 × 10 mm (No. 3001, Falcon Plastics, Oxnard, California); for preparation of spleen cells: 100 × 20 mm (No. 3003, Falcon)

2.7. Pipettes, plastic, 1 ml (No. 7506, Falcon), 5 ml (No. 7529, Falcon), 10 ml (No. 7530, Falcon)

2.8. Biopette gun (No. 0010-29, Schwarz-Mann)

2.9. Biotips, 1 ml (No. 0010-30, Schwarz-Mann)

2.10. Syringe, Hamilton, gastight, 2.5 ml (No. 1002) with repeating dispenser (No. PB600-1, Hamilton Co., Whittier, California)

2.11. Syringe, Cornwall, 1 ml

2.12. Conical centrifuge tubes, 50 ml (No. 2070, Falcon)

2.13. Plastic counting tubes (Beckman Biovials No. 566353)

2.14. Sodium chromate, ^{51}Cr-labeled, specific activity 200–500 mCi/mg (^{51}Cr, New England Nuclear Corp., Boston, Massachusetts)

2.15. Roswell Park Memorial Institute (RPMI) medium 1640 [No. 1876, Grand Island Biological (GIBCO), Grand Island, New York]

2.16. Penicillin and streptomycin, 200X (NIH Media Unit)

2.17. Fetal bovine serum (FBS), heat inactivated (56°C, 30 min) (No. 614H1, GIBCO)

2.18. Glutamine, 3% (NIH Media Unit)

2.19. HEPES buffer, 1 M (NO 17-737, Microbiological Associates, Bethesda, Maryland)

2.20. Hanks' balanced salt solution (BSS) with Ca and Mg (NIH Media Unit)

2.21. Complete medium for assay: RPMI 1640 + 10% FBS + penicillin (100 units/ml) + streptomycin (100 μg/ml) + glutamine (0.3 mg/ml) + HEPES buffer (20 mM)

2.22. Trypan blue solution in ACK lysing buffer (in g/liter): trypan blue, 4; ammonium chloride, 8.3; potassium bicarbonate, 1; potassium EDTA, 0.037.

2.23. Trypsin, 0.1% crystalline (Worthington Biochemical Co., Freehold, New Jersey)

3. Method

3.1. Preparation of attacker cells and tumor cells from solid tissues: Tissues are minced in petri dish (100 $\times$ 20 mm) with scissors and forceps and a single-cell suspension in BSS is prepared. When necessary, solid tissues and tumor cells from tissue culture monolayers are disaggregated by brief treatment with 0.1% trypsin.

3.2. Attacker cells and tumor cells washed in 50 ml of BSS and centrifuged at 250 g for 10 min.

3.3. Attacker cells and cells to be tested for inhibition are resuspended in complete medium (see 2.21). An aliquot of cell suspension is diluted 1:100 in the trypan blue solution and the concentration of viable cells is counted. (This solution lyses erythrocytes so that only nucleated cells are counted.) The concentration is adjusted to 1 $\times$ 10^7/ml.

3.4. To label the target cells, 1 ml of the cell suspension is placed in a 50 ml conical tube, to which 0.15 ml of ^{51}Cr is added. This mixture is incubated 45 min at 37°C in a shaking water bath. The cells are then washed twice with 50 ml of complete medium. The number of viable cells is then counted and the concentration adjusted to 5 $\times$ 10^5/ml.

3.5. The usual ratio of attacker cells:labeled target cells in the inhibition assay is 200:1. However, with strong systems, lower ratios, e.g., 50:1, may be more sensitive to inhibition. For an A/T ratio of 200:1, 0.5 ml of attacker cells (at 1 $\times$ 10^7/ml) and 0.5 ml of the appropriate dilutions of inhibitor cells (quadruplicates for each dilution) are added to each petri dish (35 $\times$ 10 mm), using a Biopette. In all the systems that we have examined, ratios of attacker cells:inhibitor cells (A/I) of 5:1, 10:1, and 20:1 have been most satisfactory. Therefore the concentrations of inhibitor cells to be used are 2 $\times$ 10^6/ml, 1 $\times$ 10^6/ml, and 5 $\times$ 10^5/ml. Labeled target cells (0.05 ml at 5 $\times$ 10^5/ml) are then added to each petri dish, using a Hamilton syringe.

3.6. In addition of the experimental groups containing attacker cells, inhibitor cells, and labeled target cells, a series of controls (all containing a total of 1.05 ml) are set up: (a) Baseline control: We have found that an "autologous" control provides the most stable baseline. This consists of unlabeled target cells in place of, and at the same concentration as, attacker cells. When quantities of target cells are limited, we use either a medium control (i.e., labeled target cells alone) or a control with unreactive lymphoid cells (e.g., thymus cells) in place of attacker cells. (b) Immune control: Immune attacker cells and labeled target cells, with no inhibitor cells added. (c) Positive inhibition control: The cells used as labeled targets are also used as inhibitor cells. (d) Negative inhibition control: Cells known to lack the relevant antigen and to lack cytotoxic reactivity are used. In an alloimmune system, and in the tumor immunity systems, normal spleen cells syngeneic to the donor usually have been used. (e) Labeled target cells alone, to determine total ^{51}Cr incorporated into cells, for use as denominator in formula for percent cytotoxicity (see 3.10).

3.7. The petri dishes are placed in metal trays on the rocker platform in a 37°C incubator, with a humidified 10% CO_2 atmosphere. The dishes are rocked continuously at 6 complete to-and-fro tilts per minute for the incubation period of 4 hr.

3.8. After incubation, the trays are removed from the incubator, and the contents of each petri dish are transferred with a Pasteur pipette to 10 X 75 glass tubes. One milliliter of medium at 0°C is added to each tube, with a Cornwall syringe, to stop the reaction. The tubes are centrifuged at 2000 g for 10 min.

3.9. The supernatants are transferred into counting vials, and the ^{51}Cr radioactivity is determined in the gamma counter by counting each tube for 5–10 min.

3.10. The percent cytotoxicity for each dish is calculated as follows:

$$\% \text{ Cytotoxicity} = \frac{\text{cpm } ^{51}\text{Cr in supernatant}}{\text{total cpm } ^{51}\text{Cr in cells at the beginning of experiment}} \times 100$$

Experimental results are expressed as

$$\% \text{ Experimental cytotoxicity} = \% \text{ cytotoxicity in experimental group} - \% \text{ cytotoxicity in baseline control group}$$

% Inhibition of cytotoxicity

$$= \frac{\% \text{ cytotoxicity in immune control} - \% \text{ cytotoxicity in group with inhibitor cells}}{\% \text{ cytotoxicity in immune control}} \times 100$$

The percent inhibition values obtained with the various concentrations of inhibitor cells are plotted against the $\log_2$ of the A/I ratios.

3.11. The criteria used to define a positive result in the inhibition assay are: (a) significant ($p < 0.05$ by student's T test) reduction in cytotoxicity compared to the immune control, and to the negative inhibition controls, at all three A/I ratios; (b) a clear dose–response relationship, with increased inhibition with greater numbers of added cells; and (c) the slope of the inhibition curve similar to that produced by the positive inhibition control. All these criteria must be met if one is to consider a result positive.

4. Critical Comments

4.1. It is important to perform this assay with an A/T ratio that gives results on or close to the linear portion of the dose–response curve. The use of a 200:1 A/T with a highly cytotoxic attacker cell population may yield results on the plateau part of the curve (i.e., with similar percent cytotoxicity at 100:1), and this will result in decreased sensitivity in the inhibition assay.

4.2. The main problem that currently exists with this assay is that of nonspecific inhibition. This is particularly seen when the assay is performed in certain vessels (e.g., tubes, Microtest wells), which contribute to cell crowding and insufficient interactions among the cells. We have obtained optimal results in the petri dishes, with gentle rocking to enhance cell–cell interactions.

4.3. The presence of relatively large numbers of cells in the culture plates tends to maintain optimal viability of the target cells. In medium controls, with low concentration of labeled target cells by themselves, the percent ^{51}Cr release is often higher. In the autologous control or a control with unreactive lymphoid cells in place of attacker cells, the viability of the target cells is better preserved, and these often give lower base line levels of ^{51}Cr release. This raises the concern that some inhibition is related to adding even more cells to the culture vessel. However, this does not appear to be a significant problem. Addition of inhibitor cells to the autologous control or to the control with unreactive lymphoid cells does not significantly reduce the ^{51}Cr release.

4.4. Even when the assays are performed under optimal conditions, some cells produce nonspecific inhibition. Some tumor cells and normal lymphoblasts (e.g., induced by mitogens) present particular difficulties in this regard. Normal lymphoid cells and erythrocytes, even in concentrations close to or exceeding the concentration of attacker cells, usually give little or no nonspecific inhibition. Size of the cells does not appear to be a sufficient explanation for this difference, since some large tumor cells are noninhibitory. The main problems with nonspecific inhibition are seen with A/I ratios of less than 5:1. The range of A/I ratios of 5:1 to 20:1 appears to offer the combination of sufficient sensitivity to detect antigens and a minimum amount of nonspecific interference.

4.5. Cells producing nonspecific inhibition tend to give flat or irregular dose–response curves when tested at A/I ratios between 5:1 and 20:1. Also, the degree of inhibition by such cells varies considerably among experiments. In contrast, the percent of inhibition produced by antigenic cells is similar from experiment to experiment. The calculation of percent inhibition permits comparison between different experiments, which have varying levels of cytotoxicity in the immune controls. Variability among tests can be further reduced by the use of cryopreserved effector, target and inhibitor cells, which have been found to work well in this assay (J. Ortaldo, H. T. Holden, and R. K. Oldham, unpublished observations).

4.6. Although quantitative inhibition curves are generated in each experiment, we do not feel that it is yet possible to use this assay to make quantitative comparisons of antigen expression among different inhibitory cells. It has been our experience and that of others (e.g., 12) that normal lymphoid cells with the relevant antigens inhibit less well than do tumor cells. It seems quite possible that the efficiency of inhibition may depend on factors other than the amount of antigen per cell. There has been a good qualitative correlation between results in the inhibition assay and results with the same cells as labeled targets. However, the inhibition assay appears to be a more sensitive detection method. Some cells that are rather resistant to rapid ^{51}Cr release cytotoxicity inhibit quite efficiently.

4.7. Another limitation of the method is that it cannot distinguish well between a monospecific antigen system and a multiple antigen system, with particular attacker and target cells. In either case, the dose–response curves may be similar. Partial inhibition could be due either to lack of one of several antigens involved in the reaction or to quantitatively less expression of one antigen. To distinguish between these possibilities, it is helpful to perform inhibition assays, using the various inhibitor cells with different labeled target cells. Selection of target cells with fewer or separate antigens recognized by the attacker cells may distinguish qualitative antigen differences among various inhibitor cell populations.

REFERENCES

1. Ortiz de Landazuri, M., and Herberman, R. B., *Nature (London), New Biol.* **238,** 18 (1972).
2. Cerottini, J.-C., and Brunner, K. T., *Adv. Immunol.* **18,** 67 (1974).
3. Nunn, M. E., Djeu, J. Y., Glaser, M., Lavrin, D. H., and Herberman, R. B., *J. Natl. Cancer Inst.* **56,** 393 (1976).
4. Herberman, R. B., Aoki, T., Nunn, M., Lavrin, D. H., Soares, N., Gazdar, A., Holden, H., and Chang, K. S. S., *J. Natl. Cancer Inst.* **53,** 1103 (1974).
5. Aoki, T., Herberman, R. B., and Liu, M., *Intervirology* **5,** 31 (1975).
6. Herberman, R. B., Nunn, M. E., and Lavrin, D. H., *Int. J. Cancer.* **16,** 216 (1975).
7. Sendo, F., Aoki, T., Boyse, E. A., and Buafo, C. K., *J. Natl. Cancer Inst.* **55,** 603 (1975).
8. Kiessling, R., Klein, E., and Wigzell, H., *Eur. J. Immunol.* **5,** 112 (1975).
9. Zarling, J. M., Nowinski, R. C., and Bach, F. H., *Proc. Natl. Acad. Sci. U.S.A.* **72,** 2780 (1975).

10. Rosenberg, E. B., McCoy, J. L., Green, S. S., Donnelly, F. C., Siwarski, D. F., Levin, P. H., and Herberman, R. B., *J. Natl. Cancer Inst.* **52**, 345 (1974).
11. Svedmyr, E., Jondal, M., and Leibold, W., *Scand. J. Immunol.* **4**, 721 (1975).
12. Bevan, M. J., *J. Immunol.* **114**, 316 (1975).
13. Sondel, P. M., and Bach, F. H., *J. Exp. Med.* **142**, 1339 (1975).
14. Bevan, M. J., *J. Exp. Med.* **142**, 1349 (1975).
15. Sendo, F., Aoki, T., and Buafo, C. K., *J. Natl. Cancer Inst.* **52**, 769 (1974).

Purification and Fractionation of Human Blood Lymphocytes. Characterization of Subclasses by Their Antibody-Dependent Cytotoxic Potential (K Cell Assay)

Hedvig Perlmann, Peter Perlmann, Ulla Hellström, and Sten Hammarström

1. Introduction

Leukocytes of several types are known to have antibody-dependent cytotoxic potential (1, 2). Lymphocytic cells with this capacity are called K cells, and this strictly operational definition will be used in the following. K cell activity *in vitro* is assumed to be the *in vitro* correlate of one of the tissue-damaging mechanisms arising in the course of an immune response to tumors, transplants, or virally modified tissue or in autoimmunity (3).

Although T cells have recently been reported to have affinity for IgM (4) and IgM antibodies may also induce cell-mediated cytotoxicity *in vitro* (5), the predominating antibody involved in K cell cytotoxicity is IgG (3). In order to display K cell activity, the effector cells must have receptors for structures in the Fc fragment of IgG. Human lymphocytes with Fc receptors are heterogeneous both in regard to the avidity of these receptors (6) and in regard to the simultaneous occurrence of other surface markers, such as surface-bound immunoglobulin, complement receptors, or receptors for sheep erythrocytes (6–8). Recent evidence indicates that several lymphocyte types, differing in regard to surface marker distribution, also have K cell activity, implying that K cells may be lymphocytes of both the thymus-dependent and the thymus-independent variety. However, it is well established that the majority of the peripheral T cells in man have no K cell activity and, further, that K cells are distinct from the cytotoxic T cells (CTL), which are independent of IgG antibodies and are important effector cells in many immune systems (2, 3).

K cells may be effector cells in systems in which the lymphocytes are isolated from *immune donors*. In these instances K cell activity *in vitro* represents a cell cooperation phenomenon between antibody-producing cells and effector cells, which utilize this antibody but do not produce it themselves (9). In these systems, the K cell assay is performed by mixing donor lymphocytes with target cells of relevant antigenicity without addition of antibody. In contrast to CTL-mediated reactions, K cell activity is easily inhibited by the addition of anti-immunoglobulin (as Fab fragments). Fractionation of the lymphocytes before the assay may give important information as to the cytotoxic mechanisms involved (3).

K cell assays are most frequently performed with effector cells from *non-immune donors,* incubated with antiserum and target cells of corresponding antigenicity. Because of the extraordinary sensitivity of these systems, this assay is very useful for the determination of antibodies against cell surface antigens, e.g., in connection with tissue typing (3). Since K cell activity is highly suscepti-ble to inhibition by immune complexes the test may be performed as an inhibition assay, with addition of antibody-coated cells or immune complex-con-taining sera to a standard system (10, 11). In addition, the K cell assay is highly useful for the functional characterization of lymphocytes in the blood or lymphoid organs of normal individuals or patients (12).

Since many cell types display antibody-dependent cytotoxicity, and different target cells vary in regard to their susceptibility to different effector cell types, a meaningful analysis requires work under strictly standardized conditions. Suit-able methods for *isolation and purification of human blood lymphocytes* are described in Section 3.1. In Section 3.2 we describe a widely used *K cell model,* consisting of ^{51}Cr-labeled chicken erythrocytes (target cells), rabbit anti-chicken erythrocyte antibodies (inducing agent), and human blood lymphocytes (effec-tor cells). The assay has been designed to permit rapid comparison of the relative cytolytic potential of different effector cell preparations. In Sections 3.2–3.6 we describe a number of simple *fractionation procedures for characterization of K cells* in regard to their surface markers and other properties. Most of these methods are based on principles previously described by many authors and outlined in other chapters of this book. Brief *interpretations* of the results obtained with these methods and some *critical comments* are given in Sections 4.1–4.5.

2. Materials

2.1. Glassware, Plastic Products, Media, and Supplements. *2.1.1. Glass-ware.* Conical incubation tubes for the cytotoxicity assay were made from Pasteur pipettes by closing the capillary end in a flame. All glassware was sterilized by dry heat at 160° for 3 hr, or autoclaved 20–30 min at 2 kg/cm^2.

2.1.2. Disposable plastic products for cell culture work from Falcon, Oxnard, California, Nunc Products, Roskilde, Denmark; Heger Plastics AB, Stallar-holmen, Sweden.

2.1.3. Media and Supplements

TH: Tris-buffered Hanks' solution (1 volume of isotonic Tris buffer, pH 7.4 + 1 volume of Hanks' balanced salt solution) (13)

TCM: complete tissue culture medium, RPMI 1640 (Biocult, Paisley, Scot-land), supplemented before use with 2 mM glutamine, 100 IU of penicillin and

100 μg of streptomycin per milliliter and, as indicated, with either heat-inactivated FBS (fetal bovine serum, Flow Co., Irvine, Scotland) or HSA (human serum albumin, Kabi, Stockholm, Sweden). When indicated, the RPMI 1640 medium is also supplemented with 20 mM HEPES buffer.

2.2. Material and Solutions for Lymphocyte Purification and Fractionation

Gelatin (Edible Compounds Ltd. Hull, England), dissolved at 3% in hot TH, used at 37°C

Carbonyl-iron powder (General Aniline & Film Co., New York, New York)

FIP: 24 parts of 9% Ficoll (Pharmacia Fine Chemicals, Uppsala, Sweden) mixed with 10 parts of 33.9% Isopaque (Nyegaard, Oslo, Norway), density 1.077 g/ml (14)

ACT: Tris-buffered isotonic NH$_4$Cl, pH 7.2; 9 parts of 0.83% NH$_4$Cl + 1 part Tris buffer, pH 7.6 (15)

TH-HSA-NaN$_3$: TH containing 0.2% HSA and 0.02% NaN$_3$.

Superbrite glass beads, type 100-5005 (3 M Co., St. Paul, Minnesota). The beads are given a negative charge by treatment with strong acid, followed by thorough washing

Nylon fibers (Fenwal Laboratories Inc., Morton Grove, Illinois)

HP: A-hemagglutinin from the snail *Helix pomatia* prepared by extraction of the albumin glands and purified by affinity chromatography on insolubilized hog blood group A+H substance (16)

HP-Sepharose: 1.5 g of freeze-dried large-sized particles (250–315 μm) of CNBr-activated Sepharose 6B (Pharmacia Fine Chemicals, Uppsala, Sweden) covalently conjugated with 3.5 mg of HP under standard conditions (17)

D-GalNAc: N-acetyl-D-galactosamine (Sigma Chemical Co., St. Louis, Missouri)

NANAase: Neuraminidase from *Clostridium perfringens*; type VI, 1–3 U/mg, NAN-lactose substrate (Sigma Chemical Co.)

2.3. Isotope

^{51}Cr: Na$_2$^{51}CrO$_4$, 0.5–1.0 mCi/ml, 3–20 μg Cr/ml (Radiochemical Center, Amersham, Bucks, England)

2.4. Erythrocytes

E$_c$: chicken erythrocytes from 10–20 week-old hen chicken, bled by heart puncture with 100 IU of heparin per milliliter of blood in the syringe. Used within 2–3 days.

E$_s$: sheep erythrocytes. Fresh sheep blood in Alsever's solution, obtained once a week.

2.5. Sera, Antibodies

a-E$_c$: heat-inactivated (56°C, 60 min) rabbit antiserum to chicken erythrocytes, prepared by repeated i.v. injections.

NRS: heat-inactivated normal rabbit serum.

a-E$_s$(IgM): Rabbit antiserum to boiled sheep erythrocyte stromata (State

Bacteriological Laboratory, Stockholm, Sweden). The IgM fraction of this serum is obtained by gel exclusion chromatography on Sephadex G-200 (Pharmacia Fine Chemicals) and is concentrated to its original volume by ultrafiltration.

Serum from C6-deficient rabbits (Rancho di Conejo, Vista, California) is used as the source of nonhemolytic complement (18). It is used fresh or kept in liquid nitrogen.

$F(ab')_2$ fragments from human IgG [Hu.$F(ab')_2$]. A commercial preparation of pepsin-fragmented human IgG, Gamma Venin (Behringwerke AG, Marburg a.L., West Germany) is purified by gel exclusion chromatography on Sephadex G-200.

Rabbit IgG antibodies to Hu.$F(ab')_2$ [Ra.IgG/a-Hu.$F(ab')_2$] are obtained by i.m. injections of 1 mg of Hu.$F(ab')_2$ in Freund's complete adjuvant. The rabbits are bled after one or two booster injections. IgG from the antiserum is obtained by precipitation with $(NH_4)_2SO_4$ at 50% saturation and passage through a DEAE-cellulose column (19). Pepsin fragments of these antibodies [Ra.$F(ab')_2$/a-Hu.-$F(ab')_2$] are prepared by digestion for 18 hr at 37°C in acetate-buffered saline, pH 4, 3 mg of pepsin (Sigma Chemical Co.) per 100 mg of protein (20).

3. Methods

3.1. Isolation and Purification of Human Blood Lymphocytes. Blood is defibrinated by shaking with glass beads ($\sim$ 5 mm) in an Erlenmeyer flask, approximately 50 ml/flask (10–20 ml of blood may be collected separately for preparation of donor's serum). Three volumes of defibrinated blood are mixed with 1 volume of 3% gelatin. The mixture is left to settle in a volumetric cylinder for 1 hr at 37°C (shorter settling times may be appropriate when patients' blood is utilized). The leukocyte-rich supernatant is withdrawn, and the cells are concentrated by centrifugation at 1200–1500 rpm (200–300 g) for 10 min at room temperature (RT). The pellet is suspended in $\sim$one-fourth of the supernatant. Phagocytic and adherent cells are removed by incubation in centrifuge tubes at 37°C and under frequent shaking, with 0.4 g of carbonyl iron powder per 10 ml of cell suspension. After 30 min the lymphocytes and erythrocytes are removed by decantation while phagocytic and adherent cells and iron particles are held back with a magnet. Decantation is repeated once. After centrifugation for 10 min at RT (1200–1500 rpm), the cells are suspended in TH + 2.5% FBS to approximately one-third of the original blood volume.

To remove erythrocytes, the cell suspension is transferred to conical centrifuge tubes, 5 ml/tube, and 2 ml of FIP is added to the bottom of the tubes with a Pasteur pipette. After centrifugation for 20 min at RT, 2800 rpm (1200 g), the supernatants including the lymphocyte layer at the interphase are withdrawn, pooled, and centrifuged for 5 min at 2500 rpm (1000 g). The cells are washed once in TH + 2.5% FBS. For removal of remaining monocytes, they are suspended in TH containing 50% autologous serum and are incubated in tissue culture flasks or tissue culture dishes at a density of 8 to 16 $\times$ 10^6 cells/ml. After 1 hr at 37°C the nonadherent cells are transferred to centrifuge tubes and are washed 3 times in TH + 2.5% FBS.

In order to release IgG (or immune complexes) adsorbed to the Fc-receptors of the lymphocytes, the cells are finally incubated overnight in air + 5% CO_2 at 37°C in TCM + 5% FBS. The cell density should not exceed 2 $\times$ 10^6 cells/ml.

Before use, lymphocytes purified as described above or further fractionated as described below, are washed once in TH + 2.5% FBS, counted and checked for viability with trypan blue. For the K cell assay the cells are finally suspended in TCM + 5% FBS, 4 $\times$ 10^6 cells/ml.

3.2. ^{51}**Cr-Labeled E$_c$.** Chicken blood, 0.1 ml, diluted 1:20 in TH + 2.5% FBS (15 to 20 $\times$ 10^6 erythrocytes) is mixed with 0.1 ml of ^{51}Cr (Section 2.3). After 1 hr at 37°C the erythrocytes are washed twice in TH + 2.5% FBS, counted, and kept as concentrated pellets until immediately before addition to the lymphocytes in the K cell assay.

3.3. Quantitative Cytotoxicity Assay (K Cell Assay). The tests are set up in duplicate in conical incubation tubes (Section 2.1); total volume of incubation mixtures 0.3 ml. All dilutions are made in TCM + 5% heat-inactivated FBS.

To 0.1 ml of lymphocytes, 4 $\times$ 10^6/ml, are added 0.1 ml of ^{51}Cr-E$_c$, 1, 2, or 4 $\times$ 10^6/ml and, as the last addition, 0.1 ml of either 0.1 ml of a-E$_c$, final dilution 10^{-5}, or similarly diluted NRS. Controls containing $\sim$ 10^6 unlabeled E$_c$ instead of lymphocytes are included.

The mixtures are incubated at 37°C in air + 5% CO_2. After 20 hr of incubation they are centrifuged for 6 min at 1200–1500 rpm (200–300 g). Two-tenths milliliter of each supernatant are withdrawn, and the radioactivities of both supernatants and residues are determined in a well-type scintillation counter. The percentage of the total radioactivity released from the cells to the supernatant in the experimental tubes, corrected by subtraction of the percentage of ^{51}Cr release in the controls, is taken as a measure of the degree of erythrolysis. The percentage of ^{51}Cr release in both lymphocyte-free and NRS controls is $\leqslant$ 2%. Variation between duplicates $\leqslant$ 3%. For assessment of the cytolytic potential of different lymphocyte preparations and comments see Section 4.2.

3.4. Depletion of E$_s$ Rosetting Lymphocytes. Purified lymphocytes, 8 $\times$ 10^6 in 0.5 ml of heat-inactivated FBS per tube, are mixed in conical centrifuge tubes with 0.5 ml of 2% E$_s$ in FBS. The mixtures are incubated for 5 min at 37°C, centrifuged for 5 min at 800 rpm (100 g), and kept at 5°C overnight. The cells are gently suspended, 2 tubes are pooled, and 2 ml of FIP are layered underneath with a Pasteur pipette. After centrifugation for 20 min at 2800 rpm (1200 g) at RT the E rosette-depleted lymphocytes are recovered from the interphase.

Before use in the K cell assay it is important to include a 1-hr adherence step in 50% serum (Section 3.1) since centrifugation in FIP leads to an enrichment of remaining monocytes (from <1% before to ⩾5% after centrifugation).

The E rosette-enriched lymphocyte fraction in the pellets may be dispersed by shaking and incubation for 30 min at 37°C for dissolution of the rosettes. It is freed from E_s by incubation for 5 min at 37°C with 9 volumes of ACT and may then be further fractionated (e.g., 3.5) or used directly in the K cell assay after centrifugation and washing.

3.5. Depletion of EAC Rosetting Lymphocytes. EA are formed by incubating 1 ml of 5% E_s for 30 min at 37°C with 1 ml of a-E_s (IgM), applied at the highest subagglutinating dose (~1:200). After two washes with TH + 2.5% FBS (ice cold), 1 volume of 5% EA is mixed with 1 volume of C6-deficient rabbit serum (diluted 1:2 or 1:4) and incubated for 30 min at 37°C. The EAC formed are washed twice with ice-cold TH + 2.5% FBS. Lymphocytes, 8×10^6 in 0.5 ml of HEPES-buffered TCM + 5% FBS, are mixed with 0.5 ml of 2% EAC in conical centrifuge tubes. The tubes are centrifuged for 5 min at 800 rpm (100 g). They are incubated for 15 min at 37°C and subsequently for at least 15 min on ice. For elimination of spontanous rosettes, the tubes are finally incubated for 5 min at 37°C and are agitated on a cell mixer. The contents of ten tubes are pooled, and the cells are concentrated by centrifugation (in round-bottomed tubes). The pellet is suspended in 5 ml of 8% HSA + 1.7 ml of 3% gelatin and the rosettes are removed by a very short centrifugation at 350 g. The EAC rosette-depleted lymphocytes in the supernatant are cautiously withdrawn, centrifuged, treated with ACT (Section 3.4) and washed for further use in the K cell assay.

3.6. Fractionation on Columns Charged with Human Immunoglobulin Complexed with Rabbit Anti-human Immunoglobulin, Added Either as Intact IgG, or as Pepsin-Fragmented F(ab′)$_2$. Superbrite glass beads (Section 2.2), 7 ml, are mixed with 1 ml of Hu.F(ab′)$_2$, 30 mg/ml, and are incubated at 4°C overnight. After 3 washes with saline, the beads are filled into a 10-ml disposable syringe equipped with a 22-gauge needle, giving a flow rate of ~0.7 ml/min. (A layer of nylon fiber prevents beads from leaking into the needle.) Three milliliters of IgG or of F(ab′)$_2$ from rabbit antihuman F(ab′)$_2$ serum, 10 mg/ml (~2 mg of antibody per milliliter), are added to the column. After 1 hr at RT the column is washed with saline followed by HEPES-buffered TCM containing 5% FBS. One milliliter of lymphocytes (6 to 12×10^6) is added and *immediately* eluted with ~ 12 ml of HEPES-buffered TCM + 5% FBS.

Columns containing beads similarly charged with FBS or HSA may be used for controls.

3.7. Fractionation on HP-Sepharose Columns. Three milliliters of HP-Sepharose are suspended in TH-HSA-NaN$_3$ and packed in a small column (0.9 × 15 cm, K9/15, Pharmacia Fine Chemicals) equipped with a 85-μm nylon net

(Nytal Seidengazefabrik AG., Thal, Switzerland). Control columns are filled with CNBr-activated Sepharose neutralized by addition of either glycine or HSA.

Since HP reacts with glycoproteins in serum, HSA is used as protein supplement in all solutions. Four milliliters of lymphocytes (25×10^6/ml) in TH + 0.2% HSA are incubated with 4 ml of NANAase (10 μg/ml) for 45 min at 37°C. Lymphocytes not treated with NANAase have no accessible HP receptors (21). After washing in TH containing 0.2% HSA, 1–1.5 ml of the NANAase-treated lymphocytes (60×10^6/ml) in TH-HSA-NaN$_3$ are added to the column. After incubation for 15 min at RT, the nonadherent lymphocytes, i.e., the cells lacking receptors for HP (17) are eluted with 60 ml of TH-HSA-NaN$_3$ at a flow rate of 6–10 ml/min. The retained cells, i.e., the cells with HP receptors, are eluted in two steps with the competitive hapten D-GalNAc in TH-HSA-NaN$_3$, 60 ml containing 0.1 mg/ml, and 60 ml containing 1 mg/ml, respectively. Passed and eluted cells are concentrated and washed with TH + 0.2% HSA to remove the hapten.

4. Interpretations and Comments

4.1. Isolation and Purification of Human Blood Lymphocytes.
Lymphocytes isolated from the blood of normal donors by the methods described in Section 3.1 are 98–99% pure and viable when tested with trypan blue. The recovery is 0.5 to 1×10^6 lymphocytes per milliliter of blood, corresponding to yields ranging from 30 to 55%. There seems to be no distortion in the proportion of the major lymphocyte subclasses present in the blood before purification (22).

Defibrination is useful when enough blood is available. Better yields of lymphocytes may be obtained by using heparinized blood. However, in the latter case, it may be necessary to remove platelets before further purification by centrifugation for 10 min at 1800 rpm (400–500 g). The cell sediment is then reconstituted to the original blood volume by addition of FBS or 8% HSA.

The final adherence step in 50% serum to remove remaining monocytes (Section 3.1) is optional and may not be required when blood of normal donors is processed. It may, however, be necessary to include this step when blood from certain patients is used. When purification and subsequent fractionation include additional FIP centrifugations, the adherence step is important since this procedure enriches remaining monocytes in the interphase layer together with the lymphocytes.

Equally good lymphocyte preparations for the K cell assay are obtained by replacing iron + magnet treatment with passage of the cells through nylon fiber columns (23). Provided this is done in a high concentration of serum or plasma (> 50%), there is no specific loss of any of the major lymphocyte subclasses on the column. This will be the case, however, when the serum concentration on the column is 10% or less (24). After nylon filtration, erythrocytes and PMN may be removed by FIP centrifugation (Section 3.1), or the erythrocytes may be lysed by ACT treatment (Section 3.4).

4.2. Quantitative Cytotoxicity Assay (K Cell Assay). E_c are convenient and easily available target cells for this assay. When obtained from chicken less than 12 weeks old, they are stable and release very little isotope spontanously even when kept in culture for several days. E_s or bovine erythrocytes may also be used, but the spontaneous isotope release is usually higher. Human erythrocytes are not susceptible to K cell-mediated lysis. All erythrocytes are highly suscepti- ble to antibody-mediated phagocytosis and lysis by monocytes and PMN, which therefore have to be removed if the activity of K cells is being assayed. In this regard, erythrocytes may differ from lymphoid target cells and tissue culture cells, which are less susceptible to phagocytosis or antibody-dependent cytolysis by monocytes or leukocytes. Moreover, lymphocytic K cells are probably also heterogeneous, and different types of target cells may differ in their susceptibil- ity to different types of K cells (3).

Under the conditions given above (Section 3.3) isotope release from E_c is maximal after 18–20 hr of incubation. With optimal antibody concentrations and target cells in excess, isotope release is directly proportional to the number of effector cells present (25). Thus, when the percentage of lysis after 20 hr is plotted against the effector cell:target cell ratio, a straight line through the origin is obtained. In the system discussed herein, the lymphocytes are the only metabolically active cells in the incubation mixture, and it is therefore most convenient to keep their number constant at the optimal concentration of 1 to 1.5×10^6/ml. The effector cell:target cell ratio may then be varied as described in Section 3.3 by adding 1, 2, or 4×10^5 ^{51}Cr-E_c to 4×10^5 lymphocytes. The extent of target cell lysis (e.g., percent isotope release) at any given ratio provides a direct measure of the relative K cell potential of a lymphocyte preparation. Actual values obtained with unfractionated lymphocytes and two fractions taken after HP-column separation (Section 3.7) are shown in Fig. 1.

For a valid comparison of different lymphocyte preparations, it is important to ascertain that the number of effector cells is indeed the limiting factor determining the extent of lysis. Deviations from linearity in the target cell excess area usually imply that the number of *active* effector cells differ at the different ratios plotted. This may be the case if the antibody concentration becomes suboptimal when the number of target cells added is varied, leading to a suboptimal engagement of K cells in the reaction. This may be the case at both too low and too high antibody concentrations (3). It should be pointed out that lymphocytes vary in regard to their avidity for IgG, and different subpopulations may require different antibody concentrations for optimal engagement in the K cell system (6). It is therefore essential to establish that the antibody concentra- tion is not a limiting factor in a comparative assay.

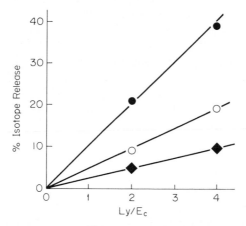

Fig. 1. Percent isotope release from ^{51}Cr-E$_c$ at different effector to target cell ratios. Each incubation tube contained 4 × 10⁵ NANAase-treated lymphocytes, 2 × 10⁵ or 1 × 10⁵. ^{51}Cr-E$_c$, and anti-E$_c$, final dilution 10^{-5}. Total volume 0.3 ml/tube. ^{51}Cr-release in NRS controls (1–2%) is subtracted. ○, Unfractionated lymphocytes; ●, lymphocytes passaged over HP-Sepharose; ■, lymphocytes eluted from HP-Sepharose with 1 mg of D-GalNAc per milliliter.

Interference between lymphocytes of different types in cell preparations that vary in regard to their composition may sometimes also affect the results of an assay. However, under the conditions described and with blood from normal donors this does not seem to be a major problem.

4.3. Depletion of E$_s$ Rosetting Lymphocytes. Depletion of E$_s$ rosetting cells (E⁺) under the conditions given is not complete. It reduces the percentage of E$_s$ rosetting lymphocytes from ~75% in the original preparations (26, 27) to ⩽ 30% in the depleted fraction, the latter comprising 5–15% of all lymphocytes added. Since the total yield of lymphocytes recovered in this fraction is small, it is usually difficult to subject it to a second cycle of E$_s$-rosette depletion. The relative concentration of cells with surface-bound immunoglobulin (SIg⁺) or complement receptors in the E$_s$-rosette depleted fraction increases 2 to 3 times, and so does its K cell activity (28, 29).

In the E⁺-enriched fraction the proportions of cells with different surface markers are reversed. Its residual K cell activity is usually ~30% of that of the E$_s$-rosette depleted fraction. It is completely removed by passing the cells through a column charged with immune complexes (IgG) (Section 3.6). The resulting fraction consists of highly purified, functionally intact T cells, completely devoid of K cell activity (23, 25, 29).

While it is obvious that the majority of the E⁺ lymphocytes (i.e., T cells) are inert in the K cell assay this does not imply that all K cells are E⁻ cells. Recent evidence suggests that K cells have receptors for sheep erythrocytes but do not form E_s rosettes that are stable enough to withstand the fractionation procedures. However, when fractionation is performed after treatment of the lymphocytes with NANAase, which stabilizes the rosettes, the K cell activity of the E_s rosette-enriched fraction is strongly enhanced (30). It remains to be established if all K cells or only part of them have E_s receptors and if these E^+ cells are indeed T cells (24).

4.4. Depletion of EAC Rosetting Lymphocytes. C6-deficient rabbit serum is a convenient source of complement (31). When serum is the source of complement, it may contain antibodies to E_s which can be removed by short absorption in the cold or in a Ca^{2+}–Mg^{2+}-free medium. However, complement receptor lymphocytes seem to bind EAC only through the C3 receptor, even in the presence of IgG antibodies (32, 33).

The risk for formation of spontaneous rosettes by using E_s for EAC-formation is small under the conditions given. It may be totally avoided by using human or bovine erythrocytes instead of E_s (22). Complement receptor lymphocytes may also be removed by passaging the cells through columns charged with particles carrying activated C3. Both human and mouse complement have been used with human lymphocytes in this way (31, 34, 35).

The lymphocyte fractions obtained by EAC rosette depletion is almost completely free of EAC^+ cells and have lost all or almost all K cell activity in the present assay. The EAC^+ cells in the pellets are also inactive and do not rerosette after lysis of the erythrocytes with ACT. K cells also seem to have receptors for both C3b and C3d (31; and unpublished). However, the results do not imply that all lymphocytes with complement receptors also have K cell potential (30). Activated C3 on the surface of the target cells does not induce K cell activity in the absence of IgG antibodies but enhances cytotoxicity when the latter are present in suboptimal concentrations (31).

4.5. Fractionation on Columns Charged with Hu.F(ab$'$)$_2$ and Either Ra.IgG/a-Hu.F(ab$'$)$_2$ or Ra.F(ab$'$)$_2$/a-Hu.F(ab$'$)$_2$. The yield of lymphocytes passaged through control columns charged with FBS or HSA is usually 80–90%. After passage through immune-complex columns with the *intact anti-immunoglobulin* used as antibody, as initially described by Wigzell *et al.* (36, 37), the yields are 50% or lower. In the passaged fraction the relative proportion of E^+ cells is increased to ~90% while SIg^+ cells, EAC^+ cells and cells with Fc receptors (Fc^+), i.e., cells forming rosettes with IgG-coated bovine erythrocytes (38), are completely or almost completely removed. At the same time, K-cell activity is also completely abolished (29). With the *fragmented anti-immunoglobulin* [Ra.F(ab$'$)$_2$/a-Hu.F(ab$'$)$_2$], i.e., in the complete absence of Fc fragments on the column, the total yield of recovered lymphocytes is usually 65–80%, with strong reduction (80–100%) of the SIg^+ cells. In contrast EAC^+ cells and Fc^+ cells show only minor relative reductions, while the proportion of E^+ cells shows a minor increase. K cell activity is either unchanged or, more often, slightly increased (28, 29).

These results suggest that B cells with a high density of SIg have no K cell activity in the test system described above. This is also suggested by passage of the lymphocytes through columns charged with ovalbumin and antiovalbumin (rabbit IgG). These columns also completely remove K cell activity and Fc^+ cells forming rosettes with IgG-carrying bovine erythrocytes, while the relative proportion of SIg^+ cells is only slightly decreased (34, and G. Pape, unpublished). It may be concluded that these immune-complex columns preferentially retain cells with high-affinity Fc receptors and that K cells active in the present system belong to this variety (6).

4.6. Fractionation on HP-Sepharose Columns. Since normal lymphocytes do not react with HP, application of this method requires that the lymphocytes be treated with NANAase, which uncovers the necessary receptor sites. The majority of the HP^+ cells in normal blood are T cells, and most, but probably not all, of them have also receptors for E_s (17, 21).

Passage of NANAase-treated lymphocytes through HP-negative control columns gives ~80% recovery. The total recovery after passage and elution from the HP-Sepharose with the competitive sugar is 60–70%, with no selective loss of any of the major lymphocyte subpopulations.

Approximately 10% of all lymphocytes pass directly through the columns. 50–55% of these cells are SIg^+ and EAC^+ while ~10% are HP^+ and ~30% are E^+. This means that only 1 and 3%, respectively, of the HP^+ cells and E_s^+ cells originally added are present in this fraction, which is strongly enriched in B cells. The lymphocytes of this fraction respond poorly to T cell mitogens but have an enhanced K cell activity (Fig. 1). For quantitative reasons, it is likely that most of these K cells are HP^- (17).

Elution of the cells retained on the column with 0.1 mg of D-GalNAc/ml gives a minor fraction (~15%) of intermediate composition. Approximately 45% of the cells are recovered by subsequent elution with 1.0 mg of D-GalNAc/ml. About 90% of these cells are HP^+ and E^+. About 10% of the HP^+ cells are SIg^+ and have also complement and Fc receptors. The surface-bound immunoglobulin on most of these lymphocytes is externally adsorbed IgG, which does not reappear after trypsinization and 24-hr culture. The lymphocytes of this fraction respond strongly to T cell mitogen while their K cell activity is weak (Fig. 1) and can be completely abolished by passage through an anti-immunoglobulin complex column as described in Section 3.5. It is presently not known if the K cells in this fraction are HP^+/E^- cells or HP^+/E^+ cells (17).

REFERENCES

1. Perlmann, P., and Holm, G., *Adv. Immunol.* **11,** 117 (1969).
2. Cerottini, J.-C., and Brunner, K. T., *Adv. Immunol.* **18,** 67 (1974).
3. Perlmann, P., *Clin. Immunobiol.* **3,** in press (1976).

4. Moretta, C., Ferrarini, M., Durante, M. L., and Mingari, M. C., *Eur. J. Immunol.* **5**, 565 (1975).
5. Lamon, E. W., Whitten, H. D., Skurzak, H. M., Andersson, B., and Lidin, B., *J. Immunol.* **115**, 1288 (1975).
6. Revillard, J. P., Samarat, C., Cordier, G., and Brochier, J., *in* "Membrane Receptors of Lymphocytes" (M. Seligmann, J. L. Preud'homme, and F. M. Kourilsky, eds.), p. 171. North-Holland Publ., Amsterdam, 1975.
7. Kurnick, J. T., and Grey, H. M., *J. Immunol.* **115**, 305 (1975).
8. Winchester, R. J., Fu, S. M., Hoffman, T., and Kunkel, H. G., *J. Immunol.* **114**, 1210 (1975).
9. Schirrmacher, V., Rubin, B., and Pross, H., *J. Immunol.* **112**, 2219 (1974).
10. Halloran, P., Schirrmacher, V., and Festenstein, H., *J. Exp. Med.* **140**, 1348 (1974).
11. Jewell, D. P., and MacLennan, I. C. M., *Clin. exp. Immunol.* 1973. **14**:219.
12. Holm, G., Björkholm, M., Mellstedt, H., and Johansson, B., *Clin. Exp. Immunol.* **21**, 376 (1975).
13. Perlmann, P., and Perlmann, H., *Cell. Immunol.* **1**, 300 (1970).
14. Böyum, A., *Scand. J. Clin. Lab. Invest.* **97**, Suppl. 21, 77 (1968).
15. Boyle, W., *Transplantation* **6**, 761 (1968).
16. Hammarström, S., and Kabat, E. A., *Biochemistry* **10**, 1684 (1971).
17. Hellström, U., Hammarström, S., Dillner, M. L., Perlmann, H., and Perlmann, P., *Scand. J. Immunol.*, Suppl. V (1976).
18. Rother, K., Rother, U., Müller-Eberhard, H. J., and Nilsson, U. R., *J. Exp. Med.* **124**, 773 (1966).
19. Weir, D. M., ed., "Handbook of Experimental Immunology," 2nd ed. Blackwell, Oxford, 1973.
20. Spiegelberg, H. L., and Weigle, W. O., *J. Exp. Med.* **121**, 323 (1965).
21. Hammarström, S., Hellström, U., Perlmann, P., and Dillner, M. L., *J. Exp. Med.* **138**, 1270 (1973).
22. Holm, G., Petterson, D., Mellstedt, H., Hedfors, E., and Bloth, B., *Clin. Exp. Immunol.* **20**, 443 (1975).
23. Perlmann, P., Perlmann, H., and Wigzell, H., *Transplant. Rev.* **13**, 91 (1972).
24. Perlmann, P., and Wåhlin, B., *in* "Proceedings of the Tenth Leucocyte Culture Conference" (V. P. Ejsvogel, D. Roos, and W. P. Zeylemaker, eds.), p. 575. Academic Press, New York, 1976.
25. Perlmann, P., Perlmann, H., Larsson, A., and Wåhlin, B., *J. Reticuloendothel. Soc.* **17**, 241 (1975).
26. Jondal, M., Holm, G., and Wigzell, H., *J. Exp. Med.* **136**, 207 (1972).
27. Yata, J., Desgranges, C., Tachibana, T., and de-Thé, G., *Biomedicine* **19**, 475 (1973).
28. Perlmann, P., Wigzell, H., Golstein, P., Lamon, E. W., Larsson, A., O'Toole, C., Perlmann, H., and Svedmyr, E. A. J., *Adv. Biosci.* **12**, 71 (1974).
29. Perlmann, H., Perlmann, P., Pape, G., and Halldén, G., *Scand. J. Immunol.*, Suppl. V (1976).
30. Perlmann, P., Biberfeld, P., Larsson, A., Perlmann, H., and Wåhlin, B., *in* "Membrane Receptors of Lymphocytes" (M. Seligmann, J. L. Preud'homme, and F. M. Kourilsky, eds.), p. 161. North-Holland Publ., Amsterdam, 1975.
31. Perlmann, P., Perlmann, H., and Müller-Eberhard, H. J. *J. Exp. Med.* **141**, 287 (1975).
32. Theofilopoulos, A. N., Dixon, F. J., and Bokisch, V. A., *J. Exp. Med.* **140**, 877 (1974).
33. Eden, A., Bianco, C., and Nussenzweig, V., *Cell. Immunol.* **7**, 459 (1973).
34. Jondal, M., Wigzell, H., and Aiuti, F., *Transplant. Rev.* **16**, 163 (1973).
35. Knapp, W., *Z. Immunitaetsforsch. Exp. Klin. Immunol.* **149**, 428 (1975).

36. Wigzell, H., and Andersson, B., *J. Exp. Med.* **129**, 23 (1969).
37. Wigzell, H., Sundqvist, K. G., and Yoshida, T. O., *Scand. J. Immunol.* **1**, 75 (1972).
38. Hallberg, T., Gurner, B. W., and Coombs, R. A., *Int. Arch. Allergy Appl. Immunol.* **44**, 500 (1973).

47

Quantitation of K Cells

Ian C. M. MacLennan, A. C. Campbell, and D. G. L. Gale

1. Introduction

Immunoglobulin can trigger a large number of different cellular mechanisms, and even if one considers those activated by the Fc portion of IgG the list remains impressive. Antibody-dependent cell-mediated cytotoxicity can be shown by neutrophils (1, 2), macrophages (1, 2), possibly by B cells (3), and by a relatively recently defined population of lymphocytes known as K cells. K cells differ from other cell types showing antibody-dependent cytotoxic activity in that they are non-glass-adherent, nonphagocytic lymphocytes which are not easily identified with immunologically competent cells (2, 4, 5). Human lymphocytes are a particularly rich source of this activity, and although several other species including rats have K cells (6), they are notably deficient in mice. In man, K cell activity is high in the blood and spleen, low in bone marrow, and very low in other lymphoid tissues, including thoracic duct lymphocytes, thymus, and lymph nodes. Marked activity has been reported for bone marrow against antibody-sensitized chicken red cells (7), but this activity may reflect contaminating immature cells of the myeloid series. Although there is no certain way of identifying K cells, available evidence indicates that this type of cytotoxic cell probably accounts for less than 5% of the total lymphocyte population in human peripheral blood.

It is important to distinguish K cells from other cells capable of producing antibody-dependent cytotoxicity. This is most conveniently done by choosing a system where K cells alone can damage the target cells. Fortunately a number of such systems exist. In measuring human and rat K cell activity we have extensively used a cell line originally derived by Chang (8) from normal human liver, which, in the presence of either human or rabbit sensitizing antibody, is resistant to lysis by macrophages or polymorphs but is highly sensitive to lysis by K cells. There are a number of other target cell combinations with this selective susceptibility to K cell-mediated lysis. These include the DBA2 mastocytoma P815 (2) sensitized with rabbit antibody and a human lymphoblastoid line sensitized with HLA antibody (5). The mouse cell line has the advantage of being relatively resistant to spontaneous lysis by human peripheral blood lymphocytes while some spontaneous cytotoxicity is apparent against Chang cells. There is increasing interest, however, in this spontaneous cytotoxicity, which is obvious in overnight cultures and appears to be mediated by cells that have many of the properties of, but are probably not identical to, K cells (9). There are some advantages in being able to measure both spontaneous and antibody-dependent cytotoxicity; these can be done in the same test, and the techniques that will be described below are easily adapted for use of either the mouse cell line mentioned or Chang cells, although experience using whole blood as a source of effector cells has only been achieved using Chang cells as targets. We do not recommend the use of chicken erythrocytes as targets since it has been clearly shown that a variety of cell types other than K cells can kill these in the presence of antibody (2). Even with the most careful separation techniques it is difficult to be certain of achieving complete elimination of nonlymphoid cells. If it is required to measure mononcyte- and macrophage-mediated cytotoxic activity selectively, this can be achieved by using human red cells sensitized with IgG anti-D or anti-A. This target system is highly resistant to K cell-mediated lysis (1, 2). The technique that we describe below for K cell quantitation can be adapted to detect certain types of immune complexes and to measure antibody against a variety of target cells including lymphocytes sensitized with antibody against histocompatibility antigens (10), virus-infected target cells sensitized with anti-virus antibody (11), and tumor cells sensitized with tumor-specific antibody (12).

1.1. Phytohemagglutinin-Induced Cytotoxicity. Cytotoxicity against target cells in the presence of phytohemagglutinin was first described by Holm *et al.* in 1964 (13). We are still uncertain about the nature of the cytotoxic cell, and in fact there is good evidence that more than one cell type may be involved. The activity can be partially, but only partially, removed by passing preparations of lymphoid cells through Fc immunoabsorbent columns (14). It is tempting to conclude that the Fc receptor-bearing part of the activity is in fact due to K cells, but this is contradicted by the finding of good K cell activity in human cord blood where PHA-induced cytotoxic activity is very low (15).

Whatever the nature of the cytotoxic cell(s), the method for measuring PHA-induced cytotoxicity can be easily incorporated into the assays described for K cells, and for this reason it is included in this chapter.

1.2. Princples of the Assay. Target cells are labeled with ^{51}Cr-labeled chromate, and cytotoxicity against the targets is measured by the release of this isotope. The relative cytotoxic activity, which is presumed to reflect the number of K cells in a test sample, can be estimated as the number required to produce a given level of cytotoxicity. K cell cytotoxic activity increases sigmoidally with log increase in the number of effector cells added (Fig. 1A) (4). A simple mathematical correction can be applied to percent ^{51}Cr release so that it becomes linearly related to the log number of effector cells added ((Fig. 1B) (4).

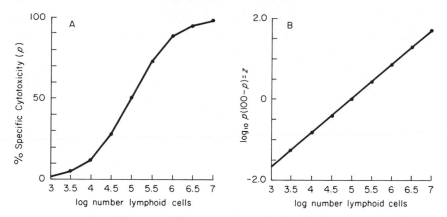

Fig. 1. (A) An idealized standard curve of $\log_{10}$ lymphoid cells added to cultures against percentage of specific cytotoxicity. This curve was derived using tube cultures with 10^4 Chang cells sensitized with rabbit anti-Chang on targets and gelatin-sedimented human peripheral blood lymphocytes as the K cell source. The position of the curve is the mean for healthy donors. In practice, as is shown in Fig. 4, there is some inhibition of cytotoxic activity when large numbers of lymphoid cells are added to cultures. (B) Logit transformation of the curve in (A).

A number of factors can give rise to erroneous results, and simple precautions which can be taken to avoid these are described below. As well as giving the assay conditions that we consider to be optimal, we have given considerable space to explaining why these conditions have been selected.

2. Materials

2.1. Target Cells. Chang liver cells are derived from normal liver (8). The assays described below have used Chang cells obtained from the American Type Culture Collection via Flow Laboratories. Chang cells can be obtained in single-cell suspension by the following simple culture procedure. The medium used is MEMS (Eagle's minimum essential medium for suspension cultures) enriched with 10% calf serum (GIBCO-Biocult); nonessential amino acids, 1% (GIBCO-Biocult); fresh glutamine, 2 mM; benzylpenicillin, 100 IU/ml; and streptomycin, 100 μg/ml. About 10^6 cryopreserved Chang cells are rapidly thawed, slowly diluted in culture medium, centrifuged once at 100 g for 5 min and resuspended in 10 ml of culture medium. This suspension is then seeded into an 8-oz medical flat bottle which is gassed with 5% CO_2 and air before being tightly closed. The culture is then incubated at 37°C for 48 hr; after which the bottle is gently shaken, the medium is removed, and the bottle is replenished with fresh medium. Regassing is carried out after this medium change but it is unnecessary after subsequent changes providing the bottle top forms a gastight seal. With medium changes every 48 hr a dense layer of cell will have developed on the glass within 6–10 days. At this stage between 2×10^6 and 5×10^6 cells can be harvested daily from such a flask by shaking the bottle and removing the medium. For optimum viability of cells, medium should be changed about 24 hr before harvesting for use in cytotoxicity cultures. When cells are not required as targets, cultures can be maintained by changing the medium about once every 48 hr. If cultures are left too long between medium changes the cells tend to come off the glass in sheets. When this happens it is best to discard cultures. By following this procedure, cultures of this sort can be maintained indefinitely, although we generally replace bottles about once every 6 weeks. In our hands, such cultures maintain consistent properties as target cells over several months, but it is wise to start new cultures from liquid nitrogen if any changes in viability or susceptibility to lysis is detected.

2.2. Anti-Chang Antibody. Rabbit anti-Chang antibody is prepared by intradermal injection over one shoulder of 10^7 Chang cells which have been thoroughly washed in phosphate-buffered saline (PBS) and emulsified in complete Freund's adjuvant. Three weeks later the rabbit is boosted with an intravenous injection of 10^7 cells in PBS. The rabbit is bled out 10 days later. Such antiserum will have a K cell-dependent anti-Chang titer of about $1:10^6$. The serum should be diluted out against Chang cells in the presence of human K cells, and the maximum kill will be seen between dilutions of about $1:10^3$ and $1:10^5$. For stability of the assay, the midpoint of this plateau is chosen as the standard sensitizing dilution. Such an antiserum can be diluted 1:10 in fetal bovine serum and stored at $-20°C$ where its shelf life is at least 5 years.

2.3. Phytohemagglutinin (PHA). Highly purified PHA is not necessary for this assay, and Wellcome reagent grade will give satisfactory results. Batches do vary in the titer inducing maximum killing, and it is best to acquire a substantial batch if long-term comparisons are required. We have found the potency of this product to be retained for at least 2 years when stored at $4°C$ in its lyophilized form. In its hydrated state, potency is retained at $4°C$ for at least 1 week. As with sensitizing antibody, a titer of PHA is used that is at the midpoint of the high plateau of induced cytotoxicity. With our current batch this is 1:300.

2.4. Culture Medium for Cytotoxicity Assays. A number of media can be used for cytotoxicity assays.

In 1-ml cultures, where 0.1 ml of whole blood is used as an effector cell source, MEM enriched with 10% fetal bovine serum and the other additives listed in Section 2.1 for MEMS is suitable.

For small volume culture using purified lymphocytes, BME (Eagle's basal medium enriched as for MEM above and buffered with HEPES buffer) is suitable.

Different batches of fetal bovine serum can give markedly different levels of cytotoxicity. Consequently, where sequential studies are being undertaken it is advisable to set aside a substantial quantity of the same batch. It is wise to avoid the use of sera containing significant amounts of IgG, as this will tend to aggregate with time and heat inactivation and inhibit cytotoxicity by blocking the Fc receptors of K cells. Any serum with anti-effector cell antibody, which, for instance, could be present in pooled AB serum, can inhibit cytotoxicity, and the degree of inhibition will vary from effector cell to effector cell. It is possible to get satisfactory killing using serum-free medium, but we have insufficient experience of such cultures to make a statement about their reproducibility.

2.5. Culture Vessels. Where 0.1 ml of whole blood is used as a source of effector cells, it is important to use 1-ml cultures; microplates are not satisfactory. We use 76×12 mm Sterilin polystyrene round-bottomed tubes. Ficoll–Triosil or gelatin-sedimented lymphocytes can be used in 200 μl cultures in round-bottomed Cook 96-well microtiter plates. In experiments where it is desirable to use very small volumes because valuable reagents, such as sensitizing antisera or inhibitory agents are being used, cultures can be scaled down to 25 μl or less. In this case there is an advantage in diluting to 250 μl with cold saline at the end of the culture period in order to reduce pipetting errors. Precautions must be taken against desiccation in such cultures, and purified lymphocytes must be used as a source of effector cells when small volumes are employed.

3. Test Procedure

3.1. Labeling Target Cells. Target cells are labeled with ^{51}Cr-labeled chromate. The $CrO_4{}^{2-}$ ions are actively taken up by the cells where they are thought to be largely converted to chromic (Cr^{3+}) ions. In this form chromium is relatively stably bound to cellular components but is released on cell lysis. Released chromium is not readily reutilized by remaining viable cells. Some degree of spontaneous release of isotope occurs. In the case of Chang cells this is in the order of 20–25% at 18 hr. This spontaneous release reflects turnover of cellular constituents and spontaneous death of labeled cells.

Uptake of isotope by cells is influenced most markedly by the following factors: (a) duration of labeling; (b) temperature of labeling; (c) specific activity of isotope; and (d) number of target cells.

For general purposes, satisfactory labeling of Chang cells will take place if 2 to 5×10^6 cells are incubated in 1 ml of HEPES-buffered basal medium with 10% fetal bovine serum at 37°C for 1 hr with 100 μl of ^{51}Cr, $Na_2{}^{51}CrO_4$ (specific activity 2–10 μg of Cr) per millicurie. Radio and chemical toxicity of ^{51}Cr-labeled sodium chromate is not critical in this range and increased labeling of cells can be achieved by increasing incubation time and decreasing the number of cells being labeled.

After incubation with isotope, the cell suspension should be diluted to 10–25 ml with a suitable washing medium, such as Hanks' balanced salt solution. About 2 ml of fetal bovine serum are then layered under the cell suspension using a

Pasteur pipette, and the target cells are centrifuged through the fetal bovine serum gradient at 200–300 g for 5 min. This leaves the free isotope in the upper layer. The supernatant is then removed, and the labeled cells are suspended in culture medium at a concentration of 2×10^5 cells/ml. No further washing is required.

3.2. Effector Cells. It is now clear that it is not necessary to purify effector cells in order to measure K cell-mediated cytotoxicity. One hundred microliters of heparinized or defibrinated whole blood in 1-ml cultures is a satisfactory source of effector cells (16). The blood can be washed first by dilution in at least 10 volumes of washing medium and centrifugation of the blood cells through a volume of fetal bovine serum equal to that of the original blood. The supernatant is then removed down to the original level of the whole blood. By the use of washed and unwashed blood, the inhibitory factors in plasma, such as immune complexes, can be assessed.

Most workers have used purified lymphocytes in assessing K cell activity, but before opting for such an approach it is as well to consider the advantages and disadvantages of purification. First, it can be argued that removal of erythrocytes, granulocytes, and macrophages will remove cells that would cause toxicity in their own right to target cells. However, in the case of Chang cells this is not so. The main problem is that of inhibition of cytotoxicity. However, as the principal elements that can cause inhibition separate with lymphoid cells and as erythrocytes and granulocytes are far less inhibitory than equal amounts of lymphocytes, there is little advantage in removing them. The best way to avoid inhibition is to keep the number of added lymphocytes to a culture down to a minimum compatible with measuring cytotoxic activity. For 1-ml cultures in 76 $\times$ 12 mm tubes, not more than 2×10^5 lymphocytes or 100 μl of whole blood should be added per culture. If higher numbers of lymphoid cells are used, it is essential to use more than one concentration to see whether any inhibition of cytotoxicity is occurring. This will be detected as a fall in the slope of log effector cell number/% specific cytotoxicity from the ideal shown in Fig. 1A. This point is discussed in detail in Section 3.7 and Fig. 4. A further disadvantage of lymphocyte purification is that this procedure inevitably yields a selected population of lymphocytes. These arguments cannot be applied to assays using target cells, such as chicken red cells, which are lysed by neutrophils and macrophages as well as K cells, in the presence of sensitizing antibody.

Details of lymphocyte purification need not be described here, and the reader is referred to the following papers for accounts of the cells involved in cytotoxicity (2, 4, 5). In summary, K cells are not glass-adherent and they are nonphagocytic. They also remain in the upper layer of Ficoll–Triosil gradients and stay in the leukocyte fraction of gelatin sediments. On the other hand, they have relatively high-affinity Fc receptors and will be removed by affinity columns exposing these determinants but not by $F(ab')_2$ anti-immunoglobulin-coated columns.

3.3. Target Cell Numbers. The accuracy of the ^{51}Cr release assay is greatest when there is substantial percentage of isotope released. For this reason, target cells should be in limiting numbers in the assays. Below 3×10^4 Chang cells per culture, the percent ^{51}Cr release in the presence of 2×10^5 human blood lymphocytes and sensitizing antibody is more or less independent of the number of target cells, i.e., percent ^{51}Cr release from 2×10^4 sensitized Chang cells is the same as that from 10^4. This clearly indicates the importance of giving absolute numbers of cells added rather than ratios. By using 2×10^4 Chang cells the reader will appreciate that there is some latitude for error in the actual number of target cells added. This obviates the necessity to make detailed viability counts of target cells. If the number of intact target cells is counted by phase contrast microscopy, this is good enough.

3.4. Length of Culture Incubation. *The kinetics of K cell lysis* is that of rapid ^{51}Cr release over a 5–7 hr period after target cells and lymphoid cells come into contact. After this, ^{51}Cr release proceeds at a rate equal to that seen in cultures without sensitizing agents but with lymphoid cells (Fig. 2). When K cells cytotoxicity is being measured, there is therefore no need to continue cultures for more than 7 hr. Although marked killing is seen within an hour or two, it is better not to harvest cultures during the rapid killing phase as results will be less

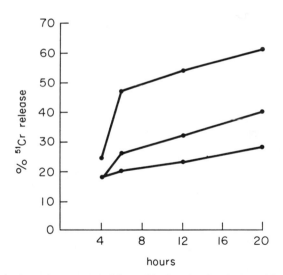

Fig. 2. Antibody-dependent cytotoxicity with length of culture. This experiment used whole blood as an effector cell source. The bottom curve shows release from Chang cells alone and the middle curve is the percent ^{51}Cr release with lymphoid cells and without sensitizing agent. The top curve shows release with effector cells and anti-Chang antibody. [Redrawn with kind permission of the Editor, from graphs published in *Clinical and Experimental Immunology* (16).]

reproducible than those taken after 7 hr. The reason for this is that the timing is far more critical and such factors as the length of time cells in the culture take to sediment are important. In conclusion, while cultures can be harvested earlier, it is often most convenient to harvest the following day at, say, 20 hr. We have adopted this timing for routine K cell quantitation assays. In the case of PHA-induced cytotoxicity the kinetics are quite different and killing continues at a more or less steady rate to at least 20 hr (Fig. 3). In order to get reasonable levels of cytotoxicity with this agent, it is desirable to leave cultures overnight, and again a 20-hr incubation period is recommended.

Spontaneous cytotoxicity proceeds at a slow rate (Figs. 2 and 3) and is also best measured after overnight culture.

3.5. Harvesting Cultures. At the end of incubation cultures are centrifuged at 200 g for 10 min at 10°C. Half the supernatant is then removed using an automatic pipette, such as fin pipette, and placed in a second tube (known as supernatant tube). In 1-ml cultures both supernatant tubes and the tube containing the residue are counted in a well scintillation counter. Percent ^{51}Cr release is then calculated by

$$\frac{2 \times (\text{counts in the supernatant tube} - \text{background})}{(\text{counts in residue and supernatant tubes}) - 2 \times \text{background}} \times 100$$

Where microplates are used, supernatant counts are compared with sample tubes containing 2×10^4 labeled Chang cells, which were prepared at the time of

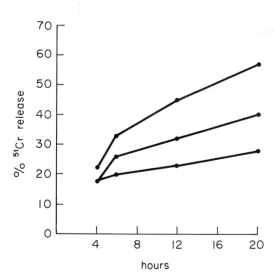

Fig. 3. As in Fig. 2, but the top line here is with effector cells and phytohemagglutinin.

setting up the cultures. The counts from these "total count tubes – background" replaces the bottom line of the formula above.

3.6. Calculation of Percent of Target Cells Killed. The best approximation to percent cells killed as a factor of crude percent ^{51}Cr release is that devised by Brunner *et al.* (17) This is generally termed specific cytotoxicity and calculated as follows:

$$\text{Specific cytotoxicity} = \frac{\text{observed } ^{51}\text{Cr release} - \text{release from target cells alone}}{\text{maximum releasable } ^{51}\text{Cr} - \text{release from target cells alone}}$$

We have calculated maximum ^{51}Cr release as the average level that cultures set up with high K-cell activity asymptotically approach with increasing numbers of effector cells. In our hands this is 87%. Other estimations can be achieved by lysing cells by freezing and thawing, use of antibody and complement, or detergent lysis. They give similar but not identical results. This calculation reduces the variation in the slope of the curve: % ^{51}Cr release/log effector cell number.

3.7. Calculating and Expressing Cytotoxic Activity in a Sample. Cytotoxic activity of a sample can be expressed as the log number of lymphoid cells required to produce 50% specific cytotoxicity. This can be calculated by fitting a standard curve, such as that shown in Fig. 1A, to experimental results and extrapolating the number of cells or volume of blood that would be required to produce 50% specific cytotoxicity. This value is inversely related to K cell activity. Where a given number of blood lymphoid cells are added to a culture, the cytotoxic activity in 1 ml of blood is expressed as the $\log_{10}$ number of lymphoid cells per milliliter of blood – the $\log_{10}$ number of cells required to produce 50% lysis. Separate curves have to be constructed for each type of cytotoxicity. In constructing such standard curves, it is important to realize that when more than 100 μl of blood or 2×10^5 lymphoid cells are added to cultures, the slope of the curve % ^{51}Cr release/log effector cell number may fall, and even reverse, as numbers are increased (see Fig. 4). Lymphoid populations with high proportional K-cell activity show the full predicted sigmoid curve.

An alternative and simpler way of calculating the cytotoxic activity of a given number of lymphoid cells or given volume of blood is to linearize the sigmoid curve: % specific cytotoxicity/log effector cell number, by logit transformation. Specific cytotoxicty (p) is converted to a value z using the following formula:

$$z = \log_{10} [p/(100-p]$$

The advantage of using this formula is that the z value is directly and linearly related to the log number of K cells in a culture assuming that there is little variation in the average cytotoxic activity of K cells from sample to sample (Fig. 1B). The z value obtained with 2×10^5 lymphoid cells gives a measure directly related to the proportion of cytotoxic cells in a sample. Activity for 1 ml of

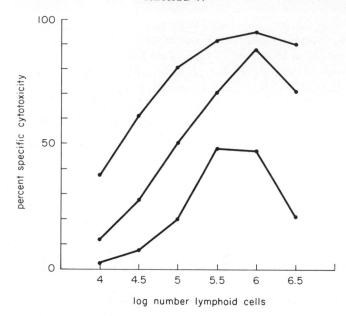

Fig. 4. Actual curves for three individual lymphoid cell preparations showing percent specific cytotoxicity against log effector cell number added. It will be seen that cytotoxicity fails to increase as very high numbers of lymphoid cells are added to cultures. The point at which inhibition occurs is more closely related to the number of lymphoid cells added to a culture than to the level of cytotoxicity reached.

blood is calculated by adding z to the $\log_{10}$ number of lymphocytes per milliliter.

3.8. Assessing the Contribution of Spontaneous Cytotoxicity to That Seen in the Presence of Sensitizing Agents. Some spontaneous cytotoxicity is usually seen against Chang cells when human peripheral blood or rat spleen is used as a source of effector cells. The question is to what extent does this spontaneous cytotoxicity falsely elevate the level of cytotoxicity seen in the presence of either antibody or phytohemagglutinin. On balance, the evidece available suggests that spontaneous cytotoxicity is not mediated by cells involved in antibody-dependent cytotoxicity although these cells have many similar characteristics. Assuming that spontaneous cytotoxicity and that seen in the presence of sensitizing agents are independent phenomena, then it can reasonably be argued that the contribution of the spontaneous cytotoxicity should be subtracted from that seen in the presence of either antibody or phytohemagglutinin.

In practice this contribution is generally extremely small. It is totally erroneous to suppose that spontaneous cytotoxicity can be allowed for by subtracting percent specific cytotoxicity without sensitizing agent from that with sensitizing agent. The same principles as were employed in quantitating K cells and the cells involved in PHA-induced cytotoxicity must be employed. That is to say, the relative number of cells required to produce a given level of killing, or z values (see Section 3.7) should be compared. It is extremely rare to find spontaneous cytotoxicity activity greater than one-third of that seen in the presence of sensitizing agents. If spontaneous cytotoxic activity is one-third as great as that in the presence of antibody, then only two-thirds of the cytotoxicity is produced by K cells. To calculate the cytotoxicity which is due to K cells alone for, say, 10^5 blood lymphocytes, one should read off the standard curve the cytotoxicity produced by 6.7×10^4 lymphocytes. At the maximum slope of antibody-dependent cytotoxicity this amounts to an error of approximately 8% specific cytotoxicity. Consequently where spontaneous cytotoxicity is less than a third of that seen in the presence of sensitizing agents we have ignored its contribution. As mentioned above, these problems can be largely overcome by using a target cell that is resistant to spontaneous lysis in the presence of lymphoid cells but sensitive to antibody-dependent K cell-mediated lysis.

4. Critical Comments

4.1. Technical Considerations in Calculating Results. Most automatic counters are fitted, or can now be fitted, with punch-tape output. Manual or semimanual calculation of results is therefore unnecessary and more likely to produce errors. By using a tape reader and a desk computer, in our case a Hewlett-Packard, we automatically calculate from the data tape; percent ^{51}Cr release, specific cytotoxicity, z value. The means of the values for replicates are also printed out.

The cost of such calculating equipment is not more than 30% of the cost of an automatic twin-channel counter.

4.2. Additional Applications of Technique. The techniques and rationale mentioned above can be applied to a wide variety of target cells, sensitizing agents, and effector cells. K cell assays are becoming increasingly used in relation to tissue typing, and in these situations cultures can be reduced to a 3-hr cross-match between transplant donor and recipient, particularly if small volumes are used.

Normal peripheral blood lymphocytes are easily used as target cells (10). When using human sera for sensitization of target cells, one of the main sources of false negative results is the presence of anti-effector-cell antibody in the serum (10). This is a particular problem in the case of serum from multiparous women or transfused donors. To some extent this problem can be overcome by presensitizing of target cells. Halloran and Festenstein (18) have used this inhibition effect as an assay for histocompatibility antigens. Recently it has become clear that virus-infected cells are susceptible to lysis by lymphoid cells in the presence of virus-specific antibody (12). Assays involving this phenomenon are likely to become increasingly used. Tumor cells, particularly leukemia cells, are readily utilizable as targets in K cell-mediated cytotoxicity assays (19, 20).

Finally, assays have been developed for assessing certain types of immune complex by their capacity to inhibit K cell-mediated cytotoxicity (21, 22). Complexes with this type of inhibitory activity, which is presumably due to blocking of Fc receptors on K cells, have been found in a number of diseases including rheumatoid arthritis, ulcerative colitis, and Crohn's disease. Penayi and Poston have recently carried out an extensive study of the optimum conditions for measuring K cell-mediated cytotoxicity inhibition (23). They have particularly noted that the sensitivity of the assay can be increased by reducing the amount of sensitizing antibody added to cultures to levels below that inducing maximum cytotoxicity.

REFERENCES

1. Holm, G., *Int. Arch. Allergy Appl. Immunol.* **43**, 671 (1963).
2. MacDonald, H. R., Bonnar, A. D., Sordat, S., and Zawodnik, S. A., *Scand. J. Immunol.* **4**, 487 (1975).
3. Chess, L., McDermont, R. P., Sondel, P. M., and Schlossman, S. F., *Prog. Immunol. II* **3**, 125 (1974).
4. MacLennan, I. C. M., *Transplant. Rev.* **13**, 67 (1972).
5. Trinchieri, G., Baumann, P., De Marchi, M., and Tokes, Z., *J. Immunol.* **115**, 249 (1975).
6. MacLennan, I. C. M., and Harding, B., *Immunology* **18**, 405 (1970).
7. Cordier, G., Samarut, C., and Revillard, J. P., *10th Leucocyte Culture Conf.,* Amsterdam, Abstracts, 1975.
8. Chang, R. S., *Proc. Soc. Exp. Biol. Med.* **57**, 444 (1954).
9. Pavie-Fisher, J., Kourilsky, F. M., Picard, F., Banzet, P., and Puissant, A., *Clin. Exp. Immunol.* **21**, 430 (1975).
10. Hersey, P., Cullen, P., and MacLennan, I. C. M. *Transplantation* **16**, 9 (1973).
11. Rager-Zisman, B., and Bloom, B., *Nature (London)* **251**, 542 (1974).
12. Hollingsworth, P. N., University of Oxford, DPhil. Thesis, 1975.
13. Holm, G., Perlmann, P., and Werner, B., *Nature (London)* **203**, 841 (1964).
14. Wisløff, F., Frøland, S. S., and Michaelsen, T. E., *Int. Arch. Allergy Appl. Immunol.* **47**, 488 (1974).
15. Campbell, A. C., Waller, C., Wood, J., Aynsley-Green, A., and Yu, V., *Clin. Exp. Immunol.* **18**, 469 (1974).
16. Gale, D., and MacLennan, I. C. M., *Clin. Exp. Immunol.* **23**, 252 (1976).
17. Brunner, K. T., Mauel, J., Cerottini, J.-C., and Chapuis, B., *Immunology* **14**, 181 (1968).
18. Halloran, P., and Festenstein, H., *Nature (London)* **250**, 52 (1974).
19. Hersey, P., MacLennan, I. C. M., Campbell, A. C. Harris, R., and Freeman, C. B., *Clin. Exp. Immunol.* **14**, 159 (1973).
20. MacLennan, I. C. M., Gale, D. G. L., and Wood, J., *Int. J. Cancer* **15**, 995 (1975).
21. MacLennan, I. C. M., *Clin. Exp. Immunol.* **10**, 275 (1972).
22. Jewell, D. P., and MacLennan, I. C. M., *Clin. Exp. Immunol.* **14**, 219 (1973).
23. Panayi, G. S., and Poston, R. N., personal communication.

48

Detection of K Cells by a Plaque Assay

Birgitta Wåhlin and Peter Perlmann

1. Introduction

The cytotoxicity of lymphocytes *in vitro* is usually defined as cytolytic potential of a given cell preparation. In order to obtain direct information on the number of effector cells present or on their nature, it is desirable to determine cytotoxicity on the level of the single effector cell as is being done for antibody-producing cells in the Jerne plaque assay. In this paper we describe a plaque assay designed to allow enumeration of antibody-dependent effector cells present in a lymphocyte preparation. The method is based on procedures recently described by Kedar *et al.* (1). In the model we will use to illustrate the method, erythrocytes forming a dense monolayer on poly-L-lysine-treated cover slips are used as target cells. When exposed to purified human peripheral blood lymphocytes in the presence of properly diluted anti-erythrocyte antibodies, clear zones (plaques) appear in the areas where erythrocytes have been lysed by the action of antibody-dependent effector cells. Counting of the number of plaques formed by a given number of lymphocytes added gives a measure of the minimum number of antibody-dependent effector cells present (2–5). Moreover, the plaque-forming lymphocytes can be studied in regard to surface markers (5), morphology, and ultrastructure (3, 4, 6).

2. Materials

2.1. Material and Solutions for Lymphocyte Purification and Processing. See Method 46.

2.2. Material and Solutions for the Plaque Assay

Petri dishes, 35 × 10 mm (No. 1008), Falcon, Oxnard, California)

Cover slips: glass, 22 × 22 mm

PLL: poly-L-lysine hydrobromide (type 1-B, MW ≥ 70.000 (Sigma Chemical Co., St. Louis, Missouri). A stock solution, 10 mg/ml, is prepared in TH (Tris-buffered Hanks' solution, pH 7.4 (see Method 46) and kept frozen. For use, it is diluted to 20 μg/ml in TH.

523

TCM: complete tissue culture medium (RPMI 1640) supplemented with glutamine, antibiotics, and heat-inactivated fetal bovine serum (FBS) (see Method 46)

Glutaraldehyde (GA): for fixation of the erythrocyte monolayers after incubation, a 25% aqueous stock solution is prepared.

HSA: human serum albumin (Kabi, Stockholm, Sweden). For use, the 20% stock solution is diluted with TH to give a 0.2% solution.

NANAase: neuraminidase from *Clostridium perfringens,* type VI, 1–3 U/mg NAN-lactose substrate (Sigma Chemical Co.)

2.3. Erythrocytes

E_c: chicken erythrocytes (see Method 46).

E_b and E_s: bovine and sheep erythrocytes, respectively, obtained once a week.

2.4. Sera, Antibodies.

Hyperimmune Rabbit Antiserum to chicken erythrocytes (a-E_c), normal rabbit serum (NRS), and the IgM fraction of antiserum to boiled sheep erythrocyte stromata, a-E_s(IgM), are prepared as described in Method 46. Hyperimmune rabbit antiserum to bovine erythrocytes (a-E_b) is prepared by three weekly i.v. injections for 3 weeks. Two milliliters of a 10% suspension are injected each time. All sera are heat inactivated at 56°C for 60 min. The IgG fraction of a-E_c or a-E_s is prepared by gel exclusion chromatography on Sephadex G-200 (Pharmacia Fine Chemicals, Uppsala, Sweden).

2.5. Reagents for Assay of Surface Markers

E_s, a-E_s (IgM), and serum from C6-deficient rabbits (see Method 46): used for building up EAC for assay of *lymphocytes with complement receptors* (EAC$^+$).

Surface-bound immunoglobulin on lymphocytes (SIg), assayed by direct staining with immunoadsorbent purified and fluorescein isothiocyanate (FITC) labeled rabbit IgG antibodies to human IgG-F(ab′)$_2$ fragments, prepared as described elsewhere (7). Fluorescein/protein molar ratio ~8.

Purified *Helix pomatia* A hemagglutinin (HP) for detection of HP receptors on NANAase-treated lymphocytes is prepared according to Hammarström and Kabat (8). FITC-conjugated HP is used, fluorescein/protein molar ratio ~4–6 (9).

3. Methods

3.1. Lymphocytes. Human peripheral blood lymphocytes from defibrinated blood are purified by gelatin sedimentation, colloidal iron uptake, Ficoll–Isopaque centrifugation and adherence. Before use in the plaque assay the cells are kept at 37°C overnight in air + 5% CO_2. The content of monocytes is $\leqslant 0.5\%$. For all details see Method 46.

For assay of surface receptors for HP the lymphocytes are treated with NANAase in TH containing 0.2% HSA as described in Method 46 (9, 10).

3.2. Erythrocyte Monolayers. Thoroughly cleaned (ethanol) cover slips are put in plastic petri dishes; 0.5 ml of freshly diluted PLL in TH (20 μg/ml) is added to the dishes to cover the cover slips only. After 45 min at room temperature (RT) the solution is removed and the cover slips are washed twice with 0.5 ml of TH, care being taken to avoid wetting the bottom of the petri dishes.

Erythrocytes (e.g., E_c or E_b) are washed twice in TH and 0.5 ml of 2.5% (E_c) or 1% (E_b) suspensions in TH ($\sim 10^8$ E) are added to each cover slip. After incubation for 45 min at RT, the nonattached erythrocytes are removed by pipetting TH into the petri dishes, followed by decantation. This is repeated several times. (Using Pasteur pipettes for the removal of TH may cause damage of the monolayers.) Approximately 1 ml of TH is finally left in the dishes. The erythrocyte monolayers may be stored at 4°C for 3–4 days.

3.3. K Cell Test by the Plaque Assay. Before use the erythrocyte monolayers are checked under the microscope, and those that are not homogeneous are discarded. TH in the dishes is decanted. A mixture of 0.5 ml of a lymphocyte suspension (e.g., 4 $\times$ 10^6/ml) in supplemented TCM and 0.5 ml of heat-inactivated anti-erythrocyte serum or its IgG fraction, properly diluted in TCM (see Section 4.3) are then added and carefully mixed by gentle agitation of the dishes. Controls containing FBS only or similarly diluted NRS are always set up. After incubation for 20 hr at 37°C in air + 5% CO_2, the monolayers are fixed by dropwise addition of 1 ml of GA (25% stock solution diluted 1:10 with distilled water). The liquid is decanted after 30 sec. Approximately 2 ml of diluted GA are slowly added once more along the walls of the dishes and decanted after 5–8 min. The monolayers are washed twice with distilled water, and enough water to cover the monolayers is left in the dishes. The lymphocytes remaining attached may be stained with Giemsa stain for microscopic inspection.

Lysis of erythrocytes is reflected by the formation of circumscribed clear zones in the monolayer. The number of plaques is counted in a phase-contrast microscope equipped with an ocular containing a grid. For rapid screening of large numbers of monolayers, the use of a monitor and television screen is recommended. Enough fields, randomly distributed over the cover slip are screened to give a reliable measure of the total number of plaques formed. Since the plaques are evenly distributed over the monolayer, screening of approximately 2 mm^2 gives a satisfactory measure of the total number of plaques. An area corresponding to 5 or more lysed erythrocytes is defined as a plaque (see Section 4.1).

The bottom area of the petri dishes used is 900 mm^2. The number of plaque-forming cells (PFC) as percentage of the total number of lymphocytes added is calculated as % PFC = $100(a \times b)/(c \times d)$, where a is the total area of dish, b is the number of plaques counted, c is the number of lymphocytes added, and d is the total area screened for counting plaques. These estimates give minimal numbers of PFC, based on the assumption that one K cell does not form more than one plaque (see Section 4.4).

3.4. Surface Markers. *3.4.1. E_s Receptors.* These tests are made with E_c or E_b monolayers. After incubation with the lymphocytes, approximately half of the medium (~ 0.5 ml) containing free and loosely attached lymphocytes are carefully removed with a Pasteur pipette. One-half milliliter of a 0.5% suspension of E_s is added to the dishes, which are incubated for 15 min at 37°C, followed by 2 hr at 4°C. The medium containing nonattached E_s is decanted and the preparations are fixed with 1% GA for 3 min as above. For microscopic observation, the cover slips are transferred to microscope slides and are covered with a drop of 50% glycerol. Rosettes formed by lymphocytes in the plaques and in plaque-free areas are counted separately under a 100X immersion lens. Lymphocytes binding $\geqslant 4$ E_s are considered as E_s-binding cells (E^+ cells).

3.4.2. Complement Receptors (EAC$^+$ Cells). E_sAC are built up with anti-E_s(IgM) and complement from C6-deficient rabbits as described in Method 46. Half a milliliter of 0.5% EAC is added to the dishes as described above for E_s binding. The dishes are incubated for 60 min at 37°C. Further processing and assessment of EAC$^+$ cells as described for E^+ cells.

3.4.3. Surface-Bound Immunoglobulin. After incubation with the lymphocytes, the monolayers are fixed for 20 sec with 0.5–1% GA. The medium is decanted, and the monolayers are carefully washed once with TH containing 0.02% NaN$_3$. Of the FITC-labeled rabbit antihuman F(ab')$_2$ reagent (250 μg of antibody protein per milliliter, containing 0.02% NaN$_3$), 0.1 ml is added and the dishes are incubated for 20 min at RT. The preparations are washed with TH + 0.02% NaN$_3$. The cover slips are transferred to slides and covered with 50% glycerol; the SIg$^+$ cells are counted in a fluorescence microscope under incident light as described elsewhere (11). At least 200 plaque-associated cells and, separately, $\geqslant 200$ cells in the plaque-free areas are counted.

3.4.4. Lymphocytes with HP Receptors. HP receptors are found only after NANAase treatment of the lymphocytes. The lymphocytes are treated with NANAase in TH containing 0.2% HSA before addition to the monolayers (see Method 46). Processing of the monolayers after incubation with the lymphocytes and staining with 0.1 ml of FITC-labeled HP (100 μg/ml) are performed exactly as described for SIg$^+$ staining (see also 11, 12).

4. Comments

4.1. Plaques. As already indicated, a clear zone corresponding to an area covered by at least 5 erythrocytes (E_c) is defined as a plaque. However, the average-sized plaque is approximately 5 times larger, and very large plaques may be formed by confluency of 2–3 smaller plaques. The plaques are irregular in shape, quite distinct from the circular plaques seen in the Jerne assay (3, 4). That plaque formation reflects lysis rather than detachment is revealed by electron microscopic observations of the clear zones, which contain cell debris and membrane material. Such studies also show that erythrocytes in contact with lymphocytes at the borders of the plaque may be swollen or fragmented (4). That plaque formation reflects lysis can also be established by making monolayers with ^{51}Cr-labeled erythrocytes and determining the relationship between ^{51}Cr release and plaque numbers. However, in order to obtain a good correlation with ^{51}Cr release, it is necessary to consider both plaque number and plaque size (12a).

4.2. Kinetics of Plaque Formation. Under the present conditions, plaque formation is a relatively rapid process and significant numbers of small-sized plaques are seen after only 2 hr of incubation. With purified lymphocytic effector cells, the number of plaques increases proportionally with time up to 20 hr of incubation (2, 4, 5). Both plaque number and plaque size increase up to that time, but only insignificantly thereafter. While the rate of plaque formation varies with both antibody concentration and lymphocyte dose, the time at which the reaction stops is independent of these variables over dilution ranges comprising 2–3 orders of magnitude (2). The cessation of plaque formation after about 20 hr most probably reflects saturation of effector cell Fc receptors with antigen–antibody complexes (13). Lymphocytes incubated on antibody-free monolayers are fully viable and form plaques when transferred to fresh monolayers in the presence of antibodies. In contrast, lymphocytes preincubated for 20 hr on antibody-coated monolayers are inactive upon transfer (12a).

The number of plaques formed at 20 hr increases with the number of lymphocytes added. At low or moderate doses, i.e., with 0.5 to 2×10^6 lymphocytes per dish, this increase is directly proportional to the lymphocyte concentration. Under the conditions given the number of E_c/mm^2 is $\sim 20,000$ while 0.5 to 2×10^6 lymphocytes added per dish make up for 500–2000 cells per mm^2 of the cover slip. Thus, the lymphocyte:erythrocyte ratios per unit area vary from 1:40 to 1:10. With smaller erythrocytes, e.g., E_b or E_s, these ratios become 2–3 times lower. When greater numbers of lymphocytes are added (up to 8×10^6/dish), the number of plaques found at 20 hr increases linearly with the logarithm of the lymphocyte dose (5) (Fig. 1).

4.3. Antibody. No plaques are formed in the absence of antibody, e.g., when rabbit serum is replaced by fetal bovine serum. With NRS, the number of plaques found at 20 hr is usually $\leqslant 5\%$ of that formed by an optimal dilution of rabbit antierythrocyte serum (5). Some rabbit sera may give higher background, probably owing to the occurrence of natural antibodies. When hyperimmune antiserum to E_c or E_b is added to the monolayers together with the lympho-

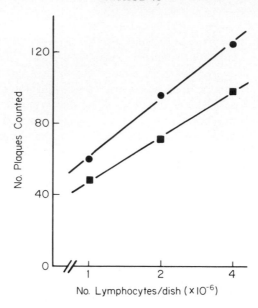

Fig. 1. K cell-dependent plaque formation. E_c monolayers; antiserum dilution 10^{-4}; duration of incubation 20 hr. Number of lymphocytes/dish ($\times 10^{-6}$); versus number of plaques
counted (total area screened for plaques = 2.15 mm^2). Lymphocytes were purified by nylon
column filtration (●) or by colloidal iron uptake and Ficoll—Isopaque centrifugation (■) (See
Method 46).

cytes, maximal plaque formation appears at high antiserum dilutions, e.g., 10^{-4}
or 10^{-5} (2, 4, 5). Lower dilutions may give a prozone (2) owing primarily to the
presence of inhibitory antibodies of IgM-type (14). No prozone is seen when the
IgG fraction of the antiserum is used. With serum suspected to contain immune
complexes or aggregates, it is advisable to pretreat the monolayers and wash
them before addition of the lymphocytes (4).

4.4. Number of Plaque-Forming Cells (PFC). Calculation of the minimal
number of PFC present in a lymphocyte preparation (see Section 3.2) is based
on several assumptions, the most important being that one effector cell forms
only one plaque. Since K cell-mediated lysis requires initial contact between
effector cells and target cells and the movement of the lymphocytes away from
the antibody coated target cells over a larger distance is restricted, it is difficult
to envisage formation of several plaques by one effector cell.

With the highly purified blood lymphocytes used herein (see Method 46) the
minimal number of PFC on an E_c monolayer ranges from 2.5 to 3.5% of the
total number of lymphocytes added (5). These numbers are obtained when the
number of lymphocytes per dish is $\leqslant 1 \times 10^6$ and antibody concentrations are

optimal. With higher numbers of lymphocytes added, the percentage of PFC decreases (5). This may be due partly to interference between the lymphocytes. However, the estimates are also subjected to various experimental errors. Thus, large plaques may have been formed by confluency of 2–3 smaller plaques, and this will lead to underestimates, particularly when high lymphocyte numbers have been applied and the plaques tend to increase in size.

That the numbers for PFC given above are on the low side becomes apparent also when bovine erythrocytes are used as target cells. These cells have no nucleus. This facilitates counting of small plaques, which are easily overlooked on E_c monolayers. With E_b monolayers, the number of PFC under optimal conditions ranges from 5 to 9%. Since surface marker studies indicate no differences between the PFC on the two types of monolayers, it is likely that the effector cells are identical. It may therefore be assumed that the actual number of erythrocyte-lysing K cells in the presence of optimal antibody concentrations comprises 10% of the cells in the purified blood lymphocyte preparations.

4.5. Nature of the Plaque-Forming K Cells. In incubation mixtures fixed and stained after completion of the experiment, one lymphocyte (or occasionally 2 or 3 lymphocytes) is found in 80% of the plaques. These lymphocytes are always seen close to the edges of the surrounding monolayers, never centrally located in the plaque. These plaque-associated cells are assumed to be the plaque-forming cells. This is supported by electron microscopic investigations (3, 4) and by studies of surface markers (5).

The results of one representative experiment performed with E_b monolayers are given in Table 1. In order to study distribution of the HP receptor, considered to be a T cell marker (9–12), plaque formation by NANAase-treated

TABLE 1
Percentage of Plaque-Forming Cells (PFC) and Surface Marker Distribution[a]

Lymphocytes	Percent PFC	Percent cells with surface marker			
		EAC^+	SIg^+	E^+	HP^+
Untreated					
Original	—	20	9	75	—
Plaque associated	5.6	35	10	3	—
On monolayer	—	17	13	20	—
NANAase treated					
Original	—	23	10	80	75
Plaque associated	6.5	47	11	9	27
On monolayer	—	21	13	27	66

[a] E_b monolayer, 2×10^6 lymphocytes/dish, 20 hr of incubation, anti-E_b diluted 10^{-3}.

lymphocytes has been included. Such lymphocytes generally give a larger number of antibody-dependent plaques than untreated lymphocytes, reflecting recruitment of additional effector cells into the system (3, 5).

For both effector cell preparations, Table 1 shows that the surface markers of the plaque-associated cells have a profile distinct from that seen in the original preparation as well as from that of lymphocytes remaining attached to the intact monolayer surrounding the plaques. The frequency of cells with different surface markers in the latter areas is very similar to that seen in the original preparation. This strongly supports the assumption that most of the plaque-associated cells represent the plaque-forming cells.

Surface marker studies indicate that PFC are heterogeneous. Generally EAC^+ cells comprise 40–60% of the plaque-associated cells. The percentage of plaque-associated SIg^+ lymphocytes ranges from 10–15%. Most of the SIg seems to be adsorbed IgG, appearing during the incubation period (B. Wåhlin, unpublished). It is unlikely that the plaque-associated SIg^+ cells are B cells since double-marker experiments show that most of them ($> 80\%$) also carry the HP marker, which has not been found on peripheral blood B cells. It is likely that these cells are identical with a subpopulation of HP^+ cells that also have Fc and complement receptors. This fraction comprises about 10% of the total HP^+ cell population in normal blood (11). It remains to be established whether or not these plaque-associated HP^+ cells, which regularly comprise $\sim$ one-third of all plaque-associated cells, are T cells or are of different ontogenetic origin.

Sheep erythrocyte-binding lymphocytes are always found associated with plaques (4, 5) but occur in higher frequency on the surrounding monolayer. The low numbers seen in Table 1 reflect the fact that the *in situ* technique used herein (see Section 3.4) detects only a minority of the E^+ cells present. Since a-E_b does not cross-react with E_s, this indicates that E_s binding is not caused by antibodies.

4.5. Other Plaque-Forming Cells. Many cell types in human blood are efficient antibody-dependent effector cells when erythrocytes are the target cells (14), and both PMN and monocytes are active in the plaque assay (5, 6). Plaque formation by isolated blood monocytes procedes at a greater rate but ceases after only about 6 hr of incubation, probably owing to their strong phagocytic activity, leading to saturation of their effector function within hours. Because of these differences in kinetics, contamination of a lymphocyte preparation with monocytes (5–10%) results in a biphasic curve when plaque formation is plotted as a function of time (5).

REFERENCES

1. Kedar, E., Ortiz de Landazuri, M., and Bonavida, B., *J. Immunol.* **112**, 1231 (1974).
2. Perlmann, P., Perlmann, H., Larsson, Å, and Wåhlin, B., *J. Reticuloendothel. Soc.* **17**, 241 (1975).

3. Perlmann, P., Biberfeld, P., Larsson, Å., Perlmann, H., and Wåhlin, B., *in* "Membrane Receptors of Lymphocytes" (M. Seligmann, J. L., Preud'homme, and F. M. Kourilsky, eds.), p. 161. North-Holland Publ., Amsterdam, 1975.

4. Biberfeld, P., Wåhlin, B., Perlmann, P., and Biberfeld, G., *Scand. J. Immunol.* **4,** 859 (1975).

5. Perlmann, P., and Wåhlin, B., *in* "Proceedings of the Tenth Leucocyte Culture Conference" (V. P. Ejsvogel, D. Roos, and W. P. Zeylemaker, eds.), p. 575. Academic Press, New York, 1976.

6. Inglis, J. R., Penhale, W. J., Farmer, A., Irvine, W. J., and Williams, A. E., *Clin. Exp. Immunol.* **21,** 216 (1975).

7. Perlmann, H., Perlmann, P., Pape, G. R., and Halldén, G., *Scand. J. Immunol.* Suppl. 5, in press.

8. Hammarström, S., and Kabat, E. A., *Biochemistry* **8,** 2696 (1969).

9. Hammarström, S., Hellström, U., Perlmann, P., and Dillner, M. L., *J. Exp. Med.* **138,** 1270 (1973).

10. Dillner, M. L., Hammarström, S., and Perlmann, P., *Exp. Cell Res.* **96,** 374 (1975).

11. Hellström, U., Hammarström, S., Dillner, M. L., Perlmann, H., and Perlmann, P., *Scand. J. Immunol.,* Suppl. 5, in press.

12. Hellström, U., Dillner, M. L., Hammarström, S., and Perlmann, P., *Scand. J. Immunol.* **5,** 45 (1976).

12a. B. Wåhlin, unpublished.

13. Perlmann, P., Perlmann, H., and Wigzell, H., *Transplant. Rev.* **13,** 91 (1972).

14. Perlmann, P., *Clin. Immunobiol.* **3,** in press.

Microcytotoxicity Assays of Cell-Mediated Tumor Immunity and Blocking Serum Factors

Ingegerd Hellström and Karl Erik Hellström

1. Introduction

A colony inhibition assay of cell-mediated immunity was introduced in the 1960s for measuring cytotoxic and growth inhibitory effects of specifically immune lymphocytes on plated target cells (1). This assay permitted a better quantitation of lymphocyte effects on target cells than did other assays available at that time. A major drawback with it was, however, that it could be used only on cells that plated well *in vitro* and that, even with such cells, it was technically demanding, both with respect to setting up the assays and counting the colonies.

Takasugi and Klein (2) introduced a microcytotoxicity assay, which differs from the colony inhibition technique in that target cells remaining attached to the surface of the wells of plastic Microtest plates are counted, rather than cells dividing and forming colonies. This assay can be used on a larger spectrum of target cells than can the colony-inhibition technique. The counting of individual target cells, rather than colonies, is also simpler.

We have modified the Takasugi–Klein assay (3), and we have used this modified assay to investigate various aspects of the immune response to both tumor antigens and normal alloantigens. Much of this work represents a continuation of our previous studies using the colony inhibition test. In particular, we have investigated the reactivity of tumor-immune lymphocytes on cultivated neoplastic cells and the blocking of such reactivity by factors present in the serum of tumor-bearing individuals. These studies have been performed in both animals and man. They have been discussed at length in two fairly recent review articles (4, 5).

A number of findings have evolved. Lymph node and spleen cells, as well as blood lymphocytes, from animals immunized with tumor cells have been found to be reactive against plated cells from the respective tumors. Lymphoid cells from tumor-bearing animals have often been found also to be reactive, but their degree of reactivity varies (5). In some systems animals with large tumors are as reactive as animals immunized with tumor cells, whereas in other cases reactivity is seen shortly after tumor transplantation and then disappears ("eclipse phenomenon").

Sera from tumor-bearing animals have been found to abrogate ("block") the cytotoxic effect of lymphocytes reactive against the tumor borne. This is most commonly demonstrated by performing microcytotoxicity assays in which the serum is left for the whole duration of the test together with lymphocytes and target cells. A blocking effect can, however, also be shown when the lymphocytes are preincubated with the tumor-bearer serum, followed by washing, before the lymphocytes are used as effector cells, as well as when the target cells are preincubated with the serum (and washed), before the lymphocytes are added (6). The blocking effect at the lymphocyte level is likely to be the more important one, since sera from tumor-immunized animals (which are resistant to tumor challenge *in vivo*) rarely block at the lymphocyte level, but more commonly do so at the target cell level (4, 5). The blocking serum effect detected by preincubating lymphocytes with tumor-bearer serum is sometimes referred to as "inhibition," while the blocking effect at the target cell level is referred to as "blocking" (4); we have, ourselves, always referred to both effects as "blocking."

The blocking serum factors are sometimes free antigens but more commonly complexes between tumor antigens and their antibodies (4, 5, 7, 8). Antisera to the respective tumor antigens can often abrogate ("unblock") the blocking serum effect (9), and they can remove blocking serum factors, when used to prepare immunoadsorbant columns through which the tumor-bearer sera are passed (8).

Sera from tumor-immunized donors can also increase ("potentiate") the reactivity detected in microcytotoxicity assays, performed as in regular tests for blocking serum activity (5). Furthermore, sera from tumor-immune and from tumor-bearing donors often contain lymphocyte-dependent antibodies, which can kill plated tumor cells in the presence of lymphoid (K) cells from nonimmune donors (10).

The microcytotoxicity assay has also been used to study immunity to human neoplasms. Findings have been reported that are essentially similar to those published from the animal studies, the major difference being that human tumors of the same histological type have been found to cross-react with each other (5). The latter conclusion has been challenged, however, (see e.g., 11), since in several studies lymphocytes from control donors have been shown to react at least as strongly as lymphocytes from patients having the respective tumor. According to some reports, there is no evidence at all for cell-mediated reactivity against tissue type-specific antigens in human neoplasms (12), while according to other (recent) reports the original claims of reactivity to tissue type-specific human tumor antigens can be confirmed, although the differences are not as absolute as was originally believed (see, e.g., 13). It is interesting that experiments performed with independent assays of cellular immunity, such as the leukocyte migration inhibition technique, give support for the presence of tissue type-specific tumor antigens in human neoplasms [see e.g., (14)].

We shall now describe in detail how the microcytotoxicity assays are presently being carried out in our laboratory.

2. Material

Both animal (mouse, rat, chicken, rabbit) and human material has been used to provide target cells. Studies performed to search for tumor specific immunity are, whenever possible, conducted also in the autochthonous system in order to minimize the impact of reactions to alloantigens. As often as is practically possible, experiments are performed in a "criss-cross" pattern, studying at the same time at least two tumors, A and B, and lymphocytes from donors immunized to either A or B, matching the target cells and the lymphocytes so that the same lymphocyte suspension will act as control with one set of target cells and as immune cells with the other. This way, the impact of various "nonspecific" effects can be decreased. Often (always for the human studies) we include normal target cells from the same patients as the tumor cells. These cells are most commonly skin fibroblasts, but normal colonic or kidney epithelial cells have also been used when studying patients with colon and kidney cancers, respectively.

The tumor target cells are grown in culture for 1–15 weeks prior to being used for the experiments. By freezing tumor cells in liquid nitrogen during their very early passage, we try to establish a stock tumor material that can be used for testing without need for long periods of propagation *in vitro*.

3. Methods

3.1. **Selection of Target Cells.** When tumor cultures are established, nonnecrotic tumors have to be used. Neoplasms that are heavily mixed with stroma cells are not suitable. Metastases are often easier to cultivate than primary neoplasms. Cultures should be selected for plating in which the cells are healthy, dividing but not growing too densely, since it is difficult to obtain a good single-cell suspension from dense cultures. Cultures are regularly checked for the absence of *Mycoplasma* infection (through the courtesy of Dr. G. E. Kenny, Department of Pathobiology, University of Washington).

3.2. **Trypsinization.** The selected culture is rinsed twice with 2 ml of 0.025% trypsin solution to remove trypsin inactivators in the culture medium. When the third rinsing is done, the trypsin is left for a short time to destroy damaged cells. Then 1 ml of trypsin is added to the target cells layer at room temperature (if the cells are especially adherent, transfer to 37°C may facilitate trypsinization). The cells should not be left with trypsin any longer than is necessary to come off the surface. As soon as the cells detach from the culture flask, a small amount of "complete Waymouth's medium" (see below) containing 30% fetal calf serum (heat inactivated at 56°C for 30 min) is added to inactivate the trypsin.

The 0.025% solution of trypsin is prepared from trypsin 1:250 dissolved in Versene. Stock Versene solution is prepared from 160 g of NaCl, 8 g of KCl, 4 g of Versene; the solution is diluted 1:10 in distilled water.

The "complete Waymouth's medium" with 30% serum is prepared by mixing 30 ml of fetal calf serum, 70% Waymouth's medium (Catalogue No. H 14, GIBCO, Santa Clara, California), 1 ml of a concentrate of penicillin–streptomycin solution containing 10^7 IU of potassium-buffered penicillin and 10 g of streptomycin per 1000 ml, 1 ml of L-glutamine solution prepared from 29.2 g of L-glutamine dissolved into 1000 ml of distilled water and 8.5 g of NaCl, 1 ml of a 100 X solution of nonessential amino acids (GIBCO, Catalogue No. 114), 1 ml of 100 mM solution of sodium pyruvate (Microbiological Associates, Bethesda, Maryland), 1.5 ml of a solution containing 75 g of NaHCO$_3$ per 1000 ml of distilled water.

The fetal calf serum is pretested for its ability to support plating of the type of target cells used for the tests.

3.3. Counting Target Cells to Be Plated. The cells are suspended carefully in a suitable amount of medium, diluted 1:10 in a isotonic trypan blue solution using a white blood cell diluting pipette, and counted in a hemocytometer to determine the number of viable (unstained) cells. The number of cells per milliliter in the suspension is calculated.

3.4. Plating. Depending upon the plating efficiency of the target cells, the number of cells plated per well generally varies between 50 and 120. The goal is to get between 50 and 200 stained cells per well in the media-control wells at the conclusion of the experiment. An appropriate dilution of target cells is prepared in a 2-oz French square bottle (Catalogue No. 4363-15, Curtin Matheson Scientific, Inc., Tukwila, Washington).

When preparing the cell suspension to be plated, we use complete Waymouth's culture medium with a pH of 7.2–7.4. The cells are stirred gently (less than 100 rpm) with a magnetic bar and stirrer, avoiding the formation of bubbles. Using a pipette or an automatic pipettor (e.g., BBL automatic pipette No. 60422, Drummond Scientific Company, Broomall, Pennsylvania), 0.2 ml of the target cell suspension is dispersed per well in a Falcon No. 3040 Microtest culture plate (Falcon Plastics, Oxnard, California). The addition of target cells to the plate is done in a defined sequence from left top (A1) to right bottom (H12). The finished plate is wiped off with a sterile paper towel, covered with Falcon No. 3041 lid, and labeled (both the plate and the lid). Plating should be accomplished rapidly to avoid dehydration and pH changes.

3.5. First Incubation. The plate is placed in a humidified 37°C incubator having an atmosphere of 5% CO_2 in air. The incubation period must be at least 4 hr, but 8–12 hr is preferable for optimal cell attachment.

3.6. Addition of Control and Experimental Group Sera to Test for Blocking ("Arming," etc.) Activity. After the incubation period, the plate is inverted and jarred to remove the culture medium. The cells will remain attached. The plate is then wiped with a sterile paper towel. A protocol is designed for each plate such that certain wells will receive control sera, others test sera, and a few no sera, but instead medium. This is done in order to minimize the influence of inequalities in different parts of the plate, so-called "row effects" (15). Principles for designation of what treatment a given well shall receive in order to minimize the influence of these "row effects" are described separately (16). Wells receiving medium only serve as controls whereby the plating efficiency can be determined. To each well 0.1 ml of test (or control) serum (or medium) is added per protocol. The sera are diluted with phosphate-buffered saline (PBS) to the desired dilutions (often 1:5 to 1:80) after they have been heat-inactivated at 56°C for 30 min.

3.7. Second Incubation. The plate is incubated for 45 min in a humidified incubator (same as 3.5).

3.8. Addition of Lymphocytes. To plates receiving sera, 0.1 ml of lymphocyte suspension per well is added as specified by protocol design. To plates not receiving sera, lymphocytes are added in 0.2 ml per well. The lymphocytes are diluted to desired cell density in complete MEM from GIBCO (Catalogue No. 7025 special). Doses between 200,000 lymphocytes per well down to 100 lymphocytes per well are commonly used. Each combination of lymphocytes and serum is tested in at least 8 replicates.

3.9. Third Incubation. The plate is incubated 45 min on a rocker; 0.05 ml of 50% inactivated fetal calf serum diluted in complete Eagle's culture medium is added.

3.10. Fourth Incubation. After 20 hr incubation at 37°C in a moist CO_2 in air atmosphere, medium is dumped off and complete MEM medium without fetal calf serum is added, 0.2 ml/well.

3.11. Fifth Incubation. The plate is incubated 16–30 hr further at 37°C in a CO_2 in air atmosphere.

3.12. Staining. The plate is washed with PBS several times very carefully and then stained with crystal violet. Stained plates can be kept for long periods of time without deterioration in quality. They are being stored after counting as a permanent record of the experiment.

3.13. Calculation of Data. All plates are coded, when the tests are set up, and they are counted without knowledge of the code. Target cells are counted as having survived the test, if they have a distinct nucleus, surrounded by cytoplasm.

Percentage "cytotoxicity" (actually, percentage of cells that have been killed by exposure to immune lymphocytes or have detached from the plastic surface and thus no longer remain attached to it, or have failed to divide, as compared to cells in the control group) is calculated by comparing the number of remaining target cells per well in the presence of immune lymphocytes with that seen in the presence of the same number of control lymphocytes. The statistical significance of these differences are determined by student's t tests. Since media wells receiving no lymphocytes are always included, calculations can also be made with respect to the number of remaining cells in these wells.

Blocking serum activity is defined as the ability of a test serum, as compared to a control serum, to abrogate cell-mediated destruction of the target cells by the same immune lymphocytes; 100% blocking activity means that a serum can completely abrogate detectable cytotoxicity, and a blocking activity beyond that implies that the number of remaining target cells per well is higher in the presence of the blocking serum and immune lymphocytes than in the presence of the same serum and control lymphocytes.

Evidence of lymphocyte-dependent antibody (LDA), sometimes referred to as "arming," activity of a test serum, as compared to a control serum, is calculated as the ability of a serum to decrease the number of target cells remaining in the presence of normal, control lymphocytes (10).

3.14. Modification of Test When Human Cells Are Studied. When human cells are used as target cells, they are treated the same way as the animal cells except for the following. The human cells are plated in complete Waymouth medium with 30% inactive fetal calf serum and incubated overnight. Media are dumped off the next morning and lymphocytes are added that have been suspended in complete Waymouth medium with HEPES buffer (GIBCO, Catalogue No. 130440) but lacking fetal calf serum, 0.2 ml of lymphocyte suspension being pipetted into each well. After 45 min incubation, 0.05 ml of 50% inactivated fetal calf serum in complete Waymouth's medium is added. The plates are incubated for 40–48 hr.

4. Effector Cell Preparation

4.1. Lymph Node Cells. Single-cell suspensions are prepared by pressing lymph nodes through a fine mesh screen, and the screen is washed in complete MEM without fetal calf serum using a volume of about 15 ml. The cells are spun down at 900–1000 rpm 10 min and washed 2 more times (total of 3 washes) in 10 ml. They are resuspended in 3–6 ml of complete MEM without serum, and counted with 1:100 dilution pipette. The viability of the cells according to trypan blue staining should be 80–90%.

4.2. Human Lymphocytes. Forty milliliters of blood are drawn and defribrinated in flasks whose bottom is covered with glass beads, 3 mm in diameter. The blood is defibrinated for approximately 10 min, or until clot is formed around the beads, and then diluted with 40 ml of PBS. The suspension is divided equally into two 90-ml centrifuge tubes, and the flask is rinsed with another 40 ml of PBS. The cells are divided equally into the 90-ml tubes so that the final dilution of blood is 1:3, and layered with 15 ml of Ficoll—Hypaque with a density of 1.077. They are then spun for 15 min at 1300 rpm. The lymphocytes are harvested by removing the lymphocyte band with a Pasteur pipette. They are diluted up to 50 ml in PBS, and spun down for 15 min at 1300 rpm. The PBS is poured off, and the pellet is resuspended in 15 ml of RPMI 1640 (GIBCO, Catalogue No. H-18) culture medium into 10% inactivated fetal calf serum. The cell suspensions are then placed in a large plastic culture flask (Falcon No. 3024) and incubated at 37°C for about 10 min. The lymphocytes are harvested from the bottles into centrifuge tubes (same as used earlier). The flasks are rinsed with another 15 ml of RPMI, and for a second time with 5 ml of RPMI. The cells are centrifuged for 15 min at 1300 rpm. They are washed one more time with 50 ml of PBS, and resuspended in 2 ml of complete Waymouth's medium with HEPES. The cells are then counted. There should be less than 5% dead cells with only 0—10% polynuclear cells present.

ACKNOWLEDGMENTS

This investigation was supported by Grants CA 19148 and CA 19149, awarded by the National Cancer Institute, Department of Health, Education and Welfare.

REFERENCES

1. Hellström, I., *Int. J. Cancer* **3**, 65 (1967).
2. Takasugi, M., and Klein, E., *Transplantation* **9**, 219 (1970).
3. Hellström, I., and Hellström, K. E., in "*In Vitro* Methods in Cell Mediated Immunity" (B. R. Bloom and P. R. Glade, eds.), p. 409. Academic Press, New York, 1971.
4. Baldwin, R. W., *Adv. Cancer Res.* **18**, 1 (1973).
5. Hellström, K. E., and Hellström, I., *Adv. Immunol.* **18**, 209 (1974).
6. Hayami, M., Hellström, I., and Hellström, K. E., *Int. J. Cancer* **13**, 43 (1974).
7. Tamerius, J., Hellström, I., and Hellström, K. E., *Int. J. Cancer* **16**, 456 (1975).
8. Tamerius, J., Nepom, J., Hellström, I., and Hellström, K. E., *J. Immunol.* **116**, 724 (1976).
9. Hellström, I., and Hellström, K. E., *Int. J. Cancer* **5**, 195 (1970).
10. Pollack, S., Heppner, G., Brawn, R. J., and Nelson, K., *Int. J. Cancer* **9**, 316 (1972).
11. Herberman, R. B., and Oldham, R. K., *J. Natl. Cancer Inst.* **55**, 749 (1975).
12. Takasugi, M., Mickey, M. R., and Terasaki, P. I., *Cancer Res.* **33**, 2898 (1976).
13. Steele, G., Sjögren, H. O., and Staudenberg, I., *Int. J. Cancer* **17**, 27 (1976).
14. McCoy, J. L., Jerome, L. F., Dean, J. H., Perlin, E., Oldham, R. K., Char, D. H., Cohen, M. H., Felix, E. L., and Herberman, R. B., *J. Natl. Cancer Inst.* **55**, 19 (1975).
15. Takasugi, M., Mickey, M. R., and Terasaki, P. I., *Natl. Cancer Inst. Monogr.* **37**, 77 (1973).
16. Brown, J., van Belle, G., and Hellström, I., *Int. J. Cancer* submitted for publication.

Blocking of Cell-Mediated Cytotoxicity

R. W. Baldwin, M. J. Embleton, and R. A. Robins

1. Introduction

An *in vitro* cell-mediated cytotoxicity assay based on that developed by the Hellströms and co-workers (1, 2) has been used extensively in our laboratory to investigate the antitumor immune responses of tumor-bearing hosts, and animals or patients receiving tumor immunization or immunotherapy (3–5). An important part of these studies has been to detect, characterize, and identify humoral factors that interfere with cell-mediated immunity. These factors are usually defined operationally as "blocking factor" when interacting at the level of the target cells, or "inhibitory factor" when tested at the level of the effector cell. Using animal models, blocking factor protecting tumor target cells against cytotoxicity has been identified as complexes of soluble tumor antigen and tumor-specific antibody (5, 6), which appear in the circulation during active tumor growth (5). Under some circumstances, sera containing excess tumor-specific antibody can block (7). Cytotoxicity can be inhibited by pretreatment of sensitized lymphoid cells with soluble antigen alone (4, 8, 9) or sera known to contain immune complexes (4, 5).

Many attempts are currently being made to investigate cell-mediated cytotoxicity to tumor cells and relate this to clinical course in cancer patients receiving conventional therapy or immunotherapy, but to date many groups have found no clear correlation (10–13). However, in studies in which blocking factors have been evaluated, a correlation seems to be emerging in that the appearance of serum-blocking factor is associated with relapse or poor prognosis, and a decrease in blocking factor is associated with a more favorable clinical course (10, 11, 14).

Another aspect of the study of blocking or inhibitory effects on cell-mediated cytotoxicity is to attempt to determine the specificity of cytotoxic reactions. It is currently believed by many workers that both normal human donors and cancer patients have lymphoid cells cytotoxic for a wide range of cultured tumor cells (15–17) contrary to earlier suggestions than human tumor cells are characterized by antigens representative of cancer of a given histological type (2, 18). Studies on antigen-mediated inhibition of lymphoid cell cytotoxicity suggest that inhibition is specific for antigen-containing extracts from the same tumor type as that of the lymphoid cell donor and the target cells (4, 9, 19). Since the antigen extracts appear to have little effect on "nonspecific" reactivity, this extra inhibition step may prove to be of great value in distinguishing between tumor-directed and nonspecific cytotoxicity against human tumors.

2. Materials

2.1. Cell cultures derived from tumors of the species under study. These are maintained in glass or plastic tissue culture flasks and should consist entirely of neoplastic cells without contamination by stromal elements.

2.2. Tissue culture media appropriate for the cells being studied. We use Eagle's minimal essential medium (MEM) supplemented with 10% calf serum, glutamine, and antibiotics (penicillin, 100 IU/ml, streptomycin, 200 μg/ml) for rat tumors, and MEM, Waymouth's 752/1, Ham's F10, or RPMI 1640 supplemented with fetal calf serum or human AB +ve plasma for different kinds of human tumor. Cultures are harvested with 0.25% trypsin (Difco) in Hanks' balanced salt solution (HBSS). Effector cells are often prepared in MEM buffered with HEPES (N-2-hydroxyethylpipera-zine-N'-2-ethanesulfonic acid, 20 mM, from Sigma or Flow).

2.3. Microtiter plates containing 96 wells of about 300 μl capacity such as Falcon 3040 or Cooke M29ART. The plates used should have flat-bottomed wells and be sterile and suitable for tissue culture.

2.4. Eppendorf pipettes or similar devices delivering volumes of 200, 100, and 50 μl.

2.5. Incubators humidified and gassed with 5% CO_2 in air, or humidified chambers if HEPES-buffered medium is used in a conventional incubator.

2.6. Solution of Ficoll (Pharmacia) and sodium metrizoate (e.g., Triosil, Hypaque, Isopaque) in concentrations appropriate to the study system.

2.7. Stainless steel or nylon mesh, cut to approximately 5-cm squares, and sterilized by autoclaving in glass petri dishes.

2.8. Heparinized or defibrinated blood from patients and controls as a source of effector cells. If heparin is used, preservative-free material should be employed.

2.9. Serum or plasma from individuals to be tested for blocking activity and from normal donors. Sera are heat-inactivated at 56°C for 30 min before use.

2.10. Soluble extracts of tumor tissue prepared by treatment of extranuclear membrane fractions with papain (8, 9) or 3 M KCl (20). Details of preparative methods for these materials are given in the references cited.

2.11. Centrifuge and sterile tubes.

2.12. 0.9% saline, methanol, 0.1% aqueous crystal violet stain.

2.13. Stereoscopic microscope, approximately ×30 magnification.

3. Methodology

3.1. Effector Cell Preparation. Rat lymph node cells are prepared by mincing aseptically removed cervical, axillary, and mesenteric lymph nodes with scissors, and gently pressing cells from the minced tissue through a stainless steel or nylon mesh in 4 ml of HEPES-MEM. The plunger of a sterile disposable syringe is a suitable tool for this purpose. The cells are washed twice (50 g for 5 min) before final resuspension, and the cells are then counted in a hemocytometer using trypan blue exclusion as a viability test.

Human mononuclear cells are prepared by layering heparinized blood over a solution containing Ficoll (6.35%, w/v) and Triosil (13.4.%, v/v), density 1.078. Usually about 10 ml of blood is layered onto 10 ml of the gradient in a 25 ml Universal bottle. The blood is centrifuged at 400 g for 20 minutes at room temperature, and the supernatant plasma and interface mononuclear cells are collected. The plasma may be stored at −20°C for use in blocking tests. The mononuclear cells are centrifuged (300 g for 10 min) then washed three times in MEM (50 g for 10 min) before final resuspension and counting by hemocytometer. Other methods of effector cell preparation have been used (15, 18), and the final choice of preparative method depends partly on the tumor system under study.

3.2. Microcytotoxicity Test. Target cells are harvested from monolayer cell cultures with 0.25% trypsin and adjusted to a cell count of 10^3/ml in the culture medium normally used for their propagation. They are plated in the wells of the microtiter plates at 100 cells (0.1 ml) or 200 cells (0.2 ml) per well, depending on the plating efficiency of the target cell line. The plates are then incubated at 37°C for between 4 and 24 hr to allow cell attachment to the bottoms of the wells. The medium is removed and replaced by lymphoid effector cells from normal or immunized animals, or, in tests with human materials, with effector cells from cancer patients or control donors. In rat tumor studies lymph node cells are used at a level of 2×10^5 to 4×10^5 cells per well, and in human tests blood mononuclear cells are used at 5×10^4 to 10^5 cells per well, again using the medium in which the target cells are normally maintained. After two further days of incubation at 37°C, the plates are rinsed with saline to remove effector cells and detached target cells. The remaining target cells are fixed with methanol, stained with 0.1% crystal violet, and counted under ×30 stereoscopic magnification. Cytotoxicity is calculated according to the following formula:

$$\% \text{ Cytotoxicity} = 100 \times \frac{C-T}{C}$$

where C is the mean number of target cells in wells exposed to control effector cells and T is the mean number of target cells in wells exposed to test mononuclear cells. At least 8 replicate wells are used for each effector cell treatment, and the statistical significance of differences between numbers of surviving target cells with test and control effector cells is calculated using the Student t test.

3.3. Blocking Test. Target tumor cells are plated as described above (Section 3.2); after cell attachment, the medium is replaced by serum to be tested for blocking. Sera are diluted 1:5 in MEM for testing, and 50 μl per well is added to the target cells. The serum and cells are incubated for 45 min at 37°C, then the serum is removed and replaced by effector cell suspension, followed by 2 days of incubation. If it is not required to distinguish between interactions at the level of the target cell and at the level of the effector cell, serum may be left in the wells at the end of 45 min of incubation. After 2 days of incubation, the plates are rinsed, fixed, and stained as in the standard microcytotoxicity assay. Both control and immune (or patient) effector cells are added to target cell wells treated with control serum, as well as to target cells treated with serum being tested for blocking activity. The percentage of cytotoxicity of immune or patient lymphoid cells compared with control effector cells is calculated separately for wells treated with test or control serum. Percent blocking is calculated by the formula:

$$\% \text{ Blocking} = 100 \times \frac{A-B}{A}$$

where A is the percent cytotoxicity against target cells treated with control serum and B is the percent cytotoxicity against target cells treated with test serum.

3.4. Inhibition Test. Target cells are plated in the same way as for the standard microcytotoxicity assay, but aliquots of effector cells are pretreated with serum or antigen extract to be tested for inhibitory activity before being added to the target cells. In rat tumor studies, lymph node cells are pretreated with serum at a dilution of 1:5 (0.5 ml of diluted serum per 5×10^6 effector cells) or various dilutions of soluble antigen up to a concentration of 2 mg/ml (1 mg per 5×10^6 effector cells). In human studies, serum is used at 0.25 ml per 10^6 cells, and soluble antigen at concentrations up to 1.5 mg/ml (2.5 mg per 10^6 effector cells). The serum or antigen and effector cells are incubated for 45 min at 37°C, then the effector cells spun down (50 g for 10 min) and resuspended in culture medium at the appropriate concentration before being added to the target cells for the usual 2-day incubation. Surviving target cells are then rinsed, fixed, stained, and counted. Both control and test effector cells are pretreated with serum or antigen preparation, and the percent inhibition is calculated using the same formula as for percent blocking (Section 3.3).

4. Comments

4.1. The large microtiter plates (i.e., 96 wells of 300-μl capacity) are preferable to Terasaki plates (10 μl per well) for blocking/inhibition tests because they are easier to manipulate (i.e., in removing and replacing medium) and there is less risk of nonspecific effects caused by adverse culture conditions. Also, human mononuclear cells prepared by the Ficoll/ Triosil method are much less nonspecifically toxic in the larger plates than in Terasaki plates.

4.2. Effector cell ratios need to be titrated in each tumor system and for each preparative method in order to determine the ratio that produces the most satisfactory levels of specific cytotoxicity compatible with minimal nonspecific cytotoxicity (i.e., cytotoxicity by control donor lymphoid cells). In our studies with rat tumors, 2×10^5 lymph node cells per well give optimum results: about 90% of rats immunized against tumors react against the immunizing tumor at this dose, whereas only 10% react against other tumors with unrelated tumor-associated antigens. Normal lymph node cells usually do not produce cytotoxic effects at this ratio compared with medium controls, but some tests show enhancement of target cell growth in wells treated with lymph node cells compared with medium alone.

In human studies the use of 5×10^4 to 10^5 mononuclear cells per well produces cytotoxicity against short-term cell lines with about 10–20% of normal donors compared with medium alone; reactivity with cancer patient donors is variable, ranging from 10% to 60% of donors in different types of cancer (3). It should be borne in mind that blocking is a competitive effect, and that if cytotoxicity is very strong, blocking effects may be difficult to demonstrate. In this case, the use of lower numbers of effector cells may allow blocking effects to be evaluated more clearly.

4.3. Target cells must be healthy tumor cells. The neoplastic nature of animal tumor cells can be tested by tumor growth in syngeneic recipients. Human cultured cells are more difficult to check, and with short-term cultures it has to be considered that some normal cells may be present in the target cell cultures. Long-term culture lines may be preferable from this viewpoint, but these, owing to *in vitro* selection, may be very different from the tumor from which they were derived. Some workers report that long-term cell lines are more susceptible to cytotoxicity than short-term cultures, giving a lesser degree of specificity with normal donor effector cells (21).

4.4. If antigen preparations are to be used for inhibition studies, the method of extraction must be shown to be suitable for the system under study. Thus, alternative tests for antigen activity should be employed to check that the materials used are indeed antigenic, otherwise interpretation of results may be invalid.

4.5. Nonspecific toxicity of antigen preparations may be a problem, which we have overcome by several methods. These include (a) using antibacterial agents (for example sodium azide) throughout the preparative procedure, with rapid dialysis and sterilization by filtration as the final step; (b) treatment of the preparation with 70% saturated ammonium sulfate and redissolving the precipitated protein, followed by dialysis and sterilization (4, 9); and (c) incubation of the antigen and lymphoid cells in the presence of normal serum at a 1:5 dilution (8).

4.6. It is important to test wells involving both normal and "sensitized" effector cells with blocking serum (or antigen) and normal serum, since the addition of serum could affect effector populations in a manner that would lead to erroneous conclusions if only one population were exposed to the serum.

REFERENCES

1. Hellström, I., and Hellström, K. E., *Int. J. Cancer* 4, 587 (1969).
2. Hellström, I., Hellström, K. E., Sjögren, H. O., and Warner, G. A., *Int. J. Cancer* 7, 1 (1971).
3. Baldwin, R. W., Embleton, M. J., Jones, J. S. P., and Langman, M. J. S., *Int. J. Cancer* 12, 73 (1973).
4. Embleton, M. J., *Br. J. Cancer* 28, (Suppl. I) 142 (1973).
5. Bowen, J. G., Robins, R. A., and Baldwin, R. W., *Int. J. Cancer* 15, 640 (1975).
6. Baldwin, R. W., Price, M. R., and Robins, R. A., *Nature (London), New Biol.* 238, 185 (1972).
7. Baldwin, R. W., Embleton, M. J., and Robins. R. A., *Int. J. Cancer* 11, 1 (1973).
8. Baldwin, R. W., Price, M. R., and Robins, R. A., *Int. J. Cancer* 11, 527 (1973).
9. Baldwin, R. W., Embleton, M. J., and Price, M. R., *Int. J. Cancer* 12, 84 (1973).
10. Hellström, I., Warner, G. A., Hellström, K. E., and Sjögren, H. O., *Int. J. Cancer* 11, 280 (1973).
11. Currie, G. A., *Br. J. Cancer* 28, 25 (1973).
12. Berkelhammer, J., Mastrangelo, M. J., Laucius, J. F., Bodurtha, A. J., and Prehn, R. T., *Int. J. Cancer* 16, 571 (1975).
13. Baldwin, R. W., *J. Natl. Cancer Inst.* 55, 765 (1975).
14. Hellström, I., Sjögren, H. O., Warner, G. A., and Hellström, K. E., *Int. J. Cancer* 7, 226 (1971).
15. Takasugi, M., Mickey, M. R., and Terasaki, P. I., *J. Natl. Cancer Inst.* 53, 1527 (1974).
16. Takasugi, M., Mickey, M. R., and Terasaki, P. I., *Cancer Res.* 33, 2898 (1973).
17. Herberman, R. B., *Isr. J. Med. Sci.* 9, 300 (1973).
18. Bubenik, J., Perlmann, P., Helmstein, K., and Moberger, G., *Int. J. Cancer* 5, 39 (1970).
19. Embleton, M. J., and Price, M. R., *Behring Inst. Mitt.* 56, 157 (1975).
20. Zöller, M., Price, M. R., and Baldwin, R. W., *Int. J. Cancer* 17, 129 (1975).
21. De Vries, J. E., Meyering, M., Van Dongen, A., annd Rümke, P., *Int. J. Cancer* 15, 391 (1975).

Leukocyte-Adherence Inhibition Test and Blocking Factors in Cancer

W. J. Halliday

1. Introduction

Leukocyte-adherence inhibition (LAI) is related, historically and conceptually, to macrophage-migration inhibition (MMI). The author's experience with the latter technique (1–3) led to the realization that improvements in rapidity and reliability would be most desirable. Accordingly, a study was made of the event supposedly taking place during the first hour of a migration experiment: the initial adherence of cells to the solid substrate. It was discovered that mouse peritoneal cells would rapidly adhere to glass and that this adherence could be inhibited, in the case of presensitized cells, by the addition of the specific antigen (4). Further work on this phenomenon was encouraged by reports of other rapid cell-mediated reactions, namely macrophage-spreading inhibition (5) and the slowing of macrophage electrophoretic mobility (6). The hypothesis arose that the cell populations contained specific antigen-reactive cells (probably lymphocytes) and nonspecific adherent indicator cells (probably macrophages).

The early work with LAI was done using mouse tumor systems (4, 7), with peritoneal cells as the cell populations and soluble tumor extracts as antigens. Specificity was related to individual tumors. With the technical procedures thus established, application to human blood leukocytes and human tumors was almost immediately successful (8–10). The adherent cells from human blood are mostly polymorphs, and specificity is related to tumor type. More recent studies have demonstrated the applicability of LAI to other antigens, such as those of fungi (11, 12) and bacteria (13), and also to hapten systems (14). The idea that LAI and MMI may be related aspects of cell-mediated immunity is reinforced by the discovery of a requirement for T cells in LAI (13, 15) and the detection of a rapidly produced lymphokine (13, 16). The biological significance of LAI is entirely conjectural; at present it is simply a convenient method of detecting *in vitro* one of the many activities of lymphocytes.

LAI has two further properties in common with MMI: the lymphocyte–antigen reactions are modified specifically by serum factors, and the tests can be converted into "two-stage" modifications. Blocking and unblocking of the LAI reaction can be readily demonstrated by suitable sera in systems utilizing mouse tumors (7), human tumors (8–10, 17), microbial antigens (11, 12), and haptens

(14). For some purposes the use of a single population to supply both reactive and indicator cells is undesirable. A supernatant can then be prepared from antigen-treated sensitized cells and tested on normal adherent cells (from another animal species if desired). This is the two-stage indirect, or split technique. These developments of the LAI test are described below.

The main advantages of the LAI technique over other methods in cell-mediated immunity are (a) rapidity, which leads to secondary advantages in that the conditions for short-term leukocyte culture are not critical; (b) use of stable soluble antigens rather than cultivated target cells; and (c) consistent results that are readily related to *in vivo* situations.

Confirmation of the reality of the LAI phenomenon has come from several other investigators (13, 18–23), who have usually attempted to modify the cell counting and washing procedures. The value of the original technique in detecting immunoreactivity in human cancer has recently been confirmed (24).

2. Materials

2.1. Materials for Preparing Human Blood Leukocytes

2.1.1. Glass bottles (25–30 ml with screw cap) containing about 300 units of sodium heparin

2.1.2. Plastic tubes (5 ml)

2.1.3. Pasteur pipettes

2.1.4. Centrifuge, bench type with swing-out head (not refrigerated)

2.1.5. Ammonium chloride solution, 0.15 M

2.1.6. Hemocytometer

2.1.7. Microscope (10X eyepieces, 10X and 40X objectives)

2.1.8. Culture medium: Eagle's basal medium with 10% fetal calf serum and 0.28 mg/ml sodium bicarbonate. The latter is only about one-fifth of the normal amount and allows the whole procedure to be conducted in air without added CO_2. Other tissue culture media may be suitable.

2.1.9. Incubator at 37°C

2.1.10. Disposable syringes (20 ml) and needles (21 gauge) for venipuncture

2.2. Materials for Preparing Mouse Peritoneal Cells

2.2.1. Disposable syringes (10 ml) and needles (18 gauge with additional holes drilled near tip, required only if mice are to be kept)

2.2.2. Hanks' balanced salt solution containing heparin (10 U/ml)

2.2.3. Mineral oil (liquid paraffin)

2.2.4. Materials as for human blood leukocytes (2.1.2–2.1.8)

2.2.5. Ice

2.3. Materials for Preparing Tumor Extracts (Antigens)

2.3.1. Small scissors and forceps

2.3.2. Stainless steel spatulas

2.3.3. Stainless steel mesh (10 X 10 cm, 80 mesh)

2.3.4. Plastic petri dishes, 60 mm diameter

2.3.5. Pasteur pipettes

2.3.6. Phosphate-buffered saline (equal parts of 0.15 M phosphate buffer, pH 7.2–7.4, and 0.85% sodium chloride solution)

2.3.7. Motor-driven glass homogenizer (plunger type, Braun or Duall)

2.3.8. Centrifuge tubes (15 ml)

2.3.9. Centrifuge tubes (high speed)

2.3.10. Centrifuge, bench type with swing-out head

2.3.11. Centrifuge, refrigerated, with high-speed attachment (International)

2.3.12. Freezer for storage at $-50°$C or lower

2.4. Serum. Serum is obtained from clotted blood and stored at $-20°$C in small tubes. It is not filtered or heat-treated. Both test sera and normal serum (from healthy donors) are required. Mouse serum is used with mouse leukocytes and human serum with human leukocytes.

2.5. Materials for LAI Test

2.5.1. Hemocytometers. Originally we used hemocytometer slides having four transverse channels, with ground-glass ridges supporting the cover slip (Arthur H. Thomas, Philadelphia). An even more convenient design has the ends of the slide thinner than the remainder, enabling the cover slip to be lowered easily with forceps onto the ridges. With practice, hemocyto-meters of any type are suitable. They are cleaned by soaking in detergent, scrubbing with a soft brush, and rinsing in distilled water several times.

2.5.2. Cover slips, No. 1, 24 mm square. These can be used straight from the original pack and discarded after use.

2.5.3. Petri dishes, 150 mm diameter, some containing filter paper circles moistened with distilled water.

2.5.3. Beakers, 150–200 ml

2.5.4. Sodium chloride solution, 0.85% (saline)

2.5.5. Microscope (10X eyepieces, 10X and 40X objectives)

2.5.6. Incubator at $37°$C (ordinary atmosphere)

2.5.7. Water bath at $37°$C

2.5.8. Plastic tubes, 5 ml, with caps

2.5.9. Tube rack

2.5.10. Pasteur pipettes

2.5.11. Forceps

2.5.12. Automatic pipette with tips (Oxford sampler) to deliver 0.05 ml

2.5.13. Culture medium as above (2.1.8)

2.5.14. Calculator

3. Methods

3.1. Preparation of Leukocyte Suspensions. *3.1.1. From Human Blood.* Venous blood (15 ml) is taken into glass bottles containing heparin. A further 5

ml may be taken at the same time and allowed to clot if serum is also required. The heparinized blood is allowed to stand undisturbed in the 37°C incubator until the erythrocytes have sedimented (30 min is often an adequate time for the blood of cancer patients, and the time should not be extended beyond 60 min). The leukocyte-rich plasma is removed into plastic tubes and centrifuged at room temperature (about 200 g for 5 min). Residual erythrocytes are removed from the deposited cells by the addition of 1 ml of ammonium chloride. After 5 min, the tubes are centrifuged again, and the leukocytes are washed twice with warm culture medium. Finally the cells are counted in a hemocytometer, and the suspension is adjusted to contain 2×10^7 leukocytes per milliliter. Clumping is avoided by the gentle dispersion of cells at each stage with a Pasteur pipette, and the gradual addition of suspending fluid. All procedures with human leukocytes are carried out at room temperature (about 22°C) or above.

3.1.2. From Human or Mouse Blood—Alternative Method for Two-Stage LAI Technique. Venous blood (0.5 ml) is taken into tubes with heparin and centrifuged; the entire cell pellet is washed twice with culture medium. The cells are then resuspended in 0.5 ml. The heparinized plasma may be kept for testing as for serum.

3.1.3. From Mouse Peritoneum. Hanks' solution (8 ml), containing heparin, is injected intraperitoneally into each mouse. If this is to be done with living anesthetized animals, it is convenient to inject and withdraw the fluid with a multiperforate needle. The cell suspension is placed in plastic tubes cooled in ice, and the leukocytes are washed twice by centrifugation with cold culture medium (about 200 g for 5 min). The use of ammonium chloride for removing erythrocytes is permissible but not usually necessary (see method above). If desired, mice may be injected with 1.5 ml of mineral oil, 2–4 days before use, to increase the cell yield. The leukocytes are finally suspended in culture medium to 2×10^7 cells/ml and stored in ice until used.

3.2. Preparation of Tumor Extracts (Antigens). Tumor tissue is trimmed free of extraneous or necrotic material. Fresh or frozen tissue may be used. The tissue (usually 3–5 g) is weighed, cut up fine with scissors, and passed through a steel mesh screen with the help of a spatula. The screened material is then washed into a homogenizer with 4 volumes of cold phosphate-buffered saline and homogenized with about 6 cycles of the motor-driven plunger. As an alternative with fibrous tumors, a blade-type homogenizer may be used. The homogenate is centrifuged at about 1000 g for 30 min at 4°C, and the supernatant is removed for further centrifugation at about 10,000–20,000 g for 30 min at 4°C. The clear supernatant, free of fat particles, is frozen at −20°C overnight, then thawed and centrifuged at 1000 g for 10 min. The supernatant is stored in 0.2-ml volumes at −50°C or lower. If the extract appears cloudy after thawing, centrifuge again before use. The total protein content of these extracts is about 10 mg/ml (Folin method), and they are diluted 1:5 with culture medium just before use.

Tumor extracts must always be tested with normal leukocytes by the standard LAI technique to ensure that they are not active in a nonspecific fashion (i.e., toxic).

3.3. Standard LAI Technique. To allow for the testing of serum for blocking and unblocking of LAI, reaction mixtures are made up to contain four components: leukocytes, antigen, serum A, and serum B, in a total volume of 0.2 ml. For the simple demonstration of LAI, the following mixtures are prepared in plastic tubes, in duplicate.

Mixture 1 (control)–leukocytes (0.05 ml) + culture medium (0.05 ml) + normal serum (0.1 ml)
Mixture 2 (test)–Leukocytes (0.05 ml) + antigen (0.05 ml) + normal serum (0.1 ml)

An unrelated antigen may be substituted for culture medium in mixture 1, to demonstrate specificity. The order of mixing is not important, but the other reagents are usually mixed while the cells are being prepared. It is convenient to use an automatic pipette or sampler.

Great emphasis is placed on the coding of the tubes by another person so that the operator is unaware of their contents until the end of the procedure.

The tubes are capped and incubated for 30 min at 37°C in a water bath, with shaking every 5 min to keep the cells suspended. With a Pasteur pipette, each mixture is then introduced into a hemocytometer with No. 1 cover slip in place, filling both sides of the counting chamber. Incubation of the hemocytometers is then done at 37°C for 1 hr in the large petri dishes containing moist filter paper. After incubation, hemocytometers are held at room temperature in the dishes, to await counting.

Cells are now counted in a pattern of 5 squares in the "red cell" area of the hemocytometer, using a magnification of 400 X. Each square (0.2 X 0.2 mm) should contain, for convenience, about 15–25 cells. All the hemocytometers of a series should be counted without delay, to give 20 initial counts for the two duplicates of each mixture.

The next step (referred to as "washing") appears to be critical and requires some dexterity and practice. The hemocytometer is held horizontally in one hand and slowly immersed in a large petri dish filled with saline at room temperature. Saline runs into the channels and the cover slip floats, to be picked up with forceps held in the other hand. Without further agitation or sideways tilting, the hemocytometer is removed from the dish and held vertically by one end, then lowered smoothly into a beaker of saline. It is immediately removed, inverted, and reimmersed. A drop of medium or saline is placed on each side of the hemocytometer, now lying horizontally on the bench, and a clean cover slip is lowered into place from one side with forceps. At this stage, hemocytometers may be left for an hour or two before recounting.

Finally, the remaining adherent cells are counted in exactly the same squares as before (initial and final counts are conveniently recorded in columns side by side).

Calculations are performed by either (a) determining the percent adherence for each square and the mean and standard deviation of 20 squares, then using student's t test to assess the significance of the difference between means, or (b) summing the initial counts for all 20 squares, then the final counts, calculating overall percent adherence and applying the χ^2 test to determine significance.

3.4. Modification of LAI by Serum Factors.　As noted above, sera of various kinds can be incorporated into the reaction mixtures, to test for factors that interfere with LAI (blocking) or abrogate blocking (unblocking). The following mixtures would be required, together with suitable controls to ensure specificity (all volumes 0.05 ml).

Mixture 3 (blocking)—leukocytes + antigen + serum A + normal serum
Mixture 4 (unblocking)—leukocytes + antigen + serum A + serum B

The procedure is now identical with the standard LAI technique. Percent adherence for Mixture 3 is then compared with that for mixture 2; that for Mixture 4 is compared with that for mixture 3. Serum B can obviously only be tested for unblocking with leukocytes, antigen, and serum A of known properties and with the prior knowledge that it (serum B) is not blocking.

3.5. Two Stage LAI Technique.　Specifically reactive cells from one source can be used with normal indicator cells from another. The method will be described for human blood leukocytes used with mouse peritoneal cells, but obviously other combinations are possible. Quantitation of CMI is achieved by titrating the soluble factor produced in the first stage; this has been described elsewhere (16), and only the qualitative test will be given here.

The two-stage technique has several advantages, apart from allowing quantitation and the comparison of several supernatants using a single batch of indicator cells: some operators find mouse peritoneal cells easier to handle and more uniform, and dividing the technique into two stages demands less time on any one day.

3.5.1. Stage 1.　Mixtures are made from equal volumes of leukocytes (usually prepared as in Section 3.1.2) and antigen diluted 1:5 (Section 3.2). The mixtures are incubated at 37°C for 30–60 min, with occasional shaking, then centrifuged at about 500 g for 5 min. Supernatants are removed and stored at −20°C until required.

3.5.2. Stage 2.　Normal peritoneal cells (Section 3.1.3) are incubated in 0.1-ml volumes with the supernatants to be tested, for 30 min at 37°C. The mixtures are then introduced into hemocytometers, incubated, counted, washed, and recounted, as in the standard technique (Section 3.3).

4. Comments

4.1. Some points mentioned above are now reemphasized: (a) always code the mixtures so that tests are done "blind"; (b) keep serum concentrations the same in mixtures which are to be compared; (c) store tumor extracts as cold as possible to avoid inactivation.

4.2. Suggestions for beginners: (a) practice the procedure with normal cells and no extracts, until counts are consistent; (b) mouse peritoneal cells, in a one-stage or two-stage technique, may be easier to handle than human leukocytes; (c) follow the above procedures first, then try variations when skill and confidence are achieved. Other methods for preparing leukocytes and tumor extracts may or may not be suitable.

4.3. Consistently good results have been obtained with a variety of tumors, with two main exceptional situations: (a) primary colonic carcinomas usually produce toxic extracts, and secondary metastatic tissue must be used for this tumor; (b) patients examined in the week or two after surgery and some other immunosuppressive procedures have inactive leukocytes.

4.4. Where possible, tumor specificity should be ensured by (a) testing reactive leukocytes against control tumor extracts, especially against appropriate normal tissue extract, preferably from the same donor as the tumor; (b) testing tumor extracts against related and unrelated leukocytes, including those from normal donors.

4.5. A positive LAI test (for leukocyte or serum activity) is one where adherence is significantly different from the appropriate control.

4.6. Some modifications of the original technique include the use of solid substrates other than glass hemocytometers: glass beads (18), plastic wells (13, 19), glass tubes (20, 23, 25); radioisotopic labeling of leukocytes (19); electronic counting of nonadherent leukocytes (18, 25); use of leukocytes from small volumes of blood (13, 16), separation of mononuclear cells from blood (13, 24, 25); and applications to various antigens (see Introduction). The ideal technique for use in routine assays has yet to be devised but may involve some combination of these modifications (25).

REFERENCES

1. Halliday, W. J., and Webb, M., *J. Natl. Cancer Inst.* **43**, 141 (1969).
2. Halliday, W. J., *J. Immunol.* **106**, 855 (1971).
3. Halliday, W. J., *Cell Immunol.* **3**, 113 (1972).
4. Halliday, W. J., and Miller, S., *Int. J. Cancer* **9**, 477 (1972).
5. Dekaris, D., Veselic, B., and Tomarlc, V., *Immunology* **20**, 363 (1971).
6. Field, E. J., Caspary, E. A., Hall, R., and Clark, F., *Lancet* **1**, 1144 (1970).
7. Halliday, W. J., Maluish, A. E., and Miller, S., *Cell Immunol.* **10**, 467 (1974).
8. Halliday, W. J., Maluish, A. E., and Isbister, W. H., *Br. J. Cancer* **29**, 31 (1974).
9. Maluish. A. E., and Halliday, W. J., *J. Natl. Cancer Inst.* **52**, 1415 (1974).

10. Halliday, W. J., Halliday, J. W., Campbell, C. B., Maluish, A. E., and Powell, L. W., *Br. Med. J.* **2**, 349 (1974).
11. Walters, B. A. J., Chick, J. E. D., and Halliday, W. J., *Int. Arch. Allergy Appl. Immunol.* **46**, 849 (1974).
12. Walters, B. A. J., Beardmore, G. L., and Halliday, W. J., *Br. J. Dermatol.* **94**, 55 (1976).
13. Holt, P. G., Roberts, L. M., Fimmel, P. J., and Keast, D., *J. Immunol. Methods* **8**, 277 (1975).
14. Noonan, F.P., and Halliday, W.J., manuscript in preparation.
15. Maluish, A.E., and Halliday, W.J., unpublished data.
16. Maluish, A.E., and Halliday, W.J., *Cell Immunol.* **17**, 131 (1975).
17. Halliday, W. J., Maluish, A. E., Little, J. H., and Davis. N. C., *Int. J. Cancer* **16**, 645 (1975).
18. Lampert, F., and Dietmair, E., *Klin. Wochenschr.* **51**, 198 (1973).
19. Pierce, G. E., and DeVald, B. L., *Int. J. Cancer* **14**, 833 (1974).
20. Holáň, V., Hašek, M., Bubeník, J., and Chutná, J., *Cell. Immunol.,* **13**, 107 (1974).
21. Hartmann, D., Lewis, M. G., Proctor, J. W., and Lyons, H., *Lancet* **2**, 1481 (1974).
22. Allardyce, R. A., and Shearman, D. J. C., *Int. Arch. Allergy Appl. Immunol.* **48**, 395 (1975).
23. Grosser, N., and Thomson, D. M. P. *Cancer Res.* **35**, 2571 (1975).
24. Powell, A. E., Sloss, A. M., Smith, R. N., Makley, J. T., and Hubay, C. A., *Int. J. Cancer* **16**, 905 (1975).
25. Rutherford, J. C., Walters, B. A. J., Cavaye, G., and Halliday, W. J., submitted for publication.

52

Immune Complexes in Human Sera Detected by the Raji Cell Radioimmune Assay

Argyrios N. Theofilopoulos and Frank J. Dixon

1. Introduction

Immune complexes (IC) appear to be one of the most important mechanisms by which immunological tissue injury is produced (1). Immunofluorescence and electron microscopy are used to demonstrate fixed IC in tissues (2, 3). Moreover, IC can be eluted from diseased tissues and the antigen and antibody recovered, identified, and quantitated (3, 4). Increasingly, detection of IC directly in biological fluids has assumed importance, and numerous attempts have been and are being made to develop immunological techniques sensitive and reliable enough for their demonstration and quantitation. Currently the presence of IC in biological fluids may be judged by (a) suggestive clinical findings such as hypocomplementemia, anticomplementary activity, alternating antigen and antibody levels, cryoglobulinemia, (b) physicoimmunochemical techniques, such as analytical and sucrose density ultracentrifugation (5), polyethyleneglycol precipitation (6), rheumatoid factor precipitation (7), (c) complement (C) techniques such as C1q precipitation (8), radioactive C1q binding (9, 10), quantitative consumption (11), and (d) cellular techniques, such as platelet aggregation (12), inhibition of macrophage uptake of IC (13). However, no single method combined the specificity, reproducibility, and sensitivity necessary for the adequate study of most IC diseases. We have, therefore, developed another method employing cellular C receptors as *in vitro* detectors of IC.

Human bone marrow (B) derived lymphocytes as well as human lymphoblastoid cells with B cell characteristics in continuous culture (HCL) can bind IC via receptors for Fc and altered C3 (14–17). Therefore, these cells can be used as *in vitro* detectors of IC in biological fluids. HCL have an advantage over peripheral B lymphocytes in that they are relatively homogeneous and easily accessible. Studies performed with several HCL of B origin showed that they carry some or all of the following: membrane bound immunoglobulin (MBIg) and receptors of IgG Fc, C3b, C3d (17, 18), C1q (19), and C4b (20). Additional studies (16, 17) demonstrated that (a) the receptors for Fc are distinct from all the C receptors; (b) IC reacted with active C bind to cells only via receptors for C, and (c) after IC have fixed C, their binding to cells is greatly enhanced. Raji cells (21) were found to be the most suitable of many studied for detecting IC *in vitro* since they are devoid of MBIg, but have IgG Fc receptors of low avidity and have a large number of receptors of C3b, C3d, and C1q (17, 19). Consequently, C receptors on Raji cells were used in an immunofluorescence assay for the detection of C fixing IC in experimental animal and human sera (22). However, this assay had the disadvantage of not being quantitative. Therefore, this method was modified so that IC in human sera could be quantitated by measuring uptake of radioactive antibody by Ig in the IC bound to Raji cells (23).

The Raji cell radioimmune assay herein described is based on the ability of these cells to bind much more IgG from a serum containing IgG-type IC with fixed C than from normal human sera (NHS). In fact, approximately 10 times more molecules of IgG bind via C receptors than Fc receptors (23). The higher binding of complexed IgG with fixed C can be explained by postulating that there is a larger number or greater affinity of Raji cells' C receptors than that of Raji cells' Fc receptors for their ligand molecules.

In calculating results from the Raji cell assay, one determines uptake of radioactive antihuman IgG by the cells previously incubated with human sera and refers this number to a standard curve of radioactive antibody uptake by cells previously incubated with increasing amounts of aggregated human gamma-globulin (AHG) in serum. AHG is an *in vitro* model of human immune complexes since they possess many of the same properties (24, 25) and bind to the same Fc and C receptors on cell surfaces (17, 26). The amount of complexes present in the test serum is expressed as micrograms of AHG equivalent per milliliter of serum. The assay's limit of sensitivity is 6 μg of AHG per milliliter of serum. With this assay only 3.3% of NHS tested exceeded a value of 12 μg AHG equivalent per milliliter. Therefore, this value (12 μg/ml) is considered as the upper limit of normal. Values higher than 24 μg AHG equivalent/ml serum were observed in patients with suspected IC diseases (23) such as serum hepatitis, sytemic lupus erythematosus, dengue hemorrhagic fever, subacute sclerosing panencephalitis, and various forms of vasculitis and malignancies.

The relationship of the results obtained by the Raji cell assay in detecting IC in sera of patients with various disorders and the results obtained by other methods as well as other clinical and experimental data supporting the specificity of the test have been presented elsewhere (23).

2. Materials and Methods

2.1. Equipment

2.1.1. Microscope

2.1.2. Cell counting chamber (any standard type)

2.1.3. Plastic Eppendorf conical tubes (1.5 ml; Brinkman Instruments, Inc., Westbury, New York, Catalogue No. 22-36-411-1)

2.1.4. Plastic racks (holders) for the Eppendorf conical tubes (Van Waters and Rogers, Los Angeles, California)

2.1.5. Eppendorf pipettes (Van Waters and Rogers) of different sizes (25, 50, 200, and 1000 μl) and Eppendorf plastic tips (for 500-μl Eppendorf pipettes or bigger, tips were obtained from Brinkman Instruments, Catalogue No. 2235090-1, and for Eppendorf pipettes smaller than 500-μl tips were obtained from Sherwood Medical Industry Inc., St. Louis, Missouri, Catalogue No. 18000)

2.1.6. Gamma counter

2.1.7. Water bath

2.1.8. Centrifuge (Model PR-6; International Equipment Co., Needham Heights, Massachusetts) capable of forces up to 2000 g

2.1.9. Beckman ultracentrifuge (Beckman Instruments, Inc., Model L5-50, SW 50.1 rotor)

2.1.10. Spectrophotometer

2.1.11. A 37°C incubator or preferably a warm room (37°C) for tissue culturing with a gyrator (New Brunswick Scientific Co., Inc., New Brunswick, New Jersey, G10 gyrotory shaker)

2.1.12. Laminar flow hood (BioQuest Biological Cabinet; Envirco, Albuquerque, New Mexico)

2.1.13. A suction unit, preferably with a probe long enough to remove most of the supernatant without disturbing the cell pellet at the bottom of the Eppendorf tube

2.1.14. Sterile disposable plastic serological pipettes and 50-ml conical tubes (Falcon, Oxnard, California)

2.1.15. Sterile Erlenmeyer flasks and stoppers of different sizes for holding tissue culture

2.2. Solutions

2.2.1. 0.15 M NaCl (physiological saline)

2.2.2. Spinner's medium, Earle's salts (Grand Island Biological Corp., Catalogue No. 138) supplemented with antibiotic–antimycotic solution and sodium bicarbonate (see below)

2.2.3. Eagle's minimum essential medium (MEM; Autopow, Flow Laboratories, Inc., Rockville, Maryland). In 800 ml of MEM the following were added under sterile conditions: 100 ml of heated (56°C, 30 min) fetal bovine serum (Catalogue No. 4-055D), 10 ml of L-glutamine (200 mM, 100X, Catalogue No. 1447650), 10 ml of nonessential amino acids (100X, Catalogue No. 6-244D), 10 ml of sodium pyruvate (100 mM, Catalogue No. 6-254D), 10 ml of antibiotic–antimycotic solution containing penicillin–streptomycin–fungizone (100X, penicillin 10,000 U/ml, fungizone 25 μg/ml, streptomycin 10,000 μg/ml Catalogue No. 524) and 25 ml of 5.6%

sodium bicarbonate (Catalogue No. 7-040D). All the above were obtained from Flow Laboratories except the L-glutamine (Associated Biomedic Systems, Inc., Buffalo, New York) and the antibiotic–antimycotic solution (Grand Island Biological Co., Grand Island, New York)

2.2.4. Trypan blue (0.5% solution in 0.85% saline (Flow Laboratories Catalogue No. 7-070D)

2.2.5. Human serum albumin (HSA; Miles Laboratories, Inc., Kankakee, Illinois)

2.2.6. Human IgG: Human Cohn fraction II (Pentex, Miles) in saline (20 mg/ml) was freed of aggregates by centrifugation at $100,000\,g$ for 90 min at $4°C$ in a Beckman ultracentrifuge using a SW50.1 rotor. Fluid in the upper third of the tube (deaggregated or 7 S IgG) was removed, and the protein concentration was determined by an automated micro-Kjeldahl method (27) or by spectrophotometry at 280 nm. The protein content was then adjusted to 6.5 mg/ml saline and stored in aliquots of 0.2 ml at $-70°C$.

2.2.7. Aggregated human gamma-globulin (AHG). AHG was prepared fresh after heating an aliquot (0.2 ml) of 7 S IgG in a water bath at $63°C$ for 30 min. However, in order to ensure uniformity in the size of AHG in later experiments, a large batch (2 ml) of AHG was prepared and aliquots of 0.1 ml of this preparation were stored at $-70°C$. Just prior to use in the assay, the AHG preparation was centrifuged at $1500\,g$ for 15 min in order to remove insoluble large aggregates. On sucrose gradients, approximately 50% of the total protein present in a solution of AHG was heavier than 7 S (9, 23).

2.2.8. Antiserum to human IgG. The antiserum was prepared in rabbits, the IgG fraction was isolated on a DEAE-52 column and brought to a concentration of 5 mg of protein per milliliter of phosphate-buffered saline (PBS). This antiserum (1 ml) was iodinated according to the procedure of McConahey and Dixon (28) with 100 μg of chloramine-T and 3000 μCi of ^{125}I and brought to 1 mg/ml PBS. The specific activity was 1 μCi cpm/μg protein.

2.2.9. Experimental sera. Sera from patients with various disorders and from normal subjects were obtained after allowing the blood to clot at room temperature for 30 min and $4°C$ for 30 min and subsequent centrifugation. Sera to be tested were used fresh or after being frozen at $-70°C$ and thawed once.

2.3. Cell Culture Conditions. Raji cells, which are derived from a Burkitt's lymphoma (21) were cultured in Eagle's MEM supplemented as above (Section 2.2.3). Cell cultures were placed in sterile Erlenmeyer flasks (cell culture volume not exceeding one-fifth of the total volume of the flask) at a cell density of 2×10^5 cells/ml, tightly stoppered, and incubated at $37°C$ (warm room) on a gyratory shaker. Receptors for Fc, C3b, and C3d are expressed equally well throughout the cell cycle (23). However, cells used in the assay were obtained 72 hr after initiation of the culture.

2.4. Raji Cell Radioimmune Assay

2.4.1. One milliliter of Raji cell suspension was removed from a 72-hr culture (cell density $\sim 1 \times 10^6$ cells/ml) under sterile conditions. Two drops of trypan blue were added; after mixing with a Pasteur pipette, the cell number and cell viability were assessed with a hemocytometer.

2.4.2. The total number of Raji cells needed was calculated on the basis that 2 $\times 10^6$ cells are required per each test. Each test serum was run in duplicate or triplicate and each point of the standard curve (see below) in duplicate. Cells were removed from the 72-hr culture and poured into 50-ml conical tubes.

2.4.3. The cells were centrifuged at 1800 rpm for 10 min at 4°C. Supernatants were removed; cell pellets were combined and resuspended in Spinner's medium to a volume of 2×10^6 cells for 200 μl.

2.4.4. Aliquots of 2×10^6 cells (200 μl) were placed into the 1.5-ml plastic Eppendorf conical tubes. One milliliter of Spinner's medium was added to each tube, and the cells were centrifuged at 1800 rpm for 10 min.

2.4.5. Supernatants were removed by using an aspirator (suction unit), and the cell pellets were resuspended in 50 μl of Spinner's.

2.4.6. Serum to be tested for IC was diluted 1:4 with 0.15 M NaCl, and 25 μl were added to the 2×10^6 cells.

2.4.7. After an incubation period of 45 min at 37°C with gentle shaking (every 5–10 min by hand), cells were washed 3 times with Spinner's medium. For the first wash, 1 ml of Spinner's was added, and the cells were centrifuged at 1800 rpm for 10 min. Supernatants were aspirated and discarded. Second and third washings were carried out by adding 200 μl of Spinner's to the cell pellet, mixing carefully with an Eppendorf pipette and adding 1 ml Spinner's. Cells were centrifuged as above and supernatants were removed.

2.4.8. After the final wash, the cells were allowed to react (30 min, 4°C) with gentle shaking (every 5–10 min by hand) with an optimum amount (see Section 3) of the ^{125}I rabbit anti-human IgG diluted 1:2 with Spinner's containing 1% HSA.

2.4.9. After incubation, the cells were washed 3 times as in step No. 7 with the exception that the Spinner's with 1% HSA was used.

2.4.10. At the final wash the supernatant was removed as close to the cell pellet as possible and radioactivity associated with the pellet was determined in a gamma counter.

2.4.11. The amount of uptake (mean of duplicate or triplicate) expressed as absolute counts or as a percentage of the input was then referred to a standard curve of radioactive antibody uptake by cells incubated with NHS containing various amounts of AHG (standard curve). The amount of IC in a serum is thereafter readily equated to an amount of AHG after correcting for the dilution factor and is expressed as micrograms of AHG equivalent per milliliter of serum.

2.4.12. The standard curve was obtained as follows: $50\mu l$ of AHG (80 μg of protein) were serially diluted in fourteen 2-fold dilutions in saline. Subsequently, to each dilution of AHG, 50 μl of a 1:2 dilution of NHS freshly obtained, stored at $-70°C$ or from a pool of 20 NHS (sources of C) were added, mixed carefully, and incubated at $37°C$ for 30 min. Thereafter, 25 μl of each mixture were added to 2×10^6 cells in duplicate (1:4 final dilutions of serum containing from 20 μg to $\sim$2 ng AHG), and incubation, washes, and counting were performed as with the test sera (steps 6 to 10). A base line of radioactive antibody uptake (background) by cells incubated with 25 μl of a 1:4 dilution of NHS or of pooled NHS, which were used as C sources in the above reference curve, was also established. Even at a concentration of 40 ng of AHG in 25 μl of serum diluted 1:4 (6 $\mu g/ml$), the uptake of radioactive antibody was considerably greater than that by cells incubated with NHS without AHG.

3. Comments

3.1. The method described above is not the only one for the detection of circulating IC; nevertheless, it has several advantages over others: (a) Its limit of sensitivity is 6–12 μg of AHG per milliliter of serum, which is far greater than the other methods described for detecting IC. (b) The Raji test is specific for C fixing IC, since excess IgG (above background binding via Fc receptors) would bind to cells only if it is altered (complexed) so that it can fix C and bind to cellular C receptors. Assays in which precipitation of C1q (8) or binding of C1q (9, 10) have been employed may detect not only IC, but also other substances, such as endotoxin and DNA. C consumption assays (11) also may give positive results with a variety of materials that can consume C or inhibit C-induced red blood cell lysis, the end point of the assay. (c) This test requires small amounts of serum, and the lymphoblasts employed are easily cultured. Other cellular techniques such as the platelet aggregation assay (12) and the macrophage inhibition assay (13) are subject to problems caused by nonreproducible platelet preparations, the necessity of isolating macrophages from guinea pigs and the interference of other than IC substances. (d) The results are reproducible (29). (e) The Raji cell assay can efficiently detect IC of even 18–11 S (23). (f) By using the appropriate fluoresceinated antisera, one can identify the antigen within the cell-bound complexes (23). (g) Apart from their ability to detect IC *in vitro,* Raji cells can concentrate antigen–antibody complexes on their surfaces, which may provide the tool by which IC can be isolated.

3.2. Critical steps of the method are the following. (a) Before attempting to detect IC in sera, one must determine the optimum amount of radiolabeled antibody to be employed in the assay. Raji cells allowed to react with NHS bind IgG only via Fc receptors. In contrast, these cells incubated with sera containing

IgG complexes with fixed C bind native 7 S IgG via Fc receptors and complexed IgG via C receptors (17). To detect the difference in radioactive antibody uptake between cells incubated in sera with or without IC, an excess of that amount of antibody needed to react with the molecules of native 7 S IgG bound via Fc receptors must be offered to the cells. The amount of antibody necessary for the Raji cell assay is established by incubating aliquots of cells with 25 μl of 1:4 NHS in saline alone or containing 20 μg of AHG and then allowing them to react with increasing amounts of ^{125}I-labeled rabbit anti-human IgG. The optimum amount of radiolabeled antibody is that in which the highest difference of uptake between cells incubated with NHS alone and cell incubated with NHS containing AHG is observed (23). (b) In order to obtain reproducible results, one should: (i) Use the same cell number (same number of available receptor sites) per test at each examination. The amount of IC bound to C receptors is linearly related with the cell number (16). (ii) Use the same preparation of AHG or preparations of AHG containing similar distribution of sizes of aggregates in the standard reference curve. Larger aggregates or IC fix more C than smaller ones and AHG or IC having more C bind best to cellular C receptors (16, 17). (iii) Use the same kind of radioactive antibody. (c) The presence of anti-lymphocyte antibodies in certain test sera (30, 31) may interfere with the results. However, our studies (23) have shown that under the conditions of the Raji cell test (interaction of test serum with cells at 37°C) anti-lymphocyte antibodies, which are mostly if not all of the cold reactive IgM type (31), are not adsorbed onto Raji cells. (d) In order to ensure that the cells in culture are indeed Raji cells (especially in laboratories carrying several HCL), periodically the cells must be checked for their characteristics. Raji cells are devoid of MBIgG, have Fc, C3b, C3d, and C1q receptors. The techniques for identifying these receptors have been described in detail (17–19).

4. Addendum

4.1. In order to reduce the time required for performing the Raji cell test, the following modifications may be introduced: Together with the ^{125}I-labeled anti-human IgG, ^{131}I-labeled bovine serum albumin may be added (Section 2.4, Step 2.4.8). After the subsequent incubation period and removal of the supernatant, no further washes are required since the specific percentage of ^{125}I cell pellet-associated counts can be calculated by subtracting the nonspecific percent of ^{131}I pellet-association counts.

4.2. Raji cells can be fixed with limited concentrations of glutaraldehyde [shown to preserve the C receptors—(A. N. Theofilopoulos and F. J. Dixon; unpublished observations) and Ref. (32)]. This treatment eliminates the requirement for cell culture facilities and may allow the routine performance of the test in clinical laboratories.

4.3. The discovery of a cell line devoid of MBIg and Fc receptors but having large numbers of C receptors may further help the specificity and sensitivity of the test, since it would eliminate the background binding of 7 S IgG to Fc receptors.

ACKNOWLEDGMENTS

This is publication No. 1063 from the Department of Immunopathology, Scripps Clinic and Research Foundation, La Jolla, California. This work was supported by Contract No. DADA 17-73-C-3137 from the United States Department of the Army, Contract No. NO1-CB-53592 from the National Cancer Institute, and The Elsa U. Pardee Foundation.

REFERENCES

1. Dixon, F. J., *J. Immunol.* **109,** 187 (1972).
2. Wilson, C. B., and Dixon, F. J., *Kidney Int.* **5,** 389 (1973).
3. Oldstone, M. B. A., *Prog. Med. Virol.* **19,** 84 (1975).
4. Koffler, D., Schur, P. H., and Kunkel, H. G., *J. Exp. Med.* **126,** 607 (1967).
5. Franklin, E. C., Holman, H. R., Müller-Eberhard, H. J., and Kunkel, H. G., *J. Exp. Med.* **105,** 425 (1957).
6. Creighton, W. D., Lambert, P. H., and Miescher, P. A., *J. Immunol.* **111,** 1219 (1973).
7. Winchester, R. J., Kunkel, H. G., and Agnello, V., *J. Exp. Med.* **134,** 286s (1971).
8. Agnello, V., Winchester, R. J., and Kunkel, H. G., *Immunology* **19,** 909 (1970).
9. Nydegger, V. E., Lambert, P. H., Gerber, H., and Miescher, P. H., *J. Clin. Invest.* **54,** 297 (1974).
10. Sobel, A. T., Bokisch, V. A., and Müller-Eberhard, H. J., *J. Exp. Med.* **142,** 139 (1975).
11. Mowbray, J. F., Hoffbrand, A. V., Holborow, E. J., Seah, P. P., and Fry, L., *Lancet* **1,** 400 (1973).
12. Myllylä, G., *Scand. J. Haematol. Suppl.* **19,** 1 (1973).
13. Onyewotu, I. I., Holborow, E. J., and Johnson, G. D., *Nature (London) New Biol.* **248,** 156 (1974).
14. Dickler, H. B., and Kunkel, H. G., *J. Exp. Med.* **136,** 191 (1972).
15. Bianco, C., Patrick, R., and Nussenzweig, V., *J. Exp. Med.* **132,** 702 (1970).
16. Eden, A., Bianco, C., and Nussenzweig, V., *Cell Immunol.* **7,** 459 (1973).
17. Theofilopoulos, A. N., Dixon, F. J., and Bokisch, V. A., *J. Exp. Med.* **140,** 877 (1974).
18. Ross, G. D., Polley, M. J., Rabellino, E. M., and Grey, H. M., *J. Exp. Med.* **138,** 798 (1973).
19. Sobel, A. T., and Bokisch, V. A., *Fed. Proc., Fed. Am. Soc. Exp. Biol.* **34,** 965 (1975).
20. Sobel, A. T., and Bokisch, V. A., *J. Exp. Med.* **140,** 1336 (1975).
21. Pulvertaft, R. J. V., *J. Clin. Pathol.* **18,** 261 (1965).
22. Theofilopoulos, A. N., Wilson, C. B., Bokisch, V. A., and Dixon, F. J., *J. Exp. Med.* **140,** 1230 (1974).
23. Theofilopoulos, A. N., Wilson, C. B., and Dixon, F. J., *J. Clin. Invest.* **57,** 169 (1976).
24. Ishizaka, K., Ishizaka, T., and Banovita, J., *J. Immunol.* **94,** 824 (1965).
25. Christian, C. L., *J. Immunol.* **84,** 112 (1960).
26. Dickler, H. B., *J. Exp. Med.* **140,** 508 (1974).
27. Ferrari, A., *Ann. N. Y. Acad. Sci.* **87,** 792 (1960).
28. McConahey, P. J., and Dixon, F. J., *Int. Arch. Allergy. Appl. Immunol.* **29,** 185 (1966).

29. Theofilopoulos, A. N., and Dixon, F. J., *in* "Manual of Clinical Immunology" (N. R. Rose, and H. Friedman, eds.). Am. Soc. Microbiol., Washington, D. C., 1976.
30. Winchester, R. J., Winfield, J. B., Siegal, F., Wernet, P., Bentwich, Z., and Kunkel, H. G., *J. Clin. Invest.* **54**, 1082 (1974).
31. Winfield, J. B., Winchester, R. J., Wernet, P., Fu, S. M., and Kunkel, H. G., *Arthritis Rheum.* **18**, 1 (1975).
32. Dierich, M. P., and Reisfeld, R. A., *J. Exp. Med.* **142**, 242 (1975).

The ^{125}I-C1q Binding Test for the Detection of Soluble Immune Complexes

Rudolf H. Zubler and Paul-H. Lambert

1. Introduction

Tests for a quantitative measurement of immune complexes may be either antigen-specific or nonspecific for the antigens involved in the complexes. Antigen nonspecific radioimmunological methods have been recently developed for the detection and quantitation of immune complexes in various biological fluids. Such methods are mainly based on the interaction of immune complexes with biological receptors for aggregated immunoglobulins or for complement-coated immune aggregates, such as the C1q component of complement (1, 2), some monoclonal rheumatoid factors (3), and Fc-receptors or C3b-receptors on various cell surfaces (4, 5).

The modified ^{125}I-C1q binding test which is described here (6) allows for a rapid quantitation of soluble immune complexes in native unheated human and animal sera. Independently of various eventual denaturing effects of heating, the testing of native samples is preferable since it was found that heat inactivation (56°C, 30 min) reduces the C1q binding activity (C1q-BA) of serum containing immune complexes (6). The principle of the test is to measure the amount of C1q that can be bound to macromolecular substances in a given biological sample. Radiolabeled C1q is mixed with the tested sample, and free C1q is separated from C1q bound to complexes by a precipitation with polyethylene glycol (PEG). This test is performed in two steps. First, the tested native serum sample is incubated with EDTA in order to prevent the integration of ^{125}I-C1q into the intrinsic C1qrs complex; second, ^{125}I-C1q and PEG (final concentration: 2.5%) are added to this mixture and further incubated for 1 hr at 4°C. Under these conditions, free C1q remains soluble, whereas C1q bound to macromolecular complexes is precipitated. The competitive effect of intrinsic C1q and the interference of some substances, such as DNA or bacterial lipopolysaccharides, known to bind C1q under certain conditions (2), are very limited in this PEG test system. However, one cannot rule out that other biological substances which bind C1q may produce false positive results.

The C1q binding test has been applied to the quantitation and further characterization of soluble immune complexes in various clinical conditions: the level of the C1q-BA in sera from patients with systemic lupus erythematosus correlated with the clinical disease activity, the anti-DNA antibody levels and the depression of some complement components (6), the C1q-BA in synovial fluids of patients with rheumatoid arthritis correlated with the intraarticular C4 depression, and the C1q-BA in the sera of these patients correlated with the presence of extraarticular disease manifestations. The C1q binding material in rheumatoid arthritis was characterized by ultracentrifugation and immuno-chemical analysis and represented mainly IgG complexes (7). The C1q-BA was also found to be elevated in the sera of patients with various forms of leprosy. The C1q binding material has been partially isolated by PEG precipitation and ultracentrifugation. It lost its C1q binding activity after incubation with an excess of *Mycobacterium leprae* antigens, suggesting that this material is formed of *M. leprae* antigens and corresponding antibodies (8). Preliminary studies indicate an increased incidence of C1q binding complexes in acute leukemia sera as compared to chronic leukemia and normal blood donor sera. In experimental systems, the C1q binding test has been applied successfully to the detection of complexes formed *in vitro* as well as those occurring in some animal models of immune complex disease (1).

In order to complete the description of the methodology, the methods for rapid purification of C1q according to Volanakis and Stroud (9) and for radiolabeling of C1q with lactoperoxydase according to Heusser *et al.* (10) as they are currently performed in our laboratory are also described here in detail.

2. Materials

2.1. Materials for the Purification of Human C1q

2.1.1. Freshly drawn human blood from a single blood donor (approx. 150 ml)

2.1.2. Chemicals: Na_2-EDTA (Titriplex III) (Merck AG, Darmstadt, Germany); NaCl, 1 N; HCl, 1 N; NaOH

2.1.3. Glassware: flasks for buffer solutions, centrifuge tubes (25 ml), pipettes (10 ml), Pasteur pipettes, 1 stick.

2.1.4. Synthetic material: 50-ml polycarbonate and 16-ml polypropylene centrifuge tubes (Sorvall Inc. Norwalk, Connecticut); dialysis membrane (Union Carbide Corp., Chicago, Illinois); 0.5 ml polypropylene tubes for storage of C1q.

2.1.5. Material for immunoelectrophoresis: rabbit anti-human C1q antiserum (OTNT 05); horse anti-total human serum (ORCO 05P) (Behring-werke, Marburg-Lahn, Germany); agarose (Fluka AG, Buchs, Switzerland)

2.1.6. Equipment: magnetic stirrer, balance, pH meter, conductivity meter (not absolutely necessary), water bath at 37°C, ice bath, cooled blood bank centrifuge, cooled centrifuge for 30,000 g (Sorvall RC2-B with SS-34 and SM-24 rotors), UV spectrophotometer, immunoelectrophoresis equipment.

2.2. Materials for Radiolabeling of C1q

2.2.1. Pure C1q

2.2.2. ^{125} I (The Radiochemical Centre, Amersham, Bucks, England; specific activity 14 μCi/μg I) for protein labeling

2.2.3. Lactoperoxidase, lyophilized, B grade (Cat. No. 427466, Calbiochem Corp., San Diego, California)

2.2.4. Chemicals: NaI, NaN$_3$, H$_2$O$_2$ ("Perhydrol" 30%, Merck), trichloroacetic acid (TCA), Veronal-buffered saline with Ca^{2+} and Mg^{2+} (VBS) (Mérieux, Lyon, France)

2.2.5. Glassware: tubes, pipettes, 2-liter recipient for dialysis

2.2.6. Synthetic material: 5-ml plastic tubes, pipette tips, gloves for handling radioactive material, dialysis membrane (see 2.1.4), 0.5-ml polypropylene tubes for storage of labeled C1q

2.2.7. Equipment: balance, ice bath, automatic pipettes for 5 and 10 μl. (Eppendorf Geratebau GmbH, Hamburg, Germany), watch; eventually cold room for dialysis, centrifuge for 1500 g, freezer at -70°C or liquid nitrogen container for storage of labeled C1q.

2.3. Materials for the ^{125} I-C1q Binding Test

2.3.1. ^{125} I-labeled C1q

2.3.2. Normal human serum (NHS), Cohn fraction II γ-globulin (Globuman, 16%, Berna, Bern, Switzerland) for test controls

2.3.3. Chemicals: polyethylene glycol (PEG) (DAB-7, MW 6000, Siegfried AG, Zofingen, Switzerland), VBS (Mérieux), boric acid, disodium tetraborate, NaCl, NaOH, trichloroacetic acid (TCA), Na$_2$-EDTA (Titriplex III) (Merck)

2.3.4. Glassware: recipients for buffer solutions, 10-ml pipettes

2.3.5. Synthetic material: pipette tips, gloves, polypropylene tubes and caps for the test (Bio-Vials, recorder No. 566353, Beckman Inc., Palo Alto, California).

2.3.6. Equipment: balance, pH meter, magnetic stirrer, water bath at 37°, 56°, and 63°C, automatic pipettes for 50 and 100 μl (Eppendorf) and 1 ml (Oxford Laboratory, Foster City, California), ice bath, cooled centrifuge for 1500 g (Universal Junior II KS, Heraeus-Christ GmbH, Osterode am Harz, Germany, with swing-out buckets for 4 times 26 tubes), gamma counter (Biogamma, Beckman).

3. Methods

3.1. Method for the Purification of Human C1q. *3.1.1. Preparation of Serum.* Freshly drawn blood is allowed to clot in 25-ml glass tubes for 1 hr at

room temperature. After another hour at 4°C the serum is obtained by centrifugation at 1500 g for 15 min at 4°C. This serum is recentrifuged at 30,000 g (e.g., 16,000 rpm with SS-34 Sorvall rotor) for 30 min at 4°C. A lipid layer on the top of the tubes is first removed by aspiration with a Pasteur pipette; the remainder of the supernatant is used for the purification of C1q either immediately or after storage of the serum at −70°C.

3.1.2. Preparation of Solutions

Solution A: prepare 500 ml of 0.1 M EDTA then adjust to pH 7.5 by addition in 1 N NaOH

Solution B: add 950 ml of distilled water to 50 ml of solution A

Solution C: add 700 ml of distilled water to 200 ml of solution A. The conductivity of this solution should correspond to that of 0.04 M NaCl; relative salt concentration (RSC) = 0.04

Solution D: 100 ml of 0.75 M NaCl 0.01 M EDTA, adjusted to pH 5.0 with 0.1 N NaOH

Solution E: prepare 2 liters of 0.1 M EDTA then adjust to pH 5.0 by addition of 1 N NaOH. Add 1 liter of distilled water to 2 liters of this adjusted solution (RSC should be 0.078)

Solution F: 100 ml of 0.3 M NaCl, 0.01 M EDTA, adjusted to pH 7.5 with 0.1 N NaOH

3.1.3. Purification of C1q

a. Serum 40 ml, is mixed with 10 ml of solution A and incubated for 10 min at 37°C in order to dissociate the C1qrs complex in the serum. Immediately thereafter the mixture is placed in the ice bath and the pH is adjusted to 7.5.

b. *From now on all steps are done in the ice bath and with ice-cooled solutions:* Slowly and while stirring gently with a glass stick, 200 ml of solution B are added to the serum−EDTA mixture (RSC should be 0.040). The final mixture is left in the ice bath for 1 hr. One should stir gently with the glass stick for 1 min every 20 min.

c. The formed precipitate is recovered after centrifugation at 12,000 g (e.g., 10,000 rpm with SS-34 Sorvall rotor) for 30 min at 4°C. One should use translucent tubes in order to find the discrete precipitate. The precipitate is extremely gently resuspended in 80 ml of solution C and recentrifuged as described. Resuspend the precipitate in 80 ml of solution C and repeat centrifugation.

d. After the second wash, the precipitate is dissolved in ± 10 ml of solution D and let stand overnight at 4°C. Thereafter this solution is centrifuged at 30,000 g for 30 min at 4°C, and the supernatant is used in the next step.

e. This supernatant is dialyzed for 2 hr against 1 liter of solution E and again for 2 hr after a change of solution E (a magnetic stirrer is used).

f. The formed precipitate is recovered after centrifugation at 12,000 g for

30 min at 4°C and resuspended in 20 ml of solution E and then recentrifuged as described. This wash is repeated once.

g. After the second wash, the precipitate is dissolved in 3 ml of solution F and let stand at 4°C for 2 hr. Thereafter this solution is centrifuged at 30,000 g for 30 min at 4°C, and the supernatant is considered as pure C1q.

3.1.4. Control of Yield and Purity. The OD_{280} is measured and an $E_{1\,cm}^{1\%}$ of 6.82 is used for calculation of the yield (it is about 1 or 2 mg from 40 ml of serum). Purity is checked by performing an immunoelectrophoresis on 1% agarose in Michaelis buffer containing EDTA (10 mM) using anti-total human serum and anti-C1q antisera.

3.2. Method for the radioiodination of C1q with Lactoperoxydase

3.2.1. The radioiodination is performed on 200 μg C1q dissolved in 500–800 μl Solution F (see 3.1.3. point g). The following reactants are added to the C1q: (a) 5 μl of the [125] I preparation (about 500 μCi); (b) 5 μl of NaI (0.006 mg/ml in VBS), (c) 5 μl of lactoperoxidase (1 mg/ml in VBS), (d) 5 μl of H_2O_2, 0.003% in VBS (Perhydrol diluted 1:10,000)

3.2.2. The tube is shaken and let stand for 15 min in an ice bath. Thereafter the reaction is stopped through the addition of: (e) 10 μl of NaI; VBS, 6 mg/ml; (f) 10 μl of NaN_3, VBS, 0.03 mg/ml; (g) 2 ml of VBS.

3.2.3. The percentage of radioactivity uptake (i.e., percent TCA-precipitable radioactivity) is calculated and should be 50–80%. The specific activity of the [125] I-C1q is therefore 1.25–2.0 μCi/μg C1q. This preparation is dialyzed against VBS for 20 hr at 4°C. Thereafter the preparation is conveniently further diluted to a final volume of about 5 ml, with VBS, and is stored in portions of 100 μl at −70°C for up to 2 months.

3.3. Method for the [125] I-C1q Binding Test. *3.3.1. Preparation of the [125] I-C1q for the Use in the Test.*

On the day of testing, a portion of the labeled C1q is thawed and diluted in 3–5 ml of VBS containing 1% (v/v) heat-inactivated serum (56°C for 30 min). The diluted supernatant is centrifuged at 18,000 g for 40 min at 4°C. The aggregate free supernatant is used in the test.

3.3.2. Preparation of Solutions. (a) EDTA, 0.2 M, adjusted to pH 7.5 with 1 N NaOH, is stored at 4°C. (b) Borate buffer, pH 8.3, containing boric acid 0.1 M, disodium tetraborate 0.025 M, NaCl 0.075 M, can be stored at 4°C. (c) A solution of 3% (w/v) PEG in borate buffer is prepared on the day of testing.

3.3.3. Preparation of Soluble Heat Aggregated Human Immunoglobulin (AHG). A solution of Cohn fraction II, 6 mg/ml NaCl 0.9%, is heated at 63°C for 20 min and thereafter centrifuged at 1500 g for 15 min. Prepare standard solutions containing 3, 0.5, and 0.1 mg of AHG per milliliter of NaCl 0.9%.

3.3.4. Performance of the [125] I-C1q Binding Test. The test is always done in duplicate, in Bio-Vial polypropylene tubes.

a. A tested serum (native serum), 50 μl, is mixed with 100 μl of EDTA solution and incubated for 30 min at 37°C. As negative controls, sera from healthy blood donors or a pool of such sera are incubated in the same way. As positive controls, 50 μl of each of various dilutions of AHG are mixed with 50 μl of heat-inactivated serum (56°C, 30 min) and 50 μl of EDTA solution and incubated in the same way.

b. After this incubation, the tubes are placed in the ice bath. Then 50 μl of the ^{125} I-C1q solution and immediately thereafter 1 ml of the PEG solution are added to the previous mixtures and the tubes are let stand without shaking or mixing for 1 hr.

c. Two TCA control tubes are prepared by mixing 50 μl of the ^{125} I-C1q solution, 150 μl of serum, and 1 ml of TCA 20%.

d. After 1 hr, all tubes are centrifuged at 1500 g for 20 min at 4°C. Thereafter, the supernatants are completely discarded, and the radioactivity is measured in the precipitates.

e. The test results are expressed as percent ^{125} I-C1q precipitated as compared with the radioactivity precipitated in the TCA control tubes; the mean of duplicated tests is calculated and represents the C1q binding activity (C1q-BA).

4. Critical Comments

4.1. Interpretation of Data. The normal range of C1q-BA measured by the ^{125} I-C1q binding test is established by testing sera from normal blood donors. In a representative experiment the mean C1q-BA of sera from 20 blood donors was 5± 1.4% (± 1 SD). The mixtures of various solutions of AHG with heat-inactivated serum represent the positive test controls. In sera mixed with an equal volume of AHG at concentrations of 3, 0.5, and 0.1 mg/ml the C1q-BA should be around 90, 55, and 30%, respectively. With several batches of C1q and various preparations of AHG, the variation in the C1q-BA measured on these positive controls is relatively limited (the variation coefficient was 6.2% for AHG 0.5 mg/ml, 10 different tests). Usually the results of C1q-BA measured on duplicate serum samples exhibit little variation (the variation coefficient for 50 duplicated samples was 3.4%). The individual values of C1q-BA are interpreted by statistical evaluation (SD) as compared to the normal range. The results can also be expressed in equivalents of AHG, but this expression gives a wrong idea of the actual amount of complexes in the tested sample since the C1q-BA will vary with the size and the nature of the detected immune complexes.

4.2. Specificity of the Method. It has been shown that complexes formed of at least 3 IgG molecules can give a positive C1q binding test (1). In human diseases it is likely that most immune complexes contain immunoglobulins that can bind C1q. However, some complexes, such as those involving only IgA antibodies, would not be detected in a C1q binding test (11). Various polyanionic and polycationic biological substances were also shown to bind C1q (12).

It is therefore surprising that single-stranded DNA, which is known to bind C1q, leads to only limited C1q precipitation in this test system (20% at an optimal concentration of 60 μg per milliliter of serum), but DNA can compete with immune complexes for the binding of C1q. No increase in C1q-BA was observed when bacterial lipopolysaccharide (LPS S. Minnesota RE 595) was added to normal human serum (6). This can be explained by the rather good solubility of DNA and LPS in PEG. The binding of C1q by calcium-dependent complexes of C reactive protein (CRP) and polycationic substances has been described (12, 13). Such complexes should not interfere with the C1q binding test, which is performed on EDTA-treated serum. It cannot be ruled out that other substances produce false-positive test results through a nonspecific binding of C1q. Indeed, the addition of heparin to normal serum or plasma can lead to an increased C1q-BA.

4.3. The Nature of C1q Binding Material. This can be further characterized by some additional investigations on such topics as the following: (a) the C1q-BA of serum containing immune complexes will be inhibited after reduction and alkylation (14); (b) possible effects of DNA can be excluded by DNase treatment of samples; (c) the size of C1q binding material can be studied by fractionation of the sample on sucrose density gradients and testing of the fractions for C1q-BA; (d) the C1q-BA of immune complexes will disappear after separation on sucrose density gradients prepared in acid buffer.

4.4. Technical Comments

a. Sera can be stored at $-20°C$ for several weeks and at $-70°C$ for several months and be frozen and thawed up to 4 times without any alteration of the C1q binding activity.

b. For testing of biological fluids or serum fractions poor in proteins, the test system should contain at least 25 μl of normal serum per tube in order to assure a minimal protein concentration for the reproducibility of the PEG precipitation.

c. Preliminary results indicated the applicability of the C1q binding test to the testing of sera from mice, monkeys, and cattle. For mice, the amount of 0.2 M EDTA added in the first step should be 200 μl instead of 100 μl.

d. It is critical to centrifuge the ^{125}I-C1q preparation immediately before its use in the test in order to clear aggregated C1q. Such aggregates are less soluble in PEG and may lead to increased nonspecific precipitation.

REFERENCES

1. Nydegger, U. E., Lambert, P.-H., Gerber, H., and Miescher, P. A., *J. Clin. Invest.* **54**, 297 (1974).
2. Sobel, A. T., Bokish, V. A., and Müller-Eberhard, H. J., *J. Exp. Med.* **142**, 139 (1975).
3. Luthra, H. S., McDuffie, F. C., Hunder, G. G., and Samayoa, E. A., *J. Clin. Invest.* **56**, 458 (1975).

4. Onyewotu, I. I., Holborow, E. J., and Johnson, G. D., *Nature (London)* **248**, 156 (1974).
5. Theofilopoulos, A. N., Wilson, C. B., and Dixon, F. J., *J. Clin. Invest.* **57**, 169 (1976).
6. Zubler, R. H., Lange, G., Lambert, P.-H., and Miescher, P. A., *J. Immunol.* **116**, 232 (1976).
7. Zubler, R. H., Nydegger, U., Perrin, L. H., Fehr, K., McCormick, J., Lambert, P. H., and Miescher, P. A., *J. Clin. Invest.* **57**, 1308 (1976).
8. Bjonvatn, B., Zubler, R. H., Lambert, P. H., Barnetson, R., and Kronvall, G., *Clin. Exp. Immunol.* in press.
9. Volanakis, J. E., and Stroud, R. M., *J. Immunol. Meth.* **2**, 24 (1972).
10. Heusser, C. M., Boesman, M., Nordin, J. H., and Isliker, H., *J. Immunol.* **110**, 820 (1973).
11. Augener, W., Grey, H. M., Cooper, N. R., and Müller-Eberhard, H. J., *Immunochemistry* **8**, 1011 (1971).
12. Siegel, J., Rent, R., and Gewurz, H., *J. Exp. Med.* **140**, 631 (1974).
13. Kaplan, M. H., and Volanakis, J. E., *J. Immunol.* **112**, 2135 (1974).
14. Wiedermann, G., Miescher, P. A., and Franklin, E. C., *Proc. Soc. Exp. Biol. Med.* **113**, 609 (1963).

Lymphocyte Transformation: Utilization of Automatic Harvesters

J. J. Oppenheim and D. L. Rosenstreich

1. Introduction

The majority of normal, mammalian peripheral lymphocytes are resting cells until they are stimulated in some fashion. This stimulation induces the lymphocyte to begin a series of changes whereby it becomes more metabolically active, increases its protein synthesis and enzyme content, and enlarges until it becomes a "blast" cell. This process, which eventually results in new DNA synthesis and cell division, is referred to as "lymphocyte transformation."

Assays of lymphocyte transformation in man have proved to be of great utility for: (a) determining and monitoring genetic and acquired states of immunological deficiency; (b) detecting serum factors that depress lymphocyte reactivity; (c) obtaining evidence of previous sensitization to pathogenens, to allergens, or to self in patients with autoimmune diseases; (d) histocompatibility typing with mixed leukocyte reactions (MLR); and (e) studying lymphocyte subpopulations, such as T suppressor cells, and the generation of mediators of cell-mediated immunity (CMI).

The basic methodology of these assays is essentially the same regardless of the species and site of origin of the lymphocytes or the type of stimulants being tested. The procedure involves collecting a lymphocyte population, culturing these cells *in vitro* for various periods of time in the presence or in the absence of selected stimulants, and assaying the changes induced by the stimulants in these lymphocyte populations in comparison to resting, unstimulated lymphocytes. In the sections to follow, we shall outline our methods for assaying *in vitro* lymphocyte transformation of human peripheral blood lymphocytes. Although the methods described will be applicable to most other lymphocyte assays, critical variables, such as the type and amount of serum, cell concentration, type of culture vessel, and duration of culture, must each be evaluated individually to optimize the assay.

The incorporation of radiolabeled thymidine into new DNA or leucine into new proteins provide the most commonly used and convenient means of assessing lymphocyte transformation because these assays yield a quantitative measure of the degree of cellular reactivity in contrast with morphological assessment of blastogenesis. Furthermore, these assays have recently been improved by being miniaturized and automated using disposable, plastic microtiter plates for culturing cells and semiautomatic harvesters to rapidly process the cultures. This approach results in greater reproducibility, speed, and economy than manual harvesting of "macrocultures." We shall therefore concentrate on reviewing the methods and materials required for culturing human lymphocytes most efficiently for automated harvesting procedures. For more detailed reviews of the methodology and relevance of assays of lymphocyte transformation, a number of comprehensive reviews (1–3) and books (4–6) are available.

2. Materials and Equipment

2.1.1. Syringes, disposable of various sizes (Pharmaseal Labs., Glendale, California) and needles, disposable butterfly (Abbott Laboratories, North Chicago, Illinois)

2.1.2. Preservative-free heparin (Eli Lilly, Indianapolis, Indiana)

2.1.3. Sterile glass culture tubes (25 × 200 mm) (Kimble, Arthur H. Thomas, Philadelphia, Pennsylvania).

2.1.4. Automatic cell counter (Coulter Counter Model D2, Coulter Electronics Inc., Hialeah, Florida)

2.1.5. Water-jacketed CO_2 incubator (Thelco, Precision Scientific, Chicago, Illinois)

2.1.6. Refrigerated centrifuge (Model PR_2, IEC Division, International Equipment Co., Boston, Massachusetts)

2.2. Solutions, Media, and Additives

2.2.1. Phosphate-buffered saline (PBS) with 0.15 M sodium chloride, 0.01 M sodium phosphate, pH 7.2

2.2.2. Ficoll, MW 400,000 (9% in doubly distilled H_2O) (Sigma Chemical, St. Louis, Missouri), Hypaque-M 90% (Winthrop Laboratories, Division of Sterling Drugs, New York, New York) or lymphoprep (Nyegard and Co., Oslo, Norway)

2.2.3. Tissue culture medium RPMI 1640 (GIBCO, Grand Island, New York)

2.2.4. Penicillin and streptomycin with 10,000 U and 10 mg/ml respectively, in stock solution (Microbiological Associates, Bethesda, Maryland)

2.2.5. Dextran (Type 200 C) (Sigma Chemical Co., St. Louis, Missouri)

2.2.6. Gentamycin, (Schering Corp., Port Reading, New York)

2.2.7. 5-Fluorocytocine (5-FC) (Hoffmann-La Roche, Nutley, New Jersey)

2.2.8. HEPES buffer 10–25 mM (Calbiochem, Rockville, Maryland)

2.3. For Determination of ^{3}H-Leucine Incorporation

2.3.1. Eagle's medium without leucine (Microbiological Associates, Bethesda, Maryland)

2.3.2. Nonessential amino acids (100X) (GIBCO, Grand Island, New York)

2.4. Tissue Culture Ware

2.4.1. Disposable sterile pipettes (Falcon Plastics, Oxnard, California)

2.4.2. Disposable sterile pasteur pipettes (Forma Scientific, Marietta, Ohio)

2.4.3. Flat-bottomed tissue-culture plates and lids (Microtest II, Falcon Plastics, Oxnard, California), or V-shaped microtiter plates especially prepared for tissue culture (Cooke Microtiter System, Alexandria, Virginia)

2.4.4. Sterile glass vials (Wheaton Glass Co., Millville, New Jersey), or plastic tissue-culture flasks (Falcon Plastics, Oxnard, California)

2.4.5. Automatic pipettes and sterile disposable tips (from Eppendorf, Hamburg, West Germany; Oxford Laboratories, Oxford, California) or Pipetman (from Rainin, Brighton, Massachusetts)

2.5. Harvesting Requirements

2.5.1. ^{14}C-Thymidine (50 mCi/mmole); ^{3}H-thymidine (2 Ci/mmole); ^{14}C-leucine (350 mCi/mmole); ^{3}H-leucine (1 Ci/mmole) in sterile aqueous solution (from Schwarz-Mann, Rockville, Maryland)

2.5.2. ^{125}I-labeled 5-iododeoxyuridine (^{125}IudR) (200 Ci/mmole, New England Nuclear, Boston, Massachusetts)

2.5.3. Hamilton syringes (Hamilton Co., Whittier, California)

2.5.4. Automatic harvesters (Mash III, Microbiological Associates, Bethesda, Maryland), Skatron Multiple Cell Culture Harvester (Flow Laboratories, Inc.), or M24 Harvester (Biomedical Research and Development Laboratories, Rockville, Maryland)

2.5.5. Glass fiber filters, 934 AH (Whatman, Inc., Clifton, New Jersey)

2.5.6. Infrared lamp (Infra Rediator, Fisher Scientific Co., Silver Spring, Maryland)

2.5.7. Scintillation fluid: (A) toluene containing 4 g of PPO and 100 mg of dimethyl POPOP/liter (Packard Instruments, Downers Grove, Illinois), (B) Liquifluor, mixed as directed with toluene (New England Nuclear, Boston, Massachusetts, (C) Aquasol (New England Nuclear), (D) Hydromix (Yorktown Research, South Hackensack, New Jersey), (E) PCS (Amersham Searle, Arlington Heights, Illinois)

2.5.8. Vial inserts and caps (Yorktown Research, South Hackensack, New Jersey)

2.5.9. Scintillation vials (Kimble, Toledo, Ohio)

2.5.10. Liquid scintillation spectrometer (Model No. 3375, Packard Instrument Co., Downers Grove, Illinois)

2.6. Commonly Used Stimulants

2.6.1. Phytohemagglutinin (PHA) (Burroughs-Wellcome Co., Tuckahoe, N.Y.). Dissolve in PBS and store at $-20°C$ at a concentration of 1 mg/ml. Higher dilutions used for routine work will be stable at $4°C$ for up to a month.

2.6.2. Concanavalin A (Con A) (Miles-Yeda Ltd., Rehovot, Israel). Handle in the same manner as PHA.

2.6.3. Pokeweed mitogen (PWM) (GIBCO, Grand Island, New York). Dilute with medium and freeze at $-20°C$ in small aliquots prior to use.

2.6.4. Purified protein derivative (PPD) (Connaught Laboratories, Toronto, Ontario, Canada). Store at $4°C$ and dilute for use.

2.6.5. Streptolysin O (SLO) (Difco Laboratories, Detroit, Michigan). Unstable unless kept at $-20°C$ in small aliquots and thawed only once.

2.6.6. *Candida albicans* (Hollister-Stier, Spokane, Washington). Use at 1:100 final dilution of glycerin saline extract and store at $4°C$.

2.6.7. Tetanus toxoid: Obtained on request from Dr. L. Levine, Massachusetts Department of Health, Boston, and used at 2 LFU/ml which contains 6 μg/ml protein nitrogen.

3. Methodology

3.1. Donors. Patients should always be tested simultaneously with normal donors to control for variables in technique. Normal subjects should be age- and sex-matched if possible and not be suffering from any acute or chronic illnesses. In donors who are allergic to penicillin, medium containing gentamycin rather than penicillin should be used. Donors should not be taking any drugs, including aspirin, which suppress lymphocyte function *in vitro*.

3.2. Preparation of Cell Suspensions. Blood (10–500 ml) is obtained by venipuncture and drawn into syringes coated with sufficient heparin to provide a concentration of 10–50 U/ml. To obtain peripheral blood leukocytes (PB WBC), the red blood cells are sedimented for 1–2 hr at $37°C$ in long narrow sterile tubes at an angle of $15°$ from the horizontal. Occasionally blood samples will require the addition of 1:4 (v/v) sterile dextran (6% in isotonic saline) for 30–60 min in order to sediment adequately.

Suspensions of leukocytes can also be prepared from lymphoid organs, such as the tonsils, thymus, and spleen as described (7). The leukocyte suspension is then pipetted into sterile centrifuge tubes, which are centrifuged at 750 g for 8–10 min to pellet the WBC and remove the plasma. The cells are then resuspended in PBS or medium, and 9 ml containing up to 10^8 WBC are carefully layered on 3 ml of Ficoll–Hypaque (2.4:1) or on premixed Lymphoprep in 15 × 125 mm sterile tubes and centrifuged for 40 min at 400 g at $20°C$ in a refrigerated centrifuge according to Böyum (8). To obtain a greater cell yield, the whole blood remaining after removal of WBC-rich plasma can be recentrifuged at 1000 g, and the buffy-coat layer of WBC in plasma is diluted 3:1 with PBS and then similarly layered onto 3 ml of Ficoll–Hypaque. The resulting layer of mononuclear lymphocytes and monocytes at the interface between the Ficoll–Hypaque and plasma is recovered, thoroughly washed with 50 ml of PBS 3 times, counted using a Coulter counter or hemocytometer, and resuspended at 1 to 2 × 10^6/ml in medium containing 10–20% autologous or pooled homologous plasma or serum. Usually autologous or pooled homologous plasma or serum will be equally effective. Heterologous plasmas, such as calf serum, should be avoided since they are themselves stimulatory.

In the case of cultures to be assayed for DNA synthesis, adequate nutritional support is provided by media ranging in complexity from Eagle's minimal essential medium (MEM) to enriched Roswell Park Memorial Institute 1640 (RPMI-1640) supplemented with 2 mM glutamine, 50 U of penicillin, and 50 μg of streptomycin per milliliter. If the medium is to be utilized over longer intervals it must be resupplemented with freshly thawed 2 mM glutamine once a month. In donors who are allergic to penicillin, one should use gentamycin (5 μg/ml). Growth of fungi or molds can sometimes be prevented by the addition of 5 μg of 5-fluorocytosine (5FC) per milliliter. Although antibiotics minimize contamination, strict sterile techniques must still be used. When cultures contain less than 10% plasma, the "nonspecific" background reactivity of lymphocytes may increase and/or the degree of reaction to stimulants may be suboptimal. In the absence of serum or plasma only reactions to the more potent mitogens can be elicited, but antigen-induced lymphoproliferative reactions fail to occur (9). In contrast, at concentrations > 40% plasma the maximal lymphoproliferative responses to both mitogens and antigens becomes progressively lower, and detection of reactivity to weaker stimulants may be lost. This may be due to the presence of nonspecific immunosuppressive factors such as α-macroglobulins or competitive binding of mitogens to other plasma constituents (10).

3.3. Macroculture Techniques. "Macrocultures" have been performed in a great variety of tubes, vials, and bottles ranging in volume from 0.5 to 500 ml. One of the crucial determinants of a successful outcome of such cultures is the final density of leukocytes or lymphocytes that settles and interact on the bottom of the culture vessel. Generally 1 to 2 $\times$ 10^6 leukocytes or lymphocytes per cm^2 leads to optimal cell survival and reactivity. At lower densities, lymphocytes (perhaps because of suboptimal cell–cell interactions or failure to "condition" the medium) will not grow well, and at higher densities lymphocytes appear to inhibit one another's growth and survival. The depth of medium that can be used to obtain optimal growth in macrocultures is less critical (ranging from 0.5 to 3 ml), which reinforces the view that cell density rather than cell concentration is the crucial factor.

3.4. Microculture Techniques. For clinical laboratory studies, we currently advocate the use of microculture techniques because they are more economical in use of tissue-culture materials, patients' blood, and space and require less labor than macrocultures. The only disadvantage of microcultures is that they are significantly less sensitive in the presence of polymorphonuclear leukocytes. Therefore, they require the time-consuming step of fractionation of leukocytes on Ficoll–Hypaque gradients to obtain mononuclear cells.

For microculture assays of DNA synthesis plastic plates that are specified for tissue-culture purposes are used. They contain 96 flat-bottomed wells which hold a volume of 0.2 ml with 1 to 2 $\times$ 10^5 mononuclear cells. Operationally, it is simplest to add the desired cell number in 0.1-ml volume of medium, as previously described, to the appropriate number of wells, followed by 0.1-ml volume of medium containing twice the desired final concentration of stimulant. Either 1-ml sterile disposable pipettes or automatic pipettes with disposable sterile plastic tips can be used to dispense the cells and stimulants. They are then covered with sterile plastic lids and incubated.

3.5. Nonspecific and Specific Lymphocyte Stimulants. Readily available T-cell mitogens that are commonly used include phytohemagglutinin (PHA, 1–5 μg/ml) and/or concanavalin A (Con A, 1–10 μg/ml). Pokeweed mitogen (PWM, 1:20 dilution) stimulates both T and B cells.

Antigens that are also commonly used to evaluate the efficacy of human lymphocyte transformation include purified protein derivative (PPD, at 20 μg/ml), streptolysin-O (SLO, 1:20 final dilution), *Candida albicans* (1:100 final dilution of glycerin saline extract), and tetanus toxoid (2 LFU/ml or 6 μg/ml). All the stimulants can be dissolved either in sterile water, PBS, or medium. The activity of these stimulants is usually best preserved by storing them in aliquots at $4°C$, except for SLO, which can only be kept frozen and thawed once; this avoids subjecting it to denaturation by repeated freezing and thawing. The concentration ranges given for each stimulant are those that generally produce maximal stimulation. Nevertheless, it is usually necessary to perform preliminary experiments in any system to determine the optimal stimulant concentration, cell concentration, and time of incubation.

In the case of the bidirectional MLR, equal numbers of leukocytes or lymphocytes from two unrelated individuals are mixed and serve as stimulants that induce an *in vitro* response to one another. In order to be able to determine the response of one subject's cells, a "unidirectional" MLR has to be performed. This can be achieved by preparing viable but nonproliferating leukocytes as stimulants. Such viable stimulator cells can be obtained either by irradiating leukocytes with 1000–4000 R or by incubating them for 25 min at $37°C$ with mitomycin C (25 μg/ml, which must then be thoroughly washed off), both of which will block proliferative responses but not the stimulating capacity of the cells. Since irradiation and mitomycin C fail to block protein synthesis, attempts to obtain unidirectional MLR's with assays of protein synthesis have been unsuccessful.

3.6. Incubation Procedures. Water-jacketed incubators usually provide more stable temperature regulation than those in which the atmosphere is circulated with fans, but both types are adequate. Incubation of cells in a humidified atmosphere of 5–10% CO_2 and air is necessary for optimal reactivity of microcultures. The presence of CO_2 maintains the bicarbonate-buffered media at the proper pH of 7.2. When macrocultures are incubated in the absence of CO_2 the cells can be grown in tightly capped vials or tubes. Microtiter plates can be closed with sealing tape. In both cases the cells can generate sufficient CO_2 when adequately stimulated. However, weak stimulants do not induce sufficient metabolic activity by the cells to support growth under these conditions. The use of HEPES buffer can stabilize the pH and partially alleviate this problem.

It takes 2–4 days of incubation to detect optimal DNA synthesis in response to mitogens, whereas optimal lymphocyte reactions to antigenic stimulants take 4.5–7 days. In fact, the maximal response to suboptimal doses of potent mitogens also occurs later, indicating an inverse relationship between the size of the reactive cell population and time when DNA synthesis becomes significantly elevated.

3.7. Assays of DNA Synthesis. The great utility and widespread use of lymphocyte assays has been made possible by the development of quantitative assays of incorporation of radioisotope precursors, which has replaced subjective evaluation of blastogenesis by laborious morphological evaluation. The uptake of tritiated thymidine (^{3}H-TdR, 0.5 μCi/well) or ^{14}C-thymidine, (0.05 μCi/well) are most commonly used to determine DNA synthesis by cells in S phase. Investigators who wish to avoid the problem of reutilization of isotope use ^{125}-labeled 5-iododeoxyuridine (^{125}IUdR) which also has the advantage that ^{125}I can be measured in a gamma rather than a beta scintillation counter (11). To ensure that the radiolabeled precursor is present in excess it is very important to add a radiolabeled precursor with low specific activity (12) (see materials). One can usually demonstrate significant incorporation by adding radiolabeled precursors 4–16 hr prior to processing. The shorter 4-hr exposure to radioisotope is preferable, but for the sake of convenience, overnight labeling is often used. Cultures are either immediately harvested or stored as described in the next section.

3.8. Assays of Protein Synthesis. A microculture as well as macroculture technique has been developed which accurately assesses lymphocyte transformation by determining radioactive leucine incorporation into proteins of responding mononuclear leukocytes. The major advantage of this technique is its speed, low incidence of contamination, and lack of requirement for serum. Only 6–48 hr of incubation are needed to assess lymphocyte competence by this method. It requires the use of leucine-free media to avoid dilution of the radiolabeled leucine precursor in these studies. The absence of leucine does not affect lymphocyte transformation (13). The medium is supplemented with antibiotics, as previously discussed, and the labile essential amino acid glutamine (2 mM). The medium can also be enriched by addition of 1 ml of a nonessential amino acid concentrate (100 X) per 100 ml of medium. Alternatively, leucine-free RPMI 1640 can be used. Under these conditions 90% of the lymphocytes remain viable for 48 hr of incubation (13). After 48 hr, in the absence of serum, the viability of lymphocyte cultures decreases drastically.

It has been observed that the incorporation of radiolabeled leucine by both unstimulated and stimulated cultures increases proportionately over a wide concentration range of 2×10^5 to 10^6 mononuclear cells per 0.1 ml. Therefore, the stimulation ratio of counts per minute (cpm) of radiolabeled leucine in experimental stimulated to control unstimulated cultures (E/C) remains stable over this range of cell concentrations. Since the amount of blood that can be used for such studies is usually limiting, only 2.5×10^5 cells per 0.1 ml are incubated for 24 hr to assay the response to potent mitogens. If necessary, as few as 10^4 cells can be used to obtain significant reactions to potent mitogens, albeit with lower E/C ratios (13).

Aliquots of 0.1 ml of the cell suspension are added to microtiter tissue culture plate with 96 V-shaped wells using automatic pipettes with sterilized disposable plastic tips. The stimulants are added to the appropriate wells in 10 μl volumes of medium or PBS at 10 times the desired final concentration. In general, five times higher concentrations of antigens and mitogens are needed to activate early protein synthesis optimally than to induce DNA synthesis. To mix the cells and stimulants, the plates can then be placed on a microshaker for 15 sec. The plates are incubated in a humidified mixture of 5–10% CO_2 in air at 37°C for 6–48 hr.

The degree of background protein synthesis in control culture decreases slowly over a 48-hr period of incubation. In contrast, mitogen-stimulated cultures show increases in protein synthesis by 4–6 hr of incubation. This continues to increase for 24 hr and plateaus by 48 hr. Optimal sensitivity of the assay and reproducibility of ± 10% SD of the mean counts per minute of replicate cultures to lower doses of mitogens is obtained by 24 hr. However, in the case of weaker antigenic stimulants and the MLR, higher cell concentrations of 10^6 per 0.1 ml and a longer incubation period of 48 hr are needed to obtain a significant difference in E/C.

At 2–3 hr before harvesting the cultures, 1–2 μCi of ^{3}H-leucine (specific activity 1–2 Ci/mmole) or 0.25 μCi ^{14}C-leucine (350 mCi/mmole) are added to each well in a volume of 0.01 ml of PBS with a repeating dispenser Hamilton syringe. The plates are reshaken and reincubated. The culture is stopped by the addition of 0.02 ml of 50% trichloroacetic acid to each well at room temperature. The plates can either be processed immediately or stored at 4°C for up to a week. Alternatively, these cultures can also be harvested immediately with automated harvesters using only water, as will be described for the microassay of DNA synthesis.

3.9. Harvesting Cultures. One of the great advantages of assays based on the incorporation of radioisotopes with automatic harvesters is that they can be rapidly processed with automated harvesting machines (14), which aspirate and wash cells on to glass fiber filters. This method results in more reproducible data and saves time and effort in comparison with other approaches. In measuring incorporation into DNA or protein, the filters can be washed many times sequentially with isotonic saline, 5% trichloroacetic acid, and absolute methanol.

However, repeated washing (6 times) of prewetted filters with either isotonic saline or water yields similar results (15). The filters retain predominantly macromolecules with incorporated radioisotope since the cells are broken up on the filter and unincorporated isotope is washed out. By the use a suction attachment of appropriate size provided with a Skatron automatic harvester, either macro- or microcultures can be harvested automatically. The MASH unit has not been adapted for harvesting macrocultures as yet. The filters are then dried overnight at room temperature or for 30 min under infrared lamps, punched out, and dropped into scintillation vials that contain scintillation fluid. Although more expensive than homemade mixtures, such as toluene with POP and POPOP, versatile commercially prepared scintillation fluids are available for counting dried or dissolved samples (PCS). For samples containing some residual water one can use Aquasol. The most economical means of counting the large number of samples generated by these easy microassays is to count the filters in small, capped vial inserts containing 3 ml of scintillation fluid, which are inserted into the larger scintillation vials. The latter, which are more expensive, remain uncontaminated and can be reutilized, and only the cheaper small inserted vials need be discarded. The scintillation vials are stored in the dark, cooled, and counted in a beta scintillation counter at the appropriate settings to determine the counts per minute. The first few samples should be recounted to ensure that the counts are stable and not falsely high owing to transient chemoluminescence.

4. Interpretation of Data and Critical Comments

Experimental points should be performed at least in duplicate and preferably in triplicate or quadruplicate. The arithmetic mean and standard error of the mean (SE) of the counts per minute (cpm) of the samples should be determined. Some laboratories correct the cpm for both degree of quenching and efficiency of their counter and express their results in disintegrations per minute (dpm). When, as usually is the case, the degree of quenching of samples within a given experiment is similar and machine efficiency constant, this additional step does not affect the interpretation of the data and can be omitted. The cpm of replicate samples, except in the case of very weak stimulants and unstimulated cultures, should vary by less than 20% from the mean. Variations in excess of 20% in replicate stimulated cultures are indicative of technical problems. It is not valid to eliminate replicate samples that vary too much from the mean unless they completely failed to incorporate radioisotope. This may be caused by bacterial contamination, cell death for unknown causes associated with evidence of alkalinity of medium (purple phenolphthalein indicator) or omission of the radiolabeled precursor.

The large changes in magnitude of thymidine incorporation by cultured lymphocytes with increasing duration of incubation are due to the exponential growth rate of the cells. Therefore, small differences in growth rate become magnified with time and result in a nonnormal distribution of data. In order to permit a proper statistical assessment of data of this type, they must be normalized. This can be achieved by logarithmic conversion of the cpm, which can then be analyzed by student's t tests or analysis of variance. The data can then be reconverted to cpm, and the geometric mean ± confidence limits expressed. Although the same approach can be used to analyze the uptake of radiolabeled leucine, analysis of the arithmetic means of uptake of radiolabeled leucine is probably adequate since the duration of culture is shorter and the response not as subject to exponential changes.

Frequently, only the ratio of experimental to control cpm (E/C) of incorporation of thymidine are shown. Although this normalizes the data to some extent, use of the E/C is based on the assumption that the degree of reactivity of control and experimental cultures will be affected by variables in the same way and will remain proportional. Unfortunately, this is sometimes not the case. (a) There may be uncontrollable prior *in vivo* excitation of immunological reactivity that elevates the response in "control" cultures and interferes with the reactivity to other stimuli as in Wiskott–Aldrich syndrome, infections mononucleosis, and leukemia. (b) Stimulants present *in vivo* may be transferred into the cultures and may be responsible for the progressive increases in proliferation in unstimulated cultures that occur with longer periods of incubation. (c) Alternatively, these lymphoproliferative reactions in control cultures may be induced by media components, cell products, or too vigorous handling, which may damage and stimulate some cells. Factors that stimulate control cultures appear to lower the E/C although the actual degree of experimental response may remain the same. Therefore, although it is more cumbersome, the control as well as experimental results always ought to be indicated to permit proper evaluation of the data.

The thymidine incorporation by unstimulated cultures is usually low because only stimulated lymphocytes go on to synthesize DNA. This low background is responsible for the sensitivity of this assay, and it has been estimated that repeated divisions of an initial clone with fewer than 10 cells in a population of 10^6 lymphocytes theoretically can result in significant increases (E/C) in thymidine uptake after 5–7 days of incubation. Provided the background cpm of thymidine incorporation are reasonably low and the variation between replicates < 20%, reproducible 3-fold or greater differences between E and C are indicative of significant lymphocyte proliferation. Smaller differences than that must be consistently reproduced many times to be indicative of a biologically meaningful reaction.

Since protein synthesis, in contrast with DNA synthesis, is an ongoing process in the resting lymphocyte, there is considerably higher uptake of radiolabeled leucine by unstimulated cultures. However, "small" increases in protein synthesis by stimulated cultures can be quite significant since the variation between replicate cultures is much smaller ($\pm$ 10%) than in the case of thymidine uptake ($\pm$ 20%). The only valid criterion for determining significant stimulation of protein synthesis depends on comparison with the corresponding unstimulated controls (E/C), but ratios of 1.5 or greater are usually significant. Repeated assays of a normal subjects lymphocyte response to a stimulant will result in considerable variation in degree of incorporation of radiolabeled leucine. However, the E/C of the normal subjects will fluctuate much less than their absolute cpm.

We recommend that the more rapid reproducible and serum-free microassay of protein synthesis be used for assaying efficacy of response to mitogens to diagnose immunodeficiency states. The assay of DNA synthesis, although slower, is more sensitive and requires fewer cells, and we therefore recommend it to detect prior antigenic sensitization and for performing the unidirectional MLR.

The technique of lymphocyte transformation provides a commonly used *in vitro* correlate of CMI. However, it must be emphasized that, unless special methods that will be described in other chapters of this book are used to fractionate lymphocytes into subpopulations, one is actually testing a heterogeneous population of lymphocytes involved in cell-mediated as well as antibody-mediated immunological activities. Furthermore, the type and degree of reactivity of these various subpopulations will vary depending on the nature of the stimulants used.

Stimulants can be characterized by whether they are thymus dependent and stimulate purified thymus-derived (T) but not bone marrow-derived (B) cells, or, conversely, whether they are thymus independent and stimulate purified B but not T cells. It must be emphasized that in the usual heterogeneous mixtures of T and B lymphocytes, T cell stimulants, such as PHA and Con A actually, activate both lymphocyte populations because they stimulate T cells to make factors that in turn enhance the reactions of B cells (7). Since both B and T cells participate in the human lymphocyte reaction to most stimulants, it is difficult to assess the function of these subpopulations of cells without going through arduous purification procedures (10a). However, since 80% of peripheral human blood lymphocytes are T cells, their proliferative reactions are indicative predominantly of T cell-mediated immunological responses. Unfortunately the best known B-cell mitogens, such as thymus-independent lipopolysaccharide endotoxins (LPS) and anti-immunoglobulin antibodies, are too limited in potency to permit evaluation of peripheral blood B lymphoproliferative reactivity in man (16). In the case of man, LPS stimulates only B cells of sensitized subjects and does so only in the presence of some T cells; it behaves, therefore, like a T-dependent B cell antigen (17).

In assessing immunocompetence of lymphocytes, it is very important to test the lymphocyte reactivity to suboptimal doses of a mitogen, such as PHA. This can be achieved by determining the dose response to five 2-fold dilutions of

PHA, which will at times detect obvious hyporeactivity of lymphocytes in subjects that have normal reactions to the optimal doses of potent stimulants. For example, in a number of immunodeficiency states (18, 19), including Wiskott Aldrich syndrome (20), the proliferative response to optimal doses of PHA will be normal, whereas, subnormal reactivity can be detected only in response to suboptimal doses of PHA.

In order to establish whether a single individual's lymphocytes are functioning within the normal range, his response should be compared to concomitantly tested normally reactive controls. His response must also be assessed relative to the 95% or 99% confidence limits of the reactivity of a large number of age-matched normal subjects, previously tested by the laboratory. However, whenever possible it is preferable to determine whether a group of patients have normally transforming lymphocytes by comparing them to concomitantly tested groups of normals using student's t tests.

One can also culture whole blood directly diluted 1:10 to 1:40 with medium. This obviously provides the simplest and most economical approach. Although in our hands this method was lacking in sensitivity (2), convincing data have been published which show marked mitogen- and antigen-stimulated proliferative reactions by such whole-blood cultures (21). Since the responses in these cultures peak later, there is the disadvantage that it takes 4 days to obtain mitogen and 7 days for antigen-induced reactions. There is the additional disadvantage that these cultures have to be decolorized with acetic acid and/or hydrogen peroxide as well as repeatedly centrifuged and washed to be harvested. There is one report, however, in which as little as 7 μg of whole blood diluted in medium has been used in microcultures (22). If this is confirmed as being a sensitive and reproducible approach, it promises to become a most effective means of assaying lymphocyte transformation.

In summary, the incorporation of radiolabeled leucine and thymidine by cultured lymphocytes provides a measure of protein and DNA synthesis by these cells. Significant increases in these parameters over background in response to stimulants correlate with, but as if often incorrectly assumed, are not necessarily indicative of the characteristic morphological changes of lymphocyte transformation or of proliferation. Failure of lymphocytes to respond normally to stimulants correlates directly with impaired *in vivo* immunological functions, and this test therefore provides one means of assessing CMI. However, some immunological defects, such as hypogammaglobulinemia and CMI defects due to selectively impaired mediator functions, will be missed by these tests. The assays are very sensitive and will detect lymphocyte responses to antigens even a long time after exposure. This indicates that the assay provides a good measure of prior sensitization, but it fails to distinguish between acute, chronic, and old antigenic sensitization. Even with these limitations recently developed microculture techniques for growing lymphocyte in conjunction with automatic harvesters should make this informative and sensitive assay sufficiently rapid, economical, and reproducible to permit utilization by all clinical immunology laboratories.

REFERENCES

1. Douglas, S. D., *Int. Rev. Exp. Pathol.* **10,** (1971).
2. Oppenheim, J. J., Dougherty, S., Chan, S. C., and Baker, J., *in* "Laboratory Diagnosis of Immunological Disorders" (G. N. Vyas, D. Stites, and G. Brecher, eds.), p. 87. Grune & Stratton, New York, 1975.
3. Oppenheim, J. J. and Schecter, B., *in* "Manual of Clinical Immunology" (N. R. Rose and H. Friedman, eds.) Am. Soc. Microbiol., Washington, D. C., in press.
4. Bloom, B. R., and Glade, P. (Eds.), "*In Vitro* Methods in Cell-Mediated Immunity." Academic Press, New York, 1971.
5. Greaves, M. F., Owen, J. J. T., and Raff, M. C. "T and B Lymphocytes, Origins, Properties and Roles in Immune Responses." American Elsevier, New York, 1973.
6. Ling, N. R., and Kay, J. E., "Lymphocyte Stimulation." Elsevier, Amsterdam, 1975.
7. Geha, R. S., and Merler, E., *Eur. J. Immunol.* **4,** 193 (1974).
8. Böyum, A., *Scand. J. Clin. Lab. Invest.* **21,** 3 (1968).
9. Kirchner, H., and Oppenheim, J. J., *Cell. Immunol.* **3,** 695 (1972).
10. Murgita, R. A., and Tomasi, T. B., Jr., *J. Exp. Med.* **141,** 440 (1975).
10a. Greaves, M., Janossy, G., and Doenhoff, M., *J. Exp. Med.* **140,** (1974).
11. Pellegrino, M. A., Ferrone, A., Pellegrino, A., and Reisfeld, R., *Clin. Immunol. Immunopathol.* **2,** 67 (1973).
12. Janossy, G., Greaves, M. F., Doenhoff, M. J., and Snajar, J., *Clin. Exp. Immunol.* **14,** 581 (1973).
13. Adkinson, N. F., Jr., Rosenberg, S. A., and Terry, W. D., *J. Immunol.* **112,** 1426 (1974).
14. Hartzman, R. J., Bach, M. L., Bach, F. H., Thurman, G., and Sell, K. W., *Cell. Immunol.* **4,** 182 (1972).
15. Hirschberg, H., and Thorsby, E., *J. Immunol. Meth.* **16,** 451 (1973).
16. Ivanyi, L., and Lehner, T., *Clin. Exp. Immunol.* **18,** 347 (1975).
17. Baker, J. J., Chan, S. P., Mergenhagen, S. E., and Oppenheim, J. J., in preparation.
18. Levy, R., and Kaplan, H. S., *N. Engl. J. Med.* **290,** 181 (1974).
19. Ziegler, J. B., Hansen, P., and Penny, R., *Clin. Immunol. Immunopathol.* **3,** 451 (1975).
20. Oppenheim, J. J., Blaese, R. M., and Waldmann, T. A., *J. Immunol.* **104,** 835 (1970).
21. Pauly, J. L., Sokal, J. E., and Han, T., *J. Lab. Clin. Med.* **82,** 500 (1973).
22. Kaplan, J. M., and Raffano, A. F., *Immunol. Commun.* **2,** 507 (1973).

Lymphocyte Transformation against Human Tumor Antigens*

J. U. Gutterman, G. M. Mavligit, C. Y. Hunter, and E. M. Hersh

1. Introduction

In vitro stimulation of lymphocytes by tumor-associated antigens have been carried out in several human tumor systems (1–8). Thus, the ability of remission lymphocytes to respond *in vitro* to autologous leukemic cells and to single-cell suspensions of various solid tumor cells, including Burkitt's lymphoma, brain tumors, lymphomas, sarcomas, melanoma, and carcinomas have been confirmed by many workers (1–8).

The question whether these reactions represent a primary recognition reaction or true immunity was answered in part by the studies of Stjernswärd and co-workers, who showed that normal kidney cells did not stimulate lymphocytes, but that tumor cells from renal cell carcinomas did (9). Similarly, our own group in studies by Mavligit and co-workers showed that, in general, normal tissues failed to stimulate autologous lymphocytes whereas tumor cells from analogous tissue did stimulate autologous lymphocytes (5).

Our own studies demonstrated that the treatment of the stimulator cells was important in detecting reactivity. Thus, viable cells stimulated better than did nonviable cells (5, 10). Tumor cells left unirradiated or irradiated stimulated significantly better than did mitomycin-treated tumor cells (5, 10). Most of the studies have been carried out with mitomycin, which might account for the greater degree of reactivity noted in the studies by Mavligit and co-workers compared to Stjernswärd and co-workers.

In addition to peripheral blood lymphocytes, lymph node lymphocytes have been used as responder cells in these assays. Stjernswärd and Vánky showed that cells from lymph nodes draining tumor could not respond to autologous tumor cells (11). They suggested that excess antigen coating responding lymphocytes probably accounted for the lack of reactivity. In contrast, our group (Ambus and co-workers) demonstrated that both peripheral blood lymphocytes and

*Supported by Grant 15009-02 from the National Cancer Institute, Bethesda, Maryland. Drs. Gutterman and Mavligit are the recipients of Research Career Development Awards (CA 71007-02 and CA00130-01, respectively) from the National Cancer Institute, Bethesda, Maryland.

lymph node lymphocytes could respond to autologous tumor cells (12). There tended to be an inverse relationship between the response of peripheral blood lymphocytes and lymph node lymphocytes to tumor cells.

The mixed lymphocyte tumor interaction (MLTI) has been predictive for prognosis in some studies in leukemia and solid tumors. Thus, among solid-tumor patients, the *in vitro* lymphocyte blastogenic response was related to the extent of disease (5). A more vigorous response was noted among patients with localized disease compared to those with disseminated metastases.

Similarly, in acute leukemia, patients with acute myeloblastic leukemia (AML) responded much more vigorously to their own tumor cells compared to adult patients with acute lymphoblastic leukemia (ALL) (4, 13–15). This correlated well with subsequent prognosis of patients with AML compared to ALL. Some studies in acute leukemia have found no correlation of reactivity with prognosis whereas others have (3, 16).

Schweitzer and co-workers found no stimulation to autologous leukemic blast cells (17). These workers felt that the MLTI was of no help to detect tumor-associated immune reactivity. However, these resuls would correlate with the results of our group and others who showed that leukemic lymphoblasts, in general, failed to stimulate autologous lymphocytes (13, 18).

As pointed out previously, the specificity of the MLTI reactions in acute leukemia has not been absolutely determined. Thus, cells from autologous remission bone marrow frequently stimulated an *in vitro* blastogenic response among autologous lymphocytes (3, 18, 19). This reaction has been useful as an immunodiagnostic tool to detect residual leukemic disease. Thus, we have shown that patients whose peripheral blood lymphocytes were stimulated by autologous remission bone marrow cells tended to relapse early compared to those patients whose remission lymphocytes failed to respond to autologous bone marrow cells (19). Vánky and co-workers showed that lymph node lymphocytes draining tumors may actually stimulate peripheral blood lymphocytes in the MLTI. This may be due to tumor antigen which has coated the draining lymph node lymphocyte population (11).

The demonstration of tumor-associated antigens on human leukemic blast cells by the MLTI reaction has also been confirmed among HLA identical siblings. Thus, Bach and co-workers and Santos and co-workers demonstrated that HLA identical leukemic sibs can respond *in vitro* to leukemic blast cells from their HLA identical leukemic sib, but not to the remission lymphocytes (20, 21). Other workers including Rudolph and co-workers showed that leukemic blast cells cannot stimulate identical twin lymphocytes (22). Similarly, Halterman and Leventhal showed that HLA identical sibling lymphocytes did not respond to leukemic blast cells from their sibs (23).

Serum studies have been useful for understanding the host–tumor relationship in the MLTI assay. Thus, our group showed that autologous serum could both facilitate as well as inhibit the response of remission lymphocytes to autologous tumor cells compared to the response carried out in allogeneic serum (4, 5, 13, 14), In acute leukemia, the presence of inhibitor serum was correlated with coating of leukemic blasts with IgG immunoglobulin (13). The inhibitory phenomena tend to disappear in remission, suggesting that the inhibitory material (whether it be antibody, antigen, or antigen—antibody complexes) was removed.

Vánky and co-workers have also demonstrated that the majority of patients with solid tumors have inhibition of reactivity in the MLTI to autologous solid tumor tissues (24). Vánky showed that the autologous inhibitory serum enhanced the blastogenic response of PHA and allogeneic lymphocytes. Studies of Vánky and co-workers showed that allogeneic sera from patients with related tumors blocked the reaction in a majority of sarcoma and carcinoma combinations. Unrelated allogeneic sera taken from tumor patients were inhibitory in only 1 of 11 sarcoma and 2 of 6 carcinoma combinations. Healthy donor sera were rarely inhibitory. Thus, as summarized recently, autologous patients' sera were inhibitory in 80% of combinations, allogeneic sera from patients with related tumors were inhibitory in 60% of combinations, sera from patients with unrelated tumors inhibited in only 18% of combination, and healthy donor sera were inhibitory in only 13% of combinations.

The role of IgG coating of tumor cells and *in vitro* blastogenic response has also been investigated. As pointed out above, leukemic myeloblasts coated with IgG stimulated vigorously in allogeneic sera, but not in autologous serum (13). In contrast, Vánky and co-workers showed that solid tumor cells coated with immunoglobulin stimulated poorly unless the immunoglobulin was eluted off the cell (25).

Extracts of human tumors also stimulate lymphocyte proliferation. Thus, Savel (26) and Jehn *et al.* (27) have reported that crude extracts will stimulate autologous and, occasionally, allogeneic lymphocytes.

Our group has used the hypertonic 3 *M* KCl extracts to stimulate lymphocytes (28–30). In general, autologous lymphocytes respond vigorously to approximately one-third of KCl extracts from solid tumors and about one-half of KCl extracts of human leukemia cells. In general, the reactivity corresponds fairly well to that seen for the respective autologous leukemic blast cells or solid tumor cells. Vánky and co-workers demonstrated that a concordant stimulation by autologous tumor biopsy cells and the KCl extracts among autologous lymphocytes (31). Six of 16 solid tumor extracts stimulated autologous lymphocytes. In general, normal allogeneic lymphocytes responded not at all or weakly to these KCl extracts, suggesting that the response involves a presensitization immune response rather than a primary recognition response. In contrast, the work of Dean and co-workers suggested that normal individuals reacted with a greater frequency and stronger blastogenic response to tumor extracts than did breast carcinoma patients (32). This is not entirely inconsistent with our results that among normal lymphocytes the only response was to breast carcinoma extracts (28). The suggestion was made that recognition of HLA or tissue antigen with these allogeneic tumor extracts was probably due to a primary recognition event as in the MLC rather than to prior *in vivo* sensitization. They question, therefore the value of unfractionated allogeneic tumor cell extracts for assessment of cell-mediated immune reactivity in breast carcinoma patients by the lymphocyte stimulation assay. The use of more purified HLA-free extracts to determine specificity of tumor patients versus the normal patients will be awaited with great interest.

Finally, the correlation of lymphocyte blastogenic response in the MLTI with other assays has been evaluated. In general, there has been fairly good correlation with delayed hypersensitivity response to KCl extracts, but not to tumor cells (28, 31). Leventhal and co-workers showed a disparity of reactivity with MLTI, cellular cytotoxicity, and MIF responsiveness (3). In general, our studies and others have shown that the leukemic blast cells which evoke a brisk MLTI response also evoke a better MIF response than ALL blasts (15, 18).

2. Materials

2.1. Glassware. All Glassware used should be sterile and dry.
Screw-capped Erlenmeyer flasks, 250 ml
Screw-capped round-bottom tubes, 16 × 125 mm
Screw-capped round-bottom tubes, 25 × 125 mm
Screw-capped round-bottom tubes, 25 × 200 mm
Glass beads, 1.2-ml ampoules
Pasteur pipettes
Scintillation counting vials
White blood cell diluters
Hemocytometer

2.2. Syringes and Needles
Plastic disposable syringes, various sizes 1 ml to 60 ml
Disposable needles, 21 and 18 or 19 gauge

2.3. Media and Solutions
MEM, Spinner-modified Eagle's minimal essential medium (Schwarz-Mann)
RPMI-1640, [Grand Island Biological Company (GIBCO)]
Medium 199, (GIBCO)
Hanks' base (Schwarz-Mann)
Tris ammonium buffer
Dextran solution, 4%
Saline solution, 0.85%
Acetic acid, 2%
Trypan blue, 0.4% (GIBCO)

Dimethyl sulfoxide (DMSO)

Penicillin and streptomycin solution (GIBCO)

L-Glutamine, 200 mM (GIBCO)

Scintillation fluid

Trichloroacetic acid solution, 5%

Methanol

^{3}H-Thymidine (Schwartz BioResearch)

Ficoll solution, 9%

Hypaque solution, 33.9%

2.4. Serum

Autologous serum isolate from blood drawn from patient or normal donor on date study is made

Allogeneic serum from one or several normal subjects pooled and stored frozen

Fetal calf serum heated at 56°C for 45 min (GIBCO)

2.5. Tumor Cells, Bone Marrow Cells

Leukemic cells stored in liquid nitrogen

Solid Tumor cells prepared fresh on day of study

Bone marrow cells prepared fresh on day of study

2.6. Tumor Antigen. This was previously prepared and stored frozen.

2.7. Normal Donor or Patient Lymphocytes. These were collected on the day of study.

2.8. Equipment

Water bath 37°–56°C

CO_2 incubator

Centrifuge, unrefrigerated (International Model UV)

Centrifuge, refrigerated

Scintillation counter

Microscope

Liquid nitrogen freezer

Liquid nitrogen refrigerator

Mesh screen

3. Methodology

3.1. Leukemic Blasts

1. Collect cells from the peripheral blood with the IBM or Aminco blood separators or with a syringe with anticoagulant.

2. Centrifuge cells at room temperature for 10 min at 1500 rpm to pack cells. Remove supernatant plasma.

3. Resuspend packed cells in 5 volumes of warm Tris-buffered ammonium chloride solution and incubate at 37°C for 15 min to lyse red cells.

4. Centrifuge suspension at 1500 rpm for 10 min, discard supernatant.

5. Cells should not be "trissed" more than three times. Wash once in Hanks' base and resuspend in RPMI-1640 medium with 20% heat-inactivated FCS.

6. Count cells and adjust concentration to 5×10^7 cells/ml.

7. Add DMSO, 10% by volume, to suspension and distribute with syringe to 1.2-ml ampoules. Flame seal.

8. Freeze cells at rate of $1°$ per minute and store at $-180°C$ until ready for use.

9. On the day of study, quick-thaw ampoule in a $37°C$ water bath. Dilute cells slowly with 10 volumes of MEM warmed to room temperature.

10. Centrifuge diluted cells at 1500 rpm for 10 min, discard supernatant, resuspend in MEM, count cells, determine viability with trypan blue stain, and adjust cell concentration to 5×10^6 ml.

3.2. Solid Tumor Cells

1. Prepare a single tumor cell suspension from fresh tumor biopsies by teasing, scraping and sieving tissue through a 60-mesh screen into medium 199 containing 1 unit/ml of penicillin, 1 μg/ml of streptomycin, and 10% FCS.

2. Wash cells once in Hanks' base, lyse red blood cells with Tris-buffered ammonium chloride as described for leukemic blasts.

3. After one wash, resuspend tumor cells in medium 199, count cells, assess viability by trypan blue dye exclusion, and adjust concentration to 5×10^6 cells/ml.

4. If more than 30% of the cells are nonviable, separate them from the viable cells on a Ficoll–Hypaque gradient mixed 24 parts of Ficoll to 10 parts of Hypaque. Carefully layer cell suspension onto gradient with syringe and centrifuge in unrefrigerated centrifuge 15 min at $1500\,g$. Collect floating fraction with a siliconized Pasteur pipette, wash twice in Hanks' base, and resuspend in medium 199. Adjust cell concentration to 5×10^6/ml.

3.3. Remission Bone Marrow Cells

1. From sternum or iliac crest, aspirate approximately 5.0 ml of bone marrow into a syringe rinsed with heparin (1:1000). Dilute sample 1:3 with sterile saline and layer onto a Ficoll–Hypaque gradient as for solid tumor cells.

2. Collect floating fraction with Pasteur pipette. Wash twice in Hanks' and resuspend in MEM warmed to room temperature. Count cells, determine viability (they should be 100% viable), and adjust concentration to 5×10^6 cells/ml.

3.4. Tumor Antigen.
Prepare tumor antigen as previously described (29). On day of study, thaw antigens and dilute with MEM, 10–1000 μg/ml.

3.5. Normal Donor of Patient Lymphocytes

1. Collect peripheral venous blood from subject to be studied with plastic syringes without anticoagulant. Transfer to sterile Erlenmeyer flasks, 60 ml/flask, and defibrinate by swirling with glass beads, for approximately 10 min until a firm clot forms around the beads.

2. Decant defibrinated blood into sterile 25 × 200 mm screw-capped round-bottom tubes and add 1 ml of 4% dextran for each 10 ml of blood. Sediment red blood cells for 20–45 min by placing the tube in a horizontal position. Collect leukocyte-rich suspension with Pasteur pipette. Centrifuge sedimented red cells for 20 min at 2000 rpm. Aspirate serum and reserve for dilution of lymphocytes. Dilute cell suspension with 2% acetic acid to lyse red blood cells in a white blood cell diluter. Count total number white cells and determine number of lymphocytes. Wash cells twice and suspend in either autologous or allogeneic serum at a concentration of 1 × 10^6 lymphocytes/ml.

3.6. Cultures

1. Set up cultures in 16 × 125 mm screw-capped glass round-bottom tubes. Add 1 × 10^6 responder lymphocytes suspended in 1.0 ml of designated autologous or allogeneic serum, and 2 ml of MEM supplemented with penicillin or streptomycin. Stimulate cultures with a dose range from 10^4 to 10^6 in half-log increments of unirradiated and irradiated (1000 rads) thawed leukemic blasts, solid tumor cells, or fresh bone marrow cells. Soluble tumor antigen may be added at a dose range of 10–1000 μg per milliliter of culture. Mix cultures with gentle agitation and incubate at 37°C in a moist atmosphere of 5% CO$_2$ and air with caps loosened 5 days for tumor antigen, 7 days for tumor cells and bone marrow cells.

2. Set up appropriate control cultures of unstimulated lymphocytes irradiated lymphocytes (4000 R) with tumor cells, bone marrow cells of tumor antigen. Additional controls of tumor cells or bone marrow cells alone may be cultured simultaneously with the test cultures.

3.7. Harvesting and Counting

1. Harvest cultures as previously described (33) by addition of 2 μCi of ^{3}H-thymidine with a specific activity of 1.9 Ci/mmole for 3 hr. Measure radioactivity by liquid scintilllation counting.

2. Lymphocyte blastogenesis is measured as the net counts per minute (cpm) of tritiated thymidine incorporation per 1 × 10^6 cultured lymphocytes with the appropriate controls subtracted from that of the stimulated cultures.

4. Critical Comments

The time of the tests is critical; thus, in order to do the MLTI on patients receiving chemotherapy it is important to carry out the tests in between courses of chemotherapy so that there has been recovery of immunosuppression of previous chemotherapy (4). Thus, we normally carry out our studies 5–10 days after the last dose of chemotherapy (4–13). Serial determination of the MLTI can be influenced by prior chemotherapy as well as surgery and other immunosuppressive treatment. Leventhal and co-workers had shown that reactivity in the MLTI peaks 10–15 days after the last dose of chemotherapy and returns to a base line of value 3 weeks later (3). Thus, any data on serial determination of MLTI must take these factors into account.

In general, we have used dextran in order to sediment erythrocytes. However, Ficoll–Hypaque separation of peripheral blood lymphocytes has been used extensively and has been reported to augment responsiveness. In general, our studies have avoided Ficoll–Hypaque with the macro-system in the MLTI. Thus, a more representative population of responding cells including lymphocytes, monocytes, as well as granulocytes are maintained for the *in vitro* reaction. It is critical to have phagocytic adherent cells in the reaction. Thus, all our studies have been done with whole leukocyte preparations.

In order to obtain good proliferation, serum must be present in the culture medium. Most of our studies have been carried out with fresh autologous human serum (33%). Some of our studies have been carried out with heat-inactivated serum and some with natural serum. We would recommend nonheated activated, since this is again more representative of the *in vivo* situation. AB-positive serum has been used successfully to measure allogeneic responses. One always has the problem of interpretation of allogeneic data because of the HL-A antibodies, anti-blood group antibodies, etc. Useful information comparing autologous and allogeneic serum have been described in the introduction.

A cultured medium utilizing MEM has been used. Other workers have shown RPMI-1640 to be excellent for short-term cultures (34). In addition, other workers have shown that medium 199 was superior to MEM in mixed leukocyte reactions (35).

Since cell contact is required for the first 36 hr of culture, round-bottom tubes have been used. This assures adequate density (36). The cell concentration of responder cells has been maintained constant at 1×10^6 cells per 3 ml of culture. By this method, adequate maintenance of pH and cell nutrition is maintained. From 5×10^4 to 2×10^6 stimulator cells have been used. This is adequate to assure good contact as well as maintain nutrition.

In general, a 1:1 or 2:1 stimulator:responder cell ratio has been found to be optimal. Higher doses of stimulator cells have been found in some studies to stimulate better (6). However, since important information regarding prognosis has been derived from 1:1 and 2:1 ratios, we have continued to use these ratios. It is conceivable that the lack of responsiveness of leukemic lymphoblasts could be enhanced by higher numbers of stimulator cells to responder cells.

As noted in the introduction, the use of viable tumor cells is critical. We have found that nonviable solid tumor cells failed to stimulate well (5). Similarly, leukemic cell preparations with less than 70% viable cells stimulate poorly. If less than 70% viable cells were obtained from liquid nitrogen freezing, we placed the tumor cells on a Ficoll–Hypaque gradient to increase stability.

Solid tumor cells left untreated or irradiated with 1-4000R stimulate well (5). Mitomycin-treated solid tumor cells stimulate lymphocytes poorly (5). Whether this is due to inadequate removal of the mitomycin after washing is unclear. We have found that untreated leukemic cells stimulate better than irradiated tumor cells. Frequently, 1000 R will significantly decrease the stimulation capacity of leukemic tumor cells. We have seen occasionally, however, a feeder-layer effect with unirradiated leukemic cells, so it is important to use as a control irradiated lymphocytes plus unirradiated leukemia cells (4) if one is to use unirradiated leukemic cells as stimulator cells.

Timed studies have shown that at 7 days the maximal MLTI responsiveness is seen with lymphocytes and autologous tumor cells. Similarly, 5–7 days seems to be optimal incubation time for soluble tumor antigens (28, 29).

We have only used mechanical means to prepare our single-cell solid-tumor suspensions, since trypsin cell-surface components can be modified with trypsin (5).

Since variability is important when using frozen leukemia cells (freezing techniques must be kept constant), the thawing must be done carefully. The cells are rapidly thawed and the DMSO eliminated rapidly. We have found that diluting the cell suspension 1:20 in a stepwise fashion appears to give better viability by preventing osmotic lysis of the cells (37).

The optimal cell concentration for tumor antigens varies from preparation to preparation. For best results, a dose–response study probably needs to be done for different individual extracts. This is a major disadvantage in the use of the currently available crude extracts. Thus, we have found that the maximal stimulation capacity of different extracts vary from 1 μg to 500 μg per 3 ml of culture with 10^6 lymphocytes.

REFERENCES

1. Fridman, W. H., and Kourilsky, F. M., *Nature (London)* 224, 227 (1969).
2. Stjernswärd, J., Vánky, F., and Klein, E., *Br. J. Cancer* 28, 72 (1973).
3. Leventhal, B. G., Halterman, R. H., and Rosenberg, E. B., *Cancer Res.* 32, 1820 (1972).
4. Gutterman, J. U., Hersh, E. M., McCredie, K. B., Bodey, G. P. Sr., and Rodriguez, V., *Cancer Res.* 32, 2524 (1972).
5. Mavligit, G., Gutterman, J. U., McBride, C. M., and Hersh, E. M., *J. Natl. Cancer Inst.* 37, 157 (1973).
6. Powles, R. L., Balchin, L. A., Fairley, G. H., and Alexander, R., *Br. Med. J.* 1, 486 (1971).
7. Stjernswärd, J., Clifford, P., Singh, S., *et al., East Afr. Med. J.* 45, 484 (1968).
8. Mavligit, G. M., Gutterman, J. U., Hersh, E. M., Rossen, R. D., Butler, W. T., McCredie, K. B., and Freireich, E. J., *Transplantation* 16, 217 (1973).
9. Stjernswärd, J., Almgard, L. E., Franzen, S., *et al., Clin. Exp. Immunol.* 6, 963 (1970).
10. Mavligit, G., Gutterman, J. U., and Hersh, E. M., *Immunol. Commun.* 3, 463 (1973)
11. Stjernswärd, J., and Vanky, F., *Natl. Cancer Inst. Monogr.* 35, 237 (1972).
12. Ambus, U., Mavligit, G. M., Gutterman, J. U., McBride, C. M., and Hersh, E. M., *Int. J. Cancer* 14, 291 (1974).
13. Gutterman, J. U., Rossen, R. D., Butler, W. T., McCredie, K. B., Bodey, G. P. Sr., Freireich, E. J., and Hersh, E. M., *N. Engl. J. Med.* 288, 169 (1973).

14. Gutterman, J. U., Hersh, E. M., Mavligit, G. M., Freireich, E. J., Rossen, R. D., Butler, W. T., McCredie, K. B., Bodey, G. P. Sr., and Rodriguez, V., *Natl. Cancer Inst. Monogr.* **37**, 153 (1973).

15. Gutterman, J. U., Mavligit, G., Freireich, E. J., and Hersh, E. M., *Adv. Biosci.* **14**, 441 (1975).

16. Leventhal, B. G., Halterman, R. H., Rosenberg, E. B. *et al.*, *Cancer Res.* **32**, 1820 (1972).

17. Schweitzer, M., Melief, C. J. M., and Eijsvogel, V. P., *Int. J. Cancer* **11**, 11 (1973).

18. Anderson, P. N., Klein, D. L., Bias, W. B., Mullins, G. M., Burke, P. J., and Santos, G. W., *Isr. J. Med. Sci.* **10**, 1033 (1974).

19. Gutterman, J. U., Mavligit, G. M., Burgess, M. A., McCredie, K. B., Hunter, C., Freireich, E. J., and Hersh, E. M., *J. Natl. Cancer Inst.* **53**, 389 (1974).

20. Bach, M. L., Bach, F. H., and Joo, P., *Science* **166**, 1520 (1969).

21. Santos, G. W., Mullins, G. M., Bias, W. B., Anderson, P. N., Graziano, K. D., Klein, D. L., and Burke, P. J., *Natl. Cancer Inst. Monogr.* **37**, 69 (1973).

22. Rudolph, R. H., Mickelson, E., and Thomas, E. D., *J. Clin. Invest.* **49**, 2271 (1970).

23. Halterman, R. H., and Leventhal, B. G., *Proc. Am. Assoc. Cancer Res.* **33**, 6 (1972).

24. Vánky, F., Klein, E., Stjernswärd, J., and Trempe, G., *Int. J. Cancer* **15**, 850 (1975).

25. Vánky, F., Trempe, G., Klein, E., and Stjernswärd, J., *Int. J. Cancer* **16**, 113 (1975).

26. Savel, H., *Cancer* **35**, 56 (1969).

27. Jehn, U. M., Nathanson, L., Schwartz, R. S., and Skinner, M., *N. Engl. J. Med.* **283**, 329 (1970).

28. Mavligit, G. M., Gutterman, J. U., McBride, C. M., and Hersh, E. M., *Proc. Soc. Exp. Biol. Med.* **140**, 1240 (1972).

29. Gutterman, J. U., Mavligit, G., McCredie, K. B., Bodey, G. P., Sr., Freireich, E. J., and Hersh, E. M., *Science* **177**, 1114 (1972).

30. Mavligit, G. M., Ambus, U., Gutterman, J. U., McBride, C. M., and Hersh, E. M., *Nature (London), New Biol.* **243**, 188 (1973).

31. Vánky, F., Klein, E., Stjernswärd, J., and Nilsonne, U., *Int. J. Cancer* **14**, 277 (1974).

32. Dean, J. H., Silva, J. S., McCoy, J. L., Leonard, C. M., Middleton, M., Cannon, G. B., and Herberman, R. B., *J. Natl. Cancer Inst.* **54**, 1295 (1975).

33. Hersh, E. M., *Transplantation* **12**, 287 (1971).

34. Valentine, F., *in* "*In Vitro* Methods in Cell-Mediated Immunity" (B. R. Bloom, and P. R. Glade, eds.). Academic Press, New York, 1971.

35. Bach, F., *in* "*In Vitro* Methods in Cell-Mediated Immunity" (B. R. Bloom, and P. R. Glade, eds.). Academic Press, New York, 1971.

36. Hersh, E. M., Harris, J. E., and Rogers, E. A., *J. Reticuloendothel. Soc.* **7**, 567 (1970).

37. Dicke, K. A., Lina, P. H. C., and Van Bekkum, D. W., *Rev. Eur. Etud. Clin. Biol.* **15**, 305 (1970).

Lymphocyte Stimulation Test for Detection of Tumor-Specific Reactivity in Humans

Farkas Vánky and Jan Stjernswärd

1. Introduction

Lymphocytes from immunized animals and humans are induced to blast transformation, division, and increased DNA synthesis when cultured with the antigen to which they are sensitized (1–4). Lymphocyte proliferation also occurs when leukocytes of two individuals with different histocompatibility antigens are mixed in cultures (5–7). The *in vitro* response of lymphocytes upon stimulation with antigen correlates with the existence of delayed hypersensitivity to the antigen in the donor, both in experimental animal systems (8, 9) and humans (10, 11).

Lymphocyte stimulation can be quantitated by evaluation of the percentage of lymphoblasts or by measurement of the increased incorporation of ^{3}H-thymidine into DNA.

The test has been adapted for measurement of cell-mediated immunity to autologous tumors (12, 13). Different laboratories have been successfully using the lymphocyte stimulation test for measuring tumor-associated immunity (14–24).

Available *in vitro* methods for assaying immunity to solid tumors in man have recently been reviewed (25). The lymphocyte stimulation test came out well, being justified by its well defined theoretical basis, its relevance to the rejection reaction and to the delayed hypersensitivity reaction *in vivo,* and its use of fresh tumor cells, reducing possible artifacts present in other assays. This paper summarizes the technique we have used to demonstrate autologous tumor stimulation (ATS).

2. Materials

2.1. Preservative-free heparin, 5000 IU/ml (Vitrum AB, Stockholm, Sweden)
2.2. Plastic syringes, 50, 20, and 1 ml (B. D. Plastipak, Becton, Dickinson and Co. Ltd., Drogkeda, Ireland)

2.3. Disposable 16 × 125 mm round-bottom screw-cap culture tubes (Labora AB Stockholm, Sweden). Tubes and caps were sterilized by dry heat for 3 hr at 160°C

2.4. Glass pipettes of different sizes

2.5. Pasteur pipettes

2.6. Graduated 10-ml centrifuge tubes (Labora AB, Stockholm, Sweden)

2.7. Graduated 50-ml centrifuge tubes (Bellco Glass Inc., Vineland, New Jersey)

2.8. RPMI-1640 medium without L-glutamine (GIBCO Biocult, Glasgow, Scotland)

2.9. L-Glutamine, 200 mM solution (GIBCO Biocult, Glasgow, Scotland) 1% by volume added to media just prior to use

2.10. Benzylpenicillin (AB KABI, Sweden) 100 IU/ml medium

2.11. Streptomycin sulfate (Glaxo Lab. Ltd., Greenford, England), 100 μg/ml medium

2.12. HEPES buffer (Flow Laboratories, England) in 0.1 mmole/ml medium

2.13. AB, Rh-positive serum from healthy male donors, heat-inactivated and added to 10% concentration in the medium

2.14. Fetal cal serum (GIBCO Biocult, Glasgow, Scotland)

2.15. Ficoll 400 (MW 400,000) (Pharmacia, Uppsala, Sweden)

2.16. Isopaque, 440 mg of I/ml, 20 ml/A (Nyegaard & Co. A.S., Oslo, Norway)

2.17. Balanced salt solution (BSS), pH 7.2–7.4

2.18. Mitomycin C, 2mg, crystalline (Sigma Chemical Co., St. Louis, Missouri)

2.19. [methyl-^{3}H]Thymidine, 5 mCi/5 ml, 5 Ci/mmole (Radiochemical Centre, Amersham, Buckinghamshire, England)

2.20. Trichloroacetic acid, 10% solution

2.21. Ethanol

2.22. Ethyl ether, anhydrous, $(C_2H_5)_2O$

2.23. Formic acid, H·COOH, 98–600%

2.24. Tuluol (analytical grade) (C_7H_8) (E. Merck, Darmstadt, Germany)

2.25. PPO, 2,5-diphenyloxazole, scintillation grade MW 22,125; and POPOP, dimethyl-POPOP, 1,4-bisI-2-(4-methyl-5-phenyloxazolyl) I-benzene scintillation grade (Packard Instruments Co., Downers Grove, Illinois). (to 3.5 liters of tuluol, add 0.39 g of POPOP and 15.2 g of PPO; this is the scintillation fluid.)

2.26. Türk solution (gentian violet solution)

2.27. Methyl blue stain

2.28. Bürker chamber for counting WBC

2.29. RBC counter pipettes

2.30. Scissors

2.31. Pincettes

2.32. Spatula

2.33. Stainless steel sieve net, 60-mesh 0.0075 inch wide, 304 stainless steel (Newark Wire Cloth Company, Newark, New Jersey)

2.34. Scintillation counting vials (Packard Instruments Co.)

2.35. Microscope slides

2.36. Cold centrifuge (IEC.PR-6000 Damon IEC Division)

2.37. A 37°C carbon dioxide incubator (ASSAB, Stockholm)

2.38. Scintillation counter

2.39. Microscope

2.40. Sheep erythrocytes in Alsever's solution (State Bacteriology Laboratory, Stockholm, Sweden)

3. Methodology

3.1. General Procedures for the Evaluation of Autologous Tumor Stimulation (ATS) by Mixed Lymphocyte Tumor Cell Interaction (MLTI) Test

3.1.1. Donors: For the purpose of investigating cellular immunity to autologous tumor it is pertinent that the donors be individuals without recent infections, who are receiving neither immunosuppressives nor radiation therapy. The blood should preferably be sampled before surgery and premedication (26). If these conditions cannot be met, all aspects of the patient's condition and therapy must be considered when interpreting the results.

3.1.2. All the following procedures are carried out in sterile conditions except the procedures following final precipitation of DNA.

3.2. Venous Blood.
Blood is drawn into a 50-ml plastic syringe containing 3.5% (v/v) of heparin solution. This produces a final concentration of about 10 units of heparin per milliliter of blood. The syringe is placed with the needle upward, and red cells are allowed to settle at room temperature by gravity for about 1–1.5 hr. The plasma containing leukocytes is removed by pushing it out through the bent needle into centrifuge tubes, 3 ml in each.

3.3. Separation of the Lymphocytes.
Three milliliters of plasma in centrifuge tubes are carefully underlayered with 3 ml of Ficoll–Isopaque (F-I). The F-I is a mixture of 104 ml of 9% Ficoll in distilled water, 20 ml (1 ampoule) of Isopaque (440 mg/ml) and 45 ml of distilled water.

Underlayering is easy to do with a long thin needle. The tubes are then centrifuged for 10 min, 600 g, 4°C. Remove the lymphocytes with Pasteur pipette from the plasma–F-I interphase, and wash three times with BSS. The lymphocytes still contain macrophages. If macrophages exceed 20%, further separation is necessary by incubation with iron powder, 0.4 g per centrifuge tube containing 5 × 10⁶ cells/ml, mixed and incubated for 30 min at 37°C. If not automatically mixed, the tubes are shaken every 5 min during the incubation.

After incubation with iron, phagocytizing cells are fixed to the bottom of the tube by a strong magnet and the floating cells are removed with a Pasteur pipette. This is the lymphocyte fraction containing no more than 5% macrophages.

The centrifuged lymphocytes are resuspended in culture medium S (RPMI-1640 medium enriched with 10% human AB+ serum) and collected in a single tube; they are then diluted to a suitable concentration for counting (usually lymphocytes from 50 ml of blood to a volume of 6 ml). The number of small lymphocytes and total leukocytes is determined by diluting 1:100 with Türk solution in a clinical RBC counting pipette, then the cells are counted in a Bürker chamber.

The cell suspension is diluted with medium S to a final concentration of 5×10^6/ml.

3.4. Tumor Cells. Tumor cell separation has to be done as soon as possible after surgery, preferably within 1 hr. All procedures are at $0°C$. Tumor tissue from surgical specimen is placed in ice-cold serum-free medium. Tumor tissue free of necrosis is chopped up with scissors until a "porridge"-like state is achieved, then passed through a stainless steel net by gentle pressure. Thereafter the suspension is diluted in medium and mixed in a glass cylinder; the cells are allowed to sediment for some minutes. The supernatant containing single cells is collected. The sedimented cell clumps are further suspended and broken up by repeatedly passing it in and out of a syringe. The two suspensions are then mixed, centrifuged at $200\,g$ for 10 min, and washed once with medium.

Cell viability is assessed by trypan blue staining. If the percentage of live cells is less than 50%, further separation of viable cells is necessary. This is done by Ficoll-Isopaque flotation as described under Section 3.3. Ten milliliters of tumor cell suspension is underlayered with 10 ml of F-I in 50-ml centrifuge tubes and centrifuged at $600\,g$ for 10 min. Suspension removed from medium–F-I interphase contains mostly live cells. The material from the bottom contains red cells, dead cells, cell clumps, and a few live cells (mostly macrophages). The cell suspension containing the live tumor cells is then diluted with medium S to a concentration of 5×10^6 ml. Tumor cells are always checked bacteriologically for aerobic and anaerobic growth. This is done to exclude that stimulation is caused by tumor-contaminating bacteria to which the patient is sensitized.

3.5. Mitomycin C Treatment of the Stimulator Cells. Tumor cells, control lymphocytes, and, whenever possible, nonmalignant cells of the same histological origin as the tumor cells, are suspended in medium S, 5×10^6/ml are incubated with 25 μg of mitomycin C (MMC) per milliliter for 30 min at $37°C$, washed 3 times in BSS, and then suspended in medium S to a concentration of 5×10^6 cells/ml.

3.6. Lymphocyte Stimulation Test. A constant number of lymphocytes (10^6) are mixed with various numbers of MMC-treated tumor cells (usually 5×10^5, 10^6, 2×10^6) in round-bottom test tubes (1.6 ml of medium S, 1 million lymphocytes in 0.2 ml of medium S, and a varying number of tumor cells, always in 0.2 ml of medium S). Each sample of the test combination is made up in triplicate. Meaningful evaluation of the test is only possible if adequate negative and positive controls are included. Therefore, each test has to include the following cultures in triplicate: Lymphocytes admixed to MMC-treated identical lymphocytes (as control for the cell concentration effect) or, when possible, suspensions of normal tissue cells of same histological origin as the tumor cells. These cells are admixed in the same concentrations as the tumor cells. Used as positive controls are PHA stimulation at 1 μg/ml dilution (0.2 ml of 10 μg/ml diluted PHA is added to 1.8 ml of medium S containing 10^6 lymphocytes) and confrontation with MMC-treated allogeneic lymphocytes. The residual DNA synthesis of the MMC-treated cells is also checked by incubating these cells alone without responding lymphocytes. The various mixtures are incubated in a humid 5% CO_2 incubator at $37°C$ for 6 days.

3.7. ^{3}H-Thymidine Incorporation. Incorporation is measured during a 16-hr pulse at the end of a 6-day incubation period. For routine experiments it is convenient to add the ^{3}H-thymidine (0.2 μCi in 0.2 ml of medium S) to each culture tube on the afternoon of day 5 to permit 16 hr of incubation with isotope and to fix the cultures on the morning of day 6. The tubes are kept at $37°$ in a humid 5% CO_2 incubator during the 16-hr pulse.

After incubation with the isotope, the tubes are centrifuged at 600 g for 10 min at $4°C$, and washed once with cold BSS, 5 ml per tube. The cells are resuspended in the drop of saline remaining in the tubes and 5 ml of 10% ice-cold trichloroacetic acid is added. After incubation at $4°C$ for 30 min, the tubes are centrifuged at 600 g for 10 min at $4°C$. The precipitate is incubated for 10 min in 3 ml of ethanol at room temperature, centrifuged at 600 g for 10 min, resuspended, and incubated for 10 min in 3 ml of ethyl ether followed by centrifugation. The ether is decanted, and the pellet is allowed to dry at room temperature or at $37°C$ in an incubator. The dry precipitated material is disolved in 0.5 ml of formic acid (20 min incubation at room temperature), and care is taken that all is transferred to the counting tubes by rinsing the culture tubes 3 times with 5 ml of the toluene solution of scintillation fluid.

3.8. Evaluation of ^{3}H-Thymidine Incorporation. The samples are counted in a liquid scintillation counter and corrected for quenching; the incorporation isotope activity is expressed as cpm $\pm$ SD. The test is considered positive when the ^{3}H incorporation in the stimulated samples is increased by at least 100% and the difference between the control and the test sample is significant. The significance of the isotope uptake expressed as counts per minute (cpm) is evaluated in the arithmetic mean values of test samples compared to the control by student's t test; p values lower than 0.05 are considered to be significant.

The reactivity index (R.I.) is calculated and expressed as the ratio between the isotope uptake (cpm) in the test sample and isotope uptake in the sample to which the identical number of autologous MMC-treated lymphocytes were added.

$$\text{R.I.} = \frac{(\text{lymphocytes} + \text{``X'' stimulator}_M) - \text{``X'' stimulator}_M}{(\text{lymphocytes} + \text{``X'' identical lymphocytes}_M) - \text{``X'' identical lymphocytes}_M}$$

where X is the number of cells and M is the MMC-treated.

By introducing the R.I., comparison of different experiments is possible. However, for judging the test conditions the cpm values have also to be considered.

3.9. Evaluation of the Response by Registration of Blast-Transformed Cells. Although the incorporation of the ^{3}H-thymidine is a convenient and objective measurement of the proliferative response, the enumeration of the percentage of thymus-derived lymphocytes which are in the blast form is a complementary test of the response, which has the advantage of excluding measurement of ^{3}H-thymidine incorporated into the tumor cells.

T lymphocytes are visualized by their capacity to form rosettes (E rosettes) with sheep erythrocytes (SRBC) (27).

3.10. E Rosetting. SRBC kept in Alsever's solution are centrifuged and washed twice with BSS. The SRBC are then suspended to 1% (v/v) concentration in heat-inactivated FCS. Test samples are also washed twice with BSS, suspended in 0.25 ml of FCS and mixed with 0.25 ml of SRBC (1% suspension in FCS). The mixture is incubated for 15 min at 37°C followed by centrifugation at 300 g for 1 min (just to spin the cell down) and 1–12 hr incubation at 0°C (ice bath). Small and large rosettes are then counted under a microscope and the results expressed as percentage of blast rosettes in total number of rosettes. T cells may be identified and followed easily during the *in vitro* incubation in the lymphocyte stimulation test by regular samples which are counted every day during the 6 days of incubation.

4. Critical Comments

4.1. The advantage of the test is that biopsy material can be used and therefore the antigen source (tumor cells) is not subject to the modification and selective conditions of tissue culture.

4.2. Another advantage of the method is that tumor membrane preparations and extracts can also be used as stimulators, giving similar results (but on a lower level) as the whole tumor cells. The solubilized tumor eliminates the major disadvantage of the test, i.e., the variability of the quality of the tumor cell suspension. Furthermore, it gives the possibility to compare the *in vitro* and *in vivo* cell-mediated immunity by using the same material for lymphocyte stimulation and for skin tests for delayed hypersensitivity reactions (24, 28–33).

4.3. The main disadvantage is the variability of the quality and the quantitative limitation of the tumor cell suspension obtained from solid tumor biopsies. Cell viability can vary between 10 and 90%, a factor that will influence the results. The quality of the cell suspension can be improved by sedimentation through Ficoll–Isopaque gradient or by trypsinization followed by 12 hr of incubation of the cells in medium S at 37°C in order to regenerate the cell membrane. In our experience both methods gave good results. However, certain tumor specimens have been found to be unfit for use, because the preparation of single-cell suspensions is not possible without the cells dying during the preparation or soon after.

4.4. The contact between the tumor cell membrane and the lymphocyte may be impeded by the *N*-acetylneuraminic acid groups of the membrane glucoproteins (14, 34, 35) or by mucinous material seen around certain types of tumors. The DNA released from the dead cells may have similar effect, leading to cell clumping. A negative ATS test may be caused by the above factors without any failure of the immune response, and thus has to be taken into consideration when evaluating the results.

4.5. The variability in the quality of the responding lymphocyte population has to be taken into consideration, too. Because platelets form clumps with the lymphocytes, the percentage of contaminating platelets may influence the test. Cell populations with 5–20% macrophages seem to be optimal. Macrophage contamination greater than 20% decreases the proliferative response, but pure lymphocyte populations show less reaction to the Ag stimulus (36) or in MLC (37) than those containing macrophages. This may be caused by enzymes, because it has been found that disintegrated macrophages are able to destroy without specificity the target cells (38). The possibility of a suppressor cell population of macrophage nature may also play a role (39) in this phenomenon.

4.6. Each tumor preparation has to be controlled bacteriologically, both for aerobes and anaerobes, before the evaluation of the results to exclude blastogenesis caused by microbes.

4.7. The culture medium RPMI-1640 has, in our hands, been found to be excellent for the test. Other types of media can also be used successfully.

4.8. In order to assure good conditions for lymphocyte proliferation, serum must be present in the medium and the pH kept at 7.2. It is well established that cell-mediated responses are influenced by serum factors, antibodies, and antigen–antibody complexes as well as antigen present in the serum (40–42). Heat-inactivated AB, Rh-positive serum samples from healthy young male donors at 10% concentration seem to work best. Higher concentrations of normal human sera may inhibit the ATS (our observation). Autologous serum inhibits the ATS even at 5% concentration. The use of FCS is not advised because of its blastogenic effect on certain human lymphocytes.

Small changes of the pH may inhibit the DNA synthesis of the lymphocytes (43). In order to stabilize the pH, HEPES buffer is added to the medium (0.01 mmole/ml). If the color of the medium indicates that the pH has changed, this has to be taken into consideration when the test is evaluated.

4.9. The variability of the ^{3}H incorporation between replicate tubes is larger when the cells have been manipulated a great deal. Values plus or minus 10% of the average are expected in an experiment. In general, the more complicated the experiment and the longer the duration of culture, the greater is the variability.

4.10. Round-bottom tubes are used for the experiment because they assure optimal cell contact and prevent the crowding effect that can occur in tubes with a conical bottom.

4.11. Although heparin has been reported to inhibit the blast transformation, we have not observed such an effect. Defibrinated blood can also be used, but if so, because of the low sedimentation rate of the erythrocytes, the lymphocytes are separated from whole blood on an F-I gradient.

4.12. DNA synthesis can be blocked in different ways (7). It has been found that both MMC treatment and X-irradiation gave good results (44, 45). It was reported (46) that residual DNA synthesis is necessary to the "one way" MLC. We also found that blastogeneic potential of the MMC treated lymphocytes was lost (completely or partially) when the DNA synthesis of the stimulators was abolished, but this did not occur when residual DNA activity was present (controlled by PHA stimulation).

4.13. The measured thymidine incorporation is influenced by the time of incubation, the amount, and the specific activity of the ^{3}H-thymidine (7, 47). Optimal for the ^{3}H-thymidine pulse is a period of 8–16 hr, if it is used at the given concentration and specific activity. High concentration, or high specific activity, may damage the blast cells by autoirradiation. Measurement of "blastogenesis" by thymidine uptake is liable to interference by DNA inhibitors as well as serum factors, including antibodies. In these situations, protein synthesis may not be affected and may be measured more satisfactorily by labeled protein precursors instead of thymidine or by counting blast-transformed lymphocytes (48).

4.14. Apart from the dose dependence of ATS, cell concentration also influences the results by the crowding phenomenon, by the modified pH, and by cell nutrition (7, 43). A cell concentration around 10^6/ml has been found optimal.

4.15. The condition of the minimal number of cells responding directly to the stimulus limits the lower level of the lymphocyte number in the test; 10^6 responding lymphocytes have been found to contain enough sensitized cells. Similarly, the number of stimulating cells is limited by the fact that the reaction is dose dependent; i.e., the response is lower when doses of antigen higher or lower than the optimal are used. The optimal ratio is never known in advance when biopsy cells are used. Therefore, several lymphocyte tumor cell ratios around 1:1 have to be tested.

4.16. Although the nature of the antigen that evokes the ATS reaction is not yet known, this assay may be valuable for the study of cellular immunity against tumor-associated antigens. The justification of the method lies in its well-defined theoretical basis, its relevance to the rejection reaction and delayed hypersensitivity reaction, and the relatively simple procedure, which reduces possible artifacts present in other assays.

REFERENCES

1. Pearmain, G., Lycette, R. R., and Fitzgerald, P. H., *Lancet* **1**, 637 (1963).
2. Rosenberg, G. L., Farber, P. A., and Notkins, A. L., *Proc. Natl. Acad. Sci. U.S.A.* **69**, 756 (1972).
3. Viza, D. C., Degari, O., Dausset, J., and Davies, D. A. L., *Nature (London)* **219**, 704 (1968).
4. Oppenheim, J. J., *Fed. Proc., Fed. Am. Soc. Exp. Biol.* **27**, 21 (1968).
5. Hirschhorn, K., Bach, F. H., Kolodny, R. L., Firschein, I. L., and Hashern, N., *Science* **142**, 1185 (1963).
6. Bain, B., Vas, M. R., and Lowenstein, L., *Blood* **23**, 108 (1964).
7. Sørensen, S. F., *Acta Pathol. Microbiol. Scand. Sect. B,* Suppl. 230, p. 32 (1972).
8. Mills, J. A., *J. Immunol.* **97**, 239 (1966).
9. Meltzer, M. S., Leonard, E. J., Rapp, H. J., and Borsos, T., *J. Natl. Cancer Inst.* **47**, 703 (1971).
10. Dowling, D. C., Quagliano, D., and Davidson, E., *Lancet* **1**, 1091 (1963).
11. Schreck, R., and Rabinowitz, Y., *Am. Rev. Respir. Dis.* **87**, 834 (1964).
12. Stjernswärd, J., Clifford, P., Singh, M., and Svedmyr, E., *E. Afr. Med. J.* **45**, 484 (1968).
13. Stjernswärd, J., Almgård, L.-E., Franxén, S., von Schreeb, T., and Wadström, L. B., *Clin. Exp. Immunol.* **6**, 963 (1970).
14. Nagel, G. A., St.-Arneandt, G., Holland, J. F., Kirkpatrik, D., and Kirkpatrik, R., *Cancer Res.* **30**, 1828 (1970).
15. Green, S. S., and Sell, K. W., *Science* **170**, 989 (1970).
16. Karmer, S. P., Mardiney, M. R., Jr., and Mangi, R. J., *J. Immunol.* **105**, 1052 (1970).
17. Powles, R. L., Balchin, L. A., Fairley, C. H., and Alexander, P., *Br. Med. J.* **1**, 486 (1971).
18. Taylor, J. F., Jurige, V., Wolfe, L., Deinhardt, F., and Kyalwazi, S. K., *Int. J. Cancer* **8**, 468 (1971).
19. Watkins, E., Jr., Ogata, Y., Andersson, L. L., Watkins, E., III, and Waters, M. F., *Nature (London), New Biol.* **231**, 83, (1971).
20. Gutterman, J. U., Hersh, E. M., McCredie, K. B., Bodey, G. P., Sr., Rodriguez, H., and Freireich, E. J., *Cancer Res.* **32**, 2524 (1972).
21. Herberman, R. B., Tivj, C. C., Kirschner, H., Holden, H., Glaser, M., Bonnard, G. D., and Laurin, D., *Prog. Immunol. II,* **3**, 285 (1974).
22. Nernoto, T., Han, T., Minowada, I., Angkur, V., Chamberlain, A., and Dao, T. L., *J. Natl. Cancer Inst.* **53**, 642 (1974).
23. Robinson, E., Sker, S., and Mekori, T., *Cancer Res.* **34**, 1548 (1974).

24. Gainor, B. J., Forbes, J. T., Enneking, W. F., and Smith, R. T., *Clinical Orthopaedics and Related Research* **111**, 83 (1975).
25. Report of a Workshop on the Immune Response to Solid Tumors in Man, (Stevenson, G. T., and Lawrence, D. J. R. eds.), *Int. J. Cancer* **16**, 887 (1975).
26. Cochran, A. J., Spilg, W. G. S., Mackie, R. M., and Thomas, C. E., *Br. Med. J.* **4**, 47 (1972).
27. Jondal, M., Holm, G., and Wigzell, H., *J. Exp. Med.* **136**, 207 (1972).
28. Littman, B. H., Meltzer, M. S., Cleveland, R. P., Zbar, B., and Rapp, W. J., *J. Natl. Cancer Inst.* **51**, 1627 (1973).
29. Jehn, W. M., Nathanson, L., Schwartz, R. S., and Skirner, M., *N. Engl. J. Med.* **283**, 329 (1970).
30. Herberman, R. B., Rosenberg, E. B., Halterman, R. H., McCoy, J. L., and Leventhal, B. G., *Natl. Cancer Inst. Monogr.* **35**, 259 (1972).
31. Vánky, F., Klein, E., Stjernswärd, J., and Nilsonne, U., *Int. J. Cancer* **14**, 277 (1974).
32. Nemoto, T., Han, T., Minowada, J., Angkur, V., Chamberlain, A., and Dao, L. T., *J. Natl. Cancer Inst.* **53**, 641 (1974).
33. Dean, J. H., McCoy, J. L., Lewis, D., Apella, E., and Law, L. W., *Int. J. Cancer* **16**, 465 (1975).
34. Currie, G. A., and Bagshawe, K. D., *Br. J. Cancer* **22**, 843 (1968).
35. Bekesi, J. G., Arneandt, G. S., Walter, L., and Holland, J. F., *J. Natl. Cancer Inst.* **49**, 107 (1972).
36. Hersh, E. M., and Harris, J. E., *J. Immunol.* **100**, 1184 (1968).
37. Gordon, J., *Proc. Soc. Exp. Biol. Med.* **127**, 30 (1968).
38. Lundgren, G., Zukosi, C. R., and Möller, G., *Clin. Exp. Immunol.* **3**, 817 (1968).
39. Glaser, M., Kirschner, H., and Herberman, R. B., *Int. J. Cancer* **16**, 384 (1975).
40. Oppenheim, J. J., *Cell. Immunol.* **3**, 341 (1972).
41. Bloom, B. R., Ceppellini, R., Cerottini, J.-C., David, J. R., Kunkel, H., Landy, M., Lawrence, H. S., Maini, R., Nussenzweig, H., Perlmann, P., Spitler, L., Rosen, F., and Zabriskie, J., *Cell. Immunol.* **6**, 331 (1973).
42. Vánky, F., Klein, E., Stjernswärd, J., and Trempe, G., *Int. J. Cancer* **16**, 850 (1975).
43. Darzynkiewicz, Z., and Jacobsson, B., *Proc. Soc. Exp. Biol. Med.* **136**, 387 (1971).
44. Bach, F. H., and Bach, M. L., *Nature (London), New Biol.* **235**, 243 (1972).
45. Lightbody, J., and Kong, Y. M., *Cell. Immunol.* **13**, 326 (1974).
46. Lindahl-Kiessling, K., and Säfwenberg, J., *Int. Arch. Allergy Appl. Immunol.* **41**, 670 (1971).
47. Bain, B., *Clin. Exp. Immunol.* **6**, 255 (1970).
48. Adkinson, N. F., Jr., Rosenberg, S. A., and Terry, W. D., *J. Immunol.* **112**, 1426 (1974).

Direct Capillary Tube Leukocyte Migration Inhibition Assay for Detection of Cell-Mediated Immunity to Human Tumor-Associated Antigens

James L. McCoy, Larry F. Jerome, Jack H. Dean, Grace B. Cannon, Robert J. Connor, and Ronald B. Herberman

1. Introduction

A number of investigators have demonstrated that the direct capillary tube leukocyte migration inhibition (LMI) assay is a good *in vitro* correlate of delayed hypersensitivity with such antigens as purified protein derivative of tuberculin (PPD) (1–4): PPD has been widely used to standardize the assay. Further, several studies have demonstrated the usefulness of the LMI test in detecting cell-mediated immunity against human tumor-associated antigens (TAA) (5–13). The method permits a detailed evaluation of specificity of the reaction, including testing of normal and benign disease controls, not generally possible in *in vivo* delayed hypersensitivity tests.

LMI assays are able to demonstrate common antigens on tumors of the same organ system including breast (5–10), melanoma (7), renal (11), lung (12), colon (13), and Ewing's sarcoma (14). In contrast to most cytotoxicity tests that require cultured target cells, the LMI assay permits use of extracts directly from fresh tumor material as well as tissue-cultured cells derived from tumor tissue (15). The patterns of specificity obtained in the LMI assay with the various histological tumor types indicate its potential usefulness in diagnosis and monitoring of cell-mediated reactivity of cancer patients.

2. Materials

2.1. Sterile plastic syringes, 50 ml

2.2. Conical centrifuge tubes, 50 ml (No. 2074, Falcon Plastics, Oxnard, California)

2.3. Heparin, 5000 units/ml (sodium heparin, preservative free; Grand Island Biological Company (GIBCO), Grand Island, New York)

2.4. Plasmagel (HTI Corporation, Buffalo, New York)

2.5. Screw-top plastic tubes, 13 × 100 mm (No. 2027, Falcon Plastics, Oxnard, California)

2.6. McCoy's 5A media, fetal bovine serum (International Biological Laboratory, Rockville, Maryland)

2.7. Penicillin and streptomycin (GIBCO, Grand Island, New York)

2.8. Capillary tubes, 25 μl, unpolished (No. 4619, Clay Adams, Parsippany, New Jersey)

2.9. Seal-Ease Clay (Clay Adams, Parsippany, New Jersey)

2.10. Sterilin plates, 12-chamber (Sterilin, Surrey, England or Microbiological Associates, Inc., Bethesda, Maryland)

2.11. Stopcock grease, Silicone Lubricant (Dow Corning, Midland, Michigan)

2.12. Glass cover slips, 22 mm diameter

2.13. Antigens: Lyophilized purified protein derivative of tuberculin (PPD) without preservatives (Parke-Davis Pharmaceutical, Detroit, Michigan). A concentration range of 10–100 μg/ml was employed. KCl extracts, 3 M, run at concentrations ranging from 0.5 to 750 μg/ml of human tumor material were prepared as previously described (10). Concentration and dialysis of the 3 M KCl extracts were performed with an Amicon-Multi-Micro Ultrafiltration System (Lexington, Massachusetts) using a UM-10 membrane. The concentrated extract was passed through a 0.2 μm Millipore filter and checked for sterility with thioglycolate media. Osmolarity of the extracts was less than 500 milliosmoles as determined by an Osmette A, automatic osmometer (Precision Systems, Inc., Sudbury, Massachusetts). Potassium concentrations were at physiological levels (4 meg/liter) as measured with Stat-ion (Technicon Corp., Tarrytown, New York). The antigens were dispensed into 1-dram glass vials (Wheaton Industries, Millville, New Jersey) at a concentration of 1 mg of protein (Lowry) per milliliter and stored at −96°C in a Revco freezer. Fresh PPD was prepared approximately every 3 months and the 3 M KCl extracts were stored up to at least 18 months without apparent loss of antigenicity.

3. Method

3.1. Whole blood (50–60 ml) is drawn from the antecubital vein of the donor into 50-ml plastic syringes containing 1 ml (5000 U) of heparin and mixed.

3.2. The blood is gently expressed from the syringe (after removing the needle) down the inside of a 50-ml plastic conical centrifuge tube containing Plasmagel (1 part Plasmagel/6 parts whole blood), placed upright in a 37°C incubator, and the erythrocytes are allowed to settle at 1 g for 1 hr.

3.3. The leukocyte-rich plasma (with some contamination with red blood cells) is carefully removed from the sedimented red cells with a 10-ml plastic pipette and placed into another 50-ml conical plastic centrifuge tube; 2–3 ml of plasma containing leukocytes just above the erythrocyte layer should not be collected.

3.4. The plasma containing the leukocytes is centrifuged at 200 g for 10 min in a PR6000 International Centrifuge at room temperature. The plasma is poured from the leukocyte pellet and the pellet is resuspended in 10 ml of warm (room temperature) McCoy's 5A media containing 10% heat-inactivated ($56°C$ for 30 min) fetal bovine serum and penicillin and streptomycin (complete media). The cells are resuspended with the aid of a Vortex mixer (at high setting) until no visible clumps remain. The leukocytes are centrifuged at 200 g for 10 min at room temperature. The supernatant is carefully aspirated by vacuum suction from the cell pellet.

3.5. Ten milliliters of complete medium are added to the cell pellet, and the cells are vigorously vortexed until no visual clumps remain.

3.6. The cell concentration is adjusted to 2×10^7 leukocytes per milliliter with complete media.

3.7. One milliliter of leukocyte suspension is added to each of a series of 13 × 100 mm plastic tubes. The tubes are centrifuged at 200 g for 5 min at room temperature.

3.8. Each tube is carefully tilted to a horizontal position and the supernatant is completely removed from the cell pellet with a Pasteur pipette by vacuum suction.

3.9. The cell pellet of each tube is resuspended with 1 ml of complete media alone (media control) or with media containing a particular concentration of antigen. The cell pellets are vigorously vortexed until no clumps remain.

3.10. The tubes are placed upright in a $37°C$ CO_2 incubator for 1 hr and then centrifuged at 200 g for 5 min at room temperature.

3.11. A 0.75-ml volume of the supernatant is gently aspirated by vacuum suction from each vertically held tube, using a Pasteur pipette, leaving 0.25 ml of complete media with and without test antigen on each cell pellet. The cell pellets are vigorously vortexed until no clumps are visible.

3.12. Capillary tubes are completely filled in replicates of four with the various cell suspensions by capillary action. The capillaries are sealed with Seal-Ease clay. Each capillary contains approximately 3×10^6 leukocytes. A total of approximately 16–40 capillaries can be prepared from 60 ml of whole blood, depending on the final leukocyte yield.

3.13. The sealed capillaries are placed in 13 × 100 mm plastic tubes and centrifuged at 200 g for 5 min at room temperature.

3.14. Each capillary is quickly scored with a vial file one-third (approximately 0.5–1.5 mm) of the way below the cell pellet–liquid interface, then broken, and the cell-containing end is immediately placed in a Sterilin plate chamber. The capillary tip containing the cell pellet is held in place in the chamber at the clay-sealed end by a small drop of stopcock grease. One capillary tube is placed in each chamber of the Sterilin plate. After 4 capillaries (the replicates from one test or medium control group) are placed in chambers, 0.4 ml of complete medium without antigen is added to each chamber. This volume of medium will form a small convex miniscus in the chamber. A cover slip is gently lowered onto the chamber and pressed into place, care being taken to leave no air bubbles within the chamber.

3.15. The Sterilin plates are incubated on a level shelf at 37°C for 18–24 hr in a humidified 5% CO_2 incubator.

3.16. After incubation, the areas of migration are observed and projected onto paper with a Reichert microscope fitted with a 1X objective and a Zeiss projection tube (Projectiv, $f = 63$ mm) and the areas are drawn. The area of each migration pattern (in cm^2) is quantitated with a planimeter.

3.17. A migration index (MI) is calculated by the formula:

$$MI = \frac{\text{mean of migration of 4 replicate capillaries in the presence of antigen}}{\text{mean of migration of 4 replicate capillaries in abscence of antigen (media control)}}$$

3.18. Statistical treatment of LMI data is best handled in two ways: (a) testing for no difference in reactivity versus an increase in patient reactivity over normal donor reactivity; and (b) describing the patient reactivity relative to that of the normal donors.

The increase in reactivity of patients is tested by comparing the patient migration index values with those of the normal donors. Nonparametric methods, such as the Wilcoxon test or the Kruskal–Wallis test, are recommended (16). These tests are sensitive to shifts in the location of distributions (e.g., to differences of means or of medians) and require less stringent assumptions about the distribution of the values than do usual theory methods (e.g., the t test or analysis of variance). Further, these methods allow differences to be studied and tested between tumor extracts as well as the differences between patients and normal donors.

The percentage, or the proportion, of "positive" patient migration index values determined by utilizing a cutoff value is used to describe the patient reactivity to the various extracts. The cutoff value is based on the normal donor observations and is selected so that 10% or less of the normal migration index values fall below the cutoff value (i.e., the cutoff is the lower tenth percentile of the normal donor observations). Migration index values falling below the cutoff are considered positive. This is based on the consideration that 10% or less would be an upper limit of "false positivity" for a potentially useful diagnostic test. The cutoff value should be determined for each individual extract unless there is little or no difference between extracts in the normal donor migration index values. In our experience, substantial differences can occur between extracts and can result in a range of cutoff values (e.g., 0.75 or lower for one extract and 0.89 or higher for another extract). This procedure always yields about 10% of the normals being positive to an extract, and therefore, the percentage of patients positive is a consistent relative measure of their reactivity to extracts.

4. Critical Comments

4.1. Plasmagel greatly facilitates the sedimentation of red blood cells from the upper leukocyte-plasma layer. This separation method yields a population of leukocytes containing lymphocytes and polymorphonuclear cells, both of which are required for the test. A 1 g sedimentation without the use of Plasmagel frequently results in a high amount of erythrocyte contamination of the plasma—leukocyte layer, especially with normal donor bloods. High red blood cell contamination can interfere with interpretation of total areas of migration by the leukocytes. Minor red blood cell contamination of the leukocyte preparation is observed with plasmagel, but does not interfere with the test. No effort is made to lyse the remaining erythrocytes.

4.2. It is critical to avoid any clumping of leukocytes during cell processing. The addition of fetal bovine serum to media used for resuspending and washing the cell pellets helps alleviate potential clumping problems. Clumping can result in poor replicate values among capillaries, presumably because of poor interaction of cells with antigen as well as impairment of migration of cells from the capillary tubes.

4.3. Cutting of capillaries approximately 0.5—1.5 mm below the cell—liquid interface appears to remove a large proportion of platelets that are sedimented on top of the leukocyte pellet during centrifugation.

4.4. Cell viability of the migrating cells out of the capillaries after 24 hr is usually 90% or greater. The viability of cells remaining in the capillary tube is usually less than 50%.

4.5. The fan of migrating cells usually form two distinct zones (inner and outer). The inner zone of cells are both mononuclear cells (45—55%) and polymorphonuclear cells (47—55%) whereas the outer zone mainly contains faster moving polymorphonuclear cells (70—80%) with a smaller number of mononuclear cells (20—30%). It is important to measure the outer zone (polymorphonuclear cells) of migration in the final analysis since the polymorphonuclear cells are largely the indicator cells whose movement is impaired by the mediator, LIF, although measuring and using the inner areas of both control and test groups usually gives comparable migration index values as obtained when using the outer areas.

4.6. The technique should be as aseptic as possible, but addition of pencillin and streptomycin to the incubation media helps to control bacterial growth. These antibiotics do not appear to interfere with migration of cells or with inhibitory reactions. Considerably less contamination has been seen with the Sterilin plates than with Sykes—Moore chambers.

4.7. A level *humidified* CO_2 incubator should be used to incubate the plates. Lack of moisture in the incubator will result in evaporation of media from the wells, resulting in a drying of chambers with formation of air bubbles, or a change in the tonicity of the media, that may result in erratic migration of cells.

4.8. The assay should be run with at least four replicates for each test group. Agreement among capillaries is usually within 10% or less.

4.9. The assay is fairly easy to perform and quite reproducible with good stocks of soluble PPD. When employing tumor extracts, the technique becomes more difficult to perform reproducibly. Technical expertise and experience becomes a more critical issue. Problems of obtaining false-negative values with the tumor antigens can occur. Good technical handling of the assay, however, can largely overcome this problem.

4.10. When 3 M KCl extracts of human tumor materials are used, broad dose response studies for each extract should be run in order to establish toxicity and reactive levels. We have employed wide ranges of these antigens and have employed some extracts as high as 750 μg/ml and others as low as 0.5 μg/ml and obtained specific reactivity.

REFERENCES

1. Thor, D., and Dray, S., *J. Immunol.* **101,** 51 (1968).
2. Rocklin, R. E., Meyers, O. L., and David, J. R., *J. Immunol.* **104,** 95 (1970).
3. Rosenberg, S. A., and David, J. R., *J. Immunol.* **105,** 1447 (1970).
4. Federlin, K., Maini, R. N., Russell, A. S., and Dumonde, D. C., *J. Clin. Pathol.* **24,** 533 (1971).
5. Anderson, V., Bjerrum, O., Bendixen, G., Schiødt, T., and Dissing, I., *Int. J. Cancer* **5,** 357 (1970).
6. Wolberg, W. H., *Cancer Res.* **31,** 798 (1971).
7. Cochran, A. J., Spilg, W. G., Mackie, R. M., and Thomas, C. E., *Br. Med. J.* **2,** 67 (1972).
8. Segall, A., Weiler, O., Genin, J., Lacour, J., and Lacour, F., *Int. J. Cancer* **9,** 417 (1972).
9. Black, M. M., Leis, H. P., Jr., Shore, B., and Zachrau, R. E., *Cancer* **33,** 952 (1974).
10. McCoy, J. L., Jerome, L. F., Dean, J. H., Cannon, G. B., Alford, T. C., Doering, T., and Herberman, R. B., *J. Natl. Cancer Inst.* **53,** 11 (1974).
11. Kjaer, M., *Eur. J. Cancer* **10,** 523 (1974).
12. Boddie, A. W., Holmes, E. C., and Roth, J. A., *Surg. Forum* **25,** 109 (1974).
13. Bull, D. M., Leibach, J. H., Williams, M. A., and Helms, R. A., *Science* **181,** 957 (1973).
14. McCoy, J. L., Cannon, G. B., Oldham, R. K., Pomeroy, T. C., and Herberman, R. B., unpublished observations, 1976.
15. McCoy, J. L., Jerome, L. F., Anderson, C., Cannon, G. B., Alford, T. C., Connor, R. J., Oldham, R. K., and Herberman, R. B., *J. Natl. Cancer Inst.* in press.
16. Hollander, M. and Wolfe, D. A., "Non-parametric Statistical Methods," p. 125. Wiley, New York, 1973.

Indirect Capillary Tube Leukocyte Migration Inhibition Assay for Cell-Mediated Immunity to Human Tumor-Associated Antigens

Bruce A. Maurer, David F. Siwarski, Gregory P. Fischetti, and Ronald B. Herberman

1. Introduction

Rocklin (1, 2) has reported that human lymphocytes secrete a mediator, leukocyte-inhibitory factor (LIF), which causes the inhibition of migration of human polymorphonuclear (PMN) leukocytes. The assay described here separates the two basic events associated with this observation, i.e., secretion of mediator by lymphyocytes and the inhibition by the mediator of the appropriate target cell. In this indirect assay, we expose a population of mononuclear (MN) cells (lymphocytes and monocytes) to antigen for the production of LIF and use purified PMN leukocytes for the migrating target cells. Other investigators (3–5) have reported the use of an indirect assay for human migration inhibitory factors. Thor *et al.* (3) and Rocklin *et al.* (4) used guinea pig macrophages as the migrating target cell for human macrophage-inhibitory factor (MIF), whereas Goldberg *et al.* (5) used human peripheral blood monocytes as the migrating target cell. These studies (3–5) used concentrates of supernatants from antigen-exposed peripheral blood leukocytes (PBL). Clausen (6) employed an indirect agarose assay in contrast to the capillary tube method (7) used by Rocklin and Thor, to demonstrate the inhibition of PBL by a factor produced by human mononuclear cells.

We have developed this indirect assay in humans using a purified protein derivative of tuberculin (PPD) system in order to correlate the assay to delayed skin reactivity and to establish the optimum conditions for mediator secretion and inhibition of PMN leukocytes. This assay has also proved to be effective for the detection of reactivity of breast cancer patients to tumor-associated antigens [from a cell line derived from a patient with breast cancer, MCF-7 (8)] and virus (mouse mammary tumor virus, MMTV). This assay provides the additional advantages relative to direct migration assays, of storage of mediator for subsequent evaluation and the quantitative evaluation of the mediator induced by incubation with antigen.

2. Materials

2.1. Syringes, 50 ml plastic (Plastipak, Becton, Dickinson and Co., Rutherford, New Jersey)

2.2. Preservative-free heparin, 5000 U/ml (Catalogue No. 568, GIBCO, Grand Island, New York)

2.3. Conical tubes, 50 ml (Falcon No. 2074, Oxnard, California)

2.4. Phosphate-buffered saline (PBS), pH 7.4, 0.15 M NaCl

2.5. Ficoll–Hypaque lymphocyte separation medium (LSM) (Catalogue No. 8410-01, Litton Bionetics, Kensington, Maryland)

2.6. Pipettes, serological glass, disposable (Corning Glass Works, Corning, New York)

2.7. Propipettor (Scientific Products, McGaw Park, Illinois)

2.8. RPMI 1640 (GIBCO, Grand Island, New York)

2.9. Gentamicin (Schering Corp., Port Reading, New Jersey)

2.10. Fetal bovine serum (GIBCO, Grand Island, New York)

2.11. Hemocytometer, Spencer Bright-Line (Catalogue No. 1490, American Optical Corp. Buffalo, New York)

2.12. Trypan blue solution (GIBCO, Grand Island, New York)

2.13. Culture tube, 10 × 75 (Catalogue No. 339-267, Curtin Matheson Scientific, Inc., Beltsville, Maryland)

2.14. Screw cap tubes, 13 × 100 (No. 2027 Falcon, Oxnard, California)

2.15. Platform rocker (Bellco, Vineland, New York)

2.16. Plasmagel (HTI Corp. Buffalo, New York)

2.17. Capillary tubes, Micropet, 25 μl (Clay Adams, Parsippany, New Jersey)

2.18. Seal-Ease Clay (Clay Adams, Scientific Products, McGraw Park, Illinois)

2.19. Sterilin chambers (Sterilin, Surrey, England; or Cooke Engineering, Alexandria, Virginia)

2.20. Silicone grease (Dow Corning Corp., Midland, Michigan)

2.21. Tubing scorer (Catalogue No. 3488, Fisher Scientific, Pittsburg, Pennsylvania)

2.22. Cover slips, 22 mm (PGC Scientific Corp., Rockville, Maryland)

2.23. Antigens: Lyophilized purified protein derivative of tuberculin (PPD) without preservatives (Parke-Davis Pharmaceutical, Detroit, Michigan) in a concentration range of 10–100 μg/ml was employed. KCl extracts, 3 M, run at concentrations ranging from 0.5 to 750 μg/ml of human tumor material were prepared as previously described (9). Concentration and dialysis of the 3 M KCl extracts were performed with an Amicon-Multi-Micro Ultrafiltration System (Lexington, Massachusetts) using a UM-10 membrane. The concentrated extract was passed through a 0.2 μm Millipore filter and checked for sterility with thioglycolate media. Osmolarity of the extracts was less than 500 mosmole as determined by an Osmette A, automatic osmometer (Precision Systems, Inc., Sudbury, Massachusetts). Potassium concentrations were at physiological levels (4 meq per liter) as measured with Stat-ion (Technicon Corporation, Tarrytown, New York). The antigens were dispensed into 1-dram glass vials (Wheaton Industries, Millville, New Jersey) at a concentration of 1 mg of protein (Lowry) per milliliter and stored at $-96°C$ in a Revco freezer. Fresh PPD was prepared approximately every 3 months, and the 3 M KCl extracts were stored up to at least 18 months without apparent loss of antigenicity.

3. Methods

3.1. Part I: Preparation of LIF-Containing Supernatants from Lymphocytes (Mononuclear Cells) from Peripheral Blood

3.1.1. Approximately 60 ml of blood is drawn from the antecubital vein into 50-ml syringes containing 5000 units of preservative-free heparin ($\cong$100 U per milliliter of blood).

3.1.2. After mixing by inverting the syringe several times, 20 ml of blood is expressed from the syringe into each of 3 plastic conical centrifuge (50 ml) tubes.

3.1.3. Blood is diluted by adding 20 ml of PBS to each tube and mixing thoroughly by stirring with a pipette.

3.1.4. Ficoll–Hypaque, 10 ml, is slowly added with a 10-ml pipette to the bottom of each tube containing diluted blood, producing a layer of diluted whole blood over a layer of Ficoll–Hypaque.

3.1.5. Centrifuging the tubes at 400 g for 30 min at room temperature produces a band of MN cells ($\sim$ 80% lymphocytes, $\cong$20% monocytes) at the interface of the Ficoll–Hypaque and plasma.

3.1.6. The plasma is aspirated to within 0.5 cm of the mononuclear band without disturbing the band. The bands of MN cells are removed with a 10-ml pipette and a propipettor, pooled, and transferred into another 50-ml conical centrifuge tube.

3.1.7. The pooled MN cells are diluted with an equal volume of PBS and centrifuged at 200 g for 10 min.

3.1.8. The supernatant is decanted, the cells are resuspended with 25 ml of complete medium (RPMI 1640 with HEPES buffer, supplemented with 50 μg of gentamicin and 0.5% fetal bovine serum, FBS).

3.1.9. Centrifuge as in Step 3.1.7, decant supernatant and resuspend cells in 10 ml of complete medium.

3.1.10. Of this cell suspension, 0.1 ml is added to 0.1-ml of trypan blue solution in a 10 $\times$ 75 mm culture tube. Cell counts are determined using a hemacytometer. The cells are usually >99% viable.

3.1.11. For each antigen or concentration of antigen to be tested, 8.0×10^6 MN cells are aliquoted into a 13×100 mm plastic screw-cap tubes. An additional tube containing 8.0×10^6 cells is added for an antigen-free medium control.

3.1.12. The cells are centrifuged at $200\ g$ for 5 min, the supernatants are aspirated, and 2.0 ml of antigen in complete medium (or medium alone, medium control) is added to the cell pellet.

3.1.13. The cells are resuspended by shaking the tubes with the cap screwed on tightly. The tubes are placed horizontally on a platform rocker (rocking through an arc of $\cong 30°$ every 10 sec) in a $37°C$ incubator for 2 hr.

3.1.14. The cells are then centrifuged at $200\ g$ for 5 min. The supernatant is removed by aspiration, and the cells are washed with 2.0 ml of complete medium and centrifuged again at $200\ g$ for 5 min. The cells are then resuspended in 2.0 ml of complete medium without antigen. Incubate for 48 hr at $37°C$ in a CO_2 incubator.

3.1.15. Centrifuge at $200\ g$ for 5 min. Decant and store supernatant at $-70°C$ unless assayed on the same day.

3.2. Part II: Assay for LIF Using Purified PMN Leukocytes

3.2.1. Obtain blood from a normal donor, as in Part I, step 3.1.1., 60 ml of blood yield approximately 1.5×10^6 PMN leukocytes per milliliter of blood.

3.2.2. Add 5.0 ml Plasmagel (prewarmed to room temperature) to 50-ml conical centrifuge tubes (Falcon 2074), add 30 ml of blood to each tube. Stir with a pipette and remove any foam from the fluid surface.

3.2.3. Let stand in $37°C$ water bath for 45–60 min.

3.2.4. Remove leukocyte-rich plasma (LRP) and put 20 ml into 50-ml conical centrifuge tubes. Add an equal volume of PBS. Stir with pipette. Add 10 ml of Ficoll-Hypaque as in Part I, step 3.1.4.

3.2.5. Centrifuge at $400\ g$ for 30 min at room temperature. Aspirate all fluid from the pellet of PMN leukocytes ($\cong 98\%$ PMN, $\cong 2\%$ mononuclear cells). PMN leukocytes are contaminated with small numbers of RBC, which do not affect migration.

3.2.6. Resuspend and pool pellets in 25 ml of complete assay medium (RPMI 1640 supplemented with gentamicin, 50 $\mu g/ml$, and 10% FBS). Centrifuge at $200\ g$ for 10 min. Decant supernatant, resuspend PMN leukocytes in 20 ml of complete assay medium.

3.2.7. Determine cell concentration as in Part I, step 3.1.10.

3.2.8. Centrifuge at $200\ g$ for 10 min and resuspend with complete assay medium at a cell concentration of $8.0 \times 10^7/ml$.

3.2.9. Transfer 1.0 ml of PMN leukocytes to a 13×100 mm plastic screw-cap tube. Fill capillary pipettes with PMN by capillary action. Seal the nonrounded end with Seal-Ease Clay to a depth of approximately 4.0 mm.

3.2.10. Four to eight capillary tubes are placed in each glass 10×75 mm culture tube and centrifuged at 200 g for 5 min. Many capillary tubes can be centrifuged at the same time using an 8-place carrier.

3.2.11. Score capillary pipettes with a tube scorer and break at a point that is approximately 1.0 mm into pellet from pellet–fluid interface.

3.2.12. Put sealed end of pipette on a small drop of silicone grease, which is placed near the inner edge of each chamber of a sterilin plate.

3.2.13. FBS is added to each supernatant to a final concentration of 10%; 0.4 ml of supernatant is added to each chamber. We usually prepare four replicates for each supernatant. A 22-mm round cover slip is used to seal each chamber. Surface tension is used to draw the cover slips over each chamber, and care is taken to avoid air bubbles.

3.2.14. Incubate at $37°C$ for 24 hr in a humidified CO_2 incubator.

3.2.15. The periphery of the area of migration is traced from a projected image of the pattern of migration using a Reichert microscope fitted with a 1X objective and a Zeiss projection tube (Projectiv, $f=63$ mm). The area of migration is determined by planimetry of the traced pattern. The average area of migration is determined from four replicate measurements.

3.2.16. A migration index (MI) is determined by the following formula:

$$MI = \frac{\text{average area of migration in presence of supernatant generated in presence of antigen}}{\text{average area of migration in presence of supernatant generated in absence of antigen}}$$

4. Interpretation of Data and Critical Comments

4.1. Since this assay is based upon an inhibition effect, care must be taken to eliminate any nonspecific inhibition, i.e., toxicity. One favorable aspect of this assay is the ability to "trigger" the lymphocytes with the subsequent removal of the antigen, thereby eliminating the possible toxic effect of the antigens on the migrating population. Thus, it is not necessary to add antigen back into supernatants generated in the absence of antigen in order to assess the effect of antigen on the migrating population. Our studies with PPD indicated that 1 hr of exposure to antigen is sufficient to "trigger" the MN cells to generate LIF.

4.2. For developmental experiments in which the human PPD system was used, the data were statistically evaluated using the student's t test for paired means. In this test, the means of the area of four replicate measurements of migration produced by supernatant generated in the presence of PPD were paired with those means produced by supernatants generated in the absence of PPD.

In contrast, the statistical treatment of LMI data from groups of individuals whether using PPD or putative human tumor-associated antigens in populations of cancer patients and normal individuals is best handled in two ways: (a) testing for no difference in reactivity versus an increase in patient reactivity over normal donor reactivity (or for PPD, an increase in reactivity of skin test-positive individuals over that in skin test-negative individuals); and (b) describing the patient reactivity relative to that of the normal donors.

The increase in reactivity of patients is tested by comparing the patient migration index values with those of the normal donors. Nonparametric methods, such as the Wilcoxon test or the Kruskal–Wallis test, are recommended (10). These tests are sensitive to shifts in the location of distributions (e.g., to differences of means or of medians) and require less stringent assumptions about the distribution of the values than do usual theory methods (e.g., the t test or analysis of variance). Further, these methods allow differences to be studied and tested between tumor extracts as well as the differences between patients and normal donors.

The percentage, or the proportion, of "positive" patient migration index values determined by utilizing a cutoff value is used to describe the patient reactivity to the various extracts. The cutoff value is based on the normal donor observations and is selected so that approximately 10% or less of the normal migration index values fall below the cutoff value (i.e., the cutoff is the lower tenth percentile of the normal donor observations). Migration index values falling below the cutoff are considered positive. This is based on the consideration that 10% or less would be an upper limit of "false positivity" for a potentially useful diagnostic test. The cutoff value should be determined for each individual extract unless there is little or no difference between extracts in the normal donor migration index values. In our experience, substantial differences can occur between extracts and can result in a range of cutoff values (e.g., 0.75 or lower for one extract and 0.89 or higher for another extract). This procedure always yields about 10% of the normals being positive to an extract, and therefore the percentage of patients positive is a consistent relative measure of their reactivity to extracts.

4.3. Our studies using a human PPD system has indicated that FBS is not required for the generation of LIF. However, in the absence of serum, viscous material sometimes develops which traps some cells, leading to a variable loss of cells during centrifugation after the 2-hr "triggering" period. However, the addition 0.5% FBS prevented this and is routinely added to the cultures for the preparation of the LIF-containing supernatant. Since PMN leukocytes do not migrate well in the absence of serum, 10% FBS is added to each supernatant prior to addition to the PMN leukocytes.

4.4. Although the methods described here indicate the use of 4.0×10^6 MN cells per milliliter of supernatant desired, our studies with the human PPD system have indicated that LIF was detected at concentrations of 1.0×10^6 MN cells per milliliter. Since this greatly affects the number of antigen combinations that may be analyzed, optimal MN cell concentrations for the particular antigen should be established.

4.5. The supernatants derived from 2-day MN cell cultures are "conditioned" and support PMN leukocyte migration better than fresh medium. The supernatants generated in the presence of antigen need to be compared to supernatants generated in the absence of antigen, and should not be compared to fresh medium controls. When quantitating LIF by titration, the experimental and the control supernatants should be diluted with the same diluent (e.g., control supernatant). We have detected LIF at a 1:20 dilution of supernatant generated from 4×10^6 MN cells from a PPD skin test-positive individual cultured for 2 days after a 2-hr "triggering" period using 25 μg of PPD.

REFERENCES

1. Rocklin, R. E., *J. Immunol.* **112**, 1461 (1974).
2. Rocklin, R. E., *J. Immunol.* **114**, 1161 (1975).
3. Thor, D. E., Jureziz, R. E., Veach, S. R., Miller, E., and Dray, S. *Nature (London)* **219**, 755 (1968).
4. Rocklin, R. E., Meyers, O. L., and David, J. R., *J. Immunol.* **104**, 95 (1970).
5. Goldberg, L. S., Louie, J. S., and Baker, M. H., *J. Immunol.* **107**, 906 (1971).
6. Clausen, J. E., *J. Immunol.* **110**, 546 (1973).
7. George, M., and Vaughn, J. H., *Proc. Soc. Exp. Biol. Med.* **111**, 514 (1962).
8. Soule, H. D., Vazques, J., Long, A., Albert, S., and Brennan, M., *J. Nat. Cancer Inst.* **51**, 1409 (1973).
9. McCoy, J. L., Jerome, L. F., Dean, J. H., Cannon, G. B., Alford, T. C., Doering, T., and Herberman, R. B., *J. Natl. Cancer Inst.* **53**, 11 (1974).
10. Hollander, M., and Wolfe, D. A., "Non-parametric Statistical Methods," p. 125. Wiley, New York, 1973.

Direct and Indirect Agarose Microdroplet Migration Inhibition Assays for Detection of Cell-Mediated Immunity to Human Tumor-Associated Antigens

James L. McCoy, Jack H. Dean, and Ronald B. Herberman

1. Introduction

Direct leukocyte migration inhibition assays employing the capillary tube method have proved to be useful in the investigation of host reactivity against tumor-associated antigens of human tumors. The leukocyte migration inhibition assay seems to detect cell-mediated immunity reactions and depends on the release from sensitized leukocytes of a soluble mediator, leukocyte inhibitory factor (LIF) (1), which impedes the movement of polymorphonuclear cells.

The capillary tube method is somewhat cumbersome to perform routinely, requires a large volume (50–60 ml) of whole blood, and uses large quantities of antigen. Further, the size of experiment that can be performed on a given test day is restricted, owing to limited leukocyte yields from some blood specimens of patients and also to the number of technical manipulations required. Thus, the number of different blood specimens and the number of different test antigens and antigen concentrations that can be run in each test are limited.

The agarose microdroplet migration inhibition assay recently described by Harrington (2, 3) in guinea pig and mouse systems may overcome many of the limitations encountered with the capillary tube method with human materials. Several different antigens, over a wide range of concentrations, can be tested with leukocytes obtained from 5–10 ml of whole blood. Further, because of its technical simplicity, a larger number of blood specimens can be tested within each experiment. We have developed this assay in our laboratory by testing skin-reactive individuals with PPD, and then have applied the method to the study of reactivity to antigen extracts of human tumors. We have employed both the direct technique, using the same human leukocyte specimen as the source of reactive cells and of migrating cells, and the indirect technique, in which mononuclear cells are incubated with antigen and the culture fluids are tested for the soluble mediator LIF, as measured by inhibition of the movement of purified human polymorphonuclear cells. The following are descriptions of the human direct and indirect agarose microdroplet assays.

2. Materials

2.1. Sterile plastic syringes, 10 ml and 50 ml

2.2. Conical centrifuge tubes, 15 ml (No. 2074, Falcon Plastics, Oxnard, California)

2.3. Heparin, 5000 U/ml (sodium heparin, preservative free, Grand Island Biological Co., Grand Island, New York)

2.4. Plasmagel (HTI Corporation, Buffalo, New York)

2.5. Snap-top tubes, 12 × 75 mm, (No. 2058, Falcon Plastics, Oxnard, California)

2.6. McCoy's 5A media, RPMI 1640, and fetal bovine serum (International Biological Laboratory, Rockville, Maryland)

2.7. Gentamicin (Schering Diagnostics, Reading, New Jersey)

2.8. HEPES Buffer (Grand Island Biological Co., Grand Island, New York)

2.9. Seakem Agarose (Marine Colloid Inc., Biomedical Systems, Rockland, Maine).

2.10. 2× Medium 199 (Grand Island, Grand Island, New York)

2.11. Drummond microdispenser, 10 μl (Drummond Scientific, Broomall, Pennsylvania)

2.12. Flat-bottom microculture plates, 96 wells (Cooke Engineering, Alexandria, Virginia)

2.13. Lids for microtest plate (Linbro No. 55, Linbro Plastics, Vineland, New Jersey)

2.14. Biopipette and Biotips (Clay Adams, New York)

2.15. Light mineral oil (Carroll Chemical Co., Smyrna, Tennessee)

2.16. Antigens: Lyophilized purified protein derivative of tuberculin (PPD) without preservatives (Parke-Davis Pharmaceutical, Detroit, Michigan); dose ranges between 5×10^{-5} and 50 μg/ml were employed). KCl extracts, 3 M, of human tumor material were prepared as previously described in (4) and in the direct capillary assay method (5) and used in dose ranges between 5×10^{-2} and 50 μg/ml.

2.17. NaCl, 0.85%, phosphate buffered, pH 7.4 (PBS)

2.18. Ficoll–Hypaque solution (Litton Bionetics Research Laboratory, Kensington, Maryland)

2.19. Glass vials, 1 dram (Wheaton Industries, Millvile, New Jersey)

3. Method

3.1. Direct Leukocyte Agarose Microdroplet Assay

3.1.1. Preparation of Agarose

3.1.1.1. A 0.4% (4 mg/ml) solution of agarose is prepared in advance: Seakem agarose is dissolved in distilled water by bringing it to a boil, accompanied by vigorous stirring. The solution is then dispensed in 1-ml volumes into 1-dram glass screw-top vials, autoclaved, and stored at 4°C until use. Prepared agarose can be satisfactorily stored for 2–3 months at 4°C if vials are tightly capped.

3.1.1.2. Immediately prior to use, a 1-ml aliquot vial of 0.4% agarose is liquefied in a boiling-water bath and then placed for a few minutes in a 37°C water bath.

3.1.1.3. An equal volume of 2X Medium 199, containing 20% heat-inactivated fetal bovine serum and 200 µg of gentamicin per milliliter (warmed to 37°C), is added to the liquefied 0.4% agarose. The final mixture now contains 0.2% agarose, 1X medium 199, 10% fetal bovine serum, and 100 µg of gentamicin per milliliter and is kept at 37°C in a water bath.

3.1.2. Preparation of Leukocytes

3.1.2.1. Whole blood (10 ml) is drawn from the antecubital vein of the donor into 10-ml plastic syringes containing 0.2 ml of heparin (5000 U/ml).

3.1.2.2. The needle is removed from the syringe, and the blood is gently expressed down the inside of a 15-ml plastic conical centrifuge tube containing Plasmagel (1 ml of Plasmagel/6 ml of whole blood), placed upright in a 37°C incubator; the erythrocytes are allowed to settle at 1 g for 1 hr.

3.1.2.3. The leukocyte-rich plasma (with some contamination by erythrocytes) is carefully aspirated from the sedimented erythrocytes with a pipette and placed into another 15-ml conical plastic centrifuge tube. A 0.5–1 ml volume of plasma containing leukocytes just above the red cell layer is not collected.

3.1.2.4. The plasma containing the leukocytes is centrifuged at 200 g for 10 min in a PR 6000 International Centrifuge at room temperature. The plasma is decanted and discarded, and the leukocyte-containing pellet is then resuspended in 10 ml of warm (room temperature) McCoy's 5A medium containing heat-inactivated (56°C for 30 min) 10% fetal bovine serum and 100 µg of gentamicin per milliliter.

3.1.2.5. The cells are resuspended with the aid of a Vortex mixer (at high setting) until no visible clumps remain. The leukocytes are again centrifuged at 200 g for 10 min at room temperature. The supernatant is aspirated and discarded.

3.1.2.6. Ten milliliters of medium are again added to the cell pellet, and the cells are vigorously vortexed until no visual clumps remain.

3.1.2.7. The cells are counted, and the cell concentration is adjusted to 2 × 10^7 leukocytes per milliliter with complete medium. The cells are now ready to be added to 0.2% agarose.

3.1.3. Mixing of Leukocytes and Agarose

3.1.3.1. One milliliter of 2 × 10^7 leukocytes is dispensed into a 12 × 75 mm plastic tube, which is then centrifuged at 200 g for 10 min. The tube is carefully tilted horizontally, and all medium is removed by a Pasteur pipette connected to a vacuum source. A 0.1-ml aliquot of 0.2% agarose (37°C) is added to the leukocyte pellet, and the tube is vigorously vortexed until no clumps of cells are evident. The tube is placed in the 37°C water bath.

3.1.3.2. Two-microliter droplets of the 0.2% agarose containing leukocytes (4 $\times$ 10^5 leukocytes/droplet) are placed into each well of a 96-well flat-bottom Microtest II plate with a Drummond microdispenser. The plate should be sitting on a flat surface at room temperature. Droplets will become solidified within 1–3 min. One tube containing 2 $\times$ 10^7 leukocytes and 0.1 ml of 0.2% agarose will yield approximately 35–40 droplets.

3.1.3.3. After the agarose droplets have been placed into the Microtest plate and let dry for 2–5 min, 0.1-ml aliquots of McCoy's 5A medium containing 10% fetal bovine serum, HEPES buffer (25 mM), and gentamicin (100 μg/ml) (complete medium) are added to at least 4 wells (media control) with a Biotip pipette. Likewise, appropriate concentrations of each test antigen in complete medium are added to at least 4 wells for each antigen.

3.1.3.4. A lid (Linbro No. 55) is placed on the plate, and the plate is placed on a level shelf of a humidified 5% CO_2 incubator at 37°C for 18–24 hr.

3.1.3.5. After incubation, light mineral oil is added just to the top of each well to enhance the image of the migration patterns that will next be evaluated.

3.1.3.6. The areas of migration of cells out of the agarose droplet in each well are observed and projected onto paper with an inverted Zeiss microscope fitted with a Zeiss straight-tube photochanger with a prism and a KDL 8$\times$ eye piece. The area of the agarose droplet itself is drawn (inner area) and the dense area of migration of the cells (outer area) is then drawn for each well. Scattered cells that may be more widely distributed throughout the wells are not included in the traced area. Most patterns are fairly symmetrical. The addition of mineral oil greatly increases the clarity of the projected image.

3.1.3.7. The area of each inner area and each outer area of migration of cells for each well is quantitated with a planimeter. The total area of migration of the cells is then obtained by subtracting the inner agarose area from the outer cell migration area for each droplet.

3.1.3.8. A migration index (MI) is calculated by the formula:

$$MI = \frac{\text{mean migration of 4 or more replicate droplets in the presence of antigen}}{\text{mean migration of 4 or more replicate droplets in the absence of antigen}}$$

3.1.3.9. The procedures used to describe and statistically analyze the results are presented in detail in the direct capillary assay method (5).

3.2. Indirect Polymorphonuclear Cell Agarose Droplet Assay

3.2.1. Preparation of Agarose. The method is identical to that described in Step 3.1.1. above.

3.2.2. Preparation of Supernatants Containing LIF

3.2.2.1. Heparinized whole blood is diluted 1:2 with PBS and gently layered over 10 ml of Ficoll–Hypaque solution in a 50-ml conical plastic centrifuge tube.

3.2.2.2. Each tube is centrifuged at 400 g for 20 min in a PR2 International Centrifuge, using gradual acceleration of the centrifuge to avoid disruption of the gradient.

3.2.2.3. The mononuclear cells concentrated at the Ficoll–Hypaque–plasma interface are carefully removed and transferred to another 50-ml conical centrifuge tube. Complete medium consisting of RPMI 1640 supplemented with HEPES buffer (25 mM), glutamine (1%), 10% heat-inactivated fetal bovine serum, and gentamicin (50 μg/ml) is added to each tube, and the tubes are centrifuged at 200 g for 10 min to sediment the mononuclear cells. Complete medium is added to the cell pellet, the tube vigorously vortexed until no clumps of cells are evident and again centrifuged at 200 g for 10 min.

3.2.2.4. The cells are resuspended in 10 ml of complete medium, counted, and adjusted to a concentration of 5 $\times$ 10^6 mononuclear cells/ml. One-milliliter volumes of the suspended cells are dispensed into 12 $\times$ 75 mm snap-capped plastic tubes.

3.2.2.5. Appropriate antigen concentrations, or complete medium alone, are added in 1-ml volumes to duplicate tubes. The tubes are incubated at 37°C in a humidified 5% CO$_2$ incubator for 2 hrs.

3.2.2.6. The tubes are then centrifuged at 200 g for 10 min to pellet the cells, and the supernatant containing the antigen is aspirated and replaced by 1 ml of complete medium without antigen. The mononuclear cell cultures are then incubated at 37°C in a humidified 5% CO$_2$ incubator for 3 days.

3.2.2.7. The tubes are then centrifuged at 200 g for 10 min, and the supernatant fluid from each lymphocyte culture is transferred to a 1-dram glass vial and stored at −96°C until the time of assay.

3.2.2.8. Twofold dilutions of culture supernatants are tested for inhibition of migration of polymorphonuclear cells, as described below.

3.2.3. Preparation of Polymorphonuclear Cells

3.2.3.1. Whole blood (20 ml) is drawn from the antecubital vein of a normal donor into a 50-ml plastic syringe containing 0.4 ml of heparin (5000 U/ml).

3.2.3.2. The blood is gently expressed from the syringe down the inside of a 50-ml conical plastic centrifuge tube containing Plasmagel (1 ml of Plasmagel/6 ml of whole blood) and allowed to settle at 1 g for 1 hr at 37°C.

3.2.3.3. The leukocyte-rich plasma layer is carefully aspirated from the top of the erythrocyte layer with a pipette. A 2–3 ml volume of plasma just above the erythrocyte layer is not collected. The leukocyte-rich plasma is then diluted with 2 parts of phosphate-buffered saline (PBS) in a 50-ml conical centrifuge tube and carefully layered onto a Ficoll–Hypaque gradient (10 ml Ficoll–Hypaque/30 ml diluted leukocytes) in a 50-ml conical plastic centrifuge tube and centrifuged at 400 g in a PR2 International centrifuge for 20 min.

3.2.3.4. The mononuclear cell layer in the Ficoll–Hypaque gradient is discarded by vacuum suction as is the remaining supernatant. The pellet of cells (largely polymorphonuclear cells with some red blood cell contamination) is saved and immediately diluted with 10 ml of McCoy's 5A medium, containing 10% heat-inactivated fetal bovine serum, HEPES buffer, and 100 μg of gentamicin per milliliter (complete medium).

3.2.3.5. This polymorphonuclear cell suspension is centrifuged at 200 g for 10 min in a PR 6000 International Centrifuge at room temperature. The plasma is discarded from the cell pellet, and the pellet is then resuspended in 10 ml of warm complete media. The cells are resuspended with vigorous vortexing until no visible clumps remain. The polymorphonuclear cells are again centrifuged at 200 g for 10 min at room temperature. The supernatant is aspirated and discarded from the cell pellet.

3.2.3.6. Ten milliliters of complete medium are again added to the cell pellet, and the cells are vigorously vortexed until no clumps are evident. The cell concentration is adjusted to 2×10^7 polymorphonuclear cells per milliliter with complete media.

3.2.4. Mixing of Polymorphonuclear Cells and Agarose. All subsequent procedures with the polymorphonuclear cells are identical to those performed for the direct agarose microdroplet assay described in Section 3.1.3. except that 0.1 ml of culture supernatants is added to each droplet in replicates of four. Control supernatants, i.e., supernatants incubated for 3 days with only antigen without mononuclear cells, or supernatants from mononuclear cells incubated for 3 days in the absence of antigen, are also added (0.1 ml) to replicate wells. These latter supernatant controls constitute the control values used in calculating the migration indices.

4. Critical Comments

4.1. Plasmagel facilitates the sedimentation of the red blood cells from the leukocyte-containing plasma. This separation procedure yields a population of cells containing lymphocytes and polymorphonuclear cells, both of which are required for the direct agarose test. Minor red blood cell contamination of the leukocyte preparation following the plasmagel procedure does not interfere with the test, and no attempts are made to lyse the remaining red cells.

4.2. A 0.2% final concentration of marine colloid (Seakem) agarose remains liquefied at 37°C and is optimal for the assay. A higher final concentration of agarose interferes with good movement of cells from the droplet, and a lower concentration of agarose results in slippage of droplets when medium is added to the wells.

4.3. The agarose droplets should be added to the Microtest plate while it is sitting at room temperature. When there is high humidity, prechilling the plate or setting the plate on an ice bath while adding the droplets may cause rapid water condensation within the wells. Addition of agarose droplets to wet wells causes a wide and nonuniform dispersion of the droplet. Addition of medium to such wells causes slippage of droplets.

4.4. The agarose droplets should be allowed to solidify at room temperature for 1–3 min, and then medium should be added rapidly thereafter, before droplets start to dry.

4.5. The 0.1 ml of medium has to be added carefully to the wells, to prevent loosening or otherwise disturbing the agarose droplet. Movement of the droplet may cause some asymmetrical migration of cells. With these precautions, good symmetrical patterns of migration usually occur at the end of the test.

4.6. Addition of at least 0.1 ml of medium to the wells containing agarose droplets is important. Addition of less than 0.1 ml of medium (e.g., 0.05 ml) will not sufficiently cover the agarose droplet, and some drying of the droplet may occur.

4.7. In performing the direct microagarose assay one can preincubate the antigen with the leukocytes prior to addition to the agarose. With some antigens this may result in more efficient interaction with the leukocytes. However, with the soluble antigen preparations that we have employed, particularly PPD, addition of antigen into the medium works well in inducing inhibition of migration of cells. The addition of antigens in the medium, rather than preincubation with cells, considerably simplifies the handling of the leukocyte suspensions, and permits the setting up of a larger number of wells with small numbers of cells.

4.8. Polymorphonuclear cells migrate very rapidly and when performing indirect agarose assays the results should be read within 16–18 hr after setting up the test. Incubation for longer periods of time may result in movement of the cells to the outer periphery of the well, making reading difficult. Direct assays employing leukocytes should be read at 18–24 hr.

4.9. A level humidified CO_2 incubator should be used to incubate the plates. Lack of moisture in the incubator may result in drying out of the wells.

4.10. In evaluating the final migration patterns, only the dense outer areas of cell migration should be drawn. Some sparse, scattered cells beyond this dense area will be observed but are omitted from this evaluation.

4.11. Use of highly soluble antigens such as PPD work well in both the direct and indirect agarose microdroplet assays. Addition of crude soluble or particulate tumor extracts made by 3 M KCl and saline extraction procedures or whole tumor cells work well in the generation of supernatants for indirect testing. These more crude antigen materials do not appear to be as effective in the direct assay with cancer patients when they are added directly to the media without a preincubation step, although reactivity can be detected. Thus, it would seem that the direct assay as described here may have more application with completely soluble antigenic materials.

4.12. One advantage of the direct assay is that results can be obtained within 18–24 hr, whereas the indirect assay requires 4 days to complete. The indirect assay, however, appears to have the advantage of being capable of using crude antigen materials or whole tumor cells in generating supernatants containing lymphokine.

4.13. As little as picogram and nanogram concentrations of PPD have been effective in causing inhibition of migration of leukocytes from some PPD skin reactive donors in the direct agarose assay. This assay should prove quite useful in broad dose–response testing with a variety of solubilized and partially purified antigens, including human tumor-associated antigens, using leukocytes from as little as 2–5 ml of whole blood.

REFERENCES

1. Rocklin, R., *J. Immunol.* **112**, 1461 (1974).
2. Harrington, J. T., and Stastny, P., *J. Immunol.* **110**, 752 (1973).
3. Harrington, J. T., *Cell. Immunol.* **12**, 476 (1974).
4. McCoy, J. L., Jerome, L. F., Dean, J. H., Cannon, G. B., Alford, T. C., Doering, T., and Herberman, R. B., *J. Natl. Cancer Inst.* **53**, 11 (1974).
5. McCoy, J. L., Jerome, L. F., Dean, J. H., Cannon, G. B., Connor, R. J., and Herberman, R. B., this volume, Method 57.

60

Clinical Detection and Monitoring of Tumor-Specific Cell-Mediated Hypersensitivity (TCMH) in Man: Examinations of Hypernephroma with Leukocyte Migration Technique*

Mogens Kjaer and Gunnar Bendixen

1. Use and Applications

Increasing evidence supporting the hypothesis that tumor-specific, cell-mediated hypersensitivity (TCMH) is important for the limitation and elimination of malignant tumor growth has raised an urgent need for methods that can be used for (a) large series of patients and (b) repeated examinations in longitudinal studies of TCMH in man. Registration of intracutaneous, delayed-type hypersensitivity to tumor antigens (1–4), lymphocyte transformation technique, and lymphocyte cytotoxicity techniques (5–8) have been employed for investigation of TCMH in man, but complicated methodology has impeded the application of the latter two principles in prospective clinical trials on tumor patients, where a large number of analyses are needed.

In vitro registration of cell-mediated hypersensitivity (CMH) in man by measuring antigen-induced migration inhibition directly on the white cell population from peripheral blood was introduced by Søborg and Bendixen in 1967 (9) and has since then been widely used in several modifications for detection of CMH to, for example, microbial, haptenic, organ-specific, or transplantation antigens. The usefulness of this technique for detection of TCMH in man was first reported by Andersen *et al.* (10), who examined a small series of patients with mammary carcinoma. A great many similar studies in various human tumors have been reported since then (11–16) and have confirmed that peripheral blood white cell migration inhibition techniques in a certain proportion of cases can detect TCMH in a considerable variety of spontaneously occurring, malignant tumors in man. So far, however, more extensive studies on a single tumor type using strictly standardized technique with dose–response titrations of antigens, definition of antigenic strength, and longitudinal examinations during a clinical course have not been made, and it has therefore been impossible to evaluate

*The present studies have been supported by The Danish Society for Cancer Research and The Danish Medical Foundation.

whether the leukocyte migration inhibition test (LMT) could be developed into a useful tool in human clinical tumor research and in the diagnosis and follow-up of the individual patient.

Renal carcinoma in man was selected as a human tumor model that could be conveniently be explored, and the technique described below has been used to answer the following questions:

a. Can TCMH against hypernephroma in man be detected by the LMT?

b. Is there autologous reactivity against antigen from the patient's own tumor, and is there allogeneic cross-reactivity between tumors from different patients?

c. Is fetal antigen reactivity involved?

d. Is the antigenic strength nearly the same or highly different in hypernephroma tissue extracts from various patients?

e. How large is the proportion of patients that exhibit TCMH toward hypernephroma antigen at the time of diagnosis, before operation?

f. Can nonreactivity be caused by general immunodeficiency of the patients, or by factors that can be removed from the reacting cells by extensive washings?

g. Is there any significant correlation between TCMH at the time of diagnosis and the clinical course and prognosis?

h. Is it possible to use registration of TCMH to monitor cancer patients during the clinical course?

The results obtained with the present techniques have to some extent been published elsewhere (17–20), and the present report makes reference to these publications and those in progress (21–24), intending especially to give an elaborated description of the techniques.

2. Materials

Material on 210 persons investigated is presented in Table 1. It comprises the following groups.

    2.1. A consecutive series of 49 patients with renal tumor, examined and followed by appointment with the hospitals in the greater Copenhagen area. Histological diagnoses were as follows: hypernephroma 41; renal pelvis transitional cell carcinoma, 2; adenopapilliferous carcinoma, 3; renal sarcoma, 3. At the initial test 32 patients were without, and 17 with, clinically detectable metastases.

    2.2. Seventeen patients with benign renal disease: renal cyst, polycystic renal disease, hypertensive nephropathia, glomerulonephritis, pyelonephritis, and hydronephrosis.

    2.3. Twenty-two patients with carcinoma of nonkidney origin comprising cases of colonic, gastric, pancreatic, mammary, bladder, and lung carcinoma, all without detectable metastases and examined before operation.

TABLE 1
Patient Material Investigated

Material[a]	Men	Women	Age (years)	Total No.
2.1. Renal malignant tumor	32	17	43–80, mean 59	49
2.2. Benign renal disease	10	7	24–78, mean 57	17
2.3. Carcinoma of nonkidney origin	15	7	42–83, mean 64	22
2.4. Various benign diseases	27	18	18–87, mean 47	45
2.5. Blood donors	51	26	20–65, mean 50	77
	135	75	–	210

[a]Numbers refer to section material is discussed in text.

2.4. Forty-five patients with various forms of nonmalignant disease, examined during admission in hospital. They had no signs of malignant or benign tumors, hypertension, or autoimmune diseases and had not received glucocorticoid or cytostatic treatment within the last 6 months.

2.5. Seventy-seven members of the blood donor group of Rigshospitalet, Copenhagen, assumed to be healthy on the basis of a questionnaire concerning earlier diseases and of a set of blood analyses made before recognition as a blood donor. Since the upper age limit of blood donors is 65 years, the mean age of this control group is somewhat lower than that of the renal carcinoma group.

2.6. Technical material and analytical preparations are mentioned in detail in the description of methods.

3. Methods

3.1. Preparation of Tumor and Normal Kidney Extracts. At the operation, immediately after removal of the kidney, tissue specimens are obtained from tumor tissue and from normal kidney tissue not macroscopically invaded by the tumor. This is aseptically performed, always within 30 min after removal of the kidney. The tissue specimens are placed at $-20°C$. On the same or the following day the tissue specimens are thawed, cut into small pieces with scissors, suspended in Hanks' balanced salt solution (HBSS) (Analytical Department, Pharmacy of Rigshospitalet, Copenhagen) and homogenized in an M.S.E. rotating knife tissue homogenizer at 15,000 rpm for 7 min. The homogenates are kept at $4°C$ overnight and then centrifuged at $1000\ g$ for 20 min. The sediment is not used in the routine investigation. The protein concentration of the supernatant is spectrophotometrically determined (Lowry's method) and adjusted at 1 mg/ml by dilution with HBSS containing penicillin G, 1500 IU/ml and streptomycin 1500 μg/ml. Microbiological culture reports of material before the addition of antibiotics are procured to ensure that the tissue extracts are without demonstrable bacterial contamination; 2.5-ml aliquots of the extracts are transferred to sterile glass ampoules and lyophilized. Immediately before use the extracts are redissolved in sterile water. The tumor and normal tissue extracts from the same patient are always prepared simultaneously in parallel procedure. No pooling of tissue extracts is performed.

3.2. Preparation of Fetal Kidney Extract. Tissue extract is prepared by the same procedure as above (Section 3.1) from pooled, human fetal kidneys originating from spontaneous or therapeutic abortions in the third trimester of gestation and without detectable malformations. Material from 4–6 fetuses was pooled in one batch.

3.3. Leukocyte Migration Capillary Tube Technique (LMCT). The LMCT is performed as described by Bendixen and Søborg (25), but micromodified according to Maini *et al.* (26) in the following way: 40 ml of peripheral blood are collected from a cubital vein with moderate hemostasis into 10 ml of Nunclon polysterol tubes (Nunc, Roskilde, Denmark), each containing 250 IU of heparin (Heparin Leo, Ballerup, Denmark) and 2.0 ml of 5% dextran 250 in NaCl, 9.0 mg/ml. The tubes are slowly inverted 10 times and placed for 1 hr at 37°C. The leukocyte-containing supernatants are transferred to soft polyethylene tubes (Thrombotest tubes, Dansk Laboratorieudstyr, Copenhagen, Denmark) and centrifuged at 225 g for 5 min. The cell pellets are resuspended at the original volume with HBSS and washed (routinely 3 times) by similar centrifugations. Care must be taken at this stage to ensure monocellular suspension during all washing procedures and in the final suspension. This is accomplished by injecting HBSS through a needle-mounted syringe upon the pellets in the tubes followed by manual or machine vibration of the tubes. After the final washing in HBSS the cell pellets are resuspended in TC 199 with penicillin, 67 IU, and streptomycin, 67 μg/ml (Difco Laboratories, Detroit, Michigan) containing 10% horse serum without preservatives (State Serum Institute, Copenhagen, Denmark; batch number is important, since all batches are not equally good). Cell suspensions from all tubes are at this stage pooled to obtain a definite and final concentration of 2.2 × 10^8 cells/ml. Aliquots of cell suspension containing 3 × 10^6 leukocytes are transferred to a suitable number of 20-μl glass capillary tubes, internal diameter 0.6 mm (Drummond Hemocaps, Drummond Scientific Supplies, Broomall, Pennsylvania). The capillary tubes are sealed by melting one end in a flame and centrifuged at 900 g at room temperature for 10 min. The capillaries are cut with a glass file just below the cell–fluid interface to avoid clotting of the tube opening by thrombocytes. Immediately after cutting, each tube is placed in a 0.5-ml culture chamber (disposable polystyrene chamber for cell migration; Sterilin Ltd., Middlesex, England) containing the same TC 199 medium with 10% horse serum as described above. The capillary tubes are fixed at the floor of the chambers by a small lump of silicone wax (Dow Corning Corp.) on the melted end of the tube. Care must be taken that the whole length of each tube rests on the chamber floor. Tissue extract preparations are added to the culture chambers according to experimental schedule; the chambers are filled to the brim with culture medium and sealed with a microscope cover slip, retained by silicone wax. All cultures in all concentrations of tissue extract employed are made in quadruplicate. After 24 hr at 37°C, the migration areas of leukocytes around the capillary tube openings are studied in a projection microscope, drawn on paper, cut, and weighed. Within one set of identical quadruplicates the variation from one culture area to another should not be permitted to exceed 5% (27). The average migration areas of a set of tissue extract-containing cultures (M_x) and a set of control cultures (M_0) containing only the culture medium, from the same blood sample, are used to calculate the migration index (MI):

$$MI = M_x/M_0$$

An MI below 1.0 accordingly indicates tissue extract-induced inhibition; and an MI greater than 1.0, tissue extract-induced stimulation of the leukocyte migration.

3.4. Cell Washing Effect. The leukocyte suspension is divided into three aliquots that are washed 3, 6, or 10 times, respectively, before the LMCT incubation described above. The tissue extract-induced alteration of migration of these differently washed leukocytes is examined in a parallel series in the individual tests to obtain information on alterations of reactivity after extensive cell washing (21).

3.5. Test Protocol. The patients are admitted consecutively to the investigation on basis of renal arteriography, irrespective of the clinical stage at the time of initial treatment. If subsequent surgery reveals carcinoma of the kidney, the patients are included in the series. If benign disease is found, the patients serve as controls. Beginning preoperatively, 3–8 tests are performed in each patient. In each patient at least two renal carcinoma extracts and corresponding normal kidney extracts are employed at concentrations of 10, 50, 100, 300, 400, and 600 μg/ml. Only, nonpooled, renal carcinoma tissue extracts with a defined antigenic strength expressed as MIS (see below) of more than 20% and corresponding normal, renal tissue are used. Over the total test period from the first preoperative to the last postoperative day at hospital 3–8 different antigens are used for each patient. After the postoperative period, the patients are followed in the outpatient clinic every third month. After completion of a series of examinations in one patient the results of the LMCT are collected and a titration curve is drawn as exemplified in Figs. 1–4. Groups of control patients (Sections 2.2, 2.3, 2.4) are tested as far as possible according to the same protocol; blood donors, however (Section 2.5), only once.

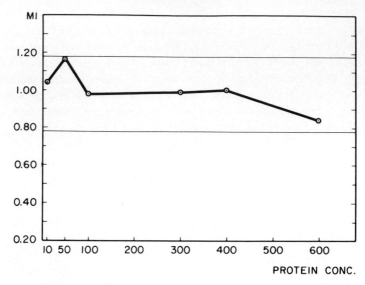

Fig. 1. Titration curve (allogeneic hypernephroma) from a patient with hypernephroma with extensive skeletal and pulmonary metastases. Grade 0.

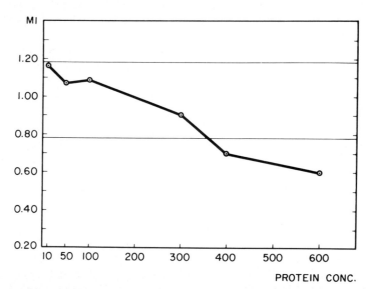

Fig. 2. Titration curve (allogeneic hypernephroma) from a patient with hypernephroma without distant metastases. Grade 1.

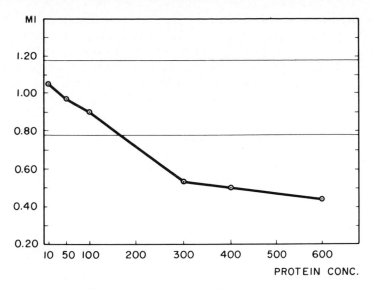

Fig. 3. Titration curve (allogeneic hypernephroma) from a patient with hypernephroma without distant metastases. Grade 2.

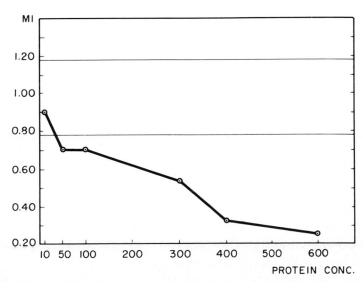

Fig. 4. Titration curve (allogeneic hypernephroma) from a patient with hypernephroma without distant metastases. Grade 4.

3.6. Definition of Antigenic Strength. The antigenic strength of each tumor extract is determined by its capacity to induce significant leukocyte migration inhibition in allogeneic combinations in hypernephroma patients without distant metastases. This capacity is expressed in this study as a migration inhibition score (MIS) (expressed as percent) for each of 24 different tumor extracts, calculated in the following way.

$$MIS = \frac{\text{number of positive tests}}{\text{total number of negative tests}}$$

As elsewhere discussed in detail (23), the MIS seems to be an *in vitro* correlate of tumor antigenicity *in vivo*. The MIS of 24 tumors examined in this way varies between 0 and 60%. In the overall examination only tumor extracts with an MIS exceeding 20% are used.

3.7. Statistical Evaluation. Significant migration inhibition is defined as the mean $\pm$ 2 SD of the MI in the control groups (Sections 2.2–2.5) using the maximal, nontoxic concentration of tumor extract, which is 400 μg/ml in both autologous and allogeneic combinations. For fetal kidney extract, 100 μg/ml was nontoxic. The ranges, as previously discussed in detail (19), are as follows: For tumor extracts, MI = 0.79 to 1.19; for fetal kidney extract, MI = 0.78 to 1.18. A numerical grading of TCMH is made for each patient based on the lowest tumor extract concentration giving significant migration inhibition/stimulation. This grading is exemplified in Figs. 1–4.

Grade 0: MI > 0.79, MI < 1.19 at all tissue extract concentrations employed except 600 μg/ml (Fig. 1)
Grade 1: MI < 0.79, MI > 1.19 at 400 μg/ml, but not at lower concentrations (Fig. 2)
Grade 2: MI < 0.79, MI > 1.19 at 400 and 300 μg/ml, but not at lower concentrations (Fig. 3)
Grade 3: MI < 0.79, MI > 1.19 at 400, 300, and 100 μg/ml, but not at lower concentrations
Grade 4: MI < 0.79, MI > 1.19 at 400, 300, 100, 50, or 10 μg/ml (Fig. 4)

This grading of TCMH (21) can be statistically correlated to clinical, histopathological, and survival data of the patients. A computerized, combined Fischer's exact probability test (modification of the Westenberg interquartile range test), Wilcoxon, Mann-Whitney, and Lepage test have been used for comparing groups of data in the present studies; level of significance = 5%.

4. Interpretation of Data and Critical Comments

4.1. Dose-Related Effect. Figure 5 shows an example of the LMCT reactivity in a patient with hypernephroma without distant metastases compared to a normal person (blood donor), using allogeneic hypernephroma extract at con-

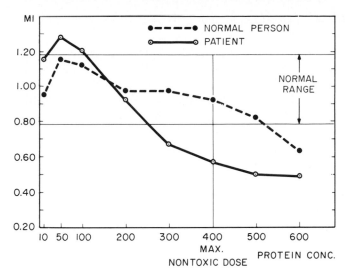

Fig. 5. Titration curves (allogeneic hypernephroma) from a patient with hypernephroma (o———o) without distant metastases and a control patient (blood donor) (●– – –●). Maximal nontoxic dose = 400 μg of protein per milliliter. Normal range at 400 μg/ml, MI = 0.79–1.19.

centrations of 10–600 μg/ml. The specifically altered reactivity of the hypernephroma patient is evident at 300 and 400 μg/ml, whereas 600 μg/ml induces a migration inhibition of both normal and patient leukocytes (19, 20). Use of allogeneic hynephroma tissue extract in prospective studies on renal carcinoma patients and controls confirm a dose-related response at 100, 300, and 400 μg/ml as compared to the control groups. A clear toxic effect is evident in all persons at 600 μg/ml (20).

4.2. Specificity of the Reaction. The following types of tissue extract were used: (a) fetal kidney tissue, pooled; (b) autologous renal carcinoma tissue; (c) autologous normal renal tissue corresponding to (b); (d) allogeneic renal carcinoma tissue; (e) allogeneic normal renal tissue corresponding to (d).

According to the above-mentioned criteria for significant reactivity, the patients tested with extracts of fetal kidney, autologous tumor, and allogeneic hypernephroma during the preoperative period showed significant reactivity in the following proportion of cases: 12/23 = 52% of patients showed reactivity toward fetal kidney tissue, 13/18 = 72% showed reactivity toward autologous tumor, and 23/49 = 47% showed reactivity toward allogeneic hypernephroma (18, 20).

Cross-reactivity in the LMCT between both fetal kidney tissue and allogeneic hypernephroma is a predominant feature in renal carcinoma patients (18–20). When the preoperative tests are compared in patients examined with all three types of tissue extract, it clearly appears that reactivity toward autologous tumor and fetal kidney tissue is fairly common in patients who have TCMH (expressed as inhibition in the LMCT) against allogeneic tissue of the same histological type (20). In some cases, positive reaction to allogeneic hypernephroma extract was found in patients with renal carcinoma histologically different from hypernephroma, e.g., transitional cell carcinoma, adeno-papilliferous carcinoma, or renal sarcoma (18, 20).

4.3. Relation between TCMH and Clinical Stage. Results of preoperative LMCT in renal carcinoma patients clearly show that significant reactivity is confined almost exclusively to patients without distant metastases, and that the same reactivity is found with extracts of allogeneic tumor tissue, autologous tumor tissue, and fetal kidney tissue extracts (18–20).

4.4. Causes of Nonreactivity in Patients with Disseminated Disease. Usually three washings were used before incubation of leukocytes in the migration chambers. By using 6 or 10 leukocyte washings before incubation, the frequency of positive reactions can be increased in patients with distant metastases, suggesting removable coating of lymphocytes by factors inhibiting their reactivity. The factor (circulating tumor antigen?) can be demonstrated in the supernatants after cell washing, and in serum from some patients with hypernephroma (17, 21, 22).

4.5. Survival. A highly significant correlation between initial, preoperative LMCT reactivity and survival after operation can be demonstrated ($p = 0.017$), suggesting that the response detected *in vitro* is directed toward rejection antigens present in the tumor (20, 24).

4.6. Monitoring. Figures 6–8 show the reactivity of a patient with renal carcinoma in the LMCT using allogeneic hypernephroma tissue extract at concentrations from 10 to 600 $\mu g/ml$, and with 3, 6, or 10 leukocyte washings before incubation in the migration chambers. At operation the patient had lymph node metastases, but no other signs of disseminated disease. In the preoperative test (Fig. 6) the response was grade 1, using 3 cell washings, but grade 3 using 6 and 10 washings. The patient was postoperatively treated with extracorporeal immunohemadsorption of circulating tumor antigen as described by Langvad *et al.* (28). After one series of treatments, the response was grade 2 at 3 cell washings and grade 3 at 6 washings (Fig. 7). After three further series, the response was still grade 2 at 3 cell washings, but grade 4 using 6 leukocyte washings (Fig. 8). The patient is still monitored, alive and tumor-free. In a preliminary way this exemplifies how the LMCT can be used for monitoring the effect of treatment in patients with renal carcinoma.

4.7. Selection of Migration Inhibition Technique. A one-step assay (25) in which the antigen-exposed, specifically reacting cell population is mixed with the migrating cell population is preferable for routine use because the procedure is less time- and resource-consuming than two-step assays (29). The use of tissue

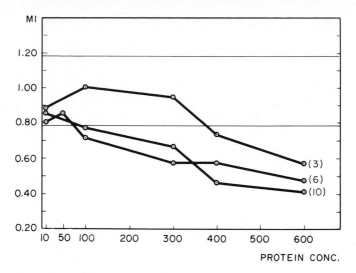

Fig. 6. Titration curves (allogeneic hypernephroma) from a patient with hypernephroma with regional lymph node but without distant metastases. Preoperative response using 3, 6, and 10 leukocyte washings before incubation in the migration chambers. At 3 washings = grade 1, at 6 washings = grade 3, at 10 = grade 3.

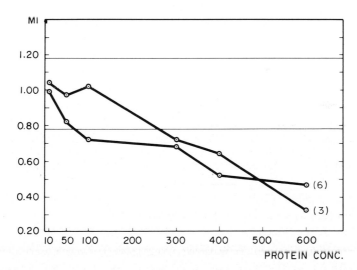

Fig. 7. Titration curves (allogeneic hypernephroma) from the patient shown in Fig. 6. Postoperative response after one series of immunehemabsorption. At 3 washings = grade 2, at 6 washings = grade 3.

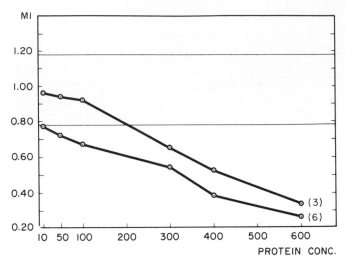

Fig. 8. Titration curves (allogeneic hypernephroma) from the patient shown in Figs. 6 and 7. Response after a total of 4 series. At 3 washings = grade 2, at 6 washings = grade 4.

extracts as antigen also speaks in favor of selecting a direct technique, since an indirect technique would anyway be hampered by admixture of crude tissue extracts with numerous unknown cell components influencing the second step. In the long run, two-step techniques would be preferable from several points of view, but would presuppose highly purified antigen preparations that are not at our disposal at the present stage of development. Therefore, the choice of method was confined to the capillary tube migration technique (LMCT) or the agarose migration technique (LMAT) (30). The LMCT in its original modification as described by Søborg and Bendixen and Bendixen and Søborg (9, 25) was found to be too cell-consuming, since it was necessary in our experimental protocol to include a comparatively large number of simultaneous cultures and therefore too large amounts of blood from the individual patient in the repeated, longitudinal studies. The micromodification of the LMCT described by Maini *et al.* (26) represents an advantage at this point and was compared to the LMAT described by Clausen (30). These studies clearly showed (31) that the LMAT with the antigenic preparations employed could not be used, since significant results were not obtained in parallel experiments with positive performance of the LMCT. Direct LMCT was therefore selected as the standard method in the investigation.

4.8. Selection of Technique for Antigen Preparation. It was considered to be of primary importance to obtain an antigen preparation that contained the tumor-specific components in a form that could be expected to react with specifically reactive lymphocytes in the test system. At this initial stage of the project, it was found advisable to avoid fractionation of the antigen-containing tumor tissue material, because such procedures might exclude fractions with antigenic activity. A similar argument behind examinations in various organ-specific, autoimmune diseases had led to development of a preparation technique, which had yielded tissue extracts with antigenic activity in the LMCT (32–34), and it was found reasonable to adopt the identical antigen preparation procedure in the present project.

4.9. General Comments. A reactivity in the LMCT to crude tissue extracts of tumor material can be interpreted in different ways. Since the difference of reactivity is significant between normal kidney tissue and tumor kidney tissue in a test system that permits autologous comparison, a different reactivity in the parallel trials must be associated with components, which are present in the tumor, not in the normal tissue. It would be reasonable to assume that such cell components were expressions of malignant transformation of cells originating from the corresponding normal parenchyma, that they were macromolecules constituting a part of the cytoplasmic matrix or membranes of the tumor cells, and that they, being macromolecules, would possess antigenic potency—in brief: tumor antigens. The clear correlation between the presence of TCMH *in vitro* and tumor disease survival supports the assumption that tumor antigens in hypernephroma are the molecular target in the immunological *in vivo* elimination of tumor cells. The LMCT detects cell-mediated hypersensitivity *in vitro,* probably owing to the release of LIF from antigen-stimulated, precommitted lymphocytes. Migration inhibition in the present system was found associated with use of tumor tissue extract in the migration cultures, unassociated with autologous and allogeneic, normal kidney extracts. The most probable explanation, therefore, is that the LMCT in the present modification detects TCMH against tumor antigen in hypernephroma tissue. Fetal kidney extract seems to contain antigenic determinants with a similar capacity, which is not very surprising since otherwise-derived fetal organs are known to contain antigenic material that can cross-react with tumor antigen from corresponding, adult tumor tissue.

It is considered of the utmost importance to perform titration with several concentrations of antigen in each test, since this is the only way to obtain convincing evidence as to the cause of migration inhibition: Is it immunologically specific, or is it "toxic"? Such titrations are indispensable, if the present assay is applied, and can be accomplished only if a micromodification of the LMCT with limited amounts of blood for each examination is employed. A further developed micromodification of the technique would be desirable.

Obviously, the "antigen" preparation used in this system is unsatisfactory. An extremely complicated mixture of proteins and cell constituents are permitted to interact in a noncontrolled way in the test system, and the significance of the reactivity and the final conclusions mainly rest upon the significant difference between the reactivity of tumor patients and the reactivity of control persons, examined in series with tissue extract preparations that come as close as possible, except for their tumorous or nontumorous origin. Better antigen preparations have to be developed, and the hypernephroma model in man as studied by the LMCT seems well fit for development work with purification and definition of tumor-associated antigenic components.

REFERENCES

1. Oren, M. E., and Herberman, R. B. *Clin. Exp. Immunol.* **9**, 45 (1971).
2. Bluming, A. Z., Vogel, C. C., Ziegler, J. L., and Kiryabwire, W. M., *J. Natl. Cancer Inst.* **48**, 17 (1972).
3. Hollinshead, A., Glew, D., Bunnag, B., Gold, P., and Herberman, R., *Lancet* **1**, 1191 (1970).
4. Hollinshead, A. C., Stewart, T. H. M., and Herberman, R. B., *J. Natl. Cancer Inst.* **52**, 327 (1974).
5. Stjernswärd, J., Vánky, F., and Klein, E., *Br. J. Cancer* **28**, Suppl. 1, 72 (1973).
6. Vánky, F., Klein, E., Stjernswärd, J., and Nilsonne, U., *Int. J. Cancer* **14**, 277 (1974).
7. O'Toole, C., Cell-mediated immunity to carcinoma of the urinary bladder in man. Clinical correlations of the response and the nature of the effector cells. Department of Immunology, Wenner-Gren Institute, Stockholm, Sweden, 1973.
8. Heppner, G., Henry, E., Stolbach, L., Cummings, F., McDonough, E., and Calabresi, P., *Cancer Res.* **35**, 1931 (1975).
9. Søborg, M., and Bendixen, G., *Acta Med. Scand.* **181**, 247 (1967).
10. Andersen, V., Bjerrum, O., Bendixen, G., Schiødt, T., and Dissing, I., *Int. J. Cancer* **5**, 357 (1970).
11. Segall, A., Weiler, O., Genin, J., Lacour, J., and Lacour, F., *Int. J. Cancer* **9**, 417 (1972).
12. Cochran, A. J., Thomas, C. E., Spilg, W. G. S., Grant, R. M., Cameron-Mowat, D. E., Mackie, R. M., and Lindop, G., *Yale J. Biol. Med.* **46**, 650 (1973).
13. Cochran, A. J., Grant, R. M., Spilg, W. G. S., Mackie, R. M., Ross, C. E., Hoyle, D. E., and Russell, J. M., *Int. J. Cancer* **14**, 19 (1974).
14. Black, M. M., Leis, H. P., Shore, B., and Zachrau, R. E., *Cancer* **33**, 952 (1974).
15. McCoy, J. L., Jerome, L. F., Dean, J. H., Cannon, G. B., Alford, T. C., Doering, T., and Herberman, R. B., *J. Natl. Cancer Inst.* **53**, 11 (1974).
16. McCoy, J. L., Jerome, L. F., Dean, J. H., Perlin, E., Oldham, R. K., Char, D. H., Cohen, M. H., Felix, E. L., and Herberman, R. B., *J. Natl. Cancer Inst.* **55**, 19 (1975).
17. Kjaer, M., *Acta Pathol. Microbiol. Scand. Sect. B* **82**, 294 (1974).
18. Kjaer, M., *Eur. J. Cancer* **10**, 523 (1974).
19. Kjaer, M., *Eur. J. Cancer* **11**, 281 (1975).
20. Kjaer, M., and Bendixen, G., *Ann. N. Y. Acad. Sci.* in press (1976).
21. Kjaer, M., *Eur. J. Cancer* in press (1976).
22. Kjaer, M., and Thomsen, M., *Acta Path. Microbiol. Scand. Sec. C.* in press (1976).
23. Kjaer, M., and Christensen, N., *Cancer Immunol. Immunotherapy* in press (1976).
24. Kjaer, M., *Eur. J. Cancer* in press (1976).
25. Bendixen, G., and Søborg, M., *Dan. Med. Bull.* **16**, 1 (1969).
26. Maini, R. N., Roffe, L. M., Magrath, J. T., and Dumonde, D. C., *Int. Arch. Allergy Appl. Immunol.* **45**, 308 (1973).
27. Kjaer, M., and Bendixen, G., Statistical analysis of the human leucocyte migration test. In preparation.

28. Langvad, E., Hydén, II., Wolf, II., and Krøjgåård, N., *Br. J. Cancer.* **32**, 680 (1975).
29. Clausen, J. E., *J. Immunol.* **110**, 546 (1973).
30. Clausen, J. E., *Acta Allergol.* **26**, 56 (1971).
31. Kjaer, M., and Sørensen, T. B., *Acta Allergol.* **31**, 141 (1976).
32. Bendixen, G., *Acta Med. Scand* **184**, 99 (1968).
33. Bendixen, G., *Gut* **10**, 631 (1969).
34. Nerup, J., Andersen, O. O., Bendixen, G., Egeberg, J., and Poulsen, J. E., *Acta Allergol.* **28**, 223 (1973).

Leukocyte Migration Inhibition in Agarose*

Lynn E. Spitler and Christine Von Müller

1. Introduction

In experimental animals, the direct migration inhibition test, utilizing peritoneal exudate cells, is a good *in vitro* correlate of delayed hypersensitivity; i.e., inhibition of migration by specific antigen correlates well with skin test reactivity to the same antigen (1). When this test is applied to man, it is necessary to modify it in some way since human peritoneal exudate cells cannot be readily obtained.

When migration inhibition tests are applied to the study of human subjects, it is often for the purpose of studying the immune response to antigens, which cannot be used for skin testing, such as tumor or various tissue antigens. In this case, it is first essential to establish that the particular test being utilized is indeed a good correlate of delayed sensitivity. This can be done by first demonstrating a correlation between skin test reactivity and inhibition of migration to standard skin test antigens in normal subjects with the particular test. Unfortunately, many investigators have reported results of migration inhibition in studies in humans without first establishing the reliability of their test.

The indirect migration inhibition test, which involves culture of peripheral lymphocytes and testing of supernatants for activity in guinea pig peritoneal exudate cells, correlates well with skin test reactivity (2, 3) but is difficult and time-consuming to perform. The leukocyte migration test represents a dramatic departure from previously described tests that used peritoneal exudate cells as the indicator cells. In this test, peripheral buffy-coat leukocytes are placed directly into capillary tubes. In this case, the migrating cell population is the polymorphonuclear leukocytes rather than macrophages, and the mediator, termed leukocyte inhibitory factor (LIF), is chemically distinct from the mediator for macrophage migration inhibition or migratory inhibitory factor (MIF) (4). Although inhibition of migration correlates well with skin test reactivity when the test antigen is particulate (5, 6), a number of investigators could not

*Supported by NIH Career Development Award (AI 43012).

confirm the correlation when soluble antigens were used (7, 8) or found a correlation only after considerable effort (9).

A modification of this test was described by Clausen (10) and involved preculturing the buffy-coat leukocytes with antigen and placing them in wells in agarose plates. We found that this test was a good *in vitro* correlate of delayed hypersensitivity in humans using three standard antigens: *Candida,* purified protein derivative of tuberculin (PPD), and streptokinase-streptodornase (SK-SD) (11). The migrating cell population is the polymorphonuclear leukocytes, and the mediator is similar, if not identical, to the LIF that produces inhibition in the capillary tube leukocyte migration test and is distinct from the inhibitor which inhibits macrophage migration (12).

The agarose plate leukocyte migration test is easy to perform, is rapid, and is a reliable correlate of delayed hypersensitivity. It is thus ideal for use in assessing cellular immunity to tumor or tissue antigens. Since the term MIF has usually been associated with macrophage migration inhibition, for purposes of clarity and accuracy it is preferable to term the mediator of this test LIF.

2. Materials (In Order of Use)

2.1. Syringe, 35 ml (Monoject, Cat. No. 535S-R)

2.2. Heparin, 1000 U/ml (Riker Laboratories)

2.3. Dextran, Type 200 c, 234,000 MW, 6% (Sigma, St. Louis, Missouri, Cat. No. D-5126)

2.4. Pediatric scalp vein needle (Abbott 19-G or 21-G)

2.5. disposable tube, 50 ml (Falcon, No. 2074)

2.6. Hanks' balanced salt solution (GIBCO, Grand Island, New York, Cat. No. 402)

2.7. Penicillin–streptomycin, 5000 U/ml, 5000 μg/ml (GIBCO, Cat. No. 506)

2.8. Syringe, 3 ml (Monoject, Catalogue No. 503S)

2.9. Centrifuge (Sorvall RC3 or IEC PR6000)

2.10. Suction bottle

2.11. Pasteur pipettes (Kimble, Catalogue No. 72020)

2.12. Centrifuge tube, 15 ml (Pyrex brand, graduated)

2.13. Medium 199, 1X (GIBCO, Catalogue No. 115E)

2.14. Laboratory microscope (Leitz, SM Lux)

2.15. Hemacytometer (Neubauer, American Optical Co., Buffalo, New York)

2.16. Horse serum (GIBCO, Catalogue No. 605)

2.17. Falcon disposable plastic tubes (Falcon No. 2054)

2.18. Eppendorf pipettes, 50, 30, 7, and 5 μl

2.19. Antigens as desired: tumor antigen, tissue antigen. Standard antigens:

Candida (Dermatophytin "O" undiluted, Hollister-Stier), PPD (Ministry of Agriculture, Fisheries & Food, Central Veterinary Laboratory, New Haw, Weybridge, Surrey, England), SK-SD (Varidase, Lederle Laboratories, American Cyanimid Co.)

2.20. Agarose: Indubiose A37 agarose (Accurate Chemical & Scientific Corp., Hicksville, New York)

2.21. Scale (Metler H2OT)

2.22. Distilled water, pyrogen-free

2.23. Beaker

2.24. Measuring pipette (Falcon No. 7530)

2.25. Sodium bicarbonate, 10X (Baker Catalogue No. 3506)

2.26. Bunsen burner and stand

2.27. Thermometer

2.28. Medium 199, 10 X (GIBCO, Catalogue No. 118E)

2.29. Tissue culture dish (Falcon, Catalogue No. 3002)

2.30. Laminar flow tissue culture hood (Pure Aire Co. Van Nuys, California)

2.31. Steel punch, 2.3 mm diameter (made by local workshop)

2.32. CO_2 incubator (Napco 3331)

2.33. Petri dish (Kimax 100 X 15, Kimble Catalogue No. 23060)

2.34. Gauze (Parke-Davis 2 X 2 inch, 12 ply)

2.35. Measuring magnifier (Bausch & Lomb, Catalogue No. 81-34-35).

3. Method

Use sterile procedure throughout.

3.1. Draw 20 ml of blood into a 35-ml syringe containing 2 ml of heparin.

3.2. Add 5 ml of 6% dextran. Mix well.

3.3. Let sediment in vertical position, needle up, at 37°C for 30–45 mins.

3.4. Add 2 ml of penicillin–streptomycin to 100 ml Hanks' solution. Use this preparation for all subsequent steps calling for Hanks'.

3.5. Add 2 ml of penicillin–streptomycin to 100 ml of Medium 199, 1X. Add horse serum to final concentration of 10%. Use this preparation in subsequent steps requiring medium 199.

3.6. Attach pediatric scalp vein needle and express buffy coat–plasma layer into 50-ml Falcon disposable tube.

3.7. Add Hanks' solution to buffy coat–plasma layer in Falcon tube to make 50 ml.

3.8. Centrifuge at 220 g (1000 rpm) for 5 min at room temperature.

3.9. Remove supernatant.

3.10. Add 5 ml of Hanks'.

3.11. Transfer to 10-ml centrifuge tube.

3.12. Add Hanks' up to 10 ml.

3.13. Centrifuge at 200 g (1000 rpm) for 5 min at room temperature.

3.14. Remove supernatant.

3.15. Add Hanks' up to 10 ml.

3.16. Centrifuge at 220 g (1000 rpm) for 5 min at room temperature.

3.17. Remove supernatant.

3.18. Add Hanks' up to 10 ml.

3.19. Remove aliquot and perform white cell count.

3.20. Centrifuge at 220 g (1000 rpm) for 5 min at room temperature.

3.21. Remove supernatant from cells.

3.22. Resuspend cells in Medium 199 at a concentration of 220×10^6 cells/ml.

3.23. Measure 50 μl of cell suspension into Falcon disposable tubes, one tube for control and one for each test antigen.

3.24. Add 5 μl of test antigen to each tube. Add 5 μl of Medium 199 to the control tube.

3.25. Mix well.

3.26. Incubate for 0.5 hr at 37°C in CO_2 incubator.

3.27. Prepare agarose as follows during preincubation of cells with antigen.

3.28. Weigh 60 mg of agarose.

3.29. Add 6 ml of distilled water to agarose.

3.30. Bring to a boil to dissolve.

3.31. Let cool to 47°C.

3.32. Add 0.6 ml of 10 $\times$ Medium 199 containing 2 ml of penicillin–streptomycin per 100 ml of medium.

3.33. Add 0.6 ml of horse serum.

3.34. Add 1 drop of 10 $\times$ sodium bicarbonate.

3.35. Pour 6 ml of the agarose preparation into Falcon tissue culture dish. Let set.

3.36. Cut holes in agarose with 2.3-mm punch. Cut 3 holes for control cells and 3 holes for each test antigen.

3.37. Place agarose plate in a moist chamber: Invert a large petri dish. Place a piece of gauze in the bottom. Put agarose plate on the gauze. Put smaller part of petri dish on top. Seal by pouring in distilled water.

3.38. Place moist chamber in a CO_2 incubator. The appearance of the plate after migration is illustrated (Fig. 1).

3.39. Prepare cells for reading after 18–24 hr of incubation: Bring distilled water to 90°C in a bowl. Float agarose plate on top of water (kept at 85°–90°C) for 2–3 min. Dip plate into the water and take out very gently, keeping water on the surface. Let stand for 3–5 min, then dip in cold distilled water. The agarose will slip out of the plate. Dip into another bowl of cold distilled water to rinse. Let dry.

3.40. Read and record 2 diameters of migration for each hole using a measuring magnifier.

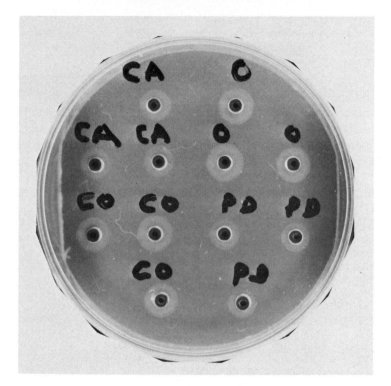

Fig. 1. Petri dish showing inhibition of leukocyte migration of peripheral buffy-coat cells. The donor in this case showed skin test reactivity to PPD and *Candida* but not to coccidioidin. Control wells are the triplicate wells marked O. Inhibition of migration is seen in the triplicate wells labeled PD and CA, but not CO. Note the uniform areas of migration and inhibition.

3.41. Calculate percent migration:

$$\frac{\text{mean area of migration of experimental wells with antigen}}{\text{mean area of migration in control wells without antigen}} \times 100$$

4. Interpretation and Comments

4.1. Less than 80% migration is often considered to indicate a positive result. Alternatively, statistical analysis can be performed in the particular study to determine when inhibition is significant.

4.2. The most difficult aspect of this test is in working out details of the technique to obtain adequate migration of the cells. Once this is worked out, one can regularly obtain adequate migration and inhibition of migration.

4.3. There is considerable difference in the agarose supplied by the various companies. Some will not support migration. Further, there is often variation in results obtained with different lots obtained from the same company.

4.4. When setting up this test with a new antigen, it is necessary to perform a dose—response curve in order to determine the appropriate dose for regular use. The dose selected must be high enough to cause inhibition in subjects who are sensitive to the antigen, but must not be so high that it causes nonspecific inhibition of cells from subjects who are not sensitive to the antigen.

REFERENCES

1. David, J. R., Al-Askari, S., Lawrence, H. S., and Thomas, L., *J. Immunol.* **93**, 264 (1964).
2. Thor, D. E., Jurreziz, R. E., Veach, S. R., Miller, E., and Dray, S. *Nature (London)* **219**, 755 (1968).
3. Rocklin, R. E., Meyers, O. L., and David, J. R., *J. Immunol.* **104**, 95 (1970).
4. Rocklin, R. E., *J. Immunol.* **112**, 1461 (1974).
5. Søborg, M., and Bendixen, G., *Acta Med. Scand.* **181**, 247 (1967).
6. Søborg, M., *Acta Med. Scand.* **182**, 167 (1967).
7. Kaltreider, H. B., Soghor, D., Taylor, J. B., and Decker, J. L., *J. Immunol.* **103**, 179 (1969).
8. Lockshin, M. D., *Proc. Soc. Exp. Biol. Med.* **132**, 928 (1969).
9. Rosenberg, S. A., and David, J. R., *J. Immunol.* **105**, 1447 (1970).
10. Clausen, J. E., *Acta Allergol.* **26**, 56 (1971).
11. Astor, S. H., Spitler, L. E., Frick, O. L., and Fudenberg, H. H., *J. Immunol.* **110**, 1174 (1973).
12. Hoffman, P. M., Spitler, L. E., Hsu, M., and Fudenberg, H. H., *Cell Immunol.* **18**, 21 (1975).

Chemotaxis of Mononuclear Cells

Ralph Snyderman and Marilyn Pike

1. Introduction

Macrophages function to localize and degrade antigenic or denatured materials, promote wound healing, and perhaps protect against the development and spread of neoplasms. These processes are essential to immunologically mediated host defense and depend upon the rapid accumulation of sufficient numbers of these cells at local tissue sites.

One mechanism that could account for the local accumulation of wandering cells, such as macrophages, is chemotaxis, the unidirectional migration of cells along a concentration gradient of a chemoattractant substance. Boyden, in 1962, developed a quantitative assay for the measurement of polymorphonuclear leukocyte chemotaxis *in vitro* (1). Subsequent modifications have expanded this assay to allow the measurement of the chemotaxis of macrophages and blood mononuclear leukocytes (MNL's) (2–6). From studies of macrophage chemotaxis *in vitro* and accumulation *in vivo* (7, 8), it has been demonstrated that these cells migrate toward chemotactic factors produced as a consequence of immunological reactions or tissue breakdown. Furthermore, dysfunctions of monocyte chemotaxis have been shown to have pathophysiological significance in some human diseases and may play an important role in neoplasia (8, 9). In the following discussion, we shall review methodology for the quantification of macrophage and monocyte chemotaxis using mouse, guinea pig, and human cells and the methods for producing chemotactic factors by activating complement or by stimulating lymphocytes.

2. Materials

2.1. Chemotaxis Chambers. These can vary in size and shape, but generally consist of a lower compartment that holds the substance being tested for chemotactic activity and an upper compartment that contains a standardized cell suspension. The two compartments are separated by a porous filter made of either cellulose nitrate or polycarbonate. Figures 1 and 2 are examples of the two types of chemotaxis chambers used by the authors: Fig. 1, modified Boyden

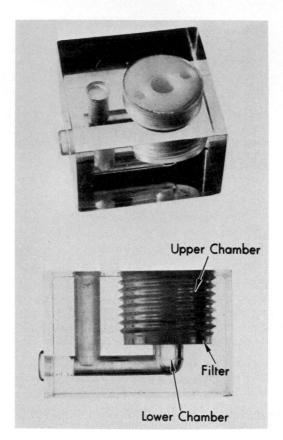

Fig. 1. Modified Boyden chemotaxis chamber. A standardized cell suspension (0.4 ml) is placed in the upper compartment of the chamber and is separated from the chemotactic stimulant or medium alone (0.85 ml) in the lower compartment by a polycarbonate or nitrocellulose filter. From Snyderman *et al.* (10).

type; Fig. 2, blind well chamber (Neuroprobe Inc., Cabin John, Maryland). A chamber similar to the modified Boyden type may also be purchased from Neuroprobe Inc., but both can be made by most good instrument shops.

2.2. Chemotaxis Filters. Two types of filters can be used to measure macrophage chemotaxis *in vitro*. Polycarbonate (Nuclepore) filters with a 5.0-μm pore size can be purchased from Wallabs Inc., San Rafael, California or Neuroprobe Inc., Cabin John, Maryland. These filters are approximately 13 μm thick and have linear through-and-through holes of uniform diameter. Cellulose nitrate filters with an 8-μm pore size can be purchased from the Sartorius Division, Brinkman Instruments, Westbury, New York. These filters are approximately 150 μm thick and have convoluted pores.

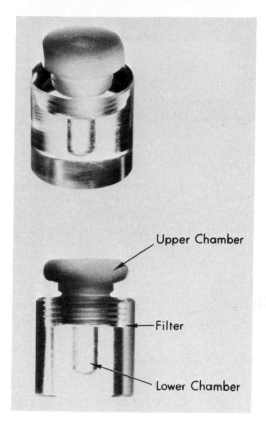

Fig. 2. Blind-well chemotaxis chamber. A standardized cell suspension (0.2 ml) is placed in the upper compartment of the chamber and is separated from the chemotactic stimulant or medium alone (0.2 ml) in the lower compartment by a polycarbonate or nitrocellulose filter.

2.3. Preparation of Human Mononuclear Leukocytes. Human peripheral blood mononuclear leukocytes (MNL's) are isolated on Ficoll–Hypaque gradients as follows: Heparinized (10 U/ml) venous blood is diluted 1:4 in isotonic saline and 35 ml of the mixture is placed in Falcon No. 2070 conical centrifuge tubes. Twelve milliliters of a mixture of Ficoll–Hypaque containing 2.4 parts of 9% Ficoll (Sigma Chemical Co., St. Louis, Missouri) and 1 part of 33.9% Hypaque (Winthrop Laboratories, Atlanta, Georgia) is slowly injected below the diluted blood with a 16-gauge, 4-inch spinal needle attached to a 50-ml syringe. The layered blood is then centrifuged at 400 g at 20°C for 35 min. The buffy coat containing 15–30% monocytes and 70–85% lymphocytes is removed with a 9-inch Pasteur pipette and no more than 10 ml of the cell suspension placed into 50-ml Falcon conical centrifuge tubes. The cells are washed twice at 4°C in 40 ml of phosphate (0.02 M)-buffered (pH 7.0) isotonic saline (PBS) and resuspended to contain 1.5×10^6 monocytes/ml in RPMI 1640 at pH 7.0 (Grand Island Biological Company, Grand Island, New York). While the cell population contains both lymphocytes and monocytes, only monocytes stick to the bottom surface of the chemotaxis filter, and they are the only cells counted by the techniques described herein.

2.4. Preparation of Mouse Peritoneal Macrophages. Mice are injected intraperitoneally with 35 μg of purified phytohemagglutinin (PHA; Burroughs Wellcome Company, Beckenham, England), contained in 2 ml of sterile isotonic saline or with 2 ml of 9% proteose peptone (w/v in water) (Difco Laboratories, Detroit, Michigan). Two days (PHA exudate) or 4 days (proteose peptone exudate) later, mice are sacrificed by cervical dislocation and the peritoneal cavities are exposed by abdominal incision. The cavities are then vigorously lavaged several times using a total volume of approximately 15 ml of Gey's balanced salt solution containing 2% bovalbumin (Flow Laboratories, Rockville, Maryland), 0.01 M HEPES buffer (Calbiochem, La Jolla, California), pH 7.0 (Gey's BSS), and 10 units of heparin per milliliter.

The peritoneal exudate cells (PEC), containing approximately 70% macrophages, 29% lymphocytes, and 1% polymorphonuclear leukocytes, are washed once in Gey's BSS and standardized to contain 2.2×10^6 macrophages/ml in Gey's BSS. Approximately 7×10^6 macrophages are obtained per mouse, and cells from syngeneic animals can be pooled.

2.5. Preparation of Guinea Pig Peritoneal Macrophages. Guinea pigs are injected intraperitoneally with approximately 25–30 ml of 0.5% (w/v) shellfish glycogen in isotonic saline. Four days later the guinea pigs are sacrificed and the peritoneal cavities are exposed and lavaged vigorously with approximately 150 ml of Gey's BSS. The exudate cells contain approximately 75% macrophages and 25% lymphocytes. After one wash, the PEC are resuspended to 1.5×10^6 macrophages per milliliter in Gey's BSS. Approximately 7×10^7 macrophages are obtained per animal.

2.6. Preparation of Human Lymphocyte-Derived Chemotactic Factor (LDCF). Human peripheral blood leukocytes are obtained by sedimentation of heparinized blood with an equal volume of sterilized 3% (w/v) dextran (T500 Pharmacia, Uppsala Sweden) in saline for 20 min at room temperature. After sedimentation, the supernatant is decanted and the cells are washed twice in sterile RPMI 1640, pH 7.2, and standardized to contain 2×10^6 total cells per milliliter in RPMI. Twenty-five milliliters of the cell suspension are placed in sterile 250-ml Falcon No. 25100 plastic tissue culture flasks to which is added 250 μg of concanavalin A (Difco Laboratories, Detroit, Michigan) contained in 5 ml of RPMI 1640. The leukocytes are incubated for 24–48 hours at 37°C in humidified air containing 5% CO_2. After incubation, the supernatant is obtained by centrifugation at 500 g for 10 min. The supernatant containing LDCF is

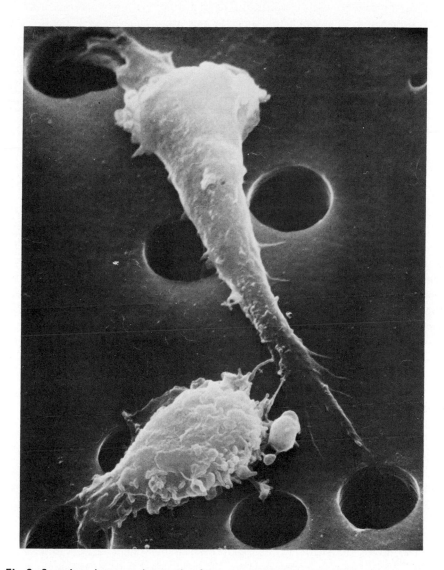

Fig. 3. Scanning electron micrograph of two normal human monocytes which have migrated in response to LDCF to the bottom surface of a polycarbonate filter. The cell at the top has completely emerged from a 5.0 μm pore and has advanced diagonally across the filter's surface. On the lower left, another cell has migrated onto the bottom surface of the membrane. × 4000. From Snyderman and Mergenhagen (11a).

number of cells per field at different depths onto the filter, one can produce migration curves that can help define the migratory behavior of the entire cell population. A method of quantifying chemotaxis using ^{51}Cr-labeled cells in a modified Boyden chamber has recently been described (14). In this method the labeled cells are placed above two filters, and, after a suitable incubation time, the lower filter is counted for gamma radiation. This procedure allows a more objective scoring of chemotaxis but is useful only when homogeneous cell populations are being used.

The methods described herein have provided extremely useful ways for analyzing factors that are chemotactic for macrophages and for factors which affect leukocyte motility. The effects of various drugs or other pharmacological agents on macrophage chemotactic responsiveness can be easily evaluated. For example, we have recently tested (15) the effect on human monocyte chemotaxis of levamisole [(−)-tetramisole], a drug reported to possess immunostimulatory properties. In these experiments, isolated MNL's were incubated with (−)-tetramisole, for 30 min at 37°C and tested for chemotactic responsiveness to LDCF, activated human serum, and a chemotactically active peptide, formylmethionyl-phenylalanine (16). Doses of (−)-tetramisole ranging from 10^{-5} M to 10^{-3} M enhanced the chemotactic responsiveness to all chemotactic factors tested by 20–148% (Table 1). When MNLs were incubated with isomers of (−)-tetramisole; (+)-tetramisole, and p-Br-(−)-tetramisole, only the latter possessed stimulatory activity, indicating that the enhancing effect was stereospecific (Table 1). To determine whether enhancement of monocyte chemotaxis by (−)-tetramisole required binding of the drug to the cells, isolated monocytes were incubated with either (−)-tetramisole alone or with (−)-tetramisole containing (+)-tetramisole and tested for chemotactic responsiveness to LDCF. Figure 4 illustrates that doses of 10^{-4} M and 10^{-3} M (+)-tetramisole reduced the enhancing effect of (−)-tetramisole. The parallel nature of the curves indicated that (+)-tetramisole inhibited the enhancing activity produced by (−)-tetramisole by competitive binding (k_D (−)-tetramisole = 1×10^{-4}, k_D (+)-tetramisole = 0.8×10^{-4}). These results demonstrate the type of data that can be produced with the chemotaxis assay and that the methods provide valuable tools for testing the effect of pharmacological agents on monocyte function.

A new area of investigation allowed by these methods is quantification of human monocyte chemotactic responsiveness and chemotactic lymphokine (LDCF) production in human diseases. We have found that the measurement of the kinetics of LDCF production is a sensitive and reproducible means for analyzing human lymphokine function (4, 5) and, in the author's experience, easier and more reproducible than most assays for lymphokine production in man. Humoral factors that may directly affect the chemotactic response of leukocytes or the activity of chemotactic factors can also be detected using the assays described here. Evaluation of all these parameters of immune effector

TABLE 1
Enhancement of Human Monocyte Chemotactic Responsiveness by (–)-Tetramisole[a]

	Chemotactic activity[c] of monocytes in response to		
Monocytes incubated with[b]	LDCF[d]	AHS[e]	fMet-Phe[f]
Medium alone	43.9±3.6	79.5±6.3	36.0±3.0
(–)-Tetramisole			
$1 \times 10^{-3}\,M$	98.0±1.0	114.8±7.3	89.4±1.7
$1 \times 10^{-4}\,M$	73.9±6.9	107.6±10.2	53.1±4.3
$1 \times 10^{-5}\,M$	59.1±0.3	95.4±1.3	44.9±5.3
p-Br-(–)-tetramisole			
$5 \times 10^{-5}\,M$	82.5±6.8	–	–
$1 \times 10^{-5}\,M$	61.7±3.5	–	–
$1 \times 10^{-6}\,M$	49.8±2.1	–	–
(+)-Tetramisole			
$1 \times 10^{-3}\,M$	49.8±5.3	–	–
$1 \times 10^{-4}\,M$	49.2±2.0	–	–
$1 \times 10^{-5}\,M$	45.5±5.6	–	–

[a]Adapted from Pike and Snyderman (15).
[b]Isolated human monocytes were suspended (1.5×10^6/ml) in medium containing various molar concentrations of the indicated isomers of tetramisole or in medium alone. After incubation (37°C for 30 min) the monocytes were placed in the upper compartment of a modified Boyden chamber and tested for chemotactic responsiveness.
[c]Chemotactic activity is expressed as the average number of monocytes migrating completely through a 5.0 μm polycarbonate filter per oil immersion field ($\times 1540$) ± SEM.
[d]Lymphocyte-derived chemotactic factor (LDCF) was obtained from supernatants of concanavalin A-stimulated lymphocyte cultures. LDCF was diluted to 15% (v/v) in RPMI 1640 for use as a chemotactic stimulant.
[e]Activated human serum (AHS) was prepared by incubation of normal serum with *Salmonella typhosa* endotoxin (1 mg/ml serum) for 60 min at 37°C followed by 56° for 30 min. AHS was then diluted to 0.5% (v/v) in RPMI 1640 for use as a chemotactic stimulant.
[f]Formylmethionylphenylalanine (fMet-Phe) was diluted to 10^{-6} moles/liter of RPMI 1640 for use as a chemotactic stimulant.

function can be expected to enhance our understanding of the pathophysiology of inflammatory, infectious, and neoplastic diseases.

A strong word of caution must, however, be added concerning the clinical application of the chemotaxis assay. Since it is biological in nature, the assay can be quite variable, especially if not routinely performed. Variability among normals should be expected, and adequate controls must be used before a patient's chemotaxis is said to be abnormal. When factors are added to cells to determine whether they affect chemotaxis, it must be determined whether the factors are chemotactic themselves or toxic to cells. If they are chemotactic, the

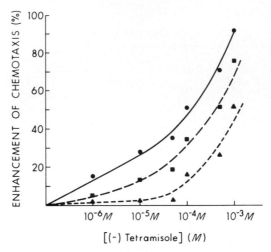

Fig. 4. Competitive inhibition of (–)-tetramisole-enhancing effect on monocyte chemotactic responsiveness by (+)-tetramisole. Isolated monocytes were incubated (37°C × 30 min) with medium containing 10^{-6} to 10^{-3} M (–)-tetramisole alone, or with 10^{-6} to 10^{-3} M (–)-tetramisole plus 10^{-3} M or 10^{-4} M (+)-tetramisole and tested for chemotactic responsiveness to LDCF (15%, v/v). K_D (–)-tetramisole = 10^{-4}, K_D (+)-tetramisole = 0.8×10^{-4}. ●——●, No (+)-tetramisole; ■— —■, $10^{-4} M$ (+)-tetramisole; ▲– – –▲, $10^{-3} M$ (+)-tetramisole.

$$\% \text{ enhancement} = \left(\frac{\text{chemotactic responsiveness of cells incubated with drugs}}{\text{chemotactic responsiveness of cells incubated with medium alone}} -1 \right) \times 100$$

From Pike and Snyderman (15).

gradient for migration will be diminished and chemotactic factors will appear to be inhibitors of directed cell movement.

It is becoming increasingly apparent that accurate means of measuring immune effector function will be necessary for our understanding of the biological role of the immune system in general, and its pathophysiological role in human disease. The chemotaxis assays and future improvements thereof can provide more tools for probing the mechanisms of a most central aspect of immune function, the accumulation of inflammatory cells.

ACKNOWLEDGMENTS

R. S. is a Howard Hughes Medical Investigator. Research supported in part by United States Public Health Service Grant R01 DEO 3738-03, Allergy Center Grant P 50 AI 12026-03, and National Cancer Institute Contract N01 CP 3313.

REFERENCES

1. Boyden, S., *J. Exp. Med.* **115,** 453 (1962).
2. Ward, P. A., *J. Exp. Med.* **128,** 1201 (1968).

3. Snyderman, R., Shin, H. S., and Hausman, M. S., *Proc. Soc. Exp. Biol. Med.* **138,** 387 (1971).
4. Snyderman, R., Altman, L. C., Hausman, M. S., and Mergenhagen, S. E., *J. Immunol.* **108,** 857 (1972).
5. Altman, L. C., Snyderman, R., Oppenheim, J. J., and Mergenhagen, S. E., *J. Immunol.* **110,** 801 (1973).
6. Wahl, S. M., Altman, L. C., Oppenheim, J. J., and Mergenhagen, S. E., *Int. Arch. Allergy Appl. Immunol.* **46,** 768 (1974).
7. Postlethwaite, A. E., and Snyderman, R., *J. Immunol.* **114,** 274 (1975).
8. Snyderman, R., Pike, M. C., Blaylock, B. L., and Weinstein, P. J., *Immunol.* **116,** 585 (1976).
9. Snyderman, R., Pike, M. C., and Altman, L. C., *Ann. N. Y. Acad. Sci.* **256,** 386 (1975).
10. Snyderman, R., Pike, M. C., McCarley, D., and Lang, L., *Infect. Immun.* **11,** 488 (1975).
11. Snyderman, R., Gewurz, H., and Mergenhagen, S. E., *J. Exp. Med.* **128,** 259 (1968).
11a. Snyderman, R., and Mergenhagen, S. *in* "Immunobiology of the Macrophage" (D. S. Nelson, ed.), p. 323. Academic Press, New York, 1976.
12. Zigmond, S. H., and Hirsch, J. G., *J. Exp. Med.* **137,** 387 (1973).
13. Zigmond, S. H., *In* "Chemotaxis, Its Biology and Biochemistry," (Sorkin, E., ed.), *Antibiot. Chemother. (Basel)* **19,** 126 (1974).
14. Gallin, J. I., Clark, R. A., and Kimball, H. R., *J. Immunol.* **110,** 233 (1973).
15. Pike, M. C., and Snyderman, R. *Nature (London)* **261,** 136 (1976).
16. Schiffman, E., Corcoran, B. A., and Wahl, S. M., *Proc. Natl. Acad. Sci. U.S.A.* **72,** 1059 (1975).

Chemotaxis under Agarose: A Method for Measurement of Spontaneous Migration and Chemotaxis of Polymorphonuclear Leukocytes and Monocytes from Human Peripheral Blood

Robert D. Nelson, Richard L. Simmons, and Paul G. Quie

1. Introduction

Directed migration of leukocytes in a chemical gradient was first observed by Leber in 1888 (1) in excised rabbit ocular tissue. Since this behavior of migratory cells provided a possible explanation for the accumulation of polymorphonuclear leukocytes (PMN's) and monocytes at sites of inflammation, attempts were made to study chemotaxis *in vitro*. This phenomenon was subsequently observed with leukocytes placed in a capillary tube (2), between a slide and cover slip (3, 4) and on a cover slip incubated in a humid atmosphere (5). These methods are all relatively simple, but they are also time consuming owing to the large number of cells that must be observed individually to obtain statistical significance.

Introduction of the membrane filter technique by Boyden in 1962 (6) greatly facilitated the study of leukocyte chemotaxis. The "Boyden chamber" consists of an upper and a lower compartment separated by a membrane filter. The cells and chemotactic agent are placed in the upper and lower compartments, respectively. Chemotaxis is measured by counting the number of cells that have traversed the filter and reached the bottom side. With this method, soluble chemotactic factors are simple to introduce and quantitation of the response is easier and more reproducible. Subsequent modifications of this technique have involved use of: a cytocentrifuge to apply the cells to the filter (7, 8); a double filter to prevent migrating cells from falling into the lower chamber (9); ^{51}Cr-labeled cells to eliminate enumeration of migrating cells (10); shorter incubation periods to permit quantitation by measurement of the advancing front (11); and filters of larger pore size to allow penetration by monocytes (12).

The methods based upon the migration of leukocytes through a filter meet with difficulties attributable to cell adhesion to the filter material and to variations in tortuosity and size of the pore channels (13). Consequently, the use of different filters may be necessary to study spontaneous and directed migration of PMN's or chemotaxis of PMN's and monocytes, thereby complicating comparisons of these events.

In this chapter we describe a new and simple method for studying human leukocyte chemotaxis *in vitro*. This method, like that introduced by Cutler (14) for guinea pig PMN's, is based upon migration of cells under agarose gel, as described by Carpenter (15) for explanted tissue fragments and used by Clausen (16) and others (17–19) to study lymphokine-mediated inhibition of leukocyte migration. Without modification, this technique permits quantitation of both spontaneous migration and chemotaxis of both PMN's and monocytes by linear movement.

The study of leukocyte migration using the agarose method also offers several additional advantages over use of the membrane filter technique. The agarose method is more rapid, easier to quantitate, requires smaller amounts of blood, and uses disposable equipment. The migrating cells can also be observed over time and photographed *in situ* or can be easily prepared for subsequent histochemical staining or electron microscopy.

2. Materials

2.1. For Isolation of Peripheral Blood Leukocytes

Anticoagulant: sodium heparin (Upjohn, Kalamazoo, Michigan, 10 U per milliliter of blood

Cell suspension medium: minimum essential medium (MEM) supplemented to contain 2 mM glutamine, 100 units of penicillin and 100 μg of streptomycin per milliliter (all from Grand Island Biological Co., GIBCO, Grand Island, New York, or equivalent)

Cell separation medium: lymphocyte separation medium (LSM) (Bionetics Laboratory Products, Kensington, Maryland or equivalent)

2.2. For Generation of Chemotactic Factors.
Bacterial chemotactic factors (BFE) are obtained from *Escherichia coli* culture filtrates by the method of Ward *et al.* (20). Zymosan-activated serum (ZAS) is prepared by the method of Ward *et al.* (21). For a list of other factors that have chemotactic properties for peripheral blood leukocytes, consult Wilkinson (22).

2.3. For Preparation of Migration Plates

Tissue culture plates: 60 X 15 mm (No. 3002, Falcon, Oxnard, California, or equivalent)

Agarose: We have used Indubiose A37 and Litex (Accurate Chemical and Scientific Corp., Hicksville, New York) and agarose for use in electrophoresis (Sigma Chemical Co., St. Louis, Missouri) with equal success. Some variation in chemotaxis using agarose preparations with different lot numbers has been observed.

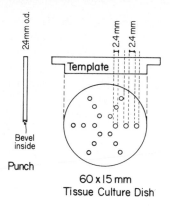

Fig. 1. Dimensions of tissue culture dish and the template and punch employed to form and align wells in the agarose gel. A maximum of six replicates of the triplicate wells are made to eliminate overlap of adjacent gradients. From Nelson *et al.* (24). Reprinted with permission from *J. Immunol.* and Williams & Wilkins Co., publisher.

Tissue culture medium: minimum essential medium (MEM), 10X (GIBCO, or equivalent); 7.5% sodium bicarbonate (GIBCO, or equivalent)

Pooled human serum: serum from 3–5 healthy donors, of any ABO type and with no history of hepatitis or blood transfusion, is pooled and decomplemented by heating at 56°C for 30 min.

Template and punch: constructed from plexiglass according to dimensions provided in Fig. 1.

2.4. For Quantitation of Migration. Cells are fixed using absolute methanol, technical grade, and buffered formalin and stained with Wright's stain. For projection and measurement of migration we use a microprojector with a 43X objective, (Tri-Simplex, Bausch and Lomb, Rochester, New York).

3. Methods

3.1. Isolation of Leukocytes. Unpurified polymorphonuclear leukocytes (WBC) are obtained by centrifugation of whole blood in 15-ml tubes at 200 *g* for 15 min. The plasma is removed and centrifuged at 750 *g* for 20 min to remove platelets. The buffy-coat leukocytes, together with the upper 0.5–1.0 cm of erythrocytes are removed and resuspended in the platelet-free plasma, and the contaminating erythrocytes are sedimented by gravity at 37°C. The WBC are recovered from the leukocyte-rich plasma by centrifugation at 200 *g* for 15 min. Removal of the majority of erythrocytes by centrifugation prior to the gravity sedimentation step results in the recovery of significantly larger volumes of leukocyte-rich plasma and numbers of WBC from most donors. The WBC are washed three times in MEM, differential counts are made using 0.01% gentian violet in 1.5% acetic acid as diluent, and the cells are resuspended in MEM at a concentration of 2.5×10^7 PMN per milliliter for culture.

To obtain purified polymorphonuclear leukocytes (PMN's) and mononuclear leukocytes (MNC), WBC are first removed as described above. The WBC are suspended at a concentration no greater than 2×10^7/ml and 8–10-ml volumes of this cell suspension are layered over 3 ml of LSM in 15-ml tubes. After centrifugation at 400 g for 35 min (23), mononuclear cells are recovered from the MEM–LSM interface and PMN's from the sediment. The cells are washed 3 times in MEM, counted, and resuspended in MEM at concentrations of 2.5×10^7 PMN's/ml and 10^8 MNC/ml for culture.

3.2. Preparation of Agarose Plates. Agarose is dissolved in sterile, distilled water at a concentration of 0.024 g/ml by heating in a boiling water bath for 10–15 min. After cooling in a 48°C water bath, the agarose is mixed with an equal volume of prewarmed (48°C) MEM diluted to 2X and supplemented to contain 20% decomplemented pooled human serum and 1.5 mg of sodium bicarbonate per milliliter. Five milliliters of the agarose medium are delivered to each culture dish, and the agarose is allowed to harden at room temperature. To prepare 20 ml of agarose medium, the formula becomes:

Agarose: 0.24 g of agarose in 10 ml of sterile, distilled water
Medium: 2.0 ml of 10X MEM, 2.0 ml of pooled human serum, 0.2 ml of
              7.5% sodium bicarbonate, and 5.8 ml of sterile, distilled water

The dishes are then transferred to the refrigerator for 30–60 min to facilitate cutting of the wells. Six series of three wells, 2.4 mm in diameter and spaced 2.4 mm apart, are cut in each plate, using the punch and template described in Fig. 1. The agarose plugs are plucked out using a hypodermic needle or can be drawn out using a disposable Pasteur pipette attached to a vacuum. Removal of the plugs by the vacuum method requires a pipette or tubing smaller than the diameter of the well; attachment of a vacuum line to the punch results in distortion of the wells. Use of the template is essential, in our experience, since it permits reproducible alignment of the wells and prevents alteration of the agarose–plastic interface, which can influence cell migration. Care must also be taken not to score the plastic with the punch since scratches become a barrier to cell migration. Adjustment of pH following refrigeration and cutting of the wells can be accomplished by placing the plates in the incubator in an atmosphere of 5% CO_2 in air for 15–30 min. During this preincubation step the plates can be stored in an inverted position to prevent the wells from filling with fluid.

3.3. Chemotaxis Assay. The center well of each 3-well series receives a 10-μl volume of the cell suspension. At the cell concentrations noted above, 10 μl will contain WBC representing 2.5×10^5 PMN's, or 10^6 MNC. Since mononuclear cell populations contain 15–30% monocytes, this number of MNC represents approximately 2.5×10^5 monocytes. The outer well receives 10 μl of chemotactic factor, i.e., bacterial factor in *E. coli* culture filtrate (BFE) or C5a in zymosan-activated serum (ZAS). The inner well receives 10 μl of the appropriate nonchemotactic, control medium, i.e., culture medium or heat-inactivated pooled human serum.

The culture dishes are incubated at 37°C in a humidified atmosphere containing 5% CO_2 in air. After incubation for 2 hr for WBC and PMN and 10–18 hr for MNC, the cells are fixed with the agarose in place by flooding the plates with 3 ml of methanol for 30 min and 3 ml of formalin for 30 min. When time is not available to complete fixation and staining, the dishes can be stored with methanol overnight at 4°C. In this situation do not use more than 3 ml of methanol, as larger volumes excessively dehydrate the agarose and make it

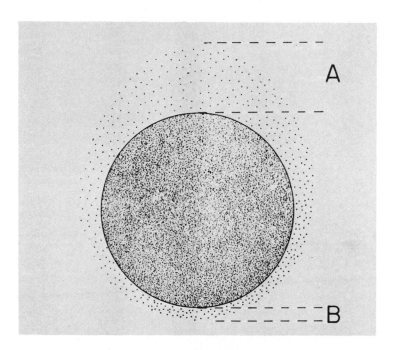

Fig. 2. Pattern of differential migration in response to chemotactic factor. Quantitation of chemotaxis is done by projecting the pattern onto a white background and measuring the linear distance the cells have migrated from the margin of the well toward the chemotactic factor (distance *A*: chemotaxis) and the distance the cells have migrated from the margin of the well toward the control medium (distance *B*: spontaneous migration). The "chemotactic index" is represented by *A/B* and the "chemotactic differential" by *A−B*. From Nelson *et al.* (24). Reprinted with permission from *J. Immunol.* and Williams & Wilkins Co., publisher.

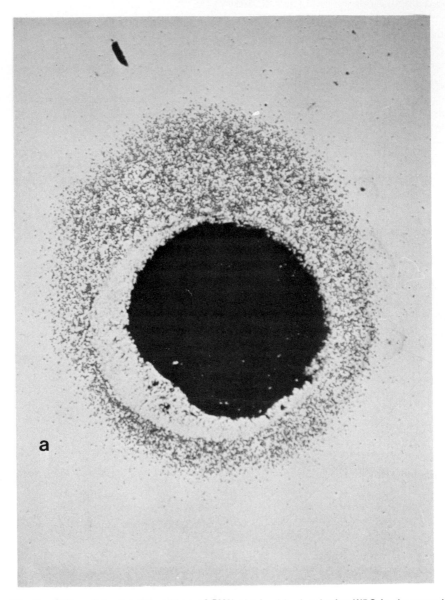

Fig. 3a. Differential migration pattern of PMN obtained by incubating WBC in the central well, BFE in the outer well, and MEM in the inner well for a period of 2 hr. Reprinted with permission from *J. Immunol.* and Williams & Wilkins, Co., publisher.

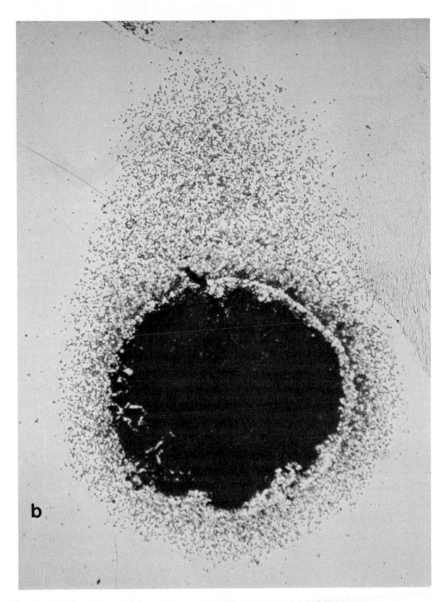

Fig. 3b. Differential migration pattern of PMN obtained by incubating WBC in the central well, ZAS in the outer well, and PHS in the inner well for a period of 2 hr. From Nelson *et al.* (24). Reprinted with permission from *J. Immunol.* and Williams & Wilkins Co., publisher.

difficult to remove intact. After fixation, the gel is removed by inverting the plate and inserting a narrow spatula along one edge. Rimming the gel is not necessary and may result in smearing of the migration patterns. The plates are rinsed with water, stained with Wright's stain, and air dried.

An alternative and faster method for removal of the gel involves floating the plate on water heated to 60°–90°C for 3–5 min. The plate is then filled with the hot water and transferred to the bench, and the agarose is poured off as it floats up (Mae, Y. H. Hsu, personal communication). Removal of the agarose gel must be preceded by chemical or heat fixation of the migrating cells.

For quantitation of chemotaxis, the migration patterns are projected onto a white background at a magnification of approximately 40X, using a microprojector. With the aid of a compass, a measurement (in cm) is made of the linear distance the cells have moved from the margin of the well toward the chemotactic factor (distance A: chemotaxis) and the linear distance the cells have moved from the margin of the well toward the control medium (distance B: spontaneous migration) (Fig. 2). A "chemotactic index," A/B, and "chemotactic differential," $A-B$, are calculated for each replicate and the mean values and standard deviations determined for $A, B, A/B$, and $A-B$.

Figures 3a and b illustrate typical migration patterns obtained for PMN's with BFE and ZAS as the chemotactic agents, respectively. Figure 4 illustrates a typical migration pattern obtained for monocytes with ZAS as the chemotactic factor. Assays of the chemotactic responses of PMN as WBC and as purified PMN's from 20 healthy donors have been performed to compare the results obtained with these two cell populations. These data are summarized in Table 1. The summary data for monocyte chemotaxis in Table 1 have been derived from 20 healthy donors.

4. Critical Comments and Interpretation of Data

4.1. Proof of Chemotaxis. That the differential migration which occurs in this system is attributable to a chemotactic response has been demonstrated by Nelson *et al.* (24). No migration is observed when the incubation temperature is reduced to 4°C, so movement of cells into the space between the agarose and plate is not due to simple diffusion. Differential migration has been demonstrated with factors known to be chemotactic for PMN's and monocytes. Reduction of the gradient of chemotactic factor by preincubation of the plate before addition of cells or by addition of chemotactic factor to both the outside well and the well receiving cells results in a reduction of the chemotactic indices, $A, A/B,$ and $A-B$. Finally, on extended incubation of PMNs, the cells migrating toward the negative control well come under the influence of the developing gradient and reverse their direction of migration.

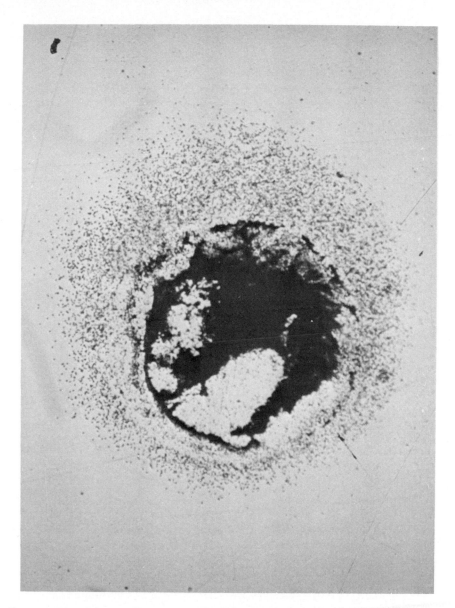

Fig. 4. Differential migration pattern of monocytes obtained by incubating mononuclear cells in the inner well, ZAS in the outer well, and PHS in the inner well for a period of 18 hr. From Nelson *et al.* (24). Reprinted with permission from *J. Immunol.* and Williams & Wilkins Co., publisher.

TABLE 1
Summary Data for Chemotaxis of PMX and Monocytes under Agarose

		A^c	B	A/B	$A-B$
WBC[a]	$\bar{x} \pm$ SD	2.9 ± 0.7	0.8 ± 0.2	3.8 ± 0.9	2.1 ± 0.6
BFE[b]	Range	$2.1 - 4.1$	$0.6 - 1.1$	$2.8 - 5.7$	$1.4 - 3.1$
PMN	$x \pm$ SD	3.2 ± 0.8	1 ± 0.2	3.3 ± 0.4	2.2 ± 0.6
BFE	Range	$1.7 - 3.9$	$0.6 - 1.3$	$2.6 - 3.7$	$1.1 - 2.8$
WBC	$\bar{x} \pm$ SD	2.8 ± 1.5	0.8 ± 0.1	3.7 ± 0.9	1.9 ± 1.4
ZAS	Range	$1.1 - 4.8$	$0.6 - 1.1$	$1.4 - 5.8$	$0.5 - 3.9$
PMN	$\bar{x} \pm$ SD	3.9 ± 1.3	1.0 ± 0.2	3.7 ± 0.9	2.9 ± 1.0
ZAS	Range	$1.3 - 4.8$	$0.7 - 1.5$	$1.0 - 4.9$	$0.6 - 4.2$
MNC	$\bar{x} \pm$ SD	5.3 ± 1.4	3 ± 1	1.8 ± 0.2	2.3 ± 0.5
ZAS	Range	$3.3 - 6.5$	$1.7 - 4.2$	$1.6 - 2.1$	$1.7 - 2.7$

[a]WBC denotes unpurified PMN; PMN denotes purified PMN; MNC denotes mononuclear cells.
[b]BFE denotes *Escherichia coli* bacterial factor; ZAS denotes zymosan-activated serum.
[c]A and B denote chemotaxis chemotaxis and spontaneous migration, respectively; A/B denotes chemotactic index; $A-B$ denotes chemotactic differential.

4.2. Optimal Cell Numbers and Incubation Time. The influence of cell number and incubation time on the migration differential have also been discussed by Nelson *et al.* (24). Using numbers of PMN's greater than 2.5×10^5 per well results in increased values for both A and B. The chemotactic differential, $A-B$, is not influenced by cell number, but the chemotactic index, A/B is greatest with 2.5×10^5 PMN's per well. When smaller numbers of PMN's are used, the migration patterns become too diffuse, making measurement of A and B more difficult.

The optimal time for termination of cultures for PMN chemotaxis has been chosen considering the relationship of the chemotactic indices to time. The numerical values of A/B and $A-B$ have been maximal at 2 hr in the majority of assays. Measurement of monocyte chemotaxis requires an incubation period greater than 2 hr due to the reduced rate of migration of these cells. Migration of monocytes is seldom observed before 6 hr of incubation. The chemotactic index, A/B, is not influenced by incubation time, although the chemotactic differential,

$A-B$, may continue to increase with incubation extended to 18 hr. We have arbitrarily chosen to terminate cultures for monocyte chemotaxis at 18 hr.

4.3. Factors Influencing Cell Migration. We have attempted to reduce the time required to obtain leukocyte-rich plasma by addition of 2.5 × 10⁶ MW dextran, but have found this treatment to reduce rates of migration. Removal of contaminating erythrocytes by hypotonic lysis does not affect cell migration. Contamination of MNC populations by platelets can, however, have an inhibitory effect on the migration of these cells.

Preliminary experiments also suggest that the anticoagulant may influence cell migration. Spontaneous migration of PMN's and monocytes has been less with heparin (1.2 and 2.9 cm) than with EDTA (1.8 and 4.4 cm) and ACD (1.5 and 4.5 cm). The chemotactic indices, A/B and $A-B$, however, are not influenced by the anticoagulant. Cells obtained from defibrinated blood do not migrate.

Our use of serum in the agarose medium is a potential source of criticism. Although three preparations of heat-inactivated pooled human serum have not been chemotactic when tested against MEM in this system, heat-stable factors with chemotactic properties could occur in some serum preparations. Agarose medium supplemented to contain 1% human serum albumin may be substituted for agarose medium containing pooled human serum. Some protein must be present to permit removal of the agarose. Concentrations of albumin or serum greater than 1 and 10%, respectively, inhibit cell migration.

4.4. Quantitation of Chemotaxis. The basis for the geometrically different migration patterns observed for PMN's using BFE and ZAS as chemotaxins is not known. Dilution of BFE and ZAS up to 50% does not alter these patterns. PMN's may, therefore, be more sensitive to the gradient of ZAS than of BFE.

Quantitation of chemotaxis and spontaneous migration with a single method makes chemotaxis under agarose a very powerful and clinically important tool. This methodology should simplify distinguishing between defects in these separate cell functions. In studies of patients, all measurements of chemotaxis, i.e., A, B, A/B, and $A-B$, are important, although the chemotactic index, A/B, may have special significance. The chemotactic index should permit identification of the patient whose PMN's or monocytes exhibit defective spontaneous migration but normal chemotaxis. For example, the chemotactic differentials (A−B) for $A = 4.0$ cm and $B = 1.0$ cm (normal spontaneous migration) and $A = 1.2$ cm and $B = 0.3$ cm (defective spontaneous migration) are 3 cm and 0.9 cm, respectively, and would suggest defective chemotaxis in the latter situation. The chemotactic indices (A/B) for both situations, however, are equivalent. Since chemotaxis denotes an increased directional migration, the cells from both donors must respond to the chemotaxin gradient to the same degree for the A/B values to be equivalent. A reduced rate of spontaneous migration simply prevents the cells from one donor from migrating normal distances.

When necessary, quantitation of chemotaxis can be accomplished more quickly by viewing the migrating cells *in situ* using a microscope with an appropriate ocular micrometer (14) or grid (25). This procedure would also permit time-course studies of a single population of migrating cells.

We have compared the use of WBC and purified PMN's for quantitation of PMN chemotaxis for clinical studies. Comparing the results obtained with these cell populations (Table 1), it appears that purification of PMN's is not necessary. Purification of PMN's reduces the variation between replicates within an experiment, which may be more of an advantage for other studies. Preliminary parallel studies comparing chemotaxis measured with the membrane filter and agarose methods indicates that concordant results are obtained with both techniques. The exception is noted above: the patient's cells, which exhibit abnormal spontaneous migration, but normal chemotaxis.

ACKNOWLEDGMENTS

The authors wish to acknowledge the technical assistance provided by Ms. Linda Walburg, Mrs. Leyla Mazoleny, Ms. Gail Hanson, and Mr. Robert McCormack in completing this study. Research supported in part by the Departments of Laboratory Medicine and Pathology, Pediatrics and Surgery, University of Minnesota School of Medicine, Minneapolis, Minnesota, and by United States Public Health Service Grants AI 12402 and CA 11605, NCI Contract No. N01-CB 43948, and grants from the Kidney Foundation of the Upper Midwest, Minnesota Heart Association, and the University of Minnesota Graduate School.

REFERENCES

1. Leber, T., *Fortschr. Med.* **6,** 460 (1888).
2. Ketchel, M. K., and Favour, C. B., *J. Exp. Med.* **101,** 647 (1955).
3. Commandor, J., *C. R. Soc. Biol.* **80,** 314 (1917).
4. McCutcheon, M., Wartman, W. B., and Dixon, H. M., *Arch. Pathol.* **17,** 607 (1934).
5. Harris, J., *J. Pathol. Bacteriol.* **66,** 135 (1953).
6. Boyden, S., *J. Exp. Med.* **115,** 453 (1962).
7. Baum, J., Mowat, A. G., and Kirk, J. A., *J. Lab. Clin. Med.* **77,** 501 (1971).
8. Hill, H. R., Mitchell, T. G., Hogan, N. A., and Quie, P. G., *J. Lab. Clin. Med.* **86,** 703 (1975).
9. Keller, H. U., Borel, J. F., Wilkinson, P. C., Hess, M. W., and Cottier, J., *J. Immunol. Meth.* **1,** 165 (1972).
10. Gallin, J. I., Clark, R. A., and Kimball, H. R., *J. Immunol.* **110,** 223 (1973).
11. Zigmond, S. H., and Hirsch, J. G., *J. Exp. Med.* **137,** 187 (1973).
12. Snyderman, R., Altman, L. C., Hausman, M. S., and Mergenhagen, S. E., *J. Immunol.* **108,** 857 (1972).
13. Keller, H. U., and Sorkin, E., *Proc. Soc. Exp. Biol. Med.* **126,** 677 (1967).
14. Cutler, J., *Proc. Soc. Exp. Biol. Med.* **147,** 471 (1974).
15. Carpenter, R. R., *J. Immunol.* **91,** 803 (1963).
16. Clausen, J. E., *Acta Allergol.* **26,** 56 (1971).
17. Astor, S. H., Spitler, L. E., Frick, O. L., and Fudenberg, H. H., *J. Immunol.* **110,** 1174 (1973).

18. Weisbart, R. H., Cunningham, J. E., Bluestone, R., and Goldberg, L. S., *Int. Arch. Allergy Appl. Immunol.* **45,** 612 (1973).
19. Ax, W., and Tantz, C., *Behring Inst. Mitt.* **54,** 72 (1974).
20. Ward, P. A., Lepow, I. H., and Neuman, L. H., *Am. J. Pathol.* **52,** 725 (1968).
21. Ward, P. A., *J. Exp. Med.* **128,** 1201 (1968).
22. Wilkinson, P. C., "Chemotaxis and Inflammation." Churchill Livingstone, London, 1974.
23. Böyum, A., *Scand. J. Clin. Lab. Invest.* **21,** Suppl. 97, 77 (1968).
24. Nelson, R. D., Quie, P. G., and Simmons, R. L., *J. Immunol.* **115,** 11650 (1975).
25. Ramsey, W. S., *Exp. Cell Res.* **70,** 129 (1972).

Cultivation, Characterization, and Identification of Human Tumor Cells

Jørgen Fogh, Maureen Goodenow, James Loveless, and Helle Fogh

1. Introduction

1.1. General Considerations. Until recently, it has been the general consensus that human tumor cells are extremely difficult to culture, and that continuous *cell lines* are very rarely established. Progress in this field of research, particularly during the last few years, now presents us with a different picture (1). Not only have numerous attempts to produce *early cultures* of human tumor cells been successful, but the number of cell lines, established by many investigators, has increased considerably. Cells from most types of tumors are available as lines for the various areas of research for which such cells are pertinent. For certain studies, the tumor cells after a short period of cultivation may be preferable. In other experiments, the number of cells required, and the need for repeated samples of similar cells, may dictate the use of established lines. We shall, therefore, in this chapter summarize our experience with early cultures, as well as with lines derived from human tumors. Collection and processing of surgical tumor specimens and effusions, and methods of cultivation of early cultures and lines as they have worked in our laboratory, will be presented and discussed.

It is of utmost importance to obtain assurance that the cultured cells are tumor cells and not, as has often been the case, cells originating from other components of the tumor specimen (2). Also, "extraneous cell contamination" during serial cultivation is a well established risk (3); for example, several of the early established lines, during many years of cultivation, may have become contaminated (with HeLa or other cells), and, therefore, may no longer represent their tumor of origin (4, 5). Consequently, in addition to confirmation of the original specimen's content of tumor cells and all possible steps to avoid culture cross-contamination, new cultures and new lines, as well as already existing lines, must be characterized by methods which can assure that the cells not only exhibit malignant properties, but also are characteristic of the tumor of origin intended for study. Only then can the cultured cells be of real value in experimental and clinical research.

There is some evidence and good reason to assume that tumor specimens obtained from patients in special therapy prior to the time of surgery (for example, chemotherapy, radiation, hormonal, or immunotherapy) may be less suitable for tissue culture attempts. Trivial factors may make the attempts less successful; for example, a long period of time elapsing between surgical removal and preparation of the tissue for culture; contamination with bacteria and fungi; exposure of the surgical specimens to disinfectants, many of which are highly cell toxic; exposure to extreme temperatures, or dehydration of the specimen prior to culture. It is not uncommon that the specimen selected for tissue culture (for example, by operating room personnel) consists only of nonmalignant tissue from the surgical specimen. As a precaution against the loss of time in working with such material, a qualified pathologist should select the specimen from which tissue culture attempts are made. Equally important, part of the specimen received in the tissue culture laboratory should be processed for examination by the pathologist in order to obtain a "confirming diagnosis." Whenever possible, this diagnosis should be obtained rapidly, and a frozen section may be in order (1).

Effusions, pleural or ascitic, may be valuable sources of malignant cells for cultivation. There are often large volumes of material containing tumor cells at high density, and multiple specimens may be obtained from a single patient. Cytologic examination will confirm the presence of tumor cells.

In spite of all precautions taken during the period of collection and preparation for tissue culture, culture attempts may not be successful. Factors relating to the individual donor, and not necessarily to type of tumor, may be pertinent. For example, in an effort with several hundred effusions from breast cancer patients, tumor cells were established in culture from only a small proportion of these, although excellent techniques were employed. However, there were cases where the same patients provided a series of effusions and cell lines were established from each of them (as many as six) (6).

1.2. Human Tumor Cell Lines. By reviewing the known lines of human tumor cells, it is apparent that some types of tumors have yielded established lines much more frequently than others (Table 1). At least 70 lines have been established from malignant melanomas, 41 from glioblastomas, 29 from breast carcinomas, 19 from lung carcinomas, 18 from cervix carcinomas, 15 from colon carcinomas, etc. In contrast, we know of very few lines from tumors of other tissues, and apparently no lines are as yet available from the prostate, stomach, tongue, and male breast, for example. For many tissues some of the more rare tumors are not represented by cell lines. Although these different numbers might be related to the relative frequencies of surgical cases, and thereby to the number of specimens available for tissue culture, there is no doubt that the infrequent establishment of lines from certain tumor types can be explained by particular problems in adapting these cells to the *in vitro* environment, problems that we have not yet identified and solved.

TABLE 1
404 Established Human Tumor Lines

Number of lines per tumor type	Carcinomas	Sarcomas	Miscellaneous tumors
70			Melanoma
41			Glioblastoma
34			Burkitt's lymphoma
29	Breast		
19	Lung		
18	Cervix		
15	Colon		
14		Osteogenic	Neuroblastoma
12			
10		Fibro	Astrocytoma, Hodgkin's
8	Bladder		
7	Renal cell	Rhabdomyo	
6	Ovary	Kaposi's; lipo	
5		Ewing's	Histocytic lymphoma
4	Endometrium, pancreas, submaxillary larynx, liver, rectum, thyroid		
3	Adrenal, bile duct, esophagus, neck, oral, stomach, testis		Giant cell tumor
2			Choriocarcinoma, embryonal carcinoma, meningioma, mesodermal mixed, paraganglioma: Wilms's tumor
1	Duodenum, gall bladder, nasal, pharynx, prostate, vulva	Angio, leiomyo, neuro, synovial	Hamartoma, islet cell tumor, mesothelioma, nephroblastoma, neurilemmoma, neurofibroma, plasmacytoma, retinoblastoma

The many lines collected in our Human Tumor Cell Line Bank are being characterized as to morphology, *in vitro* cytopathology, chromosomal characteristics, capacity to produce tumors in nude mice, G6PD isozyme type, susceptibility to poliovirus, and growth characteristics. This characterization is progressing rapidly (see Section 3, Results), and a number of lines have already qualified by most, or all, criteria as malignant cells with characteristics consistent with derivation from the reported human tumor.

1.3. "Approved Early Cultures" of Human Tumor Cells. Since certain investigations require very early cultures ("distance" between time of surgery and present state of culture may be expressed as number of culture passages or period of time in weeks or months; more correctly it should reflect the number of cell divisions), an effort has been made in our laboratory to preserve, in liquid nitrogen, samples of cells derived from human tumors as soon as an appropriate number of cells is available. Whereas microscopic morophological observations may indicate whether the cultures actually contain tumor cells, some or all of the characterization methods (see Section 2.9) have been applied and, in many cases, have confirmed the presence of tumor cells. Some of these "approved early cultures" have developed into established tumor lines; others have not.

2. Materials and Methods

2.1. Collection of Solid Tumor Specimens. Portions of surgically removed tumor specimens, as selected by the pathologist, are rapidly transported to the tissue culture laboratory. In the pathology laboratory, contact of the specimen with fixatives and disinfectants is completely avoided and sterile instruments are essential. Sterile petri dishes are used when specimens can be cultured immediately; sterile screw-cap jars containing tissue culture medium are more suitable for those specimens that cannot be prepared for culture within 0.5 hr after surgery. The volume of medium is at least five times the tumor specimen volume. Penicillin, 500 U/ml, streptomycin, 500 μg/ml, and fungizone, 30 μg/ml, are added to prevent bacterial and fungal contamination. If culture initiation is delayed beyond a few hours, the specimen is kept at 4°C. The shortest possible time between collection and processing obviously is advantageous.

2.2. Evaluation and Preparation for Culture. The tumor specimen is transferred sterilely to a petri dish containing a few milliliters of tissue culture medium with antibiotics (see Table 2, Wash). Further steps of preparation depend upon the characteristics of the specimen as to size, consistency, color, presence of fat or necrotic areas, and anatomical site. Fatty, bloody, and necrotic portions are eliminated prior to further processing. A representative portion, or portions, of the specimen (a few cubic millimeters) is selected for "confirming diagnosis" and fixed in buffered neutral formalin. The remaining

TABLE 2
Antibiotics for Cultivations of Cells from Human Tumor Specimens[a]

Site of tumor	Wash	Initial culture	Continuous culture
Lung, skin	A	D	G
Esophagus, mouth, nose, pharynx, urinary	B	E	G
Gastrointestinal, gynecological	C	F	G

[a]A = penicillin, 250 u/ml; gentamicin, 250 μg/ml. B = penicillin, 250 u/ml; gentamicin, 250 μg/ml; amphotericin B, 50 μg/ml. C = penicillin, 250 u/ml; gentamicin, 250 μg/ml; amphotericin, 50 μg/ml; clindamycin, 100 μg/ml; chloramphenicol, 50 μg/ml. D = penicillin, 100 u/ml; streptomycin, 100 μg/ml. E = penicillin, 100 u/ml; streptomycin, 100 μg/ml; amphotericin B, 3 μg/ml. F = penicillin, 100 u/ml; streptomycin, 100 μg/ml; amphotericin, 3 μg/ml; clindamycin, 10 μg/ml; chloramphenicol, 5 μg/ml. G = penicillin, 100 u/ml; streptomycin, 100 μg/ml.

part of the specimen is transferred to a second petri dish and washed in several milliliters of tissue culture medium with antibiotics. This washing is particularly necessary for specimens which may be assumed to be contaminated with bacteria and fungi.

2.3. Initiation of Culture. The size and consistency of the specimen determine the method(s) to be used. Enzymatic treatment combined with physical agitation is required to release cells from hard specimens. Soft tumor tissue is cultured as explants or from cells spilled into the fluid as the specimen is cut into small pieces or slices. The choice of medium and concentration of serum for cultures initiated from various types of tumors is listed in Table 3.

2.3.1. Explants. In preparation for explant cultures the tumor specimen is transferred into another petri dish containing a small amount of medium with antibiotics in "initial culture" concentrations (see Table 2). The specimen is minced into pieces of 1–2 mm^3 with a scalpel. The small pieces are carefully placed into culture flasks (5–8 explants per T-30 flask; 8–15 explants per T-60 flask, evenly spaced) to which tissue culture medium has been previously added. This transfer is most easily accomplished by using a Pasteur pipette with a rubber bulb. Culture flasks are handled gently during all following procedures; if not, explants may not attach to the container surface. Cultures are incubated at 36°–37°C.

2.3.2. Spilled Cells. During the mincing of the specimen, many cells are discharged into the medium. This suspension is collected for culture, and cell density, cell sizes, and appearance are evaluated microscopically in a hemacytometer in order to determine the number of tumor cells. The cells are seeded in culture flasks with medium, serum, and antibiotics at densities of 3 × 10^5 to 10^6 cells per milliliter of fluid. They are incubated at 36°–37°C.

TABLE 3
Preferred Medium and Serum Combinations for
Culture of Individual Tumor Types

Tumor type	Medium	% Fetal bovine serum
Carcinoma		
Bladder	TC-512[a] or MEM[b]	26
Breast	MEM or PAP[c]	26
Cervix	PAP or MEM	26
Gastrointestinal	MEM	26
Lung	PAP	26
Ovary	PAP	26
Pancreas	RPMI 1640[d]	26
Renal cell	PAP, MEM or McCoy's 5A[e]	26
Testis	MEM	26
Sarcoma		
Ewing's	McCoy's 5A or RPMI 1640	20–26
Fibro	PAP or McCoy's 5A	10–20
Osteo	MEM or McCoy's 5A	15–26
Rhabdomyo	MEM or McCoy's 5A	15–20
Miscellaneous		
Lymphoma	RPMI 1640 or McCoy's 5A	15
Melanoma	MEM	10–20
Neural	MEM	10–20

[a]See Ref. (7).
[b]See Ref. (8).
[c]See Ref. (9).
[d]See Ref. (10).
[e]See Ref. (11).

2.3.3. Enzymic Treatment/Spinner. Tumor specimens are cut into small pieces and transferred to a trypsinizing flask containing a Teflon stirring bar. An appropriate amount (25 times the tumor volume), of trypsin, at a concentration of 0.25% in calcium- and magnesium-free phosphate-buffered saline, is added. The flask is placed on a magnetic stirring plate at 37°C, and the contents are stirred at a low to moderate speed. At frequent intervals aliquots of the trypsinized cell suspension are removed to determine the number of cells released. The rate of cell release varies among tumors. Extended exposure to the trypsin may be disadvantageous; therefore, it is better to collect the suspended cells and to replace with fresh trypsin frequently in order to obtain the highest number of viable tumor cells from any specimen. To inactivate trypsin, a small amount of serum is added to the collected cell suspension; cells are sedimented by low-speed centrifugation, tumor cells are counted and seeded in appropriate containers at a concentration of 3×10^5 to 10^6/ml and incubated at $36°-37°C$.

2.3.4. Other Methods. Various methods for preparation of human tumor specimens which have been used successfully by other investigators include the following: enzymic separation of the tissue with collagenase (9, 12) or pronase (13–15) and physical separation of tumor cells from stromal cells by Ficoll gradient centrifugation (16). Other cultivation techniques have included the use of perforated cellophane (17, 18); stainless steel grids with tea-bag paper (19, 20); cultivation in agar media (21, 22); growth support by feeder layers (23, 24); microcultures (25, 26). In addition, a variety of media (9, 27) and buffer systems (28, 29) have been employed. Since in most cases only successful attempts have been reported, there is at this time no real basis for comparing the efficiencies of these various techniques.

2.4. Collection, Evaluation, and Processing of Effusions. Collected aseptically, the effusion is rapidly transferred to the tissue culture laboratory. After gentle agitation to disperse the cells, 10–20 ml is fixed with an equal volume of 50% ethanol for cytological evaluation. Bloody and discolored fluid and excessive coagulation may be disadvantageous for culture attempts. Within limits, the presence of red blood cells usually does not interfere with tumor cell attachment; however, very bloody effusions may be processed as follows in order to eliminate the red blood cells: (a) erythrocytes may be removed by slow-speed (70 g) sedimentation of the tumor cells or (b) the pellet resulting from centrifugation at 125 g for 10 min may be resuspended in 9 volumes of sterile distilled water for 60 sec with constant stirring. One volume of 10X concentrated phosphate-buffered saline is added. This suspension is immediately recentrifuged at 125 g for 10 min. After the fluid has been decanted, the pellet is resuspended in a few milliliters of medium and the number of tumor cells per volume is determined from counts in a hemocytometer. Cells are seeded in the medium/serum combination of choice, usually at concentrations of 10^6 cells/ml. Penicillin, 100 U/ml, and streptomycin, 100 μg/ml, serve to protect against contamination. If the fluid does not appear bloody, the cells are sedimented directly from the specimen by centrifugation at 125 g for 10 min.

2.5. Early Observation and Care of Cultures. Minimal disturbance during the first days of cultivation is essential to permit attachment of cells or explants to the surface of the culture vessel. While fluid changing is generally avoided during the first weeks, small amounts of medium with serum or serum alone are added to adjust pH and to supplement nutrients depleted from the medium. Cells which do not attach to the flask surface are never discarded. When the fluid volume becomes too great for the particular culture flask, medium is decanted into a centrifuge tube and the cells are sedimented. Part of the supernatant or "conditioned medium" is added back to the original culture flask and is supplemented with no more than 1 volume of fresh medium and serum. The sedimented cells are resuspended in a small volume of supernatant; the cells may be seeded into a new culture flask with an equal volume of fresh medium and serum or placed back into the original flask if cell attachment there has not been adequate. The developing monolayers are usually not transferred during the first weeks of cultivation.

Whereas some cultures do not contain living cells of tumor cell morphology beyond the first days or weeks, in other cultures they continue to be present in different proportions to the nontumorous stromal or other cells. This quantitative relationship varies among culture attempts from tumors of different origin, among attempts from tumors of similar origin, and even among individual cultures originating from the same tumor specimen. Occasionally, tumor cells divide rapidly, fill up the primary culture within days and, after subsequent transfers, continue to divide readily. More frequently, though, the increase in cells during the early culture period occurs more slowly, and it is not uncommon that cultures appear essentially nondividing for months. During this "adaptation period" cells of tumor cell morphology may be present in some areas (for carcinomas cells frequently in colonies) or they may be dispersed throughout the culture. Floating cells may represent part of the population. A competition between those tumor cells that have, and those that do not have, the capacity to adapt to the culture environment, and between tumor and nontumor cells, for space and nutrition, occurs during this period. The stromal cells may win this battle, and after a few weeks or months there may be no indication of dividing cells of tumor cell morphology. Yet, there have been cultures which after many months of "stalemate" suddenly contain distinct colonies of epithelial tumor cells with the capacity to transfer and divide in subcultures.

In order to build up the supply of cultured tumor cells, they must be transferred to other larger containers in which they must divide. In many cases this task is easy, sometimes it is not. The capacity of the cells to transfer is part of the adaptation to culture, and it appears to be related to the capacity of the tumor cells to divide in this environment. Certain cultures are more easily transferred by scraping and/or subculturing of spontaneously detached cells than by treatment with enzymes or Versene.

In general, when culture flasks are 60–80% confluent, subculturing is attempted as follows: half of the medium and serum is decanted, and a portion of the cells is scraped from the surface of the culture flask using a Pasteur pipette with a rubber bulb. The cells are aspirated in the volume of fluid left in the flask and seeded into a new culture flask. Large clumps of cells may be broken apart by gentle aspiration, but dispersion into single cell suspension is neither necessary nor always beneficial. A small amount of fresh medium and serum is added to the culture flask, and once attachment and proliferation have begun, more medium and/or serum may be added.

Some cultures are transferred as well, or better, with 0.25% trypsin with or without 0.01% EDTA. At this stage, subculturing may not result in increased culture areas but is necessary in order for cells to adapt to transfer.

2.6. Cell Line Establishment. An established cell line has the capability of continuous cell division and of being repeatedly subcultured. When, and if, this stage of culture is arrived at is not easily predicted during the first period. Rate of cell division is not of absolute value for prediction since some cell lines, even after long times and many culture passages, maintain a very slow increase in cell population. However, the rare culture which from the initiation, and during the first culture passages, continues to divide readily is very likely to develop into an established line. The more cautious investigator may require a population increase representing more than 50 doublings of the original cell population (which may be only a single or a few cells). The more experienced human tumor cell culturist may predict an establishment at an earlier time when cell division has assumed a reasonable constant rate, and tumor cells are definitely outgrowing nontumor cells in the subcultures.

2.7. Cultivation of Cell Lines. From the time of establishment of a cell line, the task of cultivation is limited to the serial subculturing in the best suitable medium and containers, in order to maintain the line alive at whatever level of cells is necessary. It is unwise to seed too few cells, since many of the slower dividing cultures are difficult to deal with under such conditions. The optimum medium and serum type and concentration is in most cases determined empirically; they vary among cell lines, and general rules are difficult to state.

2.8. Freezing Methods. Practically all human tumor cells, in early culture and as cell lines, are capable of surviving freezing in liquid nitrogen (30). For details of procedure see the chapter by Shannon and Macy (31).

Cultures of cells, actively dividing at the time of harvest are trypsinized, sedimented by centrifugation, resuspended in several milliliters of medium plus serum, and counted. Cell concentration is adjusted to 2.0 to 3.0 × 10^6 per milliliter in medium/serum with 10% glycerol or 5–10% dimethyl sulfoxide as preservative. A sterile syringe with a 22-gauge, 1.5-inch sterile needle is used for dispensing 1.0 ml of cell suspension per sterile 1.5-ml glass ampoule with aluminum foil cover. Ampoules are sealed using the Kahlenberg Globe ampoule sealer (Kahlenberg-Globe Equipment Co., Sarasota, Florida), labeled with tape, and held at 4°C to allow the cells to absorb the cryopreservative before being placed in the freezing chamber of the Linde Liquid Nitrogen Biological Freezing System (Linde BF-4, Union Carbide Corp., Linde Division, New York, New York) which is precooled to 4°C. A thermocouple probe is placed in an unsealed "dummy" ampoule containing the same cell suspension as that being frozen. The flow of nitrogen is regulated to freeze the cells at a precisely controlled rate (1.0–1.5°C/min) until the temperature of the cells is lowered to −100°C. The ampoules are then transferred from the freezing chamber to a liquid nitrogen refrigerator. To assure that the freezing has been successful, the contents of several ampoules are tested for viability.

2.9. Characterization of Cultures. *2.9.1. Cell Morphology.* Cells that grow as monolayers are recultured on cover slips in Leighton tubes. When cultures are approximately 75% confluent, examination of living cells is made by Nomarski interference-contrast microscopy (32) at several magnifications, and of fixed cells after staining. We use routinely hematoxylin and eosin staining (32); other methods may be useful for specific cytological details or reactions. The Nomarski technique, also applicable to cells growing in suspension, provides a three-dimensional view of the living cells unaffected by preparation and fixation. Examination of cellular morphology and cultural texture by these methods is performed periodically during the development of the culture to monitor cellular relationships and changes in cell size and shape, nuclear—cytoplasmic ratio, shape and location of nucleus, number of nucleoli, etc. (33).

2.9.2. In Vitro Cytopathology. Cells grown to 75% confluency on 3 × 1 inch microscope slides in large Leighton culture tubes are rinsed several times with phosphate-buffered saline and fixed with 70% ethanol. In addition, a suspension of cells is prepared by trypsinization of a monolayer culture. After inactivation of trypsin with serum, the cells are sedimented, resuspended in 3.8 ml of phosphate-buffered saline, and fixed with 5.0 ml of 70% alcohol. The fixed preparations are evaluated by the cytologist after Papanicolaou staining to assess the malignancy and nature of the cultured cells (34, 35).

2.9.3. Tumor Production in Nude Mice. Cells from actively dividing cultures are scraped from the flask into 2—4 ml of medium and sedimented by centrifugation at 150 *g* for 10 min. The supernatant is decanted and the cells are drawn into a 1-ml tuberculin syringe with 22- or 25-gauge needle. Athymic Nu/Nu mice, male or female, approximately 1 month old, of Rex/Trembler origin, backcrossed to BALB/c of Swiss 3 times, are inoculated subcutaneously on the dorsal side between the shoulder blades with 10^6 to 20×10^6 cells (36). Tumors of approximately 1 cm^3 are excised; a portion of the specimen is fixed in neutral buffered formalin in preparation for examination by the pathologist.

2.9.4. Chromosome Analysis. The steps in the chromosome preparation procedure used are similar for cells derived from various types of tumors. However, reagents, concentrations, and times of exposure may vary among the different cell types. In general, Colcemid is added to the cultures to a final concentration of 0.05 to 0.1 μg/ml, followed by incubation at 37°C for 1—4 hr. Cells are then trypsinized and sedimented at 180 *g*, the pellet is slowly resuspended in a hypotonic solution consisting of a mixture of potassium chloride and sodium citrate for 15 min at 37°C and fixed at 4°C with alcohol—acetic acid, 3:1, three times. Each fixation period lasts 30 min. Metaphase preparations are prepared by a method based on the suspension technique developed by Moorhead and colleagues (37). The preparations on the slides are stained with aceto-orcein or Giemsa stain for chromosome counts and observation of abnormalities, or they are banded with trypsin, followed by orcein or Giemsa staining, or with quinacrine dehydrochlorate, for more detailed determinations of individual chromosomes.

2.9.5. Susceptibility to Poliovirus. Three monolayer culture tubes of similar cell density are rinsed several times with culture medium without serum and inoculated as shown in Table 4. Cultures are incubated at 37°C. Pronounced cytopathic effect only in tube A indicates suspectibility of the cells to poliovirus.

2.9.6. Growth Studies. For cell lines, the aim is to establish a routine permitting subcultivation on a weekly basis. During the early period of culture, the transfer factor, i.e., culture area (or medium volume for suspension cultures) in subculture over same in parent culture, is determined by gradual increase. For example, initially this factor may be limited to 1.5 or 2. If the subculture in less than 1 week has reached a degree of confluency greater than that of the parent culture, the transfer factor can be increased. Eventually, the weekly transfer factor becomes a constant. Cell population increase is determined more correctly from "growth curves" based upon counts, with 24-hr intervals, of tube cultures seeded (at time 0) with equal number of cells (for example 10^4/ml).

More special parameters, including plating efficiency, saturation density, mitotic index, growth in suspension and as colonies with special morphology in agar, may be helpful in determining the "*in vitro* malignancy" of the cells.

2.9.7. Tests for Mycoplasma and Other Contaminants. Cultures to be tested for mycoplasma, and/or other contaminants, are carried for at least a week without antibiotics, which may inhibit the growth of the contaminant.

a. Cultivation of mycoplasma in special broths and agars: The following artificial media (agar dispensed in 35-mm plastic petri dishes) have been used:

TABLE 4
Test for Poliovirus Susceptibility of Human Tumor Cells

Tube	Serum-free medium (ml)	Normal rabbit serum (ml)	Poliovirus antiserum[a] (ml)	Poliovirus[b] (ml)
A	1.9	0.1	—	0.05
B	1.9	—	0.1	0.05
C	1.9	0.1	—	—

[a]Neutralizing 100 $TCID_{50}$ at a minimum titer of 1:1000.
[b]Type 1; titer approximately 10^8 $TCID_{50}$/ml.

Bye agar (38), Bye broth (38), TC PPLO agar (39), containing 15% heat-inactivated human serum; in some tests horse or calf serum has been substituted for the human serum. These three media have also been used for testing with yeast hemin extract (Baltimore Biological Laboratory, Baltimore, Maryland) added in a concentration of 5% of the total volume. Routinely, agar has been incubated in an atmosphere of 5% CO_2 in nitrogen.

b. Method for direct microscopical demonstration of mycoplasma in cultured cells: Cultures of FL cells, seeded at very low density in Leighton tubes with inserted rectangular coverslips, in antibiotic-free LY medium with 20% human serum, are used as indicator cells. They are inoculated, usually 3 days later, with the sample to be tested. After additional incubation the cultures are prepared for microscopic examination as follows: the coverslip is removed from the culture container and placed in a small petri dish containing 3 ml of 0.6% sodium citrate solution. One milliliter of distilled water is added, dropwise with a 1-ml pipette, to make the concentration of sodium citrate 0.45%. Ten minutes later, 4 ml of Carnoy's fixative (1 part glacial acetic acid, 3 parts absolute ethyl alcohol) is added, dropwise with a 2-ml pipette, in order to make the fixation gradual. The coverslip is transferred to another petri dish containing 3 ml Carnoy's fixative. Ten minutes are allowed for fixation. The coverslip is taken out and left until absolutely dry. The cells are then stained for 5 min with orcein stain (2% natural orcein and 60% glacial acetic acid), and after three washes in absolute alcohol are mounted in Euparol (Flatters and Garnett, Ltd., Manchester, England). The slides are examined under phase optics at magnifications from 200 X to 5100 X. Micrographs are taken with Zeiss photomicroscope. For recognition of mycoplasma, bacteria, and fungi, see previous publications (40, 41).

c. Standard bacteriological and mycological media may be used in tests for bacterial and fungal contaminations.

2.9.8. G6PD Isozyme Type. A monolayer of cells is rinsed 3 times with physiological saline solution; cells are removed from the culture flask with trypsin or by scraping, sedimented by low speed centrifugation at 4°C, counted, and resuspended in cold distilled water at a concentration of 1×10^7 cells/ml. Frozen cell material may be used after thawing and 3 times washing in cold saline solution prior to lysis. Cells are lysed by three cycles of rapid freezing, in acetone/Dry Ice or liquid nitrogen, and thawing. Debris may be sedimented by centrifugation at 1300 g for 10 min at 4°C. Supernatant is transferred to plastic ampoule (Nunc) and stored at 4°C for several hours, or −80°C for long term.

Thirteen percent starch gel with Tris–EDTA–borate buffer system at pH 8.6 is used for the electrophoresis (42). After applying test material and controls (HeLa, type A; and Detroit 562, type B), the gel is placed at 4°C and electrophoresis is carried out at 5 V/cm for approximately 18 hr. The gels are sliced and stained with a standard nitrotetrazolium staining mixture in agar overlay. G6PD type is determined by comparing mobility of bands of test lines with HeLa and Detroit 562 cell controls.

3. Results

This section summarizes some of our results on cultivation and characterization of early cultures and cell lines derived from human tumors. Most early cultures and 23% of the established cell lines were initiated in this laboratory. Characteristics of 31 of our lines have been previously reported (1).

3.1. Rate of Achievement in Establishing Early Cultures and Cell Lines. Since our experience with culture of human tumor cells was obtained over many years, it would be improper to evaluate the overall effort by relating all attempts to successes. Progress can be demonstrated as follows: in 1965 we established 4 human tumor cell lines out of attempts with 143 tumors (2). In sections of these specimens obtained directly from surgery, carcinoma cells were present in 96 specimens, sarcoma cells in 19, nonmalignant tumor cells in 5, but tumor cells could not be observed in 23 of the specimens. Only 4% of the carcinomas and 22% of the sarcomas yielded growth of tumor cells which could be transferred more than 5 times; 16% carcinomas, 22% sarcomas, and two-thirds of the nonmalignant tumors gave abundant tumor cells in primary culture or early passages. Sparse tumor cell growth in the primary culture was obtained from 20% of the carcinomas, 22% of the sarcomas, and one-third of the nonmalignant tumors. Primary cultures contained only stromal cells in 48% of the cultures from carcinomas and 12% of the cultures from sarcomas, and no cells were attaching in primary cultures for 12% of the carcinomas and 22% of the sarcomas.

In contrast, lately we have established lines or cultures which in our judgment will become lines, at a much higher percentage from several types of tumors emphasized in the study; i.e., carcinomas of the female genitalia, colon, lung, and breast. Osteogenic sarcomas have been successful in more than one-half of the cases.

3.2. Characterization of "Approved Early Cultures." Samples of this culture type (see Section 1.3) have been collected in our laboratory from the following types of tumors: *carcinomas*: bladder, breast, cervix, colon, kidney, liver, lung, ovary, prostate, rectum, salivary gland, testis, thyroid; *sarcomas*: Ewing, fibro, fibro/rhabdomyo, leiomyo, osteogenic; *miscellaneous tumors*: brain and other nervous tissue, giant cell tumor, Hodgkin's disease, melanoma, mesodermal mixed. With only limited material available in many cases, it is critical to decide on the allocation for characterization and storage, respectively. Since storage is needless unless there is evidence of tumor cells, a number of cultures are available only in small amounts in the frozen state.

3.3. Characterization of Cell Lines. The collected 282 cell lines are being characterized in a continuously ongoing effort. At this time, 215 lines are frozen mycoplasma-free, in liquid nitrogen. 173 lines have been tested for tumor production in nude mice (36). While morphological studies and *in vitro* cytopathology have been concluded for 190 lines, G6PD type has been determined on 166 lines (43), chromosome analysis is available for 81 lines, and polio sensitivity tests are completed for 61 of the lines. All the lines have been tested for mycoplasma and other contaminants.

3.3.1. Cell Morphology. Morphological comparison of cells of many lines from different tumors have shown that although most cultures from carcinomas contain epithelial-like cells, some of these lines consist of cells classified as mixed to fibroblastlike morphology. Similarly, a small number of sarcoma lines contain cells of epithelial-like morphology.

3.3.2. In Vitro Cytopathology. In most cases this examination has been confirming as to the specific cell type indicated by the diagnosis of the human tumor of origin. In some cases, however, the *in vitro* cytopathology diagnosis was not specific: i.e., there were cells that could be recognized as tumor cells, but their specific type was questioned. Generally the cultured cells appeared moderately well differentiated or poorly differentiated in the cytological smears (36). There have been cell lines for which *in vitro* cytopathology diagnosis differed from the (presumed) tumor of origin, indicating a diagnostic error as to the tumor of origin, a switch of specimens or an "extraneous" cell contamination during cultivation. A summary of general cytologic differences between cultured human tumor cells and the special characteristics of cells derived from epidermoid carcinoma, adenocarcinoma, soft tissue sarcomas, malignant bone tumors, and malignant melanoma has been previously published (35).

3.3.3. Tumor Production in Nude Mice. Sixty percent of 173 lines have produced progressively growing tumors in the nude mouse. Table 5 shows the proportion of tumor-producing to non-tumor-producing lines for the four major categories of tumors. Epidermoid carcinoma lines show the highest rate of tumor production (73%); sarcoma lines the lowest (33%).

TABLE 5
Tumor Production (+NMT) and Nontumor
Production (−NMT) Lines in Nude Mice by
Different Categories of Human Tumors

Tumors of origin	+NMT	−NMT
Epidermoid carcinoma	22	8
Adenocarcinoma	31	20
Sarcoma	8	16
Miscellaneous tumors	42	26

3.3.4. Chromosome Analysis. Chromosome analysis has shown great variation in chromosome numbers among all the cell lines and even among metaphases within each line. Some lines had pronounced modal numbers, others not (1, 44). Chromosome abnormalities also varied in frequency among the lines, as did the occurrence of new chromsomes. All lines examined have shown departure from diploidy, either in chromosome number, morphology, or the number of chromosomes per classification group. Certain features in terms of numbers, abnormalities, new chromosomes, and karyotypes, appear to be characteristic of individual cell lines. However, since individual tumors from the same tissue, and individual lines from the same type of tumor, show differences in chromosome number, abnormalities and new chromosomes, classical chromosome techniques have not permitted the identification of cell line cells with tumor type. There is a possibility that specific intrachromosomal changes may be pinpointed by the new banding techniques, and that some of the changes may be specific for the cells from one particular type of tumor.

3.3.5. Susceptibility to Poliovirus. Sixty-five cell lines tested have shown susceptibility to poliovirus.

3.3.6. Growth Studies. Rates of cell division differ greatly among human tumor cell lines, even among those from similar tumor types. For example, the weekly transfer factor varied among carcinoma lines as follows: breast and colon, 1.5–10; kidney and ovary, 1.5–5; cervix, 4–20. The range for melanomas and osteogenic sarcomas was 2–5. Culture environment and period of time in culture may influence this factor. Whereas most of the lines produce monolayers, with nearly all cells attached to the culture vessel, other lines consist of cells that are partly attached, partly suspended. Some lines consist of suspended cells only.

Studies of more specific growth parameters are in progress.

3.3.7. Mycoplasma Tests, Prevention, and Elimination. No early culture of human tumor cells in our laboratory has ever been found to be contaminated with mycoplasma. All lines established here over the last 12 years have also been mycoplasma-free. Out of 213 lines collected from other laboratories, 43 were found by us to be mycoplasma contaminated. At this time, mycoplasmas have been eliminated from 35 of these lines, in most cases by the method described by Gori and Lee (45).

The prevention measures taken in our laboratory have been reported elsewhere (41, 46).

3.3.8. G6PD Isozyme Type. G6PD typing, primarily aimed at identifying possible HeLa cell contamination, has shown that contamination of the human tumor cell lines in our collection has not been extensive. The results for 166 cell lines, studied so far, are shown in Table 6. Of these lines, 46 were established in our laboratory. Of all the lines, 87% were G6PD type B and 13% type A, as HeLa. 86% of all type B lines and 55% of type A lines were obtained from the

TABLE 6
Reported Donor Race and G6PD Type
for 166 Human Tumor Cell Lines

Race	B	A
Caucasian	124	18
Negroid	2	3
Other	2	
Unknown	16	1

cell line originator. The lines known not to be contaminated with HeLa include epidermoid carcinomas, adenocarcinomas, sarcomas and many miscellaneous tumors.

4. Discussion

We have specified the methods of tumor specimen preparation and cultivation that have worked in our hands and led to cultures or cell lines consisting of tumor cells. We have also indicated factors or conditions that are disadvantageous for the culture attempts. This list is not exhaustive. There are other events, random and accidental, that occur in a tissue culture laboratory and work against our aims. The solution to these problems can only be learned by practical experience, and the experienced worker in this field has the advantage of being capable of dealing with them in a more rapid and proficient way. Tissue culture has increasingly become a scientific discipline. However, there will always be aspects of intuition and art involved without which theoretical knowledge and technical proficiency may not be fully expressed in terms of the results obtained. Other investigators have also been successful. One condition seems to apply commonly to the more productive "cell line originators," i.e. a close collaboration between surgery, pathology, and tissue culture laboratory. This collaboration together with regular attendance to the needs of the cultures—but without "operating when unnecessary"—may be the most important reasons behind productive efforts.

We have emphasized the importance of characterization, which serves to assure that the cultured cells are the tumor cells wanted for study, not nontumor cells from the surgical specimen or "extraneous" cell contaminants. In addition, characterization reveals properties relevant to the choice of cells for particular experiments; for example, when large amounts of cells are needed, a fast-growing cell line is preferable. Monolayer cultures with cells attaching to the culture vessel, rather than suspension cultures, may be desired for certain purposes, etc. Negative tests for bacterial, fungal, and mycoplasmal contaminants are obvious requirements.

Determination of cell morphology by regular and special microscopic methods is important. For the experienced tissue culture researcher, certain cell appearances, interrelationships, and growth patterns are convincing. However, there are cultures in which the cell morphology is most difficult to interpret. The similarity between epithelial tumor cells and mesothelial cells, and the difficulties in distinguishing certain sarcoma cells from nonmalignant fibroblastic stromal cells are among the pitfalls. Difficulties are enhanced in cultures of low growth potential. Thus, no culture should be considered as consisting of tumor cells on the basis of plain morphological evaluation by the tissue culturist.

The pathologist is needed for the characterization of the original human tumor specimen, the tumor produced in the nude mouse, and the "*in vitro* cytopathology" examination of the cultured cells. We have stressed the importance of obtaining the diagnosis of the actual specimen processed in the tissue culture laboratory to avoid the waste of time in maintaining cultures derived from nonmalignant portions of the specimen. Slides of the original tumor are also important for a comparison with *in vitro* cytopathology preparations and with slides or nude mouse tumors, in order to identify a cell culture or line. Extensive data (36) have shown the closely identical histological morphology for the patient's surgically excised tumor and the human tumor grown in the nude mouse. There is similarity even when nude mouse tumors are produced with cell lines cultured for years. In most cases the histological grade is also the same for the human and nude mouse tumor; rarely the nude mouse tumor is more poorly differentiated than the human tumor of origin. Therefore, a nude mouse tumor which differs distinctly in histological morphology indicates a mix-up, presumably an "extraneous" cell contamination. Classification of tumors, whether or not human tumor slides are available, is based upon the classification used in surgical pathology at Memorial Hospital. It can be confirmed with certainty that a tumor (human and/or nude mouse) is an adenocarcinoma, an epidermoid carcinoma, or one of many miscellaneous tumors; for example, melanoma, sarcoma, neuroblastoma. However, the tissue type (lung, colon, duodenum, etc.) depends upon the information obtained at time of surgery and in many cases cannot be determined from tumor sections. The *in vitro* cytopathology examination also permits type-specific indentification (epidermoid carcinoma, adenocarcinoma, melanoma, sarcoma, etc.) with high degree of certainty. For cell lines that do not produce tumors in nude mice, the identification is limited to this method and a comparison with the human tumor slide, when available. When culture origin is an effusion, a cytological examination of this fluid takes the place of the solid tumor as base reference. (The collaboration of Dr. Steven Haydu, Department of Pathology, Memorial Hospital, has been invaluable in helping prove the importance of these methods.)

Many of our human tumor cell lines and early cultures have produced tumors in the nude mouse. How are we to evaluate the lines which have not produced tumors? These lines have been tested with similar inocula, and for many of them, the period of observation (time from inoculum to death of the mouse) has been longer than that required for tumors to grow to a proper size for diagnosis for the tumor-producing lines. Some lines, negative in initial attempts, have produced tumors after repeated testing, indicating variation in immunodeficiency among mice. It is conceivable, therefore, that the percentage of tumor-positive lines may be increased by (a) increasing inoculum, (b) increasing lifetime of mice, (c) increasing the number of mice inoculated per cell line, (d) attempting other routes of inoculation, and (e) further increasing the immunodeficiency by special treatments. Although it is highly desirable to establish tumor production with cultured cells derived from tumor cells we cannot exclude, at least at this stage, that certain cultures may be incapable of tumor production in this artificial host and still consist of tumor cells.

The purpose of chromosome analysis is to (a) search for abnormalities (number of chromosomes, aberrations, markers, and karyotypes) that may distinguish the cells examined from normal cells, since it is the consensus that no malignant cell is normal in all these respects; (b) attempt to establish special characteristics of a culture or cell line for the purpose of identification; and (c) exclude that "extraneous" cell contamination has occurred, especially with cells of other species or with HeLa cells. Eighty-one cell lines and many early human tumor cell cultures studied in our laboratory have shown great variation in chromosome numbers and abnormalities, also among metaphases within one line or culture. This variation is characteristic of malignancy. Still, there are features of individual lines (modal number, special markers, karyotypic changes, etc.), which, at least when combined with other characteristics, serve as identification. Based upon this analysis, many lines can conclusively be excluded as being HeLa cell contaminants. Those which bear resemblance to HeLa in terms of chromosome numbers and markers must be examined by G6PD typing; when the type is A and the donor race recorded as Caucasian, other methods involving the pathologist's evaluation and, perhaps, chromosome analysis by banding techniques, should be employed. Although this latter method has been reported as a nearly conclusive procedure for tracking contamination with HeLa cells (5), we reserve a final opinion in this matter until many more cultures, including some after long-term cultivation and mycoplasma contamination, have been examined. An attempt to correlate specific chromosomal changes in the tumor-producing lines versus the nontumor-producing lines has, so far, been mainly negative (44).

Changes may occur in the chromosomes of normal cells after a period of cultivation. The full extent of this phenomenon, as it may apply to many different kinds of human cells, is not yet known. Mycoplasma contamination has been proved to cause chromosomal aberrations in several types of cultured cells, normal and transformed (47, 48).

Susceptibility to poliovirus assures that the cultured cells are human or monkey cells and, therefore, serves to exclude that "extraneous cell contamination" with cells of other species has occurred. Growth studies supply practical information as to cell population increase *in vitro* and, when the more special methods are employed, may support the conclusion that cultured cells are of malignant origin; for example, a high cloning efficiency, mitotic index, and saturation density. Obviously, these methods are not applicable for identification in terms of type of tumor cells.

The "HeLa cell scare" (49) has made it imperative to determine the G6PD type of any human tumor cell line to exclude contamination with the type A HeLa cells. We found 18 lines reported to be of Caucasian origin to be G6PD type A and for that reason suspected to be HeLa cell contaminants. However, many of these lines differ from HeLa in other respects. For example, chromosomal numbers for several of the lines are different from those of HeLa, and nude mouse and *in vitro* cytopathology diagnosis also differ between some of these lines and HeLa. We have initiated further attempts to determine cell line identity by examining, with starch gel electrophoresis, a combination of enzymes known to have high frequencies of isozyme polymorphisms.

Mycoplasma contamination must be excluded by all means since, in addition to chromosome changes, these contaminants may change the cultures in numerous respects, and, therefore, severely affect experimental results. Mycoplasma-affected cell changes include cytological, biochemical, genetic, and immunological alterations, as well as changes in virus susceptibility. In addition, mycoplasmas may modify mammalian cell surfaces to make them capable of hemadsorption, and they can agglutinate several types of red blood cells. Attachment of mycoplasmas to the host cells and various host cell reactions have interfered with electron microscopic studies of cells and virus–cell interactions. The existence of mycoplasma viruses is now general knowledge. For a full picture, the reader is referred to review articles on this subject (50, 51).

The information obtained from the characterization of human tumor cell cultures applies to all subsequent studies with the cells, by the originator, or by others who may employ them in their research. Consequently, exact and detailed recording becomes pertinent. We consider the list of properties of early human tumor cell cultures, as shown in Table 7, to be most useful for sequential recording during the first period of cultivation. For the collection of established cell lines, we have found it advantageous to initiate a computerized file of data, since the information (clinical background, data obtained by us, data obtained from others) may be obtained randomly. Table 8 shows the printout of data on an individual cell line. The program permits for the printing of summary listings of individual characteristics of all lines in the collection. As new lines are added and additional characterization data are obtained, the computer file is updated and the information available on individual lines can be provided to interested investigators.

TABLE 7
Chart for Biweekly Evaluation of Early Cultures

CULTURE DESIGNATION _____   SURGICAL DIAGNOSIS _____

INITIATION DATE _____   PATHOLOGY DIAGNOSIS _____

	Date								
	Passage								
	Method								
Tumor Cell Morphology	Epith.								
	Fibro.								
	Stell.								
	Spher.								
	Other								
Tumor Cell Frequency	None								
	Few								
	50/50								
	Many								
Culture Type	All								
	Mono.								
	Susp.								
	Mix								
Culture Appearance	Disp.								
	Colon.								
	Pile								
Tumor Cell Division	None								
	Slow								
	Med.								
	Fast								
	Cloning Efficiency								
	Maximum Density								
	Mitotic Index								
	Division Time								

5. Summary

Cultivation of human tumor cells has been facilitated by new and better techniques and many established cell lines, representative of numerous tumor types, are now available. Some tumors have yielded lines more frequently than others. Our methods of preparation and cultivation, which have led to many

TABLE 8

Computer Printout of Current Data on One Cell Line

```
                    HT-29
TUMOR DIAGNOSIS    PATHOLOGY RELIABILITY-CONFIRMATICN CN SPECIMEN
    ADENOCARCINOMA,COLCN;PRIMARY

    PATIENT DATA- AGE-  44  SEX- FEMALE  RACE- CAUCASIAN    BLOOD TYPE- A+
        TREATMENT-
        LINE ORIGINATOR-J. FOGH          ON 11 06 64  PREVIOUS MEDIUM- 512
PREVIOUS SERUM-15% FETAL CALF      PREVIOUS SUPPLEMENTS        AND
    REFERENCES 1  FOGH & TREMPE,IN HUMAN TUMOR CELLS IN VITRC,ED. FOGH,PLENUM,1975
               2
               3

OBTAINED FROM-              ON              AT P.           HIGHEST P. HERE-0146
CONTAMINATION-  NONE          WHICH WAS ELIMINATED BY               CN
NOW FREE OF CONTAMINATIONS-          TRANSFERRED BY- 0.25% TRYPSIN AND 0.01% EDTA
    CURRENT MEDIUM-  MCCOY S      OR 512     CURRENT SERUM-  15% FETAL CALF
    WITH        AND          ANTIBIOTICS-PENICILLIN     AND STREP.
GROWN AS MONOLAYER , TRANSFERRED 1 TO 004.0 WK.  MORPHCLOGY-EPITHELIAL-LIKE
DOES    PRODUCE TUMORS IN                         G6PD TYPE    BY PREVICUS LAB
DOES    PRODUCE TUMORS IN CORT.HAMSTR AND NUDE MICE G6PD TYPE B BY HTCB LAB
SUSCEPTIBILITY POLIOVIRUS 1 —         PREVIOUS LAB   POSITIVE- HTCB LAB
CHROMOSOME —     PASS.9-HYPOTRIPLOID.PASS.122-HYPC TO HYPERTRIPLOID.ABN.INCL.DIC.,
    AC.FRAGM.,MIN.,SEC.CONSTR.LARGE SUBMETA AND LARGE META OR POLY-
    CENTRIC MAR.+A,+B,+C,+D,+E,+F,+G.

IN VITRO       P.119-IN VITRO CYTOPATH.-ALL,ADENOCARCINOMA CF CCLCN CELLS
CYTOPATHOLOGY- NUDE M.TUMCR-ADENOCARCINCMA,MUCINOUS,CONSISTENT WITH COLCNIC
NUDE MOUSE     PRIMARY
DIAGNOSES.

IMMUNOLOGICAL  E.M.VERY BUSY CELLS,MICROVILLI,MUCHMICROFILA.OFTEN BUNCHED; LARGE
VIRAL          VACUOLATED,FEW INTACT MITO.W.DARK GRANULES;SMOOTH & ROUGH E.R. W.
E.M. AND       SOME DILATED CISTERNAE;MANY FREE RIBO:SCME LIPID DROPLETS;FEW
GROWTH         LYSO.;MANY BAGS OF CELLULAR DEBRIS;NUCLEI LARGE W.NUCLECLI,FREQ.
STUDIES.       INVAG.OF CYTOSOL. NO VIRUS PARTICLES SEEN,ACC.TO SARKAR.
```

tumor cell cultures and 64 established lines from solid tumors and effusions, are described. We have found that high concentrations of fetal calf serum, up to 26%, in various media, are highly favorable for the selective growth of epithelial tumor cells. Different methods have been useful for other investigators, and 218 lines have been collected from outside laboratories. Cell line establishment may not be apparent until many months after initiation of cultures. It is critical that early cultures and established lines be characterized to assure the presence of tumor cells of the proper type and to assess the properties necessary for individual experimental purposes. A major part of this paper concerns our characterization methods and interpretation of data obtained. These methods include evaluations of cell morphology, *in vitro* cytopathology, tumor production in nude mice, chromosomal changes, suceptibility to poliovirus, growth in culture, G6PD isozyme type, and tests for mycoplasma and other culture contaminants. Our results obtained from characterizing and identifying many cultures and cell lines are presented and discussed.

ACKNOWLEDGMENTS

This work was supported in part by NIH Contract NO1-CB-43854 and NCI Grant CA-08748. Tumor specimens were obtained from Dr. Yashar Hirshaut's Procurement Service and from the Department of Pathology at Memorial Sloan-Kettering Cancer Center. We are indebted to the many investigators who provided us with cell lines from numerous tumors and therefore made it possible to conduct this comparative study. We are grateful to Dr. Donald Armstrong for the information used in Table 2 and to William Wright, Tom Orfeo, Linda Williams, Deborah Milder, Gwendolyn Holmes, and Shirley DeVore of this laboratory for their participation in this study. Special thanks to Peter Silberstein for his dedicated effort in establishing our computerized data program.

REFERENCES

1. Fogh, J., and Trempe, G., *in* "Human Tumor Cells *in Vitro*" (J. Fogh, ed.), p. 115. Plenum, New York, 1975.
2. Fogh, J., and Allen, B., *In Vitro* **2**, 125 (1966).
3. Stulberg, C. S., in "Contamination in Tissue Culture" (J. Fogh, ed.), p. 2. Academic Press, New York, 1973.
4. Gartler, S. M., *Natl. Cancer Inst. Monogr.* **26**, 167 (1967).
5. Nelson-Rees, W., Zhdanov, V. M., Hawthorne, P. K., and Flandermeyer, R. R., *J. Natl. Cancer Inst.* **53**, 751 (1974).
6. Cailleau, R., Yount, B., Olivé, M., and Reeves, W. J., *J. Natl. Cancer Inst.* **53**, 661. (1974).
7. Fogh, J., Anderson, H. C., Allen, B., Petursson, G., Saunders, E. L., and Dalldorf, G., *Cancer Res.* **24**, 416 (1964).
8. Eagle, H., *Science* **130**, 432 (1959).
9. Leibovitz, A., *in* "Human Tumor Cells *in Vitro*" (J. Fogh, ed.), p. 23. Plenum, New York, 1975.
10. Moore, G. E., Gerner, R. E., and Franklin, W. A., *J. Am. Med. Assoc.* **199**, 519 (1967).
11. McCoy, T., Maxwell, M., and Kruse, P. F., *Proc. Soc. Exp. Biol. Med.* **100**, 115 (1959).

12. Lasfargues, E. Y., *in* "Collagenase" (I. Mandl, ed.), p. 83. Gordon & Breach, New York, 1972.
13. Gwatkin, R. B. L., and Thomson, J. L., *Nature (London)* **201**, 1242 (1964).
14. Sullivan, J. C., and Schafer, I. A., *Exp. Cell Res.* **43**, 676 (1966).
15. Houba, V., *Experientia* **23**, 572 (1967).
16. Sykes, J. A., *in* "Human Tumor Cells *in Vitro*" (J. Fogh, ed.), p. 1. Plenum, New York, 1975.
17. Evans, V. J., and Earle, W. R., *J. Natl. Cancer Inst.* **16**, 1375 (1947).
18. Sinkovics, J. G., Dreyer, D. A., Shirato, E., Cabiness, J. R., and Shellenberger, C. C., *Tex. Rep. Biol. Med.* **29**, 227 (1971).
19. Jensen, F. C., Gwatkin, R. B. L., and Biggers, D., *Exp. Cell Res.* **34**, 440 (1964).
20. Feller, W. F., Stewart, S. E., and Kantor, J., *J. Natl. Cancer Inst.* **48**, 1117 (1972).
21. McAllister, R. M., and Reed, G., *Pediat. Res.* **2**, 356 (1968).
22. Macpherson, I., *in* "Tissue Culture, Methods and Applications" (P. F. Kruse, and M. K. Patterson, eds.), p. 276. Academic Press, New York, 1973.
23. Aaronson, S. A., Todaro, G. J., and Freeman, A. E., *Exp. Cell Res.* **61**, 1 (1970).
24. Lasfargues, E. Y., Coutinho, W. G., and Moore, D. H., *J. Natl. Cancer Inst.* **48**, 1101 (1972).
25. Lazarus, H., Tegeler, W., Mazzono, H. M., Leroy, J. G., Boone, B. A., and Foley, G. E., *Can. Chemother. Rep.* **50**, 543 (1966).
26. Bassin, R. H., Plata, E. J., Gerwin, B. I., Mattern, C. F., Haapala, D. K., and Chu, E. W., *Proc. Soc. Exp. Biol. Med.* **141**, 673 (1972).
27. Waymouth, C., *in* "Growth, Nutrition and Metabolism of Cells in Culture" (G. H. Rothblat, and V. J. Cristofalo, eds.), Vol. 1, p. 11. Academic Press, New York, 1972.
28. Eagle, H., *Science* **174**, 500 (1971).
29. Shipman, C., *in* "Tissue Culture, Methods and Applications" (P. F. Kruse, and M. K. Patterson, eds.), p. 709. Academic Press, New York, 1973.
30. Mazur, P., Leibo, S. P., Farrant, J., Chu, E. H. Y., Hanna, M. G., and Smith, L. W., *in* "The Frozen Cell" (G. E. W. Wolstenholme, and M. O'Connor, eds.), p. 69. Churchill, London, 1970.
31. Shannon, J. E., and Macy, M. L., *in* "Tissue Culture, Methods and Applications" (P. F. Kruse, and M. K. Patterson, eds.), p. 712. Academic Press, New York, 1973.
32. Fogh, J., and Sykes, J. A., *In Vitro* **7**, 206 (1972).
33. Rose, G. G., "Atlas of Vertebrate Cells in Tissue Culture." Academic Press, New York, 1970.
34. Bean, M. A., and Hajdu, S. I., *in* "Human Tumor Cells *in Vitro*" (J. Fogh, ed.), p. 333. Plenum Press, New York, 1975.
35. Hajdu, S. I., Bean, M. A., Fogh, J., Hajdu, E. O., and Ricci, A., *Acta Cytol.* **18**, 327 (1974).
36. Fogh, J., and Hajdu, S. I., *J. Cell Biol.* **67**, 117a (1975).
37. Moorhead, P. S., Nowell, P. C., Mellman, W. J., Battigs, D. M., and Hungerford, D. A., *Exp. Cell Res.* **20**, 613 (1960).
38. Barile, M. F., Yagochi, R., and Eveland, W. C., *Am. J. Clin. Pathol.* **30**, 171 (1958).
39. Carski, T. R., and Shepard, C. C., *J. Bacteriol.* **81**, 626 (1961).
40. Fogh, J., and Fogh, H., *Proc. Soc. Exp. Biol. Med.* **117**, 899 (1964).
41. Fogh, J., and Fogh, H., *Ann. N. Y. Acad. Sci.* **172**, 15 (1969).
42. Ruddle, F. H., and Nichols, E. A., *In Vitro* **7**, 120 (1971).
43. Fogh, J., Wright, W., and Loveless, J., *Fed. Proc., Fed. Am. Soc. Exp. Biol.* **35**, 1133 (1976).
44. Fogh, J., Hajdu, S., Fogh, H., and Loveless, J. D., *Proc. Annu. Cell Genetics Conf. 1974*, p. 12.

45. Gori, G., and Lee, D., *Proc. Soc. Exp. Biol. Med.* **117**, 918 (1964).
46. Fogh, J., Barile, M., and Hopps, H., *News Letter (Tissue Culture Assoc.)* **8**, 15 (1974).
47. Fogh, J., and Fogh, H., *Proc. Soc. Exp. Biol. Med.* **119**, 233 (1965).
48. Fogh, J., and Fogh, H., *Ann. N. Y. Acad. Sci.* **225**, 311 (1973).
49. Nelson-Rees, W., and Flandermeyer, R. R., *Science* **191**, 96 (1976).
50. Barile, M. F., *in* "Contamination in Tissue Culture" (J. Fogh, ed.), p. 132. Academic Press, New York, 1973.
51. Fogh, J., *in* "Contamination in Tissue Culture" (J. Fogh, ed.), p. 175. Academic Press, New York, 1973.

Growth of Human Tumors in the Nude Mouse

Carl O. Povlsen and Jørgen Rygaard

1. Introduction

The nude mouse, suffering from congenital thymic aplasia, has opened new and wide perspectives in the study of transplanted human tumors. The lack of a cell-mediated immune response in the nude mouse entails that it will readily and permanently accept xenografts of normal and malignant tissues (1–8).

The need for a simple *in vivo* model for the study of transplanted human tumors is urgent, and many attempts have been made to meet this need. Transplantation of such tumors has been performed utilizing privileged sites in immunologically competent animals, e.g., the anterior eye chamber in rodents (9), the brain of various laboratory animals (10), and the hamster cheek pouch (11). Human tumors have also been transplanted into animals made immunologically incompetent by means of assorted procedures, e.g., irradiation, cortisone treatment (12), and treatment with anti-thymocyte or anti-lymphocyte serum (13). The latter agents have also been used in combination with neonatal thymectomy and potentially lethal irradiation, followed by bone marrow transplantation (14). Attempts have also been made to transplant tumors into embryos and neonatal animals in which immunological competence has not yet been established (15).

While all the systems mentioned have been utilized to investigate various aspects of tumor biology, the models themselves have proved difficult to work with. The percentage of tumor takes has been low in most instances. Further, using these models only a few tumors have been serially passaged. Thus, the need for a suitable model for the transplantation of human tumors is still acute.

We wish to describe our experience in transplanting human tumors into nude mice. The nude mouse has been shown to be a suitable host for a wide spectrum of human malignant tumors. These have included adenocarcinomas from the colon and rectum (2, 3), epidermoid carcinomas (4), Burkitt's lymphoma (16), malignant melanomas (17), and carcinomas of the uterine corpus and the breast (8). These tumors have been implanted directly without prior *in vitro* culturing. As shown by Giovanella and co-workers (7, 18) and Ozzello *et al.* (19) the injection of cell suspensions, derived from cultures of human malignant tumors, both carcinomas and sarcomas, will also induce tumor formation in nude mice. The tumors can be transplanted serially. The human tumor/nude mouse system provides a unique opportunity to study various aspects of the biology of tumors, isolated from their host of origin. This would include studies of growth, metabolism, genetics, and immunology. Of greater importance, potential anticancer agents can now be tested against transplanted *human* tumors, and conversely, an individual human tumor can be tested for its susceptibility to available anticancer agents.

2. Materials

2.1. Recipients of Tumor Grafts. Recipient animals in our studies have been 6–8 week-old nude mice, of both sexes, bred at the Pathological-Anatomical Institute, Copenhagen Municipal Hospital (PAI), and at Gammel Bomholtgaard, Laboratory Animals Breeding and Research Center, Ry, Denmark (BOM). Details concerning the genetic background and principles of breeding and husbandry will be given under Methods (Section 3), and the immunodeficiency disorder of the nude mouse will be described in the next paragraph.

The Mouse Mutant Nude. The hairless mouse mutant nude was first described by Flanagan (20). In 1968, Pantelouris (21) discovered that the nude mouse lacked a thymus and showed leukopenia. Rygaard (1) confirmed the absence of the thymus and demonstrated that the leukopenia was a specific lymphopenia. He also found low immunoglobulin levels in nude mice and observed that heterotransplants of normal rat skin were accepted permanently by nude mice.

De Sousa *et al.* (22) found a pronounced lymphocytic depletion in the thymus-dependent areas of lymph nodes, Peyer's patches and spleens of nude mice. Pantelouris and Hair (23) demonstrated, in histological studies, two thin strands of tissue with fine central lumina at the site of the thymus. They interpreted this to be a thymic rudiment, lacking a lymphocyte population. Wortis *et al.* (24) showed that this "rudiment" was not populated with lymphocytes when it was transplanted under the renal capsule of normal mice. It was shown that the bone marrow of nude mice contained a stem cell population that could repopulate thymic epithelium from sublethally irradiated normal mice (25). Thus it is probable that the defects in the nude mouse are due to the lack of a functional thymic epithelium.

In the peripheral blood of nude mice there is a pronounced lymphopenia with lymphocyte counts about $1400/\mu l$ (26). Raff and Wortis (27) observed that in lymphoid tissues of nude mice few θ-positive lymphocytes could be demonstrated. Sprent (28) found that thoracic duct lymphocytes from nude mice were practically all B lymphocytes. There were a few null cells, but no T lymphocytes, present.

Humoral immune responses in nude mice were limited to the production of IgM (29). Only thymus-independent antigens such as lipopolysaccharide (LPS), Vi antigen and pneumococcal polysaccharide gave rise to antibody formation, whereas nude mice were not stimulated by so-called thymus-dependent antigens (30).

The nude mouse showed no cell-mediated immune response following sensitization with oxazolone (31) or in response to transplants of normal or malignant tissues derived from allogeneic or xenogeneic donors (1, 5, 6, 32–36). Successful heterotransplantation of human fetal organs was reported by Povlsen *et al.* (37). The results of transplanting human tumor tissue will be described in Section 4. There are now several investigations clearly showing that nude mice are far more sensitive to both experimental and accidental infections than are normal mice. This is reflected in the relationship between life-span and quality of microbiological milieu. In good conventional conditions nude mice may live 5–7 months (6), while life-span under spf conditions was extended to 18 months (38). From reports by other authors, e.g., Outzen *et al.* (39) it can be inferred that nude mice in germfree conditions will have a nearly normal life-span.

2.2. Tumor Material. Tumors in our own material were derived from patients undergoing surgery in various hospitals in Copenhagen. One single tumor was obtained at biopsy from a 7-year-old African girl. The special conditions relating to this tumor were described elsewhere (16). We have now transplanted a total of 102 human malignant tumors in nude mice. The origin of tumors and their histology and fate in nude mice are presented in Table 1.

TABLE 1

Human Tumors Transplanted in Nude Mice (Copenhagen Series)

Type of tumor	Takes/attempts	Serial transplants/takes
Adenocarcinoma of gastrointestinal tract	14/19	12/14
Malignant melanoma	14/32	7/14
Epidermoid carcinoma (head and neck, lung, penis, cervix uteri vulva)	7/12	4/7
Carcinoma testis	0/5	–
Carcinoma ovarii	1/3	–
Carcinoma mammae	1/5[a]	–
Hodgkin's lymphoma	0/5	–
Leukemia	0/9	–
Miscellaneous tumors	7/12	3/7
Total	44/102	26/42

[a]Survival, not actual growth.

3. Methods

3.1. Breeding and Husbandry of Nude Mice. Mice, used in our experiments were either bred and reared at the PAI or purchased from BOM.

Breeding was begun at the PAI in December 1968 with two heterozygous pairs obtained from Drs. R. C. Roberts and D. S. Falconer, The Institute of Animal Genetics, Edinburgh, Scotland. Various breeding schemes have been used in parallel at the PAI and BOM since 1969 (1, 40).

Initially, male heterozygous carriers of the *nu* gene were crossed with noninbred NMRI/BOM$_f$ females. At present the gene is under transfer or transferred to three inbred strains of mice: BALB/c/A/BOM$_f$, C3H/bi/BOM$_f$, and C57/B1/6/BOM$_f$. About 95% of the nude mice in this study had a BALB/c background (50–99% of the genome).

The mice at PAI were kept at a room temperature of $27°±1°C$; relative humidity $55±5\%$. The rooms were ventilated with filtered air exchanged 8 times per hour. At BOM, room temperature was $24°±1°C$, air exchange 15 times per hour, and the relative humidity was as the PAI. In both places Makrolon cages, type II, were used. Feed pellets with mineral and vitamin additives were produced and autoclaved at BOM. Sterile wood granulate was used for bedding, and tap water was supplied *ad libitum*.

Breeding and maintenance of stock mice at BOM was conducted under strict spf-conditions behind a personal barrier, whereas at PAI only one of the three animal rooms had a personal barrier. The husbandry methods in both centers, and their effects on breeding and keeping, were described in detail elsewhere (40).

3.2. Anesthetics. In early experiments ether was used as anesthetic. However, the anesthetic of choice during later years has been propanididum (Epontol, Bayer, Leverkusen, Western Germany) 0.5 mg/g body weight intraperitoneally. The duration of anesthesia was 5–6 min, but when required the same dose was repeated several times during the course of surgery.

3.3. Inoculation Methods. Tumors of our material have in all cases been inoculated directly into mice without prior culturing. Time between tumor removal and inoculation in nude mice varied from 20 to 90 min. All transplantation procedures were performed under strict sterile conditions.

3.3.1. Primary Transplantation of Solid Tumors. In primary implantations of solid tumor material, 2–8 nude mice were inoculated.

During early transplantation experiments 0.5 ml of a tumor cell suspension mechanically disintegrated in saline or tissue culture medium was injected subcutaneously in the lateral abdominal wall. In all later transplantation experiments mice were inoculated with solid blocks of tumor tissue, measuring $2 \times 2 \times 3$ mm, in the subcutaneous space of the flank.

Incisions, 6–8 mm, were made in the skin of the flank of the recipient mouse with a small pair of scissors, penetrating the panniculus musculosus. With the scissors closed, a 1 cm-deep pouch was formed in the subcutaneous space. The tumor implant was carefully selected from nonnecrotic areas. In the case of tumors of the gastrointestinal tract, tumor tissue was dissected free from the serosal aspect of the specimen, extreme care being taken to avoid penetration to the lumen. To obtain viable and noninfected tumor material, metastases of lymph nodes or organs were generally preferred.

The carefully selected tumor implant was then gently pushed into the preformed pouch and was situated at least 8 mm away from the incision. The incision was then closed with sutures or tissue adhesive, e.g., Histoacryl (Braun, Melsungen, Western Germany). Occasionally a lump of tumor tissue was selected by the surgeon and transported to the laboratory for inoculation. During transplant the specimen was kept in phosphate-buffered saline with penicillin and streptomycin added, kept on ice. During the implantation procedure tumor specimen and tumor blocks were kept moist with sterile saline.

3.3.2. Primary Inoculation of Leukemias. From 7 patients suffering from different types of leukemia 0.1 ml of bone marrow aspirate or peripheral blood with heparin added as an anticoagulant was injected intravenously, intraperitoneally, or subcutaneously in nude mice (at least 2 mice per route of administration were employed). From 2 leukemic patients group of 4 nude mice were inoculated subcutaneously with solid tissue blocks measuring 1 × 2 × 2 mm, originating from leukemic infiltration of the skin and from tumor-involved lymph nodes of the neck.

3.3.3. Serial Transplantation of Solid Tumors. In serial transplantations up to 50 nude mice were inoculated with material taken from a single nude mouse. The donor and recipient mouse were anesthetized at the same time. The skin overlying the donor tumor was dissected away, allowing free inspection for nonnecrotic areas. Solid blocks, measuring 2 × 2 × 3 mm, were removed and implanted in recipient animals as described.

3.4. Observation. *3.4.1. General.* After the inoculation of tumor tissue, mice were observed daily for tumor growth. Animals inoculated with peripheral blood or bone marrow had blood samples taken once a week for white blood cell count and differential counts in smear preparations. All animals were autopsied except in cases where results could not be interpreted because of cannibalism or severe cadaverosis. At autopsy the skin of the inoculation site was dissected free to allow for gross inspection of the tumor. Axillary and inguinal lymph nodes were examined. The thorax and abdomen were opened and the organs were examined, particularly for the presence of metastases. The upper mediastinum was inspected for thymic tissue.

3.4.2. Measurement of Tumor Growth. Tumors were measured twice weekly in two dimensions (length and breadth) with a slide caliper. Tumor size was expressed in square millimeters (length × breadth). This expression was preferred because the third dimension could not be measured with accuracy. The animals were weighed at the time of measurement, and their general condition was evaluated.

3.5. Histological Examinations. For histological examination tissue was taken from tumors or tumor remnants in the first transplant generation. From serially grown tumors one to three randomly chosen tumors of each transplant generation was prepared for microscopy. Microscopically changed organs or enlarged regional lymph nodes were also prepared for histology. Tissue was fixed in formalin and embedded in paraffin, 7-μm sections were cut and stained with hematoxylin and eosin and van Gieson—Hansen. Other appropriate staining methods were applied according to tumor type, e.g., Lillie's stain for melanin in melanotic tumors.

3.6. Chromosome Analysis. Chromosome analyses of tumor tissue from *nude* mice were carried out by a direct method without prior cultivation. The mice were given 0.2 ml of an 0.04% Colcemid solution intravenously 4 hr before operation. A block of viable tumor tissue weighing approximately 30 mg was removed surgically and comminuted in a few drops of heparinized saline containing 1 μg/ml of Colcemid (Ciba Pharmaceutical Products, Inc., Summit, New Jersey). The tissue was transferred to micro test tubes, containing 2 ml of tissue culture medium (TCM 199, Flow) and 0.2 ml of an 0.04% Colcemid solution. The suspension was then incubated in a water bath at 37.5°C for 2 hr.

Hypotonic treatment, fixation, and preparation of slides were carried out applying the methods normally followed in the laboratory (41). In cases where the individual chromosomes could be classified definitely, a thorough analysis was made. In other cases screening was performed, i.e., determination of chromosomal type with or without concurrent counting.

3.7. Preparation by Thymus Grafting. Whole thymus glands from neonatal (<24 hr old) BALB/c/BOM$_f$ mice were implanted subcutaneously in the lateral abdominal wall in nude recipients 4–5 weeks old. Transplantations were made irrespective of donor/recipient sex. Of all thymus-grafted animals, 10–20% died 2–3 weeks after thymus grafting at the present state of backcrossing, probably due to a graft-versus-host reaction.

3.8. Cancer Chemotherapy Studies. The general experimental plan utilized in our laboratory in cancer chemotherapy studies was as follows: The animals in each treatment group and corresponding control animals were inoculated with tumor tissue derived from one donor mouse. Distribution of sexes in the treatment and control groups was similar. Chemotherapy was begun when tumor growth was ascertained, in general when the tumor diameter reached 5 mm. The period between tumor inoculation and institution of chemotherapy ranged between 14 and 20 days. Experiments were usually concluded 31–32 days after the day on which treatment was begun.

All chemotherapeutic agents were administered intraperitoneally. The doses were selected with reference to toxicity studies in which the LD_{10} and LD_{50} were determined for each agent.

4. Results and Comments

We shall briefly describe the fate of tumor grafts, stressing findings confirming the human nature of the mouse-grown tumors, and potential applications of the human tumor/nude mouse model.

4.1. Fate of Tumor Grafts. The percentage of successful tumor graftings in the first transplant generation was 43 (see Table 1). If only the group of solid tumors is considered, the percentage of take was 50. In our series it has not been possible to transplant successfully Hodgkin's lymphoma and different types of leukemia.

It is also seen from Table 1 that a high percentage of tumors (26 out of 42) can be grown serially. Until now (November, 1975) an adenocarcinoma of the colon has been maintained for 62 generations during a 6-year period. The rate of take in serial transplantations of established tumors was high, reaching 90–100%. Tumor take was observed following inoculation of both cell suspensions and solid tumor blocks from surgical specimens. Apart from early transplantations, we preferred implantation of solid tumor blocks. It has been argued that the degree of accuracy is less with this method as compared to cell suspensions. It should be remembered, however, that it is extremely difficult or impossible to prepare monocellular suspensions from surgical specimens. The number of tumor cells is impossible to assess with reasonable accuracy owing to admixture of other cell types and cell death.

It may also be of importance that the architecture of tumor parenchyma and stroma is preserved in solid tumor blocks. In our hands they were readily vascularized provided the size of the implant did not exceed the dimension mentioned.

The percentage of take and the number of tumors that can be serially grown in our series was in good accordance with the findings of others (8). Other investigators (7, 19) reported the occurrence of solid tumors following inoculation of cell suspensions derived from cultured cell lines, originating from human malignant tumors. Both carcinomas and lymphomas of human origin were successfully transplanted by this procedure.

4.2. Mode of Growth. After a latency period of 8–40 days, a nodule appeared at the site of the inoculation. Tumors would grow as spherical nodules, increasing gradually in size until the death of the animal. Spontaneous regressions were not observed. The growth rate of different tumors varied considerably. However, the individual tumors showed a constant growth rate in the performed passages. Tumor growth could easily be followed by simple measurements as described.

In our nude mouse recipients tumors grew locally. The skin overlying the tumor was not adherent, and the tumor moved freely over the abdominal muscle layers. Metastatic spread to lymph nodes or organs was never observed in our laboratory. This is in accordance with the findings of Sordat et al. (8). In contrast, Giovanella and co-workers (7, 42) found metastases from both directly implanted tumors and tumors originating from cell suspensions. The explanation for this discrepancy is not obvious. Possible explanations include genetic differences, differences in living conditions, and the possible selection of highly malignant cell lines after long-term in vitro culture.

Microscopically, mouse-grown tumors showed close similarity to the human donor material, even after 6 years of transplantation. Tumors grew as local, well demarcated processes in the subcutaneous space at the site of inoculation. They were surrounded by a layer of condensed connective tissue. Two tumors (a Burkitt's lymphoma and a malignant melanoma) tended to infiltrate the subcutaneous fatty tissue and the muscle. Microscopic examinations of lymph nodes and organs never revealed metastases.

As a rule, when the tumor size increased, the amount of centrally located necrotic tissue also increased, leaving a layer of viable tumor tissue at the periphery. This should be kept in mind when transplanting tumors serially.

The above-mentioned investigators have similarly described the accordance between human donor material and mouse-grown tumor and the constancy of mouse-grown tumors during passages. Sordat and co-workers (8) on the basis of electron microscopic studies have also reported a strict resemblance of mouse-grown tumors with human material.

4.3. Further Characterization of Mouse-Grown Tumors. Early and late passages of mouse-grown tumors were studied by chromosome analysis (18, 42–45). In all cases cells with a human chromosome pattern were found. Comparisons of early and late passages of individual tumors showed a constant chromosome number. There was no evidence of interspecies hybridization or total species shift in the human tumor/nude mouse system in contrast to findings reported in other transplantation models (46).

Isozyme studies of a serially grown Burkitt's lymphoma showed the mouse-grown tumor to be of the same glucose-6-phosphate dehydrogenase (G-6-PD) and phosphoglucomutase$_1$ (PGM$_1$) phenotype as directly examined biopsy material (16). In the same Burkitt's lymphoma, IgM activity was demonstrated on cell membranes from both mouse-grown tumor and biopsy material from the patient. Sera of tumor-bearing nude mice contained anti-human species-specific antibodies, but no detectable antibody to Epstein–Barr virus.

Sordat *et al.* (8) demonstrated carcinoembryonic antigen (CEA) in human colonic tumor transplanted in nude mice. Epstein and Kaplan (45) found membrane-bound immunoglobulins in human lymphoma lines inoculated intracerebrally in nude mice. All these parameters indicate that human tumors grown in nude mice preserve their human characteristics.

4.4. Reconstitution of Immune Responses. Immunological competence can be established in nude mice after transplantation of neonatal thymus, but also by injection of, e.g., spleen cells (47). In our study of the effect of grafting with neonatal congenic thymus (48) we found that nude mice, supposed to be fully immunologically competent, would reject transplants of three different serially grown tumors. Transplantation of one of the tumors—a malignant melanoma—to nude mice, supposed to be in the process of developing immunological competence, revealed the various stages of rejection. Also tumors already established in nude mice will be rejected after subsequent thymus grafting (unpublished observation). Similar findings were reported by Schmidt and Good (49). Human tumors, transplanted in thymus-grafted nude mice, seem to be a suitable model in the study of developing immunological competence.

4.5. Cancer Chemotherapy Studies. A method for "sensitivity testing" of solid human tumors with anticancer agents in similarity with methods applied in bacteriology would be of great potential value. The human tumor/nude mouse system represents one such model. The following tumors and agents have been tested in our laboratory.

A *malignant melanoma* responded well to treatment with 1-(chloroethyl)-3-cyclohexyl-1-nitrosourea (CCNU) and 5-(3,3-dimethyl-1-triazeno)imidazole-4-carboxamide (DTIC) whereas 5-fluorouracil (5-FU) showed no effect (50). An epidermoid carcinoma responded to treatment with fleomycin (51). A Burkitt's lymphoma regressed completely after administration of cyclophosphamide to the tumor-bearing nude mice (52).

These results are in full accordance with clinical experience and indicate that the responsiveness of the tumors to various anticancer agents can be preserved after transplantation in nude mice. The potential value in primary and secondary screening of anticancer agents is being investigated.

4.6. Concluding Remarks. The human tumor/nude mouse system fulfills a number of criteria that can be set for a suitable heterotransplantation model.

4.6.1. Nude mice accept a high percentage of human solid tumors.

4.6.2. Many tumors can be grown serially in the system.

4.6.3. Tumor growth can be followed by simple measurements

4.6.4. Tumors show a constant and predictable growth pattern.

4.6.5. Human characteristics are preserved in mouse-grown tumors as judged by microscopic examination, chromosome analysis, isozyme and immunological examination.

4.6.6. Extensive studies are possible, as nude mice are bred relatively easily.

4.6.7. Nude mice demand no meticulous and costly preparations or continuous immunosuppressive treatment, which might interfere with tumor growth.

The major obstacle for the widespread use of the model is the high sensitivity of the nude mouse to infectious disease, owing to the immune deficiency, which results in a shortened life-span. However, these difficulties can partly be overcome by keeping the nude mouse in a highly protected milieu, thus extending life-span and the period available for tumor growth, treatment, and observation.

ACKNOWLEDGMENT

The original work on which this review is based was supported by The Danish Medical Research Council, The Danish Cancer Society, and the P. Carl Petersen Foundation. We wish to thank Dr. William P. Weidanz for helpful suggestions in the preparation of the manuscript and Mrs. A. Klitlund for expert secretarial assistance.

REFERENCES

1. Rygaard, J., *Acta Pathol. Microbiol. Scand.* **77**, 761 (1969).
2. Rygaard, J., and Povlsen, C. O., *Acta Pathol. Microbiol. Scand.* **77**, 758 (1969).
3. Povlsen, C. O., and Rygaard, J., *Acta Pathol. Microbiol. Scand., Sect. A* **79**, 159 (1971).
4. Povlsen, C. O., and Rygaard, J., *Acta Pathol. Microbiol. Scand., Sect. A* **80**, 713 (1972).
5. Manning, D. D., Reed, N. D., and Shaffer, C. F., *J. Exp. Med.* **138**, 488 (1973).
6. Rygaard, J., "Thymus & Self. Immunobiology of the Mouse Mutant Nude." Wiley, New York, 1973.
7. Giovanella, B. C., Stehlin, J. S., and Williams, L. J., *J. Natl. Cancer Inst.* **52**, 921 (1974).
8. Sordat, B., Fritsché, R., Mach, J.-P., Carrel, S., Ozzello, L., and Cerottini, J.-C., "Proceedings of the First International Workshop on Nude Mice," p. 269. Fischer, Stuttgart, 1974.
9. Green, H. S. N., *Cancer* **5**, 24 (1952).
10. Lumb, G., *Br. J. Cancer* **8**, 434 (1954).
11. Bradford Petterson, W., *Cancer Res.* **28**, 1637 (1968).
12. Toolan, H. W., *Cancer Res.* **13**, 389 (1953).
13. Philips, B., and Gazet, J.-C., *Br. J. Cancer* **24**, 92 (1969).
14. Detre, S. I., and Gazet, J.-C., *Br. J. Cancer* **28**, 412 (1973).
15. Southam, C. M., Burchenal, J. H., Clarkson, B., Tanzi, A., Mackey, R., and McComb, V., *Cancer* **23**, 281 (1969).
16. Povlsen, C. O., Fialkow, P. J., Klein, E., Klein, G., Rygaard, J., and Wiener, F., *Int. J. Cancer* **11**, 30 (1973).
17. Povlsen, C. O., *Acta Pathol. Microbiol. Scand., Sect. A* **84**, 9 (1976).
18. Giovanella, B. C., Yim, S. O., Morgan, A. C., Stehlin, J. C., and Williams, L. J., *J. Natl. Cancer Inst.* **50**, 1051 (1973).
19. Ozzello, L., Sordat, B., Merenda, C., Carrel, S., Hurlimann, J., and Mach, J. P., *J. Natl. Cancer Inst.* **52**, 1669 (1974).
20 Flanagan, S. P., *Genet. Res.* **8**, 295 (1966).
21. Pantelouris, E. M., *Nature (London)* **217**, 370 (1968).

22 De Sousa, M. A. B., Parrott, D. M. V., and Pantelouris, E. M., *Clin. Exp. Immunol.* **4,** 637 (1969).

23. Pantelouris, E. M., and Hair, J., *J. Embryol. Exp. Morphol.* **24,** 615 (1970).

24. Wortis, H. H., Nehlsen, S., and Owen, J. J., *J. Exp. Med.* **134,** 681 (1971).

25. Pritchard, H., and Micklem, H. S., *Clin. Exp. Immunol.* **14,** 597 (1973).

26. Rygaard, J., and Povlsen, C. O., *Acta Pathol. Microbiol. Scand., Sect. A* **82,** 48 (1974).

27. Raff, M. C., and Wortis, H. H., *Immunology* **18,** 931 (1970).

28. Sprent, J., "Proceedings of the First International Workshop on Nude Mice," p. 11. Fischer, Stuttgart, 1974.

29. Crewther, P., and Warner, N. L., *Aust. J. Exp. Biol. Med. Sci.* **50,** 625 (1972).

30. Reed, N. D., Manning, J. K., Baker, P. J., and Ulrich, J. T., "Proceedings of the First International Workshop on Nude Mice," p. 95. Fischer, Stuttgart, 1974.

31. Pritchard, H., and Micklem, H. S., *Clin. Exp. Immunol.* **10,** 151 (1972).

32. Pennycuik, P. R., *Transplantation* **11,** 417 (1971).

33. Kindred, B., *Eur. J. Immunol.* **1,** 59 (1971).

34. Rygaard, J., *Acta Pathol. Microbiol. Scand., Sect. A* **82,** 80 (1974).

35. Rygaard, J., *Acta Pathol. Microbiol. Scand., Sect. A* **82,** 93 (1974).

36. Rygaard, J., *Acta Pathol. Microbiol. Scand., Sect. A* **82,** 105 (1974).

37. Povlsen, C. O., Skakkebaek, N. E., Rygaard, J., and Jensen, G., *Nature (London)* **248,** 247 (1974).

38. Stutman, O., *Excerpta Med. Found. Int. Congr. Ser.* **349,** Vol. 1, p. 275 (1974).

39. Outzen, H. C., Custer, R. P., Eaton, G. J., and Prehn, R., *J. Reticuloendothel. Soc.* **17,** 1 (1975).

40. Rygaard, J., and Friis, C. W., *Z. Versuchtierk.* **16,** 1 (1974).

41. Visfeldt, J., *Riso Report* **117,** 33, 80, 106 (1966).

42. Giovanella, B. C., and Stehlin, J. S., "Proceedings of the First International Workshop on Nude Mice," p. 279. Fischer, Stuttgart, 1974.

43. Visfeldt, J., Povlsen, C. O., and Rygaard, J., *Acta Pathol. Microbiol. Scand., Sect. A* **80,** 169 (1972).

44. Povlsen, C. O., Visfeldt, J., Rygaard, J., and Jensen, G., *Acta Pathol. Microbiol. Scand., Sect. A* **83,** 709 (1975).

45. Epstein, A. L., and Kaplan, H. S., *Cancer* **34,** 1851 (1974).

46. Goldenberg, D. M., Pavia, R. A., and Tsao, M. C., *Nature (London)* **250,** 648 (1974).

47. Kindred, B., *J. Immunol.* **107,** 1291 (1971).

48. Povlsen, C. O., and Rygaard, J., *Acta Pathol. Microbiol. Scand., Sec. C* **83,** 413 (1975).

49. Schmidt, M., and Good, R. A., *J. Natl. Cancer Inst.* **55,** 81 (1975).

50. Povlsen, C. O., and Jacobsen, G. K., *Cancer Res.* **35,** 2790 (1975).

51. Povlsen, C. O., Jacobsen, G. K., and Rygaard, J., "The Laboratory Animal in Drug Testing" (5th ICLA Symposium), p. 63. Fischer, Stuttgart, 1973.

52. Povlsen, C. O., and Rygaard, J., "Proceedings of the First International Workshop on Nude Mice," p. 285. Fischer, Stuttgart, 1974.

Establishment of Permanent Human Lymphoblastoid Cell Lines *in Vitro*

Kenneth Nilsson

1. Introduction

During the last decade, tissue culture techniques have been developed to cultivate human hematopoietic tissue in short- and long-term culture. From early studies with malignant (1–4), and later with normal, lymphoid tissue (5–8), it became evident that cells with a lymphoblastoid morphology had the capacity for infinite growth *in vitro*. The frequency of "lymphoblastoid transformation," as the event of spontaneous establishment of such lines *in vitro* originally was termed (1), was low except when cultures were initiated from blood of patients with acute mononucleosis (9–11) or when nonneoplastic lymph nodes were cultivated by the Spongostan grid culture technique (12).

Epstein-Barr virus (EBV) soon became incriminated as the agent causing this "immortalization" of lymphoid cells [for a review see Ref. (13)]. Lymphoblastoid cell lines (LCL) could be obtained only from EBV seropositive adult donors, and no lines became established from cord blood (14) or fetal tissue (8, 15) except when exposed to Millipore-filtered supernatant from EBV-producing cell lines. Later all LCL were found to carry EBV-related antigens and/or EBV genome [for a review see (16)]. Recent studies have disclosed EBV receptors on most, if not all, human B lymphocytes (17), and EBV has been shown to stimulate cellular DNA synthesis in infected cells (18). Taken together, these and other data clearly establish that EBV can immortalize B lymphocytes to infinitely growing LCL. The precise mechanism by which EBV can immortalize B lymphocytes is unknown. Multiple copies of EBV genome seem to become partly integrated in the cellular DNA (19), but that the continuous presence of EBV genome is required for permanent growth of the LCL has as yet not been shown.

LCL have been widely employed as human models for studies of various lymphoid cell functions, such as production of migration-inhibitory factor (MIF), lymphotoxin, and a reversible inhibitor of lymphocyte activity [for a review see Ref. (20) and Table 1]. Also LCL seem to be satisfactory tools for studies on surface molecules, such as HLA (21), β_2-microglobulin (21, 22) and concanavalin A (Con A) receptors (23, 24). Finally LCL's may be ideal for studies on various types of inborn errors of metabolism *in vitro*. Lines have been reported from patients with Lesh–Nyhan syndrome (25), ganglioside storage disease (26), citrullinemia, maple syrup urine disease, galactosemia, and fructose 1,6-diphosphate deficiency (27). In all these lines the enzyme deficiency of the donor was present.

Lymphoblastoid cell lines have many advantages over other types of nonneo-plastic human cells: they have an infinite life span; they are easy to cultivate in large masses; they have a chromosomal and phenotypic stability during continu-ous cultivation which is better than that of many other human cell types, e.g., skin fibroblasts. For many lines certain functional characteristics, such as im-munoglobulin production, has remained unaltered for more than 10 years (28).

Early work with EBV as an agent causing immortalization of human lymphoid cells was hampered by the lack of a good source of EBV. Most spontaneously established human LCL produced only minute amounts of "transforming" EBV and mostly only during the first few months of continuous cultivation (15). Only a few relatively efficient, although comparatively laborious, methods to establish LCL by use of EBV from lysed human LCL cells have been reported (8, 15, 29, 30). It was therefore of great practical importance when Miller and Lipman (31) succeeded in converting marmoset lymphocytes by human EBV and found a high and apparently continuous production of immortalizing EBV in the derived cell line (B95-8). The availability of the B95-8 virus has made it possible to establish LCL with a 100% success rate from virtually all fetal and adult hematopoietic tissue. This article will describe in detail the procedure for establishment *in vitro* of LCL by use of B95-8 virus. It will also briefly review the characteristics of the derived lines.

2. Materials

2.1. Preparation of B95-8 Supernatant Containing EBV.

Initiate a culture of B95-8 cells (31) in RPMI 1640 or F-10 medium (GIBCO, Grand Island, New York) supplemented with 10–20% fetal or newborn calf serum and antibiotics (100 IU/ml of penicillin, 50 μg/ml of streptomycin) at a cell density of 3×10^5 to 5×10^5 cells/ml in any type of culture vessel, but most practical in a glass or plastic tissue culture bottle. Incubate this culture at 37°C for 1 week with change of half the medium at days 3 and 7. Incubate the culture during a second week without further medium renewal at 32°–34°C to enhance EBV produc-tion.

At the end of this incubation period EBV is prepared from the supernatant as follows: (a) Remove cells by centrifugation at 400 g for 10 min. (b) Filter the supernatant through a 0.45-μm Millipore filter. (c) Store 2-ml portions of the supernatant at $-70°C$ to $-90°C$. (d) When necessary check the stock for sterility (bacteria, fungi, mycoplasma). The immortalizing capacity of B95-8 supernatant stored in this manner will remain intact for at least 6, and probably 12, months.

2.2. Separation of Peripheral Blood Lymphocytes. Collect 10–30 ml of heparinized blood (10–20 IU of heparin per milliliter) and separate the mononuclear cells from red blood cells by a one-step gradient density centrifugation (32) (e.g., in Ficoll–Paque, Pharmacia, Uppsala, Sweden). Wash the cells (lymphocytes with admixture of monocytes and a few granulocytes) three times in phosphate-buffered saline (PBS) or serum-free medium (RPMI 1640 or F-10).

2.3. Feeder Cells. In situations where the number of lymphoid cells available for transformation is low (e.g., from small children), the presence of suitable feeder cells will enhance the survival of immortalized lymphoblastoid cells and thus increase the efficiency of establishment. The following types of feeder cells have been used with success in our laboratory: (a) adult human skin fibroblasts at a late serial passage, phase II cells (12), (b) human glia cells (33). Both types of cells are grown to from confluent, topoinhibited monolayers in 50-ml Erlenmeyer flasks to which the lymphoid cells infected by EBV (see Section 3.1) later can be added.

3. Procedure

3.1. Infection of Cells. After the last washing, the lymphocytes are resuspended in fresh RPMI 1640 or F-10 medium supplemented with 10–20% fetal or newborn calf serum and antibiotics at a concentration of 4×10^6 cells/ml. One milliliter samples of this suspension are transferred to sterile glass of plastic 12×100 ml test tubes with screw caps. To each tube one 0.2-ml aliquot of B95-8 supernatant is added and the tube is incubated at $37°C$ for 1 hr. One milliliter of the above fresh medium is then added, and the culture is ready for continuous cultivation.

When only a small amount of lymphocytes ($< 5 \times 10^5$ cells) is available, feeder cells can be employed to ensure successful establishment. The cells (in 0.5 ml medium) are exposed to 0.2 ml of B95-8 supernatant in a sterile test tube for 1 hr and then transferred to a 50-ml Erlenmeyer flask containing a confluent monolayer of feeder cells and 20 ml of fresh medium. Addition of B95-8 EBV (0.2 ml) to the Erlenmeyer flask at day 2 and 4, in connection with medium renewal, may improve the rate of establishment although this has not been studied systematically.

3.2. Incubation of Infected Cells. The test tubes with unscrewed caps and the Erlenmeyer flasks are incubated at $37°C$ in a humidified 5% CO_2-in-air atmosphere. Half of the medium is replaced twice a week.

3.3. Events during the Process of Establishment. Depending slightly on the initial amount of lymphocytes, EBV immortalized lymphoblastoid cells, growing in characteristic free-floating round clumps, can be easily detected at week 3 or 4. By cytological methods cells with a lymphoblastoid morphology can be detected after only a few days of incubation. The establishment of LCL is heralded by increased acidity in the medium.

In Erlenmeyer flask cultures established LCL are detected in inverted microscope mostly after 4–6 weeks. Since one of the characteristics of single lymphoblastoid cells on feeder cells is peripoletic activity, they remain for a long time "hidden" closely attached beneath, or on the upper surface of the feeder cells. Eventually, when a great part of the feeder layer is covered by peripoletic lymphoblastoid cells, typical LCL clusters can be detected also in this type of culture (Fig. 1). The lymphoblastoid cells can, however, be released from the feeder cells at an earlier stage by trypsinization (0.25% trypsin) and transferred to culture vessels without feeder cells.

3.4. Maintenance of Established LCL. LCL can be maintained as nonstirred suspension cultures in Erlenmeyer flasks, plastic or glass tissue culture flasks, or as roller cultures. Optimal cell concentration to initiate cultures is 2×10^5 to 5×10^5 cells/ml and cells will grow to a maximal density approximately 10^6 cell/ml. One-third of the medium (see Section 3.1) is changed twice a week. LCL

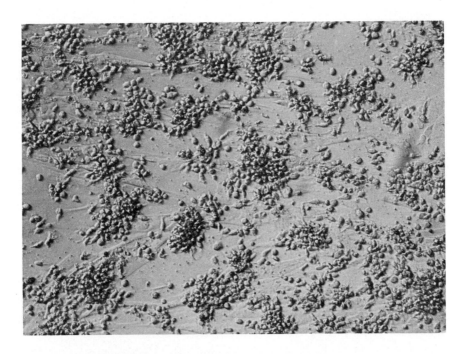

Fig. 1. Growth of human lymphoblastoid cells on a monolayer of human skin fibroblasts.

can grow exponentially in sealed culture flasks without CO_2, but only when the cell concentration is in the range 2×10^5 to 10×10^5 cells/ml.

4. Comments

4.1. Establishment of LCL from Other Sources Than Peripheral Blood. Without use of B95-8 virus LCL become spontaneously established at a high frequency ($> 90\%$) from solid lymphoid tissue (lymph nodes, spleen, and bone marrow) of EBV-infected donors provided that fragmented tissue is cultivated with a modified Trowell–Jensen grid culture—the Spongostan grid culture (Fig. 2) (12). The efficiency of this technique can be further improved by infection of the explanted tissue by B95-8 supernatant. However, it is also possible, although more laborious, to prepare single-cell suspensions of a *lymph node* or *spleen,* and in the latter case, after removal of red blood cells by gradient centrifugation, to employ the same method described above (Sections 3.1 and 3.2). Aspirated *bone marrow* samples should immediately transferred to tissue culture medium containing 10–20 IU/ml of heparin. Mononuclear cells can then be separated by gradient centrifugation (Section 2.2), and LCL can be established in the test tube cultures (Sections 3.1 and 3.2.).

From *cord blood* LCL can be established in test tubes by B95-8 EBV as detailed for peripheral blood lymphocytes.

4.2. General Technical Comments. The technique used to separate lymphocytes from blood does not seem to be critical for a high efficiency of immortalization by EBV. Useful alternative methods are (a) gravity sedimentation in Plasmagel followed by removal of remaining red blood cells by exposure to

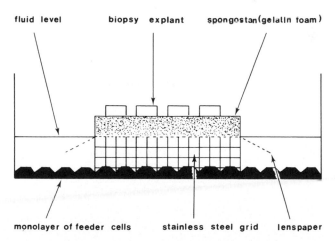

Fig. 2. The Spongostan grid organ culture for cultivation of human hematopoietic tissue.

ammonium chloride (34), (b) gravity sedimentation of red cells by addition of dextran (35), (c) centrifugation on a gradient of sucrose and a mixture of methyl cellulose and Hypaque (36).

Apart from the B95-8 cell line, the QIMR-WIL LCL, derived from a patient with myeloid leukemia, seems to be a good source for immortalizing EBV (8). However, the QIMR-WIL cells do not release EBV in an amount similar to that of the B95-8 cells. Therefore a cell lysate, not unconcentrated supernatant, is used for the establishment of LCL (8, 35, 37, 38).

The type of culture vessel widely used is the test tube, but microtest plate cultures with $0.15-0.8 \times 10^6$ cells in $0.15-0.20$ ml of medium have been described (35-37).

The initial concentration of lymphocytes in tube cultures can be varied within the range of 10^6 to 5×10^6 cells/ml. The observation of Pope (38) that lymphocyte samples from blood can be cultured *in vitro* for at least 2 weeks before exposure to EBV without a reduction in the frequency of establishment may be of practical importance.

The length of the lag period (normally 3-4 weeks) before establishment of LCL is dependent on the amount of EBV but also on the number of B lymphocytes incubated. Very short lag periods (1-2 weeks) have been noted in Erlenmeyer flasks containing feeder cells and 5×10^6 lymphocytes exposed twice to B95-8 EBV.

4.3. Characteristics of LCL. All recently established LCL are similar regardless of tissue of origin. Table 1 summarizes various characteristics of fresh (< 3 months of continuous culture) LCL. In older lines (> 1 year), secondary chromosomal alterations have been reported (39, 40), which may be followed by changes of morphology and/or functional characteristics (41). It is therefore essential to perform any studies with fresh LCL.

TABLE 1
Summary of Documented Characteristics of Human Lymphoblastoid Cell Lines

Morphology (41)	
Cell type	Lymphoblastoid
Cell shape	Highly variable (round, ovoid, elongated, pear shaped)
Cell diameter (μm)	Mean 13, range 8-22
Cell surface	Variable; most have a few slender villi located at one cell pole; a minority are symmetrically covered by short, thin villi
Nucleus	Round-ovoid; finely granular chromatin; 2-4 large pleomorphic nucleoli

(continued)

TABLE 1—*(continued)*

Cytoplasm	Moderately well developed endoplasmic reticulum; a moderate number of free polyribosomes
Nucleocytoplasmic ratio	High
Time-lapse cinematography	Highly mobile cells; pronounced capacity for locomotion on fibroblast surfaces

In vitro (41)

Dependence on complete medium (type RPMI 1640, F-10)	No
Dependence on feeder cells or conditioned medium	No
Growth in clumps	Yes
Attachment to feeder cells	Yes, strong (peripolesis)
Growth in agarose	Yes, low cloning efficiency (approx. 5%)
Population doubling time (hr)	24–84 hr
Maximum cell density (cells/ml)	$1.1.2 \times 10^6$

Cytochemistry (42)

α-Naphthylacetate esterase (ANAE)	Sparse–strong[a]
Naphthol AS-D, acetate esterase	Sparse
Naphthol AS-D chloroacetate esterase	Sparse
β-Glucuronidase	Sparse
Oil Red O	Negative
Periodic acid-Schiff	Negative
Acid phosphatase	Negative
Peroxidase	Negative

Surface receptors (43) (% positive cells)

SRBC	0
C3 (EAC)	60–95
Fc (EA)	1–5
Ig	70–95

Lymphoid functions (20)

Secretion of Ig	Yes ($1–3$ g per 10^6 cells in 24 hr)
Production of MIF	Yes
Production of "lymphotoxin"	Yes
Production of interferon	Yes

β_2-Microglobulin production (22)	300–400 g per 5×10^5 cells in 65 hr
Phagocytosis (44)	Yes, weak
EBV genome (16)	Always
Karyotype (40)	Normal diploid
Clonality (45)	Polyclonal shortly after establishment
HLA expression (46)	Typical "broad" reactivity with alloantisera

[a]The ANAE reactivity is dependent on the type of fixation procedure employed.

TABLE 2
Defining Features of Lymphoblastoid Cell Lines (LCL)

Basic cell type	Lymphoblast
Growth pattern	
Suspension	Large cell clumps
On feeder cells	Isolated cells or clumps strongly attached to feeder cells
Mobility	
Suspension	Mainly by uropods
On feeder cells	Rapid locomotion (periopolesis)
Immunoglobulin (Ig) production	Secretion of complete molecules into the medium and presence of membrane-localized Ig
Epstein–Barr virus genome	Present
Karyotype	Normal diploid[a]
Clonality shortly after establishment	Polyclonal

[a]Note that secondary chromosomal changes occur during continuous culture (> 1 year). These are sometimes followed by morphological and/or functional alterations.

By the use of a battery of morphological and functional markers, it is possible to distinguish LCL from malignant hematopoietic lines (41). This is essential when an LCL for some reason (e.g., as control cells in studies of tumor antigens on the malignant cell population) should be established from blood of a patient with hematopoietic malignancy and doubt may occur whether nonneoplastic (LCL) or malignant cells have become established. In Table 2, the defining features for LCL have been listed.

REFERENCES

1. Benyesh-Melnick, M., Fernbach, D. J., and Lewis, R. T., *J. Natl. Cancer Inst.* **31,** 1311 (1963).
2. Iwakata, S., and Grace, J. T., *N. Y. State J. Med.* **64,** 2279 (1964).
3. Foley, G. E., Lazarus, H., Farber, S., Uzman, B. G., Boone, B. A., and McCarthy, R. E., *Cancer* **18,** 522 (1965).
4. Moore, G. E., Ito, E., Ulrich, K., and Sandberg, A. A., *Cancer* **19,** 713 (1966).
5. Moore, G. E., Gerner, R. E., and Franklin, H. A., *J. Am. Med. Assoc.* **199,** 519 (1967).
6. Gerber, P., and Monroe, J. H., *J. Natl. Cancer Inst.* **40,** 855 (1968).
7. Nilsson, K., Pontén, J., and Philipson, L., *Int. J. Cancer* **3,** 183 (1968).
8. Pope, J. H., Horne, M. K., and Scott, W., *Int. J. Cancer* **3,** 857 (1968).
9. Pope, J. H., *Nature (London)* **216,** 810 (1967).
10. Diehl, V., Henle, G., Henle, W., and Kohn, G., *J. Virol.* **2,** 663 (1968).
11. Glade, P. R., Kare, J. A., Moses, H. L., Whang-Peng, J., Hoffman, P. F., Kammermeyer, J. K., and Chessin, L. N., *Nature (London)* **217,** 564 (1968).
12. Nilsson, K., *Int. J. Cancer* **8,** 432 (1971).
13. Miller, G., *Yale J. Biol. Med.* **43,** 358 (1971).
14. Chang, R. S., Hsieh, M.-W., and Blankenship, W., *J. Natl. Cancer Inst.* **47,** 479 (1971).

15. Nilsson, K., Klein, G., Henle, G., and Henle, W., *Int. J. Cancer* **8**, 443 (1971).
16. zur Hausen, H., *Biochim. Biophys. Acta* **417**, 25 (1975).
17. Greavas, F. M., Brown, G., and Rickinson, A. B., *Clin. Immunol. Immunopathol.* **3**, 514 (1975).
18. Gerber, P., and Hoyer, B. H., *Nature (London)* **231**, 46 (1971).
19. Adams, A., and Lindahl, T., *Proc. Natl. Acad. Sci. U.S.A.* **72**, 1477 (1975).
20. Glade, P. R., and Papageorgiou, P. S., *In Vitro* **9**, 202 (1973).
21. Tanigaki, N., and Pressman, D., *Transplant. Rev.* **21**, 15 (1974).
22. Nilsson, K., Evrin, P. E., and Welsh, K. I., *Transplant. Rev.* **21**, 53 (1974).
23. De Salle, L., Manukata, N., Pauli, R. M., and Strauss, B. S., *Cancer Res.* **32**, 2463 (1972).
24. Glimelius, B., Nilsson, K., and Pontén, J. *Int. J. Cancer* **15**, 888 (1975).
25. Choi, K. W., and Bloom, A. D., *Science* **170**, 89 (1970).
26. O'Brien, J. S., Okada, S., Ho, M. W., Fillerup, D. L., Veath, M. L., and Adams, K., *Fed. Proc., Fed. Am. Soc. Exp. Biol.* **30**, 956 (1971).
27. Sheeter, S., Spector, E., and Bloom, A. D., *Birth Defects* **9**, 138 (1973).
28. Nilsson, K., unpublished observation.
29. Miller, G., Enders, J. F., Lisco, H., and Kohn, H. I., *Proc. Soc. Exp. Biol. Med.* **132**, 247 (1969).
30. Henle, W., Diehl, V., Kohn, G., zur Hausen, H., and Henle, G., *Science* **157**, 1064 (1967).
31. Miller, G., and Lipman, M., *Proc. Natl. Acad. Sci. U.S.A.* **70**, 190 (1973).
32. Böyum, A., *Scand. J. Clin. Lab. Invest.* **21**, Suppl. 97 (1968).
33. Pontén, J., *in* "Tissue Culture, Methods and Applications" (P. F. Kruse and M. K. Pattersson, eds.), p. 50. Academic Press, New York, 1973.
34. Gerber, P., Nkrumak, F. K., Pritchett, R., and Kieff, E., *Int. J. Cancer* **17**, 71 (1976).
35. Rickinson, A. B., Jarvis, J. E., Crawford, D. H., and Epstein, M. A., *Int. J. Cancer* **14**, 704 (1974).
36. Pope, J., Scott, W., and Moss, D. J., *Nature (London), New Biol.* **246**, 140 (1973).
37. Moss, D. J., and Pope, J. H., *J. Gen. Virol.* **17**, 233 (1972).
38. Pope, J. H., Scott, W., Reedman, B. M., and Walters, M. K., *in* "Recent Advances in Human Tumor Virology and Immunology." (Proc. First Int. Symp. Princess Takamatsu Cancer Res. Fund) (W. Nakahara, K. Nishioka, T. Hirayama, and Y. Ito, eds.), p. 177. University of Tokyo Press, Tokyo, 1971.
39. Huang, C. C., and Moore, G. E., *J. Natl. Cancer Inst.* **43**, 1119 (1969).
40. Zech, L., Haglund, U., Nilsson, K., and Klein, G., *Int. J. Cancer* **17**, 47 (1976).
41. Nilsson, K., and Pontén, J., *Int. J. Cancer* **15**, 321 (1975).
42. Sundström, C., unpublished results.
43. Huber, C., Sundström, C., Nilsson, K., and Wigzell, H., submitted for publication.
44. Kammermeyer, J. K., Root, R. K., Stites, D. P., Glade, P. R., and Chessin, L. N., *Proc. Soc. Exp. Biol. Med.* **129**, 522 (1968).
45. Béchet, J.-M., Fialkow, P., Nilsson, K., and Klein, G., *Exp. Cell Res.* **89**, 275 (1974).
46. Lindblom, B., and Nilsson, K., *Symp. Ser. Immunobiol. Stand. 18th Int. Symp. Hl-A Reagents,* p. 124. Karger, Basel, 1973.

67

Cryopreservation of the Functional Reactivity of Normal and Immune Leukocytes and of Tumor Cells

Howard T. Holden, Robert K. Oldham,
John R. Ortaldo and Ronald B. Herberman

1. Introduction

Our knowledge and understanding of the cellular immune mechanisms that play a role in disease have progressed at a rate comparable to the rate at which assays have been developed that are capable of measuring these cell-mediated reactions. These *in vitro* and *in vivo* tests have been used to study the mechanisms of cell-mediated immunity, to assess immunological competence and to determine the level of the immune response to particular antigens, e.g., bacterial antigens, viral antigens, tumor-associated antigens. Within most of the assays, quantitative comparison of the responses has been possible as long as the testing was done on the same day. However, when comparing results of tests performed on different dates, it has been very difficult to determine whether the differences in reactivity were caused by biological or clinical changes or by altered assay conditions. Serologists have approached this problem by standardizing their reagents and using internal standards within each test. This approach is more difficult when intact cells are employed, since their viability, antigenicity, and functional reactivity must be preserved for extended periods of time.

Recent studies have indicated that cryopreservation can maintain not only cell viability and antigenicity of target cells but also preserve functional reactivity of effector cells, so that these cryopreserved cells can be employed repeatedly over long periods as standard reagents. Frozen cells have been shown to be functionally active in mitogen stimulation assays with human lymphocytes (1–4) and with mouse spleen cells (5), in the mixed lymphocyte reaction with human lymphocytes (6, 7), and in direct cell-mediated cytotoxicity with human (4, 8, 9), mouse (10, 11), and rat cells (12). The ability to produce MIF with human (7) and mouse cells (13) and the ability to form E rosettes with human lymphocytes (3, 7, 14, 15) can also be recovered after freezing. Cyropreserved human lymphocytes can also be stimulated to become cytotoxic effector cells (7).

Some studies have also shown that repeated sampling from the same population of cryopreserved lymphocytes as effectors and/or frozen cells as a source of antigen gives quite reproducible results (4, 10, 14, 16, 17). It is also possible to cryopreserve lymphocyte samples obtained at different time points and then test all the samples on the same day. Finally, the number of tests that are technical failures because of poor effector and/or stimulator-target cells can be considerably reduced when cyropreserved cells are employed as targets, a source of antigen and a source of effector cells.

2. Materials and Equipment

2.1. Planar liquid nitrogen, gas-phase, programmed freezer (Model R-201, G. V. Planar Company Ltd., Middlesex, England) or suitable controlled rate freezing apparatus (see Section 4.1)

2.2. Liquid Nitrogen Refrigerator (Linde Division, Union Carbide, New York)

2.3. Water bath, 37°C

2.4. Centrifuge

2.5. Liquid nitrogen

2.6. Glass vials, 1 dram with rubber lined screw-cap tops (Wheaton Scientific, Millville, New Jersey), Nunc polypropylene serum test tubes (Vangard International, Red Bank, New Jersey), or suitable storage vials or ampules

2.7. Pipettes, plastic, 1 ml (No. 7506), 5 ml (No. 7529), and 10 ml (No. 7530) (Falcon, Oxnard, California)

2.8. Conical centrifuge tubes, 50 ml (No. 2070, Falcon)

2.9. Petri dishes, plastic, 100 × 20 mm (No. 3003, Falcon)

2.10. Roswell Park Memorial Institute (RPMI) medium 1640 [No. 1876, Grand Island Biological Company (GIBCO) Grand Island, New York]

2.11. Fetal calf serum (FCS), heat inactivated (No. 614H, GIBCO)

2.12. Hanks' balanced salt solution, BSS (NIH Media Unit)

2.13. Dimethyl sulfoxide, DMSO (Eastman Kodak Company, Rochester, New York)

2.14. Ficoll-Hypaque, LSM Solution (Litton Bionetics, Inc., Kensington, Maryland)

2.15. Heparin, preservative-free (Fellows Medical Manufacturing Co. Inc., Anaheim, California)

2.16. 2× DMSO mixture is made as follows: To 6 ml of fetal calf serum add 10 ml of 1640 medium containing 20% serum (20%–1640). Add, with mixing, 4 ml of DMSO. (Be sure to add this last.) Cool immediately on ice. See Section 4.7 for additional information on serum.

3. Methods

3.1. Preparation of Lymphoid Cells *3.1.1. Animal Lymphocytes.* Spleen and lymph node cell suspensions are prepared by mincing the organs with scissors in cold BSS in a petri dish (100 mm). After filtering the suspension through two thicknesses of gauze, it is centrifuged at 200 g for 10 min. The cells are resuspended in 20%-1640 and placed on ice.

3.1.2. Human Lymphocytes. Sixty milliliters of peripheral blood are drawn into a syringe containing 2000 U of heparin. This blood is diluted twofold with BSS and carefully placed on a Ficoll–Hypaque gradient as described by Böyum (18). After centrifugation at 400 g for 20 min the band of cells at the interface is harvested, washed twice in 20%-1640, and placed on ice.

3.2. Preparation of Tumor Cells *3.2.1. Ascites.* Animals with ascitic tumors are killed, the peritoneal cavity opened and the ascitic fluid removed with a pasteur pipette. These cells are then washed twice with BSS, resuspended in 20% of 1640, and placed on ice.

3.2.2. Tissue Culture. Monolayers of cells are washed with BSS and then trypsinized to disperse the cells and remove them from the substrate. The cells are washed, resuspended in 20%-1640, and placed on ice.

3.3. Once the cells have been prepared and cell counts have been performed, the suspensions should be adjusted to 2 times the desired final concentration in 20%-1640. (Cell concentrations between 1×10^6/ml and 2×10^8/ml have been employed with no apparent differences in percent recovery.) The cell suspensions should then be cooled to 4°C.

3.4. An equal volume of the cold 2X DMSO mixture is added with mixing to the cell suspension in a rapid, dropwise fashion, with mixing, over a 30-sec interval. The cells are then dispensed in 1.0–2.0-ml aliquots into cold, screw cap vials and kept at 4°C until they are ready to be frozen. The cells should be frozen as soon as possible after the addition of the 2X DMSO Mixture.

3.5. The vials are then transferred in a wire test tube rack to the precooled freezing compartment (4°C) of the Planar freezer. A thermocouple probe is placed inside a sample vial containing the same volume, cell type, and cell number as found in the experimental vials. This probe is connected to a continuous recorder which gives a permanent record of the cooling rate inside the vial. A controller probe is taped to the outside of the sample vial and this regulates the rate of influx of nitrogen vapors into the chamber. After equilibration at 4°C, the freezing apparatus is cooled at a rate of −1°C/min to between −30 and −50°C and then rapidly to at least −80°C. The vials are then removed from the freezing compartment and quickly transferred to a liquid nitrogen freezer for storage and stored in vapor phase.

3.6. Recovery of Frozen Cells. Immediately after removing the cells from the freezer they should be thawed rapidly with shaking in a 37°C water bath. Just before the last ice crystal has melted, the vial is removed and placed on ice. The cell suspension is held on ice for 2 minutes and then transferred to a 50 ml conical tube. The tube is kept at room temperature (20°–22°C) and the dilution procedure to remove the DMSO is initiated immediately. Using 20% of 1640 at room temperature, 1/50 of the original volume is added to the cell suspension in a dropwise manner with mixing. At 5-min intervals, doubling volumes of medium are added until a final 1:10 dilution of the original cell suspension is achieved. When the volume to be added is greater than 0.3 ml, mixing should take place over a 1-minute interval. (For most cells, an abbreviated dilution procedure can be employed. See Section 4.11.) The cell suspension is then centrifuged at 200 g for 10 min and resuspended gently in 20% of 1640. Cells must be handled with a minimum of mechanical force so as to prevent injury, since these cells are more sensitive than fresh cells to these stresses (see Section 4.12).

4. Critical Comments

4.1. Several different features are important in selecting an apparatus for freezing. The instrument must be able to maintain a controlled temperature decrease of −1°C/min, and in addition there must be some compensation for the heat of fusion. For reproducible freezing it is useful to have a recording probe in one of the sample vials so that the precise freezing rates for all runs can be compared and controlled. After the cells have been frozen, the temperature of the vials should not be allowed to increase above −30°C while they are being transferred from the freezer to the liquid nitrogen refrigerator as this can cause additional freezing damage. Therefore a freezing apparatus that uses liquid nitrogen and can reduce the temperature to −80°C or below is preferred. Suitable freezers are made by Planar, Cryoson (Oxford Instruments Inc., Annapolis, Maryland), Cryo-med (Mt. Clemens, Michigan), and Linde Division of Union Carbide (New York). The Virtis Company (Gardiner, New York) makes a relatively inexpensive alcohol bath, controlled rate (−1°C/min) freezer that brings samples to −30°C but the vials must be immediately transferred to the liquid nitrogen refrigerator after they have been frozen. Some investigators have frozen lymphocyte cell suspensions in a low temperature freezer (19); however, this is not as controlled and as reproducible as using a controlled rate freezing apparatus and may not be a suitable method for all types of cells.

4.2. In some cases, clumping occurs after recovering cells that have been frozen. This can be prevented by using EDTA (final concentration 0.1%) in the freezing medium and in the diluting medium (20).

4.3. In order to obtain maximum recovery of the cells after freezing it is best to start with cells that are in the best physiological condition. Samples should have a high percent viability and be capable of performing fresh the function that will be required of them after they are frozen.

4.4. The optimal rate of freezing appears to be between −1 and −2°C/min. Recovery decreases at rates of −0.3 and −4°C/min.

4.5. DMSO is toxic to most types of cells, especially at concentrations at which it is employed as a cryoprotective agent. The toxicity can be reduced if the cells are kept at lower temperatures during the exposure period. For this reason it is important to keep all the reagents containing DMSO at 4°C (this would include the 2X DMSO mixture as well as the cells before and after addition of the 2X DMSO mixture) and to carefully monitor the thawing procedure to prevent any unnecessary warming. DMSO toxicity is a function of both temperature and time. After 30 minutes in 10% DMSO there is little evidence of toxicity at room temperature but if the temperature is increased to 37°C, viability and functional reactivity are adversely affected after 30 min.

4.6. For most cells (human, mouse, rat) the DMSO concentration that gives the best results is between 7.5 and 10.0%. Concentrations below this usually do not provide sufficient cryoprotection while higher concentrations have a tendency to be more toxic.

4.7. High concentrations of serum are probably not required to protect cells during freezing in the presence of DMSO. Although the final concentration as outlined in this protocol is 30%, this is probably unnecessary (except for added insurance), and the concentration could probably be reduced to around 10% for most cells. The type of serum does not appear to be important, and most sera may be employed in the place of FCS.

4.8. Another critical step in the recovery of frozen cells is the slow removal of the DMSO from the cells after they have been thawed. If medium is added too rapidly to the cells, many of them are functionally inactivated or killed (probably by the osmotic shock caused by the steep DMSO gradient between the outside and inside of the cell). The dilution method described here is designed for very fragile cells and the rate may be accelerated depending on the type of cell and the function one is trying to preserve. (For mouse lymphocytes slow dilution is important until the DMSO concentration reaches 4%. Below this level medium may be added rapidly without deleterious effects.) The addition temperature is also important. It would appear that the diluting is best performed at room temperature rather than at 4°C. The temperature effects are especially noticeable if a more rapid method of dilution is employed. Although the cells are kept at room temperature during the dilution process, the length of time is short enough so as not to allow DMSO toxicity. Rat and human cells are more sensitive to dilution at low temperatures than mouse cells (even with optimum dilution procedures) for with the latter the differences in recovery between room temperature and 4°C are not as dramatic.

4.9. Some laboratories have found that cryopreserved cells can be maintained at −70°C in an electrical freezer or on dry ice for several months without loss of certain activity (21). However, for prolonged storage the cells should be kept in a liquid nitrogen refrigerator (below $-120°C$). (We routinely store our frozen specimens at the lower temperature, even for short intervals.)

4.10. We have routinely used screw-cap, glass vials for storage of cryopreserved material because they are easier to work with than glass ampoules, especially when large numbers of samples are prepared for freezing. They should be stored in the vapor phase of the liquid nitrogen refrigerator to prevent entry of liquid nitrogen into the vial. In the event that this does occur, caution should be exercised so that upon warming the vial does not explode. This can be prevented by opening the vial immediately after removal from the liquid nitrogen refrigerator and pouring out the liquid nitrogen.

4.11. Recently we have been employing a modified dilution procedure to prepare frozen cells. It appears to be suitable for many cell types (lymphocytes, tumor cells, tissue culture cells) but has the advantage of requiring less preparation time. Thaw the frozen cells and prepare them for dilution as described in Section 3.6. Using 20% of 1640 at room temperature add one-twentieth of the original volume to the cell suspension, dropwise, with mixing. Wait 1 minute. Repeat the addition, doubling the volume each time, until achieving a DMSO concentration of 4%. (With an initial volume of 1.0 ml, this occurs after 5 additions, when the total volume is 2.5 ml.) Wait 5 minutes. Add enough medium to achieve a final 1:10 dilution. Centrifuge at 200 g for 10 min and resuspend gently in 20% of 1640.

4.12. Cells that have been thawed must be handled with greater care than their fresh counterparts. Minimum centrifugation speeds must be employed (around 200 g) and the cells must not be subjected to excessive mechanical stresses such as vigorous mixing or rapid pipetting (especially with small-bore pipettes), nor should they be exposed to extreme pH conditions (physiological values are optimal for cell survival). In addition, if the cells that have recently been thawed are to be held for any extended period of time before they are to be placed in an assay, they should be kept at room temperature and not at $4°C$. Depending on the cell type and origin, holding at $4°C$ reduces viability and functional reactivity.

REFERENCES

1. Mangi, R. J., and Mardiney, M. R., Jr., *J. Exp. Med.* **132**, 401 (1970).
2. Farrant, J., Knight, S. C., and Morris, G. J., *in* "Cryopreservation of Normal and Neoplastic Cells" (R. S. Weiner, R. K. Oldham, and L. Schwarzenberg, eds.), p. 27. INSERM, Paris, 1973.
3. V. P. Eijsvoogel, du Bois, M. J. G. J., Wal, R. v. d., Huisman, D. R., and Raat-Koning, L., *in* "Cryopreservation of Normal and Neoplastic Cells" (R. S. Weiner, R. K. Oldham, and L. Schwarzenberg, eds.), p. 101. INSERM, Paris, 1973.
4. Golub, S. H., Sulit, H. L., and Morton, D. L., *Transplantation* **19**, 195 (1975).
5. Strong, D. M., Ahmed, A., Sell, K. W., and Greiff, D., *Cryobiology* **11**, 127 (1974).

6. Segall, M., and Bach, M. L., *in* "Cryopreservation of Normal and Neoplastic Cells" (R. S. Weiner, R. K. Oldham, and L. Schwarzenberg, eds.), p. 107. INSERM, Paris, 1973.
7. Fackton, M. A., Strong, D. M., Miller, J. L., and Sell, K. W., *Cryobiology* **12**, 421 (1975).
8. Oldham, R. K., and Simmler, M. C., *in* "Cryopreservation of Normal and Neoplastic Cells" (R. S. Weiner, R. K. Oldham, and L. Schwarzenberg, eds.), p. 161. INSERM, Paris, 1973.
9. O'Toole, C., *Natl. Cancer Inst. Monogr.* **37**, 19 (1973).
10. Holden, H. T., Oldham, R. K., and Herberman, R. B., *Fed. Proc., Fed. Am. Soc. Exp. Biol.* **33**, 806 (1974).
11. Holden, H. T., Oldham, R. K., Ortaldo, J. R., and Herberman, R. B., *J. Natl. Cancer Inst.,* in press.
12. Ortaldo, J. R., Holden, H. T., and Oldham, R. K., *Cryobiology* **12**, 574 (1975).
13. Almaraz, R., Thor, D., and Harrington, J., *Proc. Am. Assoc. Cancer Res.* **16**, 125 (1975).
14. Dean, J. H., Djeu, J. Y., Silva, J. S., Oldham, R. K., Graw, R., McCoy, J. L., and Herberman, R. B., *Cryobiology* **12**, 572 (1975).
15. Bernheim, J. L., *in* "Cryopreservation of Normal and Neoplastic Cells" (R. S. Weiner, R. K. Oldham, and L. Schwarzenberg, eds.), p. 147. INSERM, Paris, 1973.
16. Terasaki, P. I., Vredevoe, D. L., and McClelland, J. D., "Histocompatibility Testing 1965, p. 267. Williams & Wilkins, Baltimore, 1966.
17. Weiner, R. S., Breard, J., and O'Brien, C., *in* "Cryopreservation of Normal and Neoplastic Cells" (R. S. Weiner, R. K. Oldham, and L. Schwarzenberg, eds.), p. 117. INSERM, Paris, 1973.
18. Böyum, A., *Scand J. Clin. Lab. Invest.* (Suppl. 97) **21**, 7 (1968).
19. Wood, N., Bashir, H., Greally, J., Amos, D. B., and Yunis, E. J., *Tissue Antigens* **2**, 27 (1972).
20. Bock, G. N., Chess, L., and Mardiney, M. R., Jr., *Cryobiology* **9**, 216 (1972).
21. Strong, D. H., Turc, J. M., and Farrant, J., *Cryobiology* **12**, 589 (1975).

Cryopreservation of Human Lymphocytes

Sidney H. Golub

1. Introduction

Studies of human cellular immunology present a number of serious logistical problems. This is especially true for investigators who are studying sequential changes in lymphocyte function as a product of changes in disease status, therapy, or some other time-related variable. Samples are often available at unpredictable times, posing difficulties when assays must be set up in advance. Furthermore, the exchange of reagents among laboratories in order to compare techniques or to resolve conflicting results is nearly impossible for cell-mediated assays. Finally, it is most difficult to standardize a cellular assay when the sources of effector cells are variable.

These problems can be overcome by using reproducible stocks of preserved lymphocytes. At present, the only means for preserving lymphocytes in a form that allows for the retention of function is cryopreservation.

Following the finding in 1964 by Ashwood-Smith (1) that viable cells could be frozen and recovered if dimethyl sulfoxide (DMSO) was used as a cryopreservative, a number of laboratories began using frozen human lymphocytes for analysis of the antigens of the HLA system (2–4). HLA typing requires only that the preserved lymphocytes be viable, that surface HLA antigens be expressed, and that the lymphocytes be susceptible to antibody and complement-mediated lysis. Several laboratories showed that the cryopreserved lymphocytes also retained their functional capacities by response to mitogens (5–9). Such studies clearly demonstrated that lymphocytes cryopreserved in DMSO by several different methods had unimpaired capacity to respond to nonspecific mitogenic stimuli. Other investigations showed that cryopreserved human lymphoid cells also responded to specific antigens and in mixed lymphocyte culture (8–12). Finally, lymphocytes recovered from liquid nitrogen storage have been used as either effector cells or target cells in cytotoxicity assays (8, 9, 13, 14). Thus, it is clear that human lymphocytes can be cryopreserved to retain function in a variety of cell-mediated assays.

Many techniques have worked successfully for cryopreservation of human lymphocytes. The method described here is one of proved usefulness and reliability in our laboratory. This same method can be used for the storage of established human tissue culture cell lines and for tissue samples. However, there are many versions of the "best" method for cryopreservation of cells, and modifications are in order for different cell types or cells from other species. Many of the technical aspects for cryopreservation were examined in detail in the excellent monograph "La Cryoconservation des Cellules Normales et Néoplastiques" (see 8, 11, 12, 14), and further details are obtainable from a recent technical study by Weiner (15).

2. Materials

2.1. Human peripheral blood lymphoid cells. We have routinely employed lymphoid cells purified on Ficoll–Isopaque gradients, although we have also found that lymphocytes purified on nylon-wool columns can be efficiently cryopreserved.

2.2. RPMI 1640 tissue culture media, supplemented with antibiotics of choice

2.3. Dimethyl sulfoxide (DMSO), reagent grade (J. T. Baker Chemical Co., Phillipsburg, New Jersey)

2.4. Human serum, either autochthonous for the cells to be frozen, pooled normal AB+ serum, or human serum depleted of γ-globulin

2.5. Screw-cap plastic vials, 2 ml (Cooke Engineering Co., Alexandria, Virginia) or some other ampoule capable of withstanding liquid nitrogen temperatures

2.6. Linde BF-4 programmable freezing apparatus (Union Carbide Co., Los Angeles, California) or comparable apparatus

2.7. Liquid nitrogen tank

2.8. Liquid nitrogen freezer

2.9. Ice bucket and ice

2.10. Water bath set at 37°C

2.11. Trypan blue dye

2.12. Hemocytometer

3. Method

3.1. Prepare the cryopreservative solution of RPMI 1640 medium (or other tissue culture medium) containing antibiotics, 10 mM HEPES buffer if desired, and 10% (v/v) DMSO. Addition of serum is not necessary, but most laboratories add 20–40% human serum. We routinely employ globulin-free human serum so as not to introduce antibodies of undesirable specificities, but autochthonous or pooled human serum are equally usable. As the serum has little cryopreservative action (15), its primary purpose is to provide some cryopreservative activity if a mistake has been made on the DMSO concentration. Also, since we routinely wash and use cells in media containing 5–20% serum, we prefer not to expose the cells to drastic changes in serum concentration during the washing procedure. Chill the cryopreservative in ice before using. Fresh cryopreservative should be used each time.

3.2. Centrifuge the cells and resuspend the cell pellet in the cold cryopreservative. Cells should be resuspended at 5×10^6 to 10^7/ml at a minimum. We have frozen at up to 200×10^6/ml without any problem.

3.3. Dispense 1-ml aliquots of the cell suspension into the vials, close the caps tightly, and place in ice.

3.4. Distribute the vials in the program freezer, and use one vial for the "pilot" vial by inserting the temperature probe. It is best to use a vial containing cells, rather than just cryopreservative, as the pilot vial.

3.5. Following the instructions of the apparatus used, introduce liquid nitrogen at a rate to yield a decline in temperature of $1°C$/min.

3.6. There will be a sudden increase of $1°-5°C$ at the phase transition (usually between $-10°C$ and $-20°C$). It is important to manually override the automatic program and introduce more liquid nitrogen to prevent excess warming of the samples. The time of override required will vary with the apparatus employed, and must be carefully worked out for the machine and cryopreservative used. Approximately 15 sec of override will usually return the freezing cycle to the $-1°C$/min rate with our apparatus, although a plateau of several minutes is not unusual.

3.7. When the temperature of the samples has reached $-50°C$, the manual override can again be used to rapidly bring the temperature down to $-100°$ to $-150°C$. This final cooling is necessary, as there is always some warming of the samples in transfer to the storage freezer.

3.8. Store the samples in the vapor phase of a liquid nitrogen freezer. The samples can be left there indefinitely, as long as precautions against freezer failure are taken. It is advisable to install a sensing alarm system if the freezer does not have one to protect the samples.

3.9. Samples to be thawed and used should be transferred promptly from the freezer to the water bath. The major advantage of the plastic vials is that they will not crack or explode as do some glass ampoules when subjected to this sudden warming.

3.10. When the last ice in the vial has melted, the sample can be diluted. This is a crucial step, and most laboratories agree that the samples should be diluted stepwise with approximately 10 volumes of medium over at least a 10-min period. The dilution medium should be at room temperature. Rapid dilution with cold medium is certainly deleterious to lymphocytes (15).

3.11. The lymphocytes can then be washed, counted, and used. A certain loss of cells must be expected, as a proportion of the cells are lost in the centrifugation process. However, the viability of the recovered cells by trypan blue exclusion should be in excess of 95%. Counting of the cells before washing may result in false-positive staining cells due to the effects of the DMSO.

4. Use and Limitations

As cryopreserved lymphocytes appear to retain function in most assays so far tested, their use is as varied as the use of freshly prepared lymphocytes. We have been particularly impressed with the usefulness of cryopreserved lymphocytes in sequential studies of cellular reactivity (9), and in the time saving involved for assays that would take excessive time if one had to begin the experiment by preparing lymphoid cell suspensions. Furthermore, cryopreservation allows the investigator to perform certain unique types of experiments. For example, one can manipulate the lymphocytes in some drastic way (e.g., transform them with an oncogenic virus) and use the cryopreserved sample as an authentic zero-time control.

However, the cryopreserved lymphocytes are not entirely indistinguishable from freshly prepared samples. Each investigator will obviously have to establish their usefulness by comparison to freshly prepared samples for each assay developed. Furthermore, there have been suggestions that freezing and thawing may select for lymphocyte subpopulations and alter the proportions of cell types in the sample. Although we have not seen any alteration in the proportion of E rosetting (T cell) lymphocytes by cryopreservation, Weiner (personal communication) observed a decline using a slightly different E rosetting assay. Also, Knight *et al.* (16) reported evidence showing a separation of cells responsive to concanavalin A from those responsive to pokeweed mitogen by adjusting the cooling rate and DMSO concentration. With the advent of multiple functional and surface markers for delineating lymphoid cell subpopulations, a proper study of the effects of freezing and thawing on subpopulations would now be possible and most welcome.

A final note concerning the cryopreservation of nonlymphoid cells is in order. The method described here is useful for peripheral blood lymphocytes and fresh or cultured human tumor cells. Alterations in the cryopreservative, cooling procedure, or other technical features may be necessary for other cell types. In many cases cryopreservation can be accomplished without the purchase of any equipment. If one wants to preserve established human tissue culture cell lines with no greater requirement than the retention of the capacity to grow in culture, many of the hardier cell lines can be simply "crash-frozen" by immersion in liquid nitrogen using DMSO or glycerol as a cryopreservative. Farrant (17) showed that placing hamster tissue culture cells at $-26°C$ for 10 min prior to crash-freezing allowing for full retention of colony forming ability *in vitro*. It is interesting to note that even human lymphocytes retained responsiveness to

PHA after this simple two-stage procedure. We found that many tissue culture cells could be effectively cryopreserved by simply wrapping the sample vial in 1–2 inches of soft Styrofoam packing material and storing it in the vapor phase of the liquid nitrogen freezer for several hours prior to crash-freezing. Because lymphocytes and tumor cells have been known to be among the most amenable cells to simple and reproducible cryopreservation, they can provide valuable and unique reagents for cellular and tumor immunologists.

ACKNOWLEDGMENTS

These investigations were supported by Grant CA12582 awarded by the National Cancer Institute, U. S. Department of Health, Education and Welfare. Dr. Golub is a recipient of NIH Career Development Award.

REFERENCES

1. Ashwood-Smith, M. J., *Blood* **23**, 494 (1964).
2. Cohen, E., and Rowe, A. W., *Vox Sang.* **10**, 543 (1965).
3. Terasaki, P. I., Vredevoe, D. L., and McClelland, J. D., *in* "Histocompatability Testing 1965" p. 267. Williams & Wilkins, Baltimore, Maryland, 1965.
4. Flynn, R., Troup, G. M., and Walford, R. L., *Int. Arch. Allergy Appl. Immunol.* **29**, 478 (1966).
5. Mangi, R. J., and Mardiney, M. R., Jr., *J. Exp. Med.* **132**, 401 (1970).
6. Stopford, C. R., MacQueen, J. M., Amos, D. B., and Ward, F. F., *Tissue Antigens* **2**, 20 (1972).
7. Wood, N., Bashir, H., Greally, J., Amos, D. B., and Yunis, E. J., *Tissue Antigens* **2**, 27 (1972).
8. Eijsvoogel, V. P., duBois, M. J. G. J., Wal, R. v. d., Huisman, D. R., and Raat-Koning, L., *in* "La Cryoconservation des Cellules Normales et Néoplastiques" (R. S. Weiner, R. K. Oldham, and L. Schwarzenberg, eds.), p. 101. (INSERM, Paris), 1973.
9. Golub, S. H., Sulit, H. L., and Morton, D. L., *Transplantation* **19**, 195 (1975).
10. Chess, L., Bock, G. N., and Mardiney, M. R., Jr., *Transplantation* **14**, 728 (1972).
11. Segall, M., and Bach, M. L., *in* "La Cryoconservation des Cellules Normales et Néoplastiques" (R. S. Weiner, R. K. Oldham, and L. Schwarzenberg, eds.), p. 107. INSERM, Paris, (1973).
12. Weiner, R. S., Breard, J., and O'Brien, C., *in* "La Cryoconservation des Cellules Normales et Néoplastiques" (R. S. Weiner, R. K. Oldham, and L. Schwarzenberg, eds.), p. 117. INSERM, Paris, 1973.
13. O'Toole, C., *Natl. Cancer Inst. Monogr.* **37**, 19 (1973).
14. Oldham, R. K., and Simmler, M. C., *in* "La Cryoconservation des Cellules Normales et Néoplastiques" (R. S. Weiner, R. K. Oldham, and L. Schwarzenberg, eds.), p. 161. INSERM, Paris, 1973.
15. Weiner, R. S., *J. Immunol. Methods* in press.
16. Knight, S. C., Farrant, J., and Morris, G. J., *Nature (London) (New Biol.)* **239**, 89 (1972).
17. Farrant, J., Knight, S. C., McGann, L. E., and O'Brien, J., *Nature (London)* **249**, 453 (1974).

3.2. Culture Conditions

3.2.1. Responding and stimulating cells are mixed together in the desired ratios in the appropriate culture vessel, depending on the number of cells cultured; e.g., 0 to 5×10^6 responding cells plus 5×10^6 stimulating cells in 4 ml of MLC medium in 13×75 mm flat-bottomed glass tubes or 6×10^6 to 25×10^6 responding cells plus 25×10^6 stimulating cells in 20 ml MLC medium in upright Falcon (3013) plastic culture flasks. The cell *ratio* and *total* cell number must be varied to determine the optimal culture conditions for each particular system in question, particularly when dealing with syngeneic MLTC cultures where the optimal responding to stimulating cell ratio may be as high as 100:1 (13). In addition, when using immune responding cells to induce $2°$ responses subcellular particulate alloantigen preparations may be substituted for intact irradiated cells as a source of stimulating alloantigen (11).

3.2.2. The cultures are then incubated in a 5% CO_2-air incubator for the optimal period (generally 5–7 days). Again, time-course studies are imperative to confirm the optimal culture conditions for any given system.

3.2.3. The cells remaining in culture are harvested by centrifugation, washed once and the viable cell number adjusted to the required concentration. These cells can then be tested for their cytolytic potential using the desired assay system, e.g., the ^{51}Cr release assay discussed in Method 38. Cell recoveries can range from 10 to 500% of the initial viable cell input, depending on the culture conditions chosen (8).

4. Comments

The generation of CTL activity *in vitro* in MLC certainly offers many advantages over the earlier studied *in vivo* models. The method described above, i.e., cells incubated in flat-bottomed culture vessels using a standard proven tissue culture medium (D-MEM), with the addition of 2-ME, appears to provide a versatile, simple, and reproducible means of obtaining high CTL responses *in vitro*. The addition of 2-ME may result in up to a 20- to 50-fold augmentation in CTL activity per culture, when measured at the peak of the response. The actual mechanism by which 2-ME enhances the induction to CTL activity remains to be clarified (14, 15).

The effective surface area provided by the culture vessels appears to be quite important; i.e., there exists an optimal relationship between the number of cells cultured and the geometry of the culture vessel. In general, flat-bottomed culture vessels (including microplates) appear to provide the most satisfactory results. On the other hand, round-bottomed tubes may be required to ensure adequate cell-to-cell contact when low numbers of responding and stimulating cells are used. It can again be stressed that optimal culture conditions should be determined for each individual system under study (dose–response curves, kinetics of the response, etc.). Culture media can also play a role, as certain commercially available D-MEM do not yield satisfactory results.

It should be noted that several other more complicated *in vitro* culture methods also appear to provide suitable conditions for the generation of murine CTL (4, 5, 7). (For a more detailed review concerning the generation of CTL *in vitro* see Ref. 3).

REFERENCES

1. Häyry, P., Andersson, L. C., Nordling, S., and Virolainen, M., *Transplant. Rev.* **12**, 91 (1972).
2. Wagner, H., Röllinghoff, M., and Nossal, G. J. V., *Transplant. Rev.* **17**, 3 (1973).
3. Engers, H. D., and MacDonald, H. R., *in* "Contemporary Topics in Immunobiology," (W. Weigle, ed.), Vol. 5, p. 145. Plenum, New York, 1976.
4. Wagner, H., and Feldmann, M., *Cell Immunol.* **3**, 405 (1972).
5. Peavy, D. L., and Pierce, C. W., *J. Exp. Med.* **140**, 356 (1974).
6. Cerottini, J.-C., Engers, H. D., MacDonald, H. R., and Brunner, K. T., *J. Exp. Med.* **140**, 703 (1974).
7. Bevan, M. J., Epstein, R., and Cohn, M., *J. Exp. Med.* **139**, 1974 (1974).
8. Fitch, F. W., Engers, H. D., MacDonald, H. R., Cerottini, J.-C., and Brunner, K. T., *J. Immunol.* **115**, 168 (1976).
9. MacDonald, H. R., Brunner, K. T., and Cerottini, J.-C., *J. Exp. Med.* **140**, 1511 (1974).
10. Andersson, L. C., and Häyry, P., *Transplant. Rev.* **25**, 121 (1975).
11. Engers, H. D., Thomas, K., Cerottini, J.-C., and Brunner, K. T., *J. Immunol.* **115**, 356 (1975).
12. MacDonald, H. R., Sordat, B., Cerottini, J.-C., and Brunner, K. T., *J. Exp. Med.* **142**, 622 (1975).
13. Plata, F., Cerottini, J.-C., and Brunner, K. T., *Eur. J. Immunol.* **5**, 227 (1975).
14. Engers, H. D., MacDonald, H. R., Cerottini, J.-C., and Brunner, K. T., *Eur. J. Immunol.* **5**, 223 (1975).
15. Harris, J., MacDonald, H. R., Engers, H. D., Fitch, F. W., and Cerottini, J.-C., *J. Immunol.* **116**, 1071 (1976).

A Sensitive Micromethod for Generating and Assaying Specifically Cytotoxic Human Lymphocytes

Joyce M. Zarling and Fritz H. Bach

1. Introduction

Human lymphocytes cultured *in vitro* with irradiated or mitomycin C-treated allogeneic cells in one-way mixed leukocyte culture (MLC) respond to alloantigens by undergoing blast transformation; they incorporate ^{3}H-TdR measured after 4–6 days in culture (1). One or two days after ^{3}H-TdR incorporation is significantly increased, cytotoxic lymphocytes can be demonstrated in the cell-mediated lympholysis (CML) assay by their ability to specifically lyse ^{51}Cr-labeled cells expressing target antigens shared with the original stimulating cells (2–7). The CML assay is an *in vitro* model of *in vivo* graft rejection. It is thymus-dependent (T) lymphocytes that proliferate and differentiate into cytotoxic cells (7, 8). It has recently been shown that the "T" cells that respond by incorporating ^{3}H-TdR in the MLC assay and the T cells that become cytotoxic cells detected in the CML assay are two distinguishable populations of lymphocytes in mouse and in man (9–12).

By the routine miniaturized MLC assay performed in microwells, it is possible to compare quantitatively the MLC response of lymphocytes from different individuals by measuring ^{3}H-TdR incorporation on day 5 into responding cells in wells each *originally* containing the same number of responding lymphocytes (13). In contrast, by the usual CML assays, sensitized lymphocytes after allogeneic stimulation are either pooled from wells or tubes or are harvested from flasks and suspended at concentrations resulting in different ratios of killer cells:target cells (2–7); thus the allogeneically induced cytotoxic response generated by an *original* given number of responder lymphocytes is not measured.

We have recently developed a micromethod for generating and assaying cytotoxic lymphocytes in microwells that enables both MLC and CML responses to be measured in replicate original culture wells (14). ^{3}H-Thymidine is added to one set of culture wells on day 5 and day 6 or 7; ^{51}Cr-labeled target cells are added to the other original culture wells and to wells containing dilutions of the stimulated cells. Since cultures are set up identically for MLC and CML assays, both MLC and CML responses of a given number of lymphocytes from different individuals can be compared. It is thus possible to identify individuals that have lymphocytes that generate low MLC responses and high CML responses and vice versa.

The CML method described here is at least as sensitive as any previously described but requires less than 10% of the amount of blood and medium necessary for existing CML methods. Both MLC and CML responses can be measured with lymphocytes from as little as 3 ml of whole blood, thus enabling the measurement of these responses in young children and patients from whom only small amounts of blood can be obtained. By means of this micromethod requiring only 10^5 responding cells per well it is possible to vary several parameters such as the ratio of stimulating cells to responding cells, day and length of CML assay, and number of different target cells. In this context, it is known that some viruses stimulate lymphocytes from virus-immune individuals to incorporate ^{3}H-TdR and leukemia cells often stimulate lymphocytes from the patients in remission or from their HLA identical siblings. However, it is not known whether, following the proliferative response, a cytotoxic lymphocyte response is generated. The micromethod described here for generating and assaying allogeneically induced cytotoxic cells may thus be useful for attempting to generate cytotoxic cells directed against virus-induced antigens and tumor antigens, where several culture parameters must be varied.

2. Materials and Methods

2.1. Purification of Lymphocytes. Lymphocytes are purified from whole heparanized blood (100 units of heparin per milliliter of blood) by Ficoll–Hypaque sedimentation (15). Volumes of blood ranging from 2 to 30 ml are diluted with equal volumes of Medium 199 and layered on a Ficoll–Hypaque gradient (specific gravity 1.077) and centrifuged for 30 min at 850 g. From volumes of blood exceeding 30 ml, buffy coats are collected and diluted with medium 199 (Grand Island Biological Co., Grand Island, New York) before layering on the Ficoll–Hypaque gradient. The lymphocytes at the interface of the gradient are collected and washed three times with serum-free Medium 199. The cells are then resuspended in "culture medium" consisting of RPMI-1640 containing 25 mM HEPES buffer (Grand Island Biological Co.), 1.2% penicillin–streptomycin, 4 mM L-glutamine, and 20% heat-inactivated human serum. Serum is pooled from 4–10 healthy males who have not had transfusions and is heat-inactivated for 1 hr at 56°C and stored at −80°C in aliquots until use.

2.2. Sensitization Procedure for MLC and CML. Cultures for both the MLC and CML assays are set up identically. Responding lymphocytes are prepared in culture medium at a concentration of 1 × 10^6 cells/ml. Stimulating cells are prepared by treating the cells (5 to 15×10^6/ml) with mitomycin C (Nutritional Biochemical Corp., Cleveland, Ohio) at a final concentration of 25 μg/ml for 30 min at 37°C, followed by three washes in Medium 199. The cells are then resuspended at 2×10^6 cells/ml in culture medium. Alternatively, stimulating cells can be prepared by exposing them to 2000 R X-irradiation. Target cells for the CML assay, performed 6 or 7 days later, are prepared by suspending 10 $\times$ 10^6 to 15×10^6 untreated lymphocytes in 4–8 ml of culture medium in upright 50-ml Falcon tissue culture flasks, (Falcon Plastics, Division of BioQuest, Oxnard, California) and incubating at 37°C in a humidified atmosphere containing 5% CO_2. The target cells are fed with 3–5 ml of fresh culture medium on days 2 and 5 (6).

For setting up cultures for both MLC and CML, 0.1 ml of responder cells (10^5) and 0.1 ml of stimulating cells (2×10^5) are placed into several replicate round-bottomed wells of Linbro microtrays (Linbro IS MRC 96TC, Linbro Scientific Co., Inc., New Haven, Connecticut). One tray is for the determination of ^{3}H-TdR incorporation (MLC), and one tray is for the CML assay. Three or four replicate wells are prepared for MLC determination, and seven or more replicate wells (depending on the number of different target cells to be used) are prepared for the CML assay. The trays are then incubated at 37°C in a humidified atmosphere containing 5% CO_2. Wells for the CML assay are fed with 0.05 ml of fresh culture medium on days 2 and 5. When the wells are full it is necessary to first remove 0.05 ml supernatant before adding this volume of fresh medium. The cells spontaneously settle to the bottom of wells and it is therefore possible to remove 0.05 ml supernatant with a dispenser designed to add or remove this volume without removing cells.

2.3. Determination of ^{3}H-Thymidine Incorporation into Lymphocytes. Five days after the beginning of culture 2 μCi of ^{3}H-TdR (specific activity 1.9 Ci/mmole, New England Nuclear, Boston, Massachusetts) are added to each well. After 8–10 hr of incubation, ^{3}H-TdR incorporation is measured by transferring the contents of the wells onto filter strips with a multiple automatic sample harvester (Otto Hiller, Madison, Wisconsin). The filters are dried and counted in a scintillation counter. The counts per minute (cpm) of ^{3}H-TdR incorporated into allogeneically stimulated cells are compared to those incorporated into responding cells cultured with mitomycin C-treated or irradiated autologous cells as previously described (13).

2.4. Determination of Cytotoxic Responses of Lymphocytes. Six or seven days after culture the CML assay is performed. First, 0.05 ml culture supernatant is removed (if necessary) from each well to allow for the addition of this volume of target cells. Cells from four replicate culture wells are pooled, and the number of viable cells per well is determined by diluting 0.1 ml of these cells with 0.1 ml of 0.1% eosin and counting. Recovery of cells sensitized to allogeneic cells ranges from 150 to 620%, the mean recovery being approximately 400%. Recovery of cells incubated with mitomycin C-treated autologous cells ranges from 50 to 100%. Viability of recovered cells always exceeds 99%.

From the remainder of the pooled culture wells different dilutions of the cells are made in fresh medium and 0.2 ml of cells at each concentration is placed into four replicate wells. Usually three dilutions of effector cells are prepared, the final dilution generally being 1:64, thus resulting in the lowest ratio of effector to target cells of 0.3:1 to 1:1. Dilutions of effector cells are tested for cytotoxicity in order to determine whether a log-linear relationship exists between the ratio of effector cells to target cells and the amount of cytotoxicity (expressed as percent of specific ^{51}Cr release) detected. This also enables a comparison to be made between the amount of cytotoxicity resulting from sensitizing low numbers of lymphocytes from different individuals with a common allogeneic cell. Cells from the remaining original sensitization wells are gently resuspended with a Pasteur pipette immediately prior to the addition of ^{51}Cr-labeled target cells. To determine spontaneous release of ^{51}Cr from target cells, 0.2 ml of medium is added to each of 4–6 wells; to determine maximal ^{51}Cr release 0.2 ml 4% Cetrimide (Fisher Chemical Co., Chicago, Illinois) is added to each well before target cells are added.

During the time when the effector cells are being resuspended and diluted, 5×10^6 target cells, in a volume of 0.2 ml of culture medium are incubated with 250 μCi of ^{51}Cr (Na$_2$ ^{51}CrO$_4$, New England Nuclear, Boston, Massachusetts). The cells are allowed to incorporate ^{51}Cr for 1 hr at 37°C (with intermittent shaking). The cells are washed three times with cold culture medium and resuspended at 2×10^5 cells/ml. Then 0.05 ml target cells (10^4 cells) are added to each well, including those containing medium alone or detergent. The microtrays are centrifuged at 140 g for 5 min and then incubated for 4–8 hr at 37°C in a humidified incubator containing 5% CO_2. At the end of the incubation period, the trays are centrifuged at 300 g for 10 min in a refrigerated centrifuge. A constant amount of supernatant is then removed from each well and transferred into tubes for determining the amount of ^{51}Cr released. This can be done with an instrument designed to remove a constant volume or more rapidly by aspirating the supernatants from the wells into tubes. An 18-gauge needle is sealed at one end, and a small hole is made approximately 3 mm above the sealed end. The opened end of the needle is attached to tubing, which is attached to another needle inserted through a cork that fits the tubes used to collect the supernatant. Another needle is inserted through the cork, attached to tubing, which in turn is attached to a vacuum pump. Thus when the needle is held in the wells, a constant amount of supernatant is aspirated from the well into the tubes, but the cells are not transferred since the needle is sealed at the bottom. The needle is then held in a beaker of water until 1–2 ml of water wash through the tubing and into the tubes. Supernatants are counted in a gamma counter. The percentage of specific ^{51}Cr release is calculated from the following formula:

$$\frac{\text{cpm test wells} - \text{cpm spontaneous release}}{\text{cpm maximum release} - \text{cpm spontaneous release}} \times 100$$

Spontaneous release of ^{51}Cr after 4 and 8 hr ranges from 10 to 14% and 14 to 25%, respectively, of the maximum cpm released. As reported previously there is no autologous killing of allogeneically sensitized cells when normal cultured lymphocytes are used as targets (6, 14) (i.e., the amount of ^{51}Cr released from A target cells incubated with AB_m effector cells does not differ from the amount of ^{51}Cr spontaneously released).

3. Interpretation of Data and Comments

3.1. **Sample Experimental Results.** To illustrate the sensitivity of the method, results from a typical experiment obtained using this micromethod are shown in Fig. 1. Lymphocytes were obtained from a normal individual (A) and 2 lymphoma patients (P_1 and P_2) and these responding lymphocytes were stimulated with allogeneic mitomycin C-treated B (B_m) cells. The MLC results (cpm

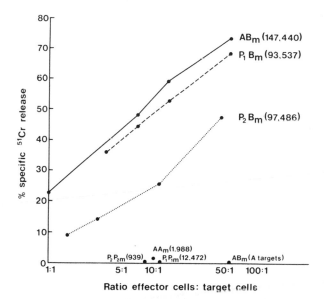

Fig. 1. Results from a typical experiment using the micromethod for generating and assaying of cytotoxic human lymphocytes. A, normal individual; P_1, P_2, lymphoma patients; B_m, mitomycin C-treated B cells. Numbers in parentheses are mixed leukocyte culture results (cpm of ^{3}H-TdR incorporation).

[3]H-TdR incorporation) are shown in parentheses next to the point representing the percentage of specific ^{51}Cr released from target cells added to the original culture wells in the CML plate. An 8-hr CML assay was performed on day 7. As shown, 73% specific ^{51}Cr release occurred from B target cells added to the original AB_m culture wells. A log-linear relationship exists between the percentage of specific ^{51}Cr release and the ratio of effector cells:target cells; significant amounts of ^{51}Cr are released at ratios as low as one effector cell per target cell. AA_m cells do not lyse B target cells and AB_m cultures are not cytotoxic for A target cells. The CML response of lymphocytes of P_1 to B_m cells was nearly the same magnitude as that of normal person A, while the CML response generated by 10^5 lymphocytes from P_2 was markedly lower. (Note that this log-linear relationship must be considered in comparing these two lines.)

3.2. Advantages. While the conventional methods for generating and assaying allogeneically induced cytotoxic cells are still useful when it is necessary to have large numbers of effector cells, we believe that the micromethod presented here offers several advantages over existing methods:

3.2.1. This method allows measurement of allogeneically induced proliferative and cytotoxic responses of 1×10^5 responding lymphocytes cultured in replicate wells. Thus it is possible to determine whether some individuals may have normal MLC responses and low CML responses and vice versa. [We have found high MLC responses and low CML responses generated by lymphocytes from some patients in remission from leukemia and lymphomas and the converse (low MLC and high CML) in a bone marrow recipient.]

3.2.2. This method enables measurement of MLC and CML responses beginning with as few as 3×10^6 lymphocytes; thus both of these responses can be measured in virtually all individuals including children and lymphopenic patients.

3.2.3. Since few lymphocytes are required per culture well, several parameters can be varied, such as the ratio of stimulating cells to responding cells, day and length of assay, and number of different target cells added.

3.2.4. Use of this method results in substantial savings of media, serum, and other reagents.

3.3. Comments. The method we have described here includes the conditions we have found maximal for generating cytotoxic responses to alloantigens, but a few additional points can be made. (a) When very few lymphocytes are available it is possible to culture 2.5×10^4 to 5×10^4 responding cells with twice that many stimulating cells. Although less cytotoxicity is detected when target cells are added to culture wells originally containing 2.5×10^4 to 5×10^4 responding cells than to culture wells originally containing 10^5 responding cells, the amount of ^{51}Cr released at the same ratio of effector cells to target cells is the same regardless of whether 2.5×10^4 or 10^5 responding cells are initially placed in culture wells (14). (b) Although we routinely performed CML assays on day 7, significant cytotoxicity can usually also be detected on days 6 or 8 (14). (c) We generally perform 8-hr CML assays because the percentage of specific ^{51}Cr release is much higher than after 4 hr whereas spontaneous release increases only minimally from 4 to 8 hr; however, significant specific ^{51}Cr release (usually 30–50%) can be detected after 4-hr CML assays (14). (d) We have found that MLC and CML responses of lymphocytes purified from blood held at room temperature for up to 20 hr and purified lymphocytes stored at 4°C overnight are not detectably different from those of freshly purified lymphocytes (14). (e) A log-linear relationship exists between the percent specific ^{51}Cr release and ratio of effector cells to target cells when normal individuals' responses lymphocytes are tested. However, when the proliferative response, and hence recovery of responding lymphocytes, is very low after culture with allogeneic cells (as we have seen in some lymphoma patients), the percentage of specific ^{51}Cr release from target cells is sometimes less in the original culture wells than when the lymphocytes are transferred to empty culture wells at the time of the CML assay. Therefore, when few cells are recovered at day 7 we transfer the contents of these wells to empty wells before adding target cells. (f) Consistent with results reported by others using the usual CML assays in mouse and man (16, 17) secondary CML responses can be detected by this micromethod by simply adding 10^5 stimulating cells to original culture wells after the primary CML response has declined (14). A stronger cytotoxic response to weak alloantigens, virus-induced cell surface antigens, or tumor-associated antigens might be detected after restimulation than after a primary sensitization.

ACKNOWLEDGMENTS

Work supported in part by NIH Grants CA-16836, AI-11576, AI-08439 and National Foundation-March of Dimes Grant CRBS 246. We thank Dr. Peter C. Raich of the University of Wisconsin Hospitals for providing us with blood from lymphoma patients, and Mark McKeough for his excellent technical assistance. This is paper No. 72 from the Immunobiology Research Center, The University of Wisconsin, Madison, Wisconsin.

REFERENCES

1. Bach, F. H., and Voynow, N. K., *Science* **153**, 545 (1966).
2. Bonnard, G. D., Lemos, L., and Chappuis, M., *Scand. J. Immunol* **3**, 97 (1974).
3. Eijsvoogel, V. P., du Bois, M. J. G. J., Meinesz, A., Bierhorst-Eijlander, A., Zeylemaker, W. P., and Schellekens, P. T. A., *Transplant. Proc* **V**, 1675 (1973).
4. Lightbody, J. J., Bernoco, D., Miggiano, V. C., and Ceppellini, R., *G. Batteriol. Virol. Immunol. Ann. Osp. Maria Vittoria Torino* **64**, 243 (1971).
5. Solliday, S., and Bach, F. H., *Science* **170**, 1406 (1970).
6. Sondel, P. M., and Bach, F. H., *J. Exp. Med.* **142**, 1339 (1975).
7. Sondel, P. M., Chess, L., MacDermott, R. P., and Schlossman, S. F., *J. Immunol.* **114**, 982 (1975).

8. Chess, L., MacDermott, R. P., and Schlossman, S. F., *J. Immunol.* **113,** 1122 (1974).

9. Bach, F. H., Segall, M., Zier, K. S., Sondel, P. M., Alter, B. J., and Bach, M. L., *Science* **180,** 403 (1973).

10. Cantor, H., and Boyse, E. A., *J. Exp. Med.* **141,** 1376 (1975).

11. Cantor, H., and Boyse, E. A., *J. Exp. Med.* **141,** 1390 (1975).

12. Wagner, H., Röllinghoff, M., and Shortman, K., "Progress in Immunology II" (L. Brent and J. Holborow, eds.), p. 111. North-Holland Publ., Amsterdam, 1974.

13. Hartzman, R. J., Segall, M., Bach, M. L., and Bach, F. H., *Transplantation* **11,** 268 (1971).

14. Zarling, J. M., McKeough, M., and Bach, F. H., *Transplantation* in press (1976).

15. Böyum, A., *Scand. J. Clin. Lab. Invest.* (Suppl. 97) **21,** 1 (1968).

16. Häyry, P., and Andersson, L., *Scand. J. Immunol.* **3,** 823 (1974).

17. Zier, K. S., and Bach, F. H., *Scand. J. Immunol.* **4,** 607 (1975).